T0294804

ALLERGY ESSENTIALS

ALLERGY ESSENTIALS

SECOND EDITION

Robyn E. O'Hehir, MD, PhD, FAHMS
Professor of Allergy, Immunology, and
    Respiratory Medicine
Monash University and Alfred Hospital
Melbourne
Australia

Stephen T. Holgate, MD, FMedSci
Clinical Professor of Immunopharmacology
Medical Faculty in Clinical and Experimental
    Sciences
Southampton General Hospital
Southampton
United Kingdom

Gurjit K. Khurana Hershey, MD, PhD
Kindervelt Endowed Chair in Asthma
    Research
Professor of Pediatrics
Director, Division of Asthma Research
Cincinnati Children's Hospital Medical Center
Director, Medical Scientist Training Program
University of Cincinnati College of Medicine
Cincinnati, Ohio
United States

Aziz Sheikh, MD, FMedSci
Professor of Primary Care Research and
    Development Director and Dean of Data
Usher Institute
University of Edinburgh
Edinburgh
United Kingdom

ELSEVIER

Elsevier
1600 John F. Kennedy Blvd.
Ste 1800
Philadelphia, PA 19103-2899

ALLERGY ESSENTIALS, SECOND EDITION

ISBN: 978-0-323-80912-2

Copyright © 2022 by Elsevier, Inc. All rights reserved.

Previous edition copyrighted 2017.

No part of this publication may be reproduced or transmitted in any form or by any means, electronic or mechanical, including photocopying, recording, or any information storage and retrieval system, without permission in writing from the publisher. Details on how to seek permission, further information about the Publisher's permissions policies and our arrangements with organizations such as the Copyright Clearance Center and the Copyright Licensing Agency, can be found at our website: www.elsevier.com/permissions.

This book and the individual contributions contained in it are protected under copyright by the Publisher (other than as may be noted herein).

Notices

Knowledge and best practice in this field are constantly changing. As new research and experience broaden our understanding, changes in research methods, professional practices, or medical treatment may become necessary.

Practitioners and researchers must always rely on their own experience and knowledge in evaluating and using any information, methods, compounds or experiments described herein. Because of rapid advances in the medical sciences, in particular, independent verification of diagnoses and drug dosages should be made. To the fullest extent of the law, no responsibility is assumed by Elsevier, authors, editors or contributors for any injury and/or damage to persons or property as a matter of products liability, negligence or otherwise, or from any use or operation of any methods, products, instructions, or ideas contained in the material herein.

Library of Congress Control Number: 2021942482

Content Strategist: Robin Carter
Content Development Manager: Meghan Andress
Publishing Services Manager: Deepthi Unni
Project Manager: Janish Paul
Design Direction: Patrick Ferguson

Printed in the United States of America

Last digit is the print number: 9 8 7 6 5 4 3 2 1

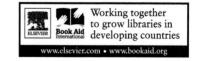

CONTRIBUTORS

Cezmi A. Akdis, MD
Professor and Director, Swiss Institute of
    Allergy and Asthma Research (SIAF),
University of Zürich, Zürich, Switzerland;
Professor, Christine Kühne Center for
    Allergy Research and Education
    (CK-CARE),
Davos, Switzerland

Mübeccel Akdis, MD, PhD
Swiss Institute of Allergy and Asthma
    Research (SIAF),
University of Zürich, Zürich, Switzerland;
Christine Kühne Center for Allergy Research
    and Education (CK-CARE),
Davos, Switzerland

Fuad M. Baroody, MD, FACS
Professor of Surgery,
Section of Otolaryngology-Head and Neck
    Surgery;
Professor of Pediatrics,
Director of Pediatric Otolaryngology;
Director, Residency Program,
Otolaryngology-Head and Neck Surgery;
The University of Chicago Medicine and The
    Comer Children's Hospital,
Chicago, IL, United States

Mark Boguniewicz, MD
Department of Pediatrics,
National Jewish Health,
Denver, CO, United States

**Simon G.A. Brown, MBBS, DA(UK),
PhD, FACEM**
Centre for Clinical Research in Emergency
    Medicine,
Harry Perkins Institute of Medical Research;
Royal Perth Hospital,
University of Western Australia,
Perth, WA, Australia

A. Wesley Burks, MD
Curnen Distinguished Professor and Chair,
Pediatrics,
University of North Carolina,
Chapel Hill, NC, United States

Anca-Mirela Chiriac, MD, PhD
Département de Pneumologie et
    Addictologie,
Hôpital Arnaud de Villeneuve,
University Hospital of Montpellier,
Institut Desbrest d'Epidémiologie et de
    Santé Publique UMR INSERM,
Université de Montpellier,
Montpellier, France

Jonathan Corren, MD
Associate Clinical Professor of Medicine,
Medicine and Pediatrics,
David Geffen School of Medicine at UCLA,
Los Angeles, CA, United States

Adnan Custovic, MD, PhD, FMedSci
Professor of Paediatric Allergy,
National Heart and Lung Institute,
Imperial College London,
London, United Kingdom

Pascal Demoly, MD, PhD
Département de Pneumologie et
    Addictologie,
Hôpital Arnaud de Villeneuve,
University Hospital of Montpellier,
Institut Desbrest d'Epidémiologie et de Santé
    Publique UMR INSERM,
Université de Montpellier,
Montpellier, France

Luz Fonacier, MD
Department of Medicine,
NYU Langone Health,
Mineola, NY, United States

David B.K. Golden, MD
Associate Professor of Medicine,
Johns Hopkins University,
Baltimore, MD, United States

Clive E.H. Grattan, MA, MD, FRCP
St John's Institute of Dermatology,
Guy's Hospital,
London,
Middlesex, United Kingdom

Oliver V. Hausmann, MD
ADR-AC GmbH,
Adverse Drug Reactions,
Analysis and Consulting,
Bern, Switzerland;
Loewenpraxis und Klinik,
St. Anna,
Lucerne, Switzerland

Gurjit K. Khurana Hershey, MD, PhD
Kindervelt Endowed Chair in Asthma
    Research
Professor of Pediatrics
Director, Division of Asthma Research
Cincinnati Children's Hospital Medical
    Center
Director, Medical Scientist Training Program
University of Cincinnati College of Medicine
Cincinnati, Ohio
United States

Stephen T. Holgate, MD, FMedSci
Professor,
Southampton School of Medicine,
Southampton,
Hampshire, United Kingdom

Lukas Joerg, MD
Department of Rheumatology,
Immunology and Allergology,
Inselspital;
Bern University Hospital;
University of Bern,
Bern, Switzerland

Catherine Lemière, MD, MSc
Professor of Medicine,
Department of Chest Medicine,
CIUSSS du Nord de l'île de Montréal-
    Hôpital du Sacré-Coeur de Montréal,
Université de Montréal,
Montreal, Canada

Donald Y.M. Leung, MD, PhD
Department of Pediatrics,
National Jewish Health,
Denver, CO, United States

Tesfaye B. Mersha, PhD
Associate Professor,
Pediatrics,
Cincinnati Children's Hospital Medical
    Center,
Cincinnati, OH, United States

Anna Nowak-Węgrzyn, MD, PhD
Professor of Pediatrics,
NYU Langone School of Medicine,
New York, NY, United States

Robyn E. O'Hehir MD, PhD, FAHMS
Professor of Allergy, Immunology, and
    Respiratory Medicine,
Monash University and Alfred Hospital,
Melbourne, Australia

Clive Robinson, BSc, PhD
Professor of Respiratory Cell Science,
Institute for Infection & Immunity,
St George's, University of London,
London, United Kingdom

Umit Sahiner
Professor, Hacettepe University,
School of Medicine,
Department of Pediatric Allergy,
Ankara, Turkey

Sarbjit S. Saini
Professor of Medicine,
Johns Hopkins University School of
    Medicine,
Baltimore, MD, United States

Hugh A. Sampson, MD
Professor of Pediatrics,
Icahn School of Medicine at
    Mount Sinai,
New York, NY, United States

Aziz Sheikh, MD, FMedSci
Professor of Primary Care Research and
    Development
Director and Dean of Data
Usher Institute
University of Edinburgh,
Edinburgh, United Kingdom

Michael G. Sherenian, MD
Assistant Professor,
Department of Pediatrics,
Cincinnati Children's Hospital Medical Center,
Cincinnati, OH, United States

Helen E. Smith, BMedSci BMBS, MSc DM
Professor,
Lee Kong Chian School of Medicine,
Nanyang Technological University,
Novena, Singapore

Geoffrey A. Stewart, BSc, PhD
Emeritus Professor,
School of Biomedical, Biomolecular and
    Chemical Sciences,
University of Western Australia;
Director,
Institute for Respiratory Health,
Perth, WA, Australia

Hille Suojalehto, MD, PhD
Adjunct Professor,
Respiratory Medicine and Allergology
    Department,
Finnish Institute of Occupational
    Health,
Helsinki, Helsinki, Finland

Paul J. Turner, FRACP, PhD, MRCPCH
Section of Inflammation,
    Repair and Development,
National Heart & Lung Institute,
Imperial College London,
London, United Kingdom

CONTENTS

Introduction to Mechanisms of Allergic Diseases

Umit Sahiner, Mübeccel Akdis, and Cezmi A. Akdis

CHAPTER OUTLINE

SUMMARY OF IMPORTANT CONCEPTS

- Allergic inflammation is a result of a complex interplay among structural tissue cells and inflammatory cells, including mast cells, basophils, lymphocytes, dendritic cells, eosinophils, and, sometimes, neutrophils.
- Cytokines are families of secreted proteins that mediate immune and inflammatory reactions at local or distant sites.
- The innate immune system first responds to early infectious and inflammatory signals, activating and instructing the adaptive immune system for antigen-specific T and B lymphocyte responses and the development of immunologic memory.
- Allergen recognition and uptake, allergic sensitization, inflammation, and disease originate in the innate immune system.
- Adaptive immune responses depend on activation of naive CD4+ T cells and differentiation into effector cells. CD4+ T

helper type 2 (Th2) cells are critical mediators of allergic inflammation.

- Production of IgE antibody is regulated mainly by Th2 cells. Activated Th2 cells trigger IgE production in B cells through a combination of signals, including secreted cytokine (interleukin [IL]-4 or IL-13) and cell surface (CD40L).
- Better understanding of the pathophysiology of allergic inflammation will enable us to identify novel therapeutic targets in the treatment of chronic allergic inflammation.

INTRODUCTION

The inflammatory process has several common characteristics shared by various different allergic diseases, including asthma, allergic rhinitis (AR) or rhinosinusitis, atopic dermatitis (AD) (eczema), and food allergy. Allergic inflammation is characterized by IgE-dependent activation of mucosal mast cells and an infiltration of eosinophils that is orchestrated by increased numbers of activated CD4$^+$ T helper type 2 (Th2) lymphocytes. In addition to these cells, various types of inflammatory cells produce multiple inflammatory mediators, including lipids, purines, cytokines, chemokines, and reactive oxygen species. Both innate and adaptive immune mechanisms and involvement of multiple cytokines and chemokines play roles.

INNATE IMMUNITY

Innate immunity is an essential part of the immune system and is the first line of defense against microorganisms and foreign bodies such as allergens. It acts by the action of a limited number of receptors specific to microbial components. As a result, both rapid immune response and activation of the adaptive immune system occurs. Starting from body surfaces, epithelial cells, dendritic cells (DCs), natural killer (NK) cells, innate lymphoid cells (ILCs), macrophages, mast cells, eosinophils, basophils, and neutrophils are main players for the innate immune response. Epithelial barrier and microbiome as well as physicochemical factors such as mucus, antimicrobial peptides (AMPs), ciliary movement, cough, and peristaltism all play a role in innate defense mechanisms.[1]

Microbial Pattern Recognition by the Innate Immune System

Microbial recognition by the innate immune system is mediated by germline-encoded receptors with genetically predetermined specificities for microbial constituents. Natural selection has formed and refined the repertoire of innate immune receptors to recognize highly conserved molecular structures that distinguish large groups of microorganisms from the host. These microbe-specific structures are called *pathogen-associated molecular patterns* (PAMPs), and the *pattern recognition receptors* (PRRs) of the innate immune system recognize these structures (Table 1.1).

Pattern Recognition Receptors

PRRs of the innate immune system can be divided into two groups: secreted receptors and transmembrane signal-transducing receptors (Table 1.1). *Secreted PRRs* typically have multiple effects in innate immunity and host defense, including direct microbial killing, serving as helper proteins for transmembrane receptors, opsonization for phagocytosis, and chemoattraction of innate and adaptive immune effector cells. AMPs are secreted PRRs that are microbicidal and rapidly acting. When secreted onto skin and mucous membranes, they create a microbicidal shield against microbial attachment and invasion.

Transmembrane PRRs are expressed on many innate immune cell types, including macrophages, DCs, monocytes, and B lymphocytes (Fig. 1.1). These PRRs are exemplified by the Toll-like receptors (TLRs) and their associated recognition, enhancing, and signal transduction proteins (Fig. 1.1). Innate immune response at the epithelial cell–related and DC-related processes are controlled by the activation of the epithelial PRR by PAMPS found in the microorganisms as well as the host-derived damage-associated molecular patterns (DAMPs). Airway epithelial cells and DCs express a wide range of TLRs, NOD-like receptors (NLRs), RIG-I-like receptors (RLRs), AIM2-like receptors (ALRs), C-type lectin receptors (CLRs), protease-activated receptors (PARs), and others.[2,3]

Cellular Responses of Innate Immunity

Microbial detection by PRRs activates the cells that express or bind them. Those in frontline positions for detection are the first responders of the innate immune system, such as tissue macrophages, fibrocytes, epithelial cells, and mast cells.

Innate immune activation also leads to multifaceted antimicrobial responses by tissue infiltrating immune cells (e.g., neutrophils, NK cells, DCs, monocytes). These responses are potent antimicrobial effectors that usually are recruited by an innate immune intermediary to induce the full weight of their response, but they can respond directly to microbial stimuli through their own surface-expressed PRRs. On reaching the infected site, neutrophils phagocytose invading microorganisms that are opsonized by complement C3 fragments (e.g., C3b, iC3b) and immunoglobulin G (IgG).[4] Recruited and activated NK cells mediate antimicrobial activities by induction of apoptosis of cell targets and cytokine secretion that promote innate immune functions and contribute to adaptive immune responses.

DCs are transformed into active antigen-presenting cells (APCs) by stimulation of the TLR and they initiate and mediate adaptive immune responses. Additionally, DCs together with interferon (IFN)-γ can induce macrophage polarization, which is important for phagocytosis.[5] DCs in the blood can be divided into two groups as myeloid DCs (mDCs) and plasmacytoid DCs (pDCs). mDCs selectively express TLR2–6 and TLR2–8 and respond to bacterial and viral infections by producing large amounts of interleukin (IL)-12. However, pDCs express TLR7 and TLR9 associated with the endosome and produce type 1 IFNs.[6] The newly described cell type native lymphoid cells have effector functions in homeostasis and inflammation. ILC1s and ILC3s are essential for defense against infection by viruses, intracellular bacteria, and parasites. However, ILC2s direct type 2 inflammation and mediate allergic inflammation, tissue repair, and anti-helminth innate immunity.[5]

TABLE 1.1   Innate Pattern Recognition Receptors in Humans

Pattern Recognition Receptors	PAMP Structures Recognized	Functions
Secreted		
Antimicrobial peptides		
α- and β-Defensins	Microbial membranes (negatively charged)	Opsonization, microbial cell lysis, immune cell chemoattractant
Cathelicidin (LL-37)		
Dermcidin		
RegIIIγ		
Collectins		
Mannose-binding lectin	Microbial mannan	Opsonization, complement activation, microbial cell lysis, chemoattraction, phagocytosis
Surfactant proteins A and D	Bacterial cell wall lipids; viral coat proteins	Opsonization, killing, phagocytosis, proinflammatory and antiinflammatory mediator release
Pentraxins		
C-reactive protein	Bacterial phospholipids (phosphorylcholine)	Opsonization, complement activation, microbial cell lysis, chemoattraction, phagocytosis
Secreted and membrane bound		
CD14	Endotoxin	TLR4 signaling
LPS binding protein	Endotoxin	TLR4 signaling
MD-2	Endotoxin	TLR4 co-receptor
Membrane bound		
Toll-like receptors	Microbial PAMPs	Immune cell activation
C-type lectin receptors		
Mannose receptor (CD206)	Microbial mannan	Cell activation, phagocytosis, proinflammatory mediator release
DECTIN-1	β-1,3-Glucan	Cell activation, phagocytosis, proinflammatory mediator release
DECTIN-2	Fungal mannose	Cell activation, phagocytosis, proinflammatory mediator release
DC-SIGN	Microbial mannose, fucose	Immunoregulation, IL-10 production
Siglecs	Sialic acid containing glycans	Cell inhibition, endocytosis
Cytosolic		
NOD-like receptors		
NOD-1	Peptidoglycans from gram-negative bacteria	Cell activation
NOD-2	Bacterial muramyl dipeptides	Cell activation
NLRP1	Anthrax lethal toxin	PAMP recognition in inflammasome
NLRP3 (cryopyrin)	Microbial RNA	PAMP recognition in inflammasome
NLRC4	Bacterial flagellin	PAMP recognition in inflammasome
RIG-I and MDA5	Viral double-stranded RNA	Type 1 IFN responses

DC-SIGN, Dendritic cell–specific intracellular adhesion molecule 3 (ICAM-3)–grabbing non-integrin; *DECTIN*, dendritic cell–specific receptor; *IFN*, interferon; *IL*, interleukin; *LPS*, lipopolysaccharide; *MD-2*, myeloid differentiation factor 2 (also called lymphocyte antigen 96 [LY98]); *MDA5*, melanoma differentiation-associated 5 (also called interferon induced with helicase domain 1 [IFIH1]); *NLR*, NOD-like receptor; *NOD*, nucleotide-binding oligomerization domain protein; *PAMP*, pathogen-associated molecular pattern; *RegIIIγ*, regenerating islet-derived 3 γ (REG3G); *RIG-I*, retinoic acid-inducible 1 (also called DDX58); *Siglecs*, sialic acid–binding immunoglobulin-like lectins; *TLR*, Toll-like receptor.

Innate Instruction of Adaptive Immune Responses

The immediate and infiltrative responses of innate immunity activate and instruct the adaptive immune system for antigen-specific T and B lymphocyte responses and the development of immunologic memory. Because the adaptive immune system essentially has a limitless antigen receptor repertoire, instruction is necessary to guide adaptive antimicrobial immune responses toward pathogens and not self-antigens or harmless environmental antigens.

Microbial pattern recognition by innate immune cells controls the activation of adaptive immune responses by directing microbial antigens linked to TLRs and other PRRs through the cellular processes leading to antigen presentation and the expression of costimulatory molecules (e.g., CD80 with CD86). This two-step activation of the immune system, an innate immune response first and then an adaptive immune response, prevents unnecessary inflammatory responses and is highly effective.[7]

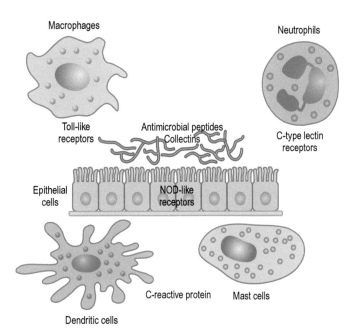

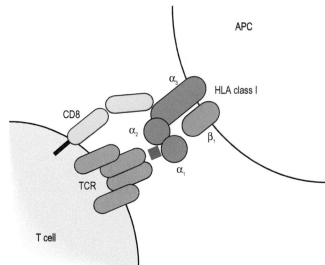

Fig. 1.1 Main categories of pattern recognition receptors and the innate immune cell types that express them. *NOD*, Nucleotide-binding oligomerization domain protein. (Adapted from Liu AH. Innate microbial sensors and their relevance to allergy. J Allergy Clin Immunol. 2008;122:846-858.)

Fig. 1.2 Interaction of a human leukocyte antigen *(HLA)* class I molecule on an antigen-presenting cell *(APC)* with a CD8⁺ T cell. The antigen receptor (i.e., T cell receptor *[TCR]*) complex *(purple)* recognizes a combination of an antigen peptide *(red)* and an HLA molecule *(brown and pink)*. The CD8 molecule *(aqua blue)* in the T cells interacts with the α_3 domain of the HLA molecule. HLA class II molecules present antigen peptides to CD4⁺ T cells in a similar manner, interacting with the TCR and the CD4 molecules.

Innate Immunity and Allergy

The innate immune system of the airways, gastrointestinal tract, and skin is continuously exposed to potential allergens. As with microbial antigens, allergens can engage innate PRRs, are processed through innate immune cells, and can lead to pathologic allergic/inflammatory immune responses. Although the circumstances leading to allergic immunity in humans are not clear, evidence suggests that allergic susceptibilities can originate in the innate immune system.[8]

ADAPTIVE IMMUNITY

Adaptive Immune Response in Allergic Disease

A remarkable property of the adaptive immune system is its memory. Immunologic memory is made possible by the clonal expansion of T and B lymphocytes in response to antigen (including allergen) stimulation. From the time the human immune system begins to differentiate in fetal life, lymphocytes possessing unique reactivity are created by the recombination of genes encoding antigen receptors expressed on the lymphocyte cell membrane. Through the expression of these receptors, T and B lymphocytes have the ability to bind to and become activated by a specific antigen, which may be natural or artificial. Interaction with antigen activates the lymphocytes and generates long-lived, antigen-specific memory T and B cell clones. When the same antigen enters the body, there is immediate recognition by these memory cells. Cellular and humoral responses to the antigen are produced more rapidly than in the first encounter, and more memory cells are generated. This process of expansion of clonal populations of uniquely reacting lymphocytes first explained the B cell origin of antibody diversity and applies to cellular (T cell) immune responses.

Main Components of the Adaptive Immune System

All cells of the immune system are derived from the pluripotent hematopoietic stem cell found in the bone marrow. This pluripotential stem cell gives rise to lymphoid stem cells and myeloid stem cells. The lymphoid progenitor cell differentiates into three types of cell, *T cell, B cell, and ILC and NK cell*, and contributes to the development of subsets of DCs. The myeloid stem cell gives rise to DCs, mast cells, basophils, neutrophils, eosinophils, monocytes, and macrophages, as well as megakaryocytes and erythrocytes. Differentiation of these committed stem cells depends on an array of cytokine and cell–cell interactions.

Features of the Adaptive Immune Response

APCs, which include DCs, monocytes, or macrophages, process and present antigen within an antigen-binding cleft of major histocompatibility complex (MHC) molecules. These events start at the APC cell surface with the capture and endocytosis of antigens, followed by a complex sequence of enzymatic activities leading to the association of antigenic peptides with MHC molecules and expression back to the cell surface. CD4⁺ T cells recognize antigenic peptides when presented in the context of a class II MHC molecule (Fig. 1.2) together with the appropriate costimulatory signals and become activated in response to monocyte-derived IL-1 and other cytokines, including autocrine stimulation by IL-2.

Subsets of Th cells dictate the cytokine production involved in three types of immune responses. Th1 response, induced by IL-12 and IFN-γ, is responsible for T cell–mediated cytotoxicity. Th2 response, induced by IL-4, IL-5, and IL-13, is responsible for the development of IgE- and eosinophil-mediated allergic disease. Th17 response leads to a characteristic neutrophilic inflammation and is pathogenic in some experimental models of autoimmunity. Transforming growth factor-β (TGF-β), IL-23, and IL-6 are essential cytokines for developing the Th17 response, which is mediated by IL-17A, IL-17F, IL-21, and IL-22.

The defensive capacity of the immune system needs a mechanism to counterbalance this proinflammatory response and to minimize unnecessary tissue damage. Several processes ensure that the different immune effector cells are not activated against host tissues and innocuous substances and that they can downregulate a response after the threat is resolved. All of these processes underlie *immune tolerance*, which is classified as central when occurring in primary lymphoid organs, or as peripheral when occurring in other tissues. Together with central and peripheral tolerance processes, a subset of T cells characterized by high levels of CD25 expression (IL-2R α chain) have been identified as regulatory T (Treg) cells because they were found to suppress the function of other T cells when present in the same site (Fig. 1.3).[9]

Mechanisms of Diseases Involving Adaptive Immunity

Distinct mechanisms of immune-mediated diseases are IgE-mediated hypersensitivity, antibody-mediated cytotoxicity, immune complex reaction, delayed hypersensitivity response, antibody-mediated activation or inactivation of biologic function, cell-mediated cytotoxicity, and granulomatous reaction.

IMMUNOGLOBULIN STRUCTURE AND FUNCTION

B Lymphocytes and the Humoral Immune Response

Engagement of the B cell receptor (BCR) by antigen initiates receptor aggregation at the cell surface followed by recruitment to lipid rafts. Lipid rafts are specialized membrane microdomains that facilitate assembly and activation of downstream signaling molecules.[10] This step places the complex in proximity to the LYN tyrosine kinase, which phosphorylates tyrosine residues in the Igα/Igβ ITAM motifs and triggers recruitment of spleen tyrosine kinase (SYK) and Bruton tyrosine kinase (BTK). Activated SYK phosphorylates and recruits the B cell linker (BLNK) protein, which provides binding sites for phospholipase Cγ2 (PLCγ2), BTK, and VAV proteins, which are guanine nucleotide exchange factors. PLCγ2 generates the second messengers inositol triphosphate and diacylglycerol, which are necessary for calcium release from intracellular stores and protein kinase C activation. BCR signal transduction also leads to activation of the mitogen-activated protein kinase (MAPK) pathway. B cell activation is further aided by a co-receptor complex that amplifies signals delivered by the BCR. The members of this complex include CD19, the complement receptor type 2 (CR2 or CD21), and CD81. The CR2 enables the complement pathway to synergize with BCR signal transduction, which enhances B cell activation. Collectively, these signaling events lead to the activation of the transcription factors known as nuclear factor of activated T cells (NFAT), nuclear factor-κB (NF-κB), and activator protein 1 (AP-1). Activation of the BCR on naive and memory B cells results in their activation and migration to the draining lymph node or other lymphatic tissue. B cells can respond to three types of antigens, and the type of antigenic exposure dictates the quality of the ensuing response.

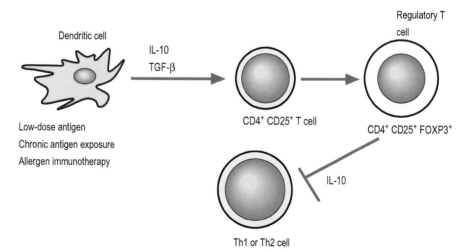

Fig. 1.3 Regulatory T cells are generated by the interaction of antigen-presenting cells and T cells, mediated by the cytokines interleukin-10 *(IL-10)* and transforming growth factor-β *(TGF-β)*. These cytokines are secreted when the antigen is presented under certain conditions, such as when administering allergen immunotherapy at very low concentration. Regulatory T cells secrete IL-10 and inhibit effector T cells that share similar antigen specificity.

Immunoglobulin Structure and Gene Rearrangement

Immunoglobulins are composed of two identical heavy chains and two identical light chains (Fig. 1.4A). Light chains lack transmembrane domains and are anchored to heavy chains by disulfide bonds. The two heavy chains are linked to each other by a distinct set of disulfide bonds. Each heavy chain or light chain has two major domains referred to as the *constant region* (C) and the *variable region* (V), with each domain responsible for a specialized function. They are denoted as C_L and V_L for the light chains and as CH and VH for the heavy chains.

Heavy-chain variable regions are encoded by one V gene, which encodes most V-region amino acids, as well as 1 of 23 diversity (D) and 1 of 6 joining (J) gene segments that are located 3′ of the V gene cluster. In contrast, light chain variable regions are encoded by only two types of genes: V genes and J genes. Whereas the J_κ genes are organized in a cluster 3′ to the V_κ gene cluster, J_λ genes are interspersed with λ constant-region genes.

Immunoglobulin diversity has four sources: multiple V(D) J genes in the germline, random assortment of heavy chains and light chains, junctional nucleotide variability introduced during pre-B cell immunoglobulin gene rearrangement, and somatic hypermutation of immunoglobulin variable regions after encounters with antigens.

Immunoglobulin Function

The five classes of antibody molecules are designated IgM, IgD, IgG, IgA, and IgE. The IgG and IgA classes have more than one member. There are four IgG (γ) sub-classes, designated as IgG1, IgG2, IgG3, and IgG4, and their constant regions exhibit 90% homology with each other. However, because each IgG sub-class constant region is encoded by a separate constant-region gene, the IgG sub-classes are closely related isotypes that exhibit a similar overall structure. The two sub-classes of IgA are similarly related to each other. There are two types of light chains: κ and λ. There are four λ sub-types but only one form of κ. The nine class and sub-classes of antibody molecules have significantly different expression levels, anatomic locations, and effector functions (Table 1.2). The five antibody classes also display characteristic structural features (Fig. 1.4B).

IMMUNOGLOBULINS AND HUMAN DISEASE

Human conditions of dysregulated immunoglobulin production include antibody deficiencies and overproduction of specific antibodies. The most serious of the three major categories of antibody deficiencies result in reduced B cell numbers and a severe decrease in all isotypes of serum immunoglobulin, as in agammaglobulinemia. This type of immunodeficiency underscores the importance of tyrosine kinases in early B cell BCR signal transduction. The second category includes selective deficiencies of IgA or IgG2 production and various genetic mutations that result in hypogammaglobulinemia, such as deficiencies in transmembrane activator and calcium-modulating cyclophilin ligand interactor (TACI). The third category includes

a number of mutations that give rise to hyper-IgM syndromes, which result from the failure of B cells to undergo class-switch recombination. These disorders highlight the critical role that CD40–CD40L interaction plays in class-switch recombination, as revealed by the lack of IgG, IgA, and IgE antibodies in these patients.

There are also some other disorders characterized by abnormalities in immunoglobulins. IgG4-related disease is a chronic inflammatory condition characterized by tissue infiltration by lymphocytes and IgG4-secreting plasma cells, varying degrees of fibrosis (scarring), and generally rapid response to oral steroids. IgG4 serum levels increased in the acute period in two-thirds of the patients. IgA nephropathy, also known as Berger disease, is a kidney disease that occurs when IgA accumulates in the kidneys and causes inflammation that damages kidney tissues. Hyperimmunoglobulinemia E syndromes (HIESs) are a heterogeneous group of immune disorders characterized by recurrent "cold" staphylococcal infections (due to inadequate accumulation of neutrophils), unusual eczema-like skin rash, pneumatoceles, and severe lung infections resulting in very high serum IgE levels.

IMMUNE TOLERANCE

Introduction

The physiopathology of immune tolerance–related diseases, such as allergies, asthma, autoimmunity, organ transplantation, tumor, chronic infections, and abortions, is complex and is influenced by factors, such as genetic susceptibility, environmental factors and route, dose, or time of the antigen exposure. Many common biologic mechanisms prevent immune responsiveness to innocuous environmental allergens and to self-antigens. Although most autoreactive T cells undergo selection and clonal deletion in the thymus, a small fraction of cells escape into the periphery. Additional immunologic control mechanisms eliminate or inactivate potentially hazardous effector cells that emerge from the thymus and move into the periphery (Fig. 1.5). Allergens enter the body through the respiratory and alimentary tract or injured skin, and the result usually is induction of tolerance in healthy individuals.[11]

Central and Peripheral Tolerance Mechanisms

The processes that constitute immune tolerance normally ensure that immune effector cells are not activated against host tissues or innocuous agents. Immune tolerance is called *central* when the response occurs in primary lymphoid organs, such as thymus or *peripheral* when it occurs in peripheral lymph nodes, Peyer's patches, tonsils, or other tissues.

Central Tolerance

T cells experience the first step of tolerance during their maturation in the thymus. Prethymic T cells reach the subcapsular region of the thymus, where they proliferate. Maturing cells move deeper into the cortex and adhere to cortical epithelial cells. The T cell receptors (TCRs) on thymocytes are exposed to epithelial MHC molecules through these contacts. Negative

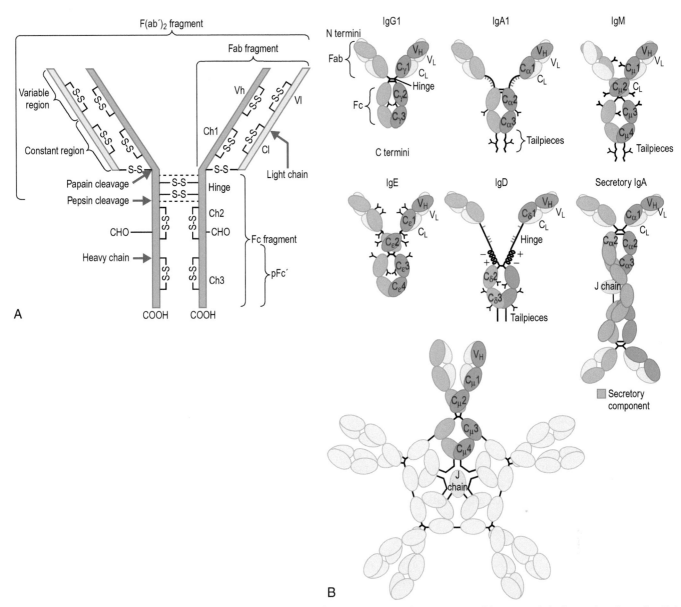

Fig. 1.4 Basic structure of immunoglobulin molecules. (A) In the monomeric structure of immunoglobulin molecules, disulfide bridges link the two heavy chains and the light chains with heavy chains. Enzymatic digestion with papain cleaves the immunoglobulin molecule into three fragments: two Fab fragments, each of which can bind a single antigen epitope, and the Fc fragment, which can bind to Fc receptors. Alternatively, pepsin digestion of immunoglobulins results in a single F(ab')₂ fragment, which remains capable of cross-linking and precipitating multivalent antigen. The Fc portion usually is digested into several smaller peptides by pepsin (pFc'). (B) Schematic structures of the five classes of antibodies. IgG1 and IgA1 are shown as examples of the basic structure of the IgG and IgA classes of antibodies. The other IgG sub-classes differ primarily in the nature and length of the hinge, and the IgA2 hinge region is very short compared with IgA1. Although membrane IgM and IgA exist as monomers, secreted IgA can exist as dimers, and secreted IgM as pentamers, when linked by an extra polypeptide called the J chain. Both multimeric forms of antibodies can be transported across mucosal surfaces by binding to the polymeric immunoglobulin receptor. Dimeric IgA coupled to the J chain and secretory component, a part of the polymeric immunoglobulin (Ig) receptor remaining after transport through epithelial cells, is shown as an example of secretory Ig. (From Delves PJ, Martin SJ, Burton DR, Roitt IM. Roitt's Essential Immunology. 12th ed. Oxford: Wiley-Blackwell; 2011:56, 62.)

selection occurs by deletion of self-reactive T cells. Autoantigens are presented by medullary thymic epithelial cells, interdigitating cells, and macrophages at the corticomedullary junction. Cells expressing CD4 or CD8 subsequently exit to the periphery. The autoimmune polyendocrine syndrome is a good example of central tolerance loss, which is caused by mutations in the AIRE gene. In this disease, self-antigens are not displayed in the

thymus, and T cells escape from deletion and negative selection and enter the peripheral circulation. T cell infiltration of the tissues and autoantibody production results in tissue destruction.[12]

Cells that have escaped negative selection in the thymus are still subject to control in the periphery, because some self-reactive CD4+ T cells that are not deleted by negative selection develop into central Treg cells. These central Treg cells circulate

TABLE 1.2   Selected Biologic Properties of Human Immunoglobulin Isotypes

Characteristics	IgG1	IgG2	IgG3	IgG4	IgM	IgA1	IgA2	IgD	IgE
Physical properties									
Molecular weight (kDa)	146	146	165	146	970[a]	160	160	170	190
Serum half-life (days)	29	27	7	16	5	6	6	–	2
Anatomic distribution									
Mean serum level (mg/mL)	5–12	2–6	0.5–1.0	0.2–1.0	0.5–1.5	0.5–2.0	0–0.2	0–0.4	0–0.002
Transport across placenta	+++	+	++	±	–	–	–	–	–
Transport across epithelium	–	–	–	–	+	+++[b]	+++[b]	–	–
Extravascular diffusion	+++	+++	+++	+++	±	++[c]	++[c]	+	+
Functional activity									
Antigen neutralization	++	++	++	++	++	++	++	–	–
Complement fixation	++	+	++	–	+++	+	+	–	–
ADCC	+	+	+	±	–	–	–	–	+
Immediate hypersensitivity	–	–	–	–	–	–	–	–	+++

ADCC, Antibody-dependent cellular cytotoxicity; –, no effect; ±, no effect or negligible degree; +, small degree; ++, moderate degree; +++, large degree.
[a]Pentameric IgM plus J chain.
[b]Dimer.
[c]Monomer.

in the periphery as mature T cells and inhibit immune or inflammatory responses against self-antigens.

Peripheral Tolerance

There are multiple mechanisms of peripheral immune tolerance (Fig. 1.5). These mechanisms prevent overactivation of immune system which cause intensive tissue inflammation. The fundamental strategy of immunotherapy for allergic diseases is to correct dysregulated immune responses by inducing peripheral allergen tolerance.

During inflammation, apoptosis of immune effector cells is induced by neighbor cells' death-inducing ligands. Immune effector cells can undergo apoptosis by expressing death receptors and ligands simultaneously. To keep tissue inflammation at low levels, effector T cells are directly tolerized by suppressive cytokines released by tissue cells. Treg cells suppress effector T cells. DCs induce tolerization of host T cells. In asthma, spatial separation of T cells and tissue cells, such as the presence of a basement membrane between the epithelium and immune cells, results in ignorance of effector mechanisms. Tissue cells in organs with immune privilege use many mechanisms to suppress or delete highly activated effector cells that could otherwise damage these tissues.

During an immune response, CD4+ T cells normally receive signals activated through engagement of the TCR, which recognizes peptides of specific antigens presented on the surface of APCs by MHC class II molecules. Costimulatory receptors, such as CD28, CD2, and inducible costimulator (ICOS) recognize ligands, such as B7 proteins, CD80, CD86, lymphocyte function–associated antigen 3 (LFA-3), and ICOS ligand (ICOSL) expressed on the surface of APCs. These costimulatory receptors contribute to activation of the T cell. When T cells receive stimulus only through the TCR without any engagement of costimulatory receptors, they enter into a state of unresponsiveness. This state has been called *T cell anergy*. In addition to Treg cells, different subgroups of regulatory B cells (Breg) play important roles in peripheral tolerance to allergens as well as immune tolerance in autoimmunity, tumor and chronic infections.

Histamine Receptors in Peripheral Tolerance

One of the primary mediators released from mast cells is histamine and this acts through histamine receptors. Histamine receptor 2 (HR2) activation mediates early desensitization of basophils. The initial decrease in basophil activity is also associated with symptom scores in grass pollen immunotherapy. H2R suppresses allergen-associated FcεRI-mediated basophil activation. HR2 mainly plays a role in immune tolerance mechanisms. Its expression increases in Th2 cells and both suppress allergen-induced T cell responses and trigger the development of peripheral tolerance by increasing IL-10 production in beekeepers.[13-15] Histamine acts through HR2 and induces IL-10 production by DCs and Th2 cells; it increases the suppressive effect of TGF-β on T cells and decreases the production of Th2 cytokines, IL-4, and IL-13, which are central Th2-type cytokines.[14,16]

Immune Effector Cells and Molecules
Treg Cells and Regulatory B cells

Although various types of cell contribute to establishing immune tolerance, CD4+FOXP3+ Treg cells play a central role in immune control in the periphery. Additionally, in peanut allergy, demethylation of FOXP3+ has been shown to be associated with tolerance development.[17] Two broad categories of Treg cells have been described: naturally occurring Treg cells and antigen-induced Treg cells that secrete inhibitory cytokines,

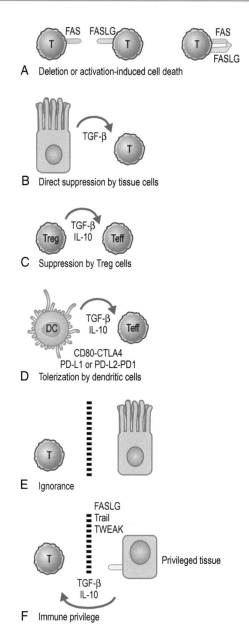

Fig. 1.5 Multiple mechanisms of immune tolerance. (A) Direct deletion of immune effector cell by expression of death-inducing ligands. (B) Direct tolerization of effector T cells by suppressive cytokines released by tissue cells. (C) Suppression of effector T cells by regulatory T cells. (D) Tolerization of host T cells by tolerizing dendritic cells. (E) Ignorance of effector mechanisms as a result of spatial separation of T cells and tissue cells, such as by basement membranes between the epithelium and immune cells in asthma. (F) Immune privilege refers to certain sites in the body that can tolerate the introduction of antigen without eliciting an inflammatory immune response. These sites include the eyes, the placenta and fetus, and the testicles. Tissue cells in these organs use many mechanisms to suppress or delete highly activated effector cells that can damage these tissues. *CTLA4*, Cytotoxic T lymphocyte–associated protein 4; *DC*, dendritic cell; *FAS*, member of the tumor necrosis factor receptor superfamily, member 6; *FASLG*, FAS ligand; *IL*, interleukin; *PD-L1*, programmed death-ligand 1; *PD-L2*, programmed death-ligand 2; *PD-1*, programmed cell death 1; *T*, T cell; *Teff*, effector T cell; *TGFβ*, transforming growth factor β; *Trail*, tumor necrosis factor (ligand) superfamily, member 10; *TWEAK*, tumor necrosis factor (ligand) superfamily, member 12; *Treg*, regulatory T cell.

such as IL-10 and TGF-β. In allergic disease, the balance between allergen-specific Treg cells and disease-promoting Th2 cells appears to determine whether an allergic or healthy immune response against allergen occurs. In healthy individuals, predominant Treg cells are specific for common environmental allergens, indicating a state of natural tolerance.

IL-10–secreting allergen-specific Breg cells have been defined in bee venom–tolerant beekeepers, and patients treated with venom immunotherapy (VIT). Breg cells are $CD73^-CD25^+CD71^+$ B cells, which are capable of suppressing allergen-specific $CD4^+$ T cells and produce allergen-specific IgG4 antibodies after allergy immunotherapy (AIT). Moreover, Breg cells produce IL-35 and TGF-β. IL-10–producing NK regulatory cells suppress allergen-stimulated T cell proliferation in patients during AIT, and these cells may take place in tolerance development as other regulatory cell types.[14,18]

T follicular helper cells (Tfh) are a newly defined cell type identified by $CXCR5^+$ surface receptor and function in B cell maturation and immunoglobulin class switching. A subgroup of Treg, defined as $CXCR5^+ FoxP3^+$ Treg cells, are called *follicular regulatory T (TFR)* cells. They act in the germinal centers of the lymph nodes and suppress T and B cell responses. TFR cells produce more IL-10 compared to TFH cells. There is plasticity between TFH and TFR cells, and this suggests that TFR cells may play essential roles in allergen-specific IgE production and suppression of Th2 responses during immune tolerance development.[13,19]

Transforming Growth Factor-β (TGF-β)

TGF-β is associated with the resolution of immune responses and the induction of Treg cell populations (Table 1.3). However, the effects of TGF-β in allergic disease are complex, with evidence of both disease inhibition and promotion. TGF-β can inhibit human Th2 responses in vitro. In a murine model, overexpression of TGF-β1 in OVA-specific $CD4^+$ T cells abolished airway hyperresponsiveness and airway inflammation induced by OVA-specific Th2 cells.

On the other hand, in a mouse model exhibiting properties of chronic asthma, blockade of TGF-β significantly reduced peribronchiolar extracellular matrix (ECM) deposition, airway smooth muscle (ASM) cell proliferation, and mucus production in the lung without affecting established airway inflammation or Th2 cytokine production. TGF-β1 may be involved in a negative feedback mechanism to control airway inflammation and repair of asthmatic airways, inducing remodeling and fibrosis to exaggerate disease development in humans.

Interleukin-10 (IL-10)

IL-10 plays a role in the control of allergy and asthma. IL-10 inhibits many effector cells and disease processes, and its levels are inversely correlated with disease incidence and severity. IL-10 is synthesized by a wide range of cell types, including B cells, monocytes, DCs, NK cells, and T cells. It inhibits proinflammatory cytokine production and Th1 and Th2 cell activation, which is likely attributable to the effects of IL-10 on APCs and its direct effects on T cell function (Table 1.3).

IL-10 levels inversely correlate with the incidence and severity of asthmatic disease in the lung. In addition, the levels of

TABLE 1.3 Functions of Interleukin-10 and Transforming Growth Factor-β

Cell Type	IL-10	TGF-β
Dendritic cells (DCs)	Inhibits DC maturation, reducing MHC class II and costimulatory ligand expression Inhibits proinflammatory cytokine secretion Inhibits APC function for induction of T cell proliferation and cytokine production (Th1 and Th2)	Promotes Langerhans cell development Inhibits dendritic cell maturation and antigen presentation Downregulates FcεRI expression on Langerhans cells
T cells	Suppresses allergen-specific Th1 and Th2 cells Blocks B7/CD28 costimulatory pathway on T cells	Promotes T cell survival Inhibits proliferation, differentiation, and effector function, including allergen-specific Th1 and Th2 cells Promotes the Th17 lineage
B cells and immunoglobulin (Ig) E	Enhances survival Promotes Ig production, including IgG4 Suppresses allergen-specific IgE	Inhibits proliferation Induces apoptosis of immature or naive B cells Inhibits most Ig class switching Switch factor for IgA Suppresses allergen-specific IgE
CD25+ Tregs	Indirect effect on the generation	Upregulates FOXP3 Promotes generation in the periphery Potential effects on homeostasis
IL-10–secreting Tregs	Promotes induction of IL-10–secreting Tregs	Can promote IL-10 synthesis
Monocytes and macrophages	Inhibits proinflammatory cytokine production and antigen presentation	Inhibits scavenger and effector functions, including proinflammatory cytokine production and antigen presentation Promotes chemotaxis
Eosinophils	Inhibits survival and cytokine production	Chemoattractant
Mast cells	Inhibits mast cell activation, including cytokine production	Promotes chemotaxis Variable effects on other functions May inhibit expression of FcεR (receptor 1)
Neutrophils	Inhibits chemokine and proinflammatory cytokine production	Potent chemoattractant

APC, Antigen-presenting cell; *FcεR*, Fc fragment of IgE receptor; *FOXP3*, Forkhead box P3 protein; *IL*, interleukin; *MHC*, major histocompatibility complex; *TGFβ*, transforming growth factor-β; *Th*, T helper cell subset; *Treg*, regulatory T cell.

IL-10 inversely correlate with skin-prick test reactivity to allergens. Beekeepers, who undergo multiple bee stings and are naturally tolerant to bee venom allergen, have a high IL-10 response. IL-10 and IL-10–producing Treg and Breg cells play essential roles in immune tolerance to allergens. In addition, the roles of Treg and Breg cells and IL-10 have been shown in many autoimmune, organ transplantation, tumor tolerance conditions.[20]

Cytotoxic T lymphocyte–associated antigen 4 (CTLA-4) and programmed death 1 (PD-1) are negative regulators of T cell function. Inhibition of these targets leads to increased activation of the immune system. While CTLA-4 is thought to regulate T cell proliferation early during an immune response, particularly in lymph nodes, PD-1 is thought to suppress T cells later, especially in peripheral tissues. In other words, CTLA-4 acts early on tolerance induction and PD-1 acts late to maintain long-term tolerance.[21]

CYTOKINES AND CHEMOKINES IN ALLERGIC INFLAMMATION

Cytokines in Allergic Inflammation
Interleukin-4 (IL-4)

In addition to T helper lymphocytes, IL-4 is derived from basophils, NK T cells, ILC2 mast cells, and eosinophils (Table 1.4).

TABLE 1.4 Sources of Interleukins IL-4 and IL-13

Cell Source	IL-4	IL-13
T helper lymphocytes		
Naive T cells	No	No
T follicular helper (Tfh) cells	Yes	No
Th2 cells	Yes	Yes
Natural killer (NK) T cells	Yes	Yes
Basophils	Yes	Yes
Eosinophils	Yes	Yes
Mast cells	Yes	Yes
Type 2 innate lymphoid cells (ILC2)	Yes	Yes

IL-4 induces immunoglobulin isotype switch from IgM to IgE. IL-4 has important influences on T lymphocyte growth, differentiation, and survival. As discussed later, IL-4 establishes the differentiation of naive Th0 lymphocytes into the Th2 phenotype.

Another important activity of IL-4 is its ability to induce expression of vascular cell adhesion molecule-1 (VCAM-1) on endothelial cells. This enhances adhesiveness of endothelium for T cells, eosinophils, basophils, and monocytes, but not

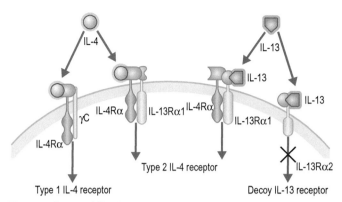

Fig. 1.6 IL-4 and IL-13 receptors. Type 1 IL-4 receptors are heterodimers of IL-4Rα interacting with the shared γC chain and bind only IL-4. Their unique expression on most T helper cells and mast cells renders these cells only responsive to IL-4. Type 2 receptors can bind both IL-4 and IL-13. They are more widely expressed and consist of heterodimers of IL-4Rα and IL-13Rα1. In addition, IL-13 can bind to the IL-13Rα2, which lacks a cytoplasmic domain and thereby functions as a decoy receptor. *IL,* Interleukin.

neutrophils, as a characteristic of allergic reactions. IL-4 receptors are present on mast cells, where they function to stimulate IgE receptor expression, along with the expression of the enzyme leukotriene C₄ (LTC₄) synthase. Functional IL-4 receptors are heterodimers consisting of the IL-4Rα chain interacting with either the shared γ chain or the IL-13Rα1 chain (Fig. 1.6). This shared use of the IL-4Rα chain by IL-4 and IL-13 and the activation by this chain of the signaling protein STAT6 serve to explain many of the common biologic activities of these two cytokines.

Interleukin-5 (IL-5)

IL-5 is the most important eosinophilopoietin and also can induce basophil differentiation. In addition to stimulating eosinophil production, IL-5 is chemotactic for eosinophils and activates mature eosinophils, inducing secretion and enhancing their cytotoxicity. IL-5 promotes accumulation of eosinophils through its ability to upregulate responses to chemokines and $\alpha_d\beta_2$ integrins on eosinophils, thereby promoting their adherence to VCAM-1–expressing endothelial cells. IL-5 prolongs eosinophil survival by blocking apoptosis.

Interleukin-9 (IL-9)

The primary source of IL-9 is the T helper lymphocyte population, including Th2 cells, with additional amounts coming from mast cells ILC2 and eosinophils. IL-9 contributes to mast cell–mediated allergic responses through its ability to stimulate production of mast cell proteases, inflammatory cytokines, and chemokines. Additionally, IL-9 primes mast cells to respond to allergens by increasing their expression of FcεRIα. IL-9 synergizes with IL-4 to enhance production of IgE and memory B cell differentiation. The same synergy leads to enhanced IL-5 production resulting in greater numbers and maturation of immature eosinophil precursors. IL-9 acts on airway epithelial cells by inducing T cell and eosinophil chemotactic factors, such as CCL11 (eotaxin), CCL2 (MCP-1), CCL3 (MIP-1α), and CCL7 (MCP-3).

Interleukin-13 (IL-13)

IL-13 is homologous to IL-4 and shares many of its biologic activities on mononuclear phagocytic cells, endothelial cells, epithelial cells, and B cells. Thus IL-13 induces IgE isotype switch and VCAM-1 expression. Biologic activities of IL-4 and IL-13 are additionally distinguished by their distinct cellular sources (Table 1.4). IL-13, acting through this hormonal mechanism, causes mucus hypersecretion and nonspecific airway hyperreactivity (AHR), and its expression results in the characteristic airway metaplasia of asthma, with the replacement of epithelial cells with goblet cells. The importance of IL-13 in presentations of asthma associated with a robust IL-13 signature is supported by the efficacy of IL-13–targeting therapies in this endotype.

Interleukin-25 (IL-25)

IL-25 is a member of the IL-17 family (IL-17E), but because of its unique spectrum of activities, it has been given this distinct nomenclature. Binding of IL-25 occurs via a heterodimer complex composed of IL-17RB and IL-17RA.[22] It is mainly derived from epithelial cells. The production of IL-25 by injured epithelial cells is an important innate immune signal driving Th2 immune deviation in the subsequent adaptive immune response. IL-25 stimulates release of IL-4, IL-5, and IL-13 from Th2 lymphocytes but, of note, also drives IL-5 and IL-13 secretion from type 2 innate lymphoid cells (ILC2).

Interleukin-33 (IL-33)

IL-33 is a member of the IL-1 superfamily (in which it is designated IL-1F11) that signals through an IL-1 receptor–related protein (originally termed ST2) and its co-receptor IL-1RAcP.[23]

IL-33 is primarily expressed by bronchial epithelial cells, with additional sources including fibroblasts and smooth muscle cells and it is also inducible in lung and dermal fibroblasts, keratinocytes, activated DCs, and macrophages. IL-33 receptors are expressed on T cells (specifically, Th2-like cells), macrophages, hematopoietic stem cells, eosinophils, basophils, mast cells, ILC2, and fibroblasts. As discussed, IL-33 enhances cytokine secretion by Th2 cells and, like IL-25, induces IL-5 and IL-13 secretion by ILC2.

It is possible to avoid food allergy development and to suppress ongoing food allergy by blocking the IL-25, IL-33, and TSLP.[24] Moreover, presence of IL-33 in the airways together with an inhaled allergen which is tolerogenic previously causes the breakdown of the tolerance.[25]

Interleukin-35 (IL-35)

IL-35 is an antiinflammatory cytokine included in the IL-12 superfamily. IL-35 is predominantly secreted by Treg and Breg cells. It consists of two chains, IL-12α chain p35 and IL-27α chain EBV-induced gene3 (Ebi3). IL-35 is involved in the development of tolerance and the production of regulatory cells that express IL-35. Bregs secrete IL-35, which has an autocrine role, to further expand Breg cells to produce more IL-35 and IL-10.[26,27] In addition to its biological function in immune cells, IL-35 is required for the maximum suppressive activity of Treg cells. IL-35 mediates the differentiation of a new subset of inducible Treg cells known as iTR35.[28] While IL-35 can inhibit the proliferation of Th1 and Th17 cells by blocking cell division, it can also hinder Th2 development through GATA3 and IL-4 suppression.[29] In addition to these effects, IL-35 mediates the transformation of Th2 cells into Treg cells, which can be reversed in the presence of IFN-γ.[30] Despite the limited number of studies in humans, it is clear that IL-35 has essential roles in the development of immune tolerance.[31]

Thymic Stromal Lymphopoietin (TSLP)

TSLP is another important contributor to Th2 immune deviation.[32] TSLP is expressed by epithelial cells of the skin, gut, and lung and primes resident DCs in such a way as to promote Th2 cytokine production by their subsequently engaged effector T cells. High levels of TSLP are found in the keratinocytes of patients with AD and in the lungs of asthmatic patients. The TSLP receptor is a heterodimer composed of a unique TSLP-specific receptor and the IL-7Rα chain (CD127). TSLP receptors are expressed primarily by DCs, but their expression by mast cells Th2 cells and ILC2 also promotes secretion of Th2 signature cytokines.

The role of IL-25, IL-33, and TSLP in promoting a Th2-associated milieu is summarized in Fig. 1.7. In this model, injured epithelium has a central role in driving allergic inflammation through its ability to produce these cytokines. TSLP acts primarily on DCs to drive them to induce a Th2-like process. In addition, both IL-25 and IL-33 act directly on mast cells to drive their repertoire of Th2-associated cytokines. More important, IL-25, TSLP, and IL-33 act on ILC2 to increase their selective production of IL-5 and IL-13. These actions on ILC2 and mast cells can occur independent of ongoing allergen exposure, suggesting a mechanism for allergen-independent perpetuation of allergic inflammation.

Chemokines in Allergic Diseases
Asthma

Asthma is a chronic inflammatory lung disease characterized by airway inflammation, mucus hypersecretion, and bronchial hyperresponsiveness. The cellular inflammatory infiltrate in asthma is composed of eosinophils, lymphocytes, mast cells, and to a varying extent, basophils and neutrophils.

Airway exposure to proteases from common allergens, such as mites and molds, disrupts airway epithelial integrity and induces epithelial TSLP production (Fig. 1.8). TSLP expands the number of basophils, prolongs eosinophil survival, and increases eosinophil production of CCL2, CXCL1, and CXCL8. Two other epithelial cytokines, IL-25 and IL-33, also are produced on allergen exposure or epithelial damage. IL-25 and IL-33 upregulate the production of TSLP by epithelial cells and mast cells; induce mast cell release of IL-4, IL-5, IL-13, CCL1, and CXCL8; promote eosinophil survival; and enhance eosinophil production of CCL2 and CCL3. Activated basophils release IL-4, IL-13, granulocyte-macrophage colony-stimulating factor (GM-CSF), and CCL3 as well as histamine and leukotriene C_4 (LTC$_4$), which causes vasodilation and increases vascular permeability. Activated eosinophils generate IL-3, IL-4, IL-5, tumor necrosis factor-α (TNF-α), LTC$_4$, platelet-activating factor (PAF), CCL3, CCL5, and CCL11. In addition to tryptase and chymase, activated mast cells are also a significant source of histamine, lipid mediators (LTB$_4$, PGD$_2$), cytokines (IL-3, IL-5, IL-13, IL-6, IL-10, TNF-α, GM-CSF), and chemokines (CCL1, CCL2, CCL3, CCL5, CCL17, CCL22, CXCL8).

Activation and differentiation of naive T cells into Th2 cells are marked by downregulation of L-selectin and CCR7 and appearance of CCR4, CCR8, CRTh2, and the BLT1 receptor

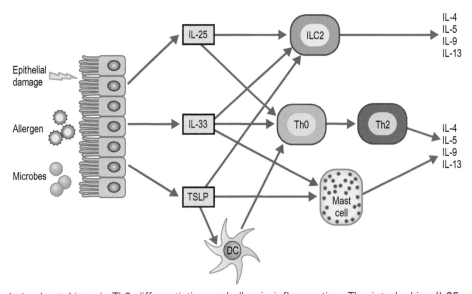

Fig. 1.7 Epithelium-derived cytokines in Th2 differentiation and allergic inflammation. The interleukins IL-25 and IL-33 and thymic stromal lymphopoietin *(TSLP)* are produced by injured epithelium and play critical roles in driving expression of Th2 cytokines. TSLP acts on dendritic cells to direct them to promote the differentiation of naive T cells into Th2 cells. By contrast, IL-25 and IL-33 act directly on the naive T cells to promote Th2 immune deviation. In addition, these three cytokines can generate a Th2 cytokine milieu independent of the adaptive immune system. TSLP and IL-33 directly induce the full repertoire of Th2 cytokine secretion from mast cells. Similarly, IL-25, TSLP, and IL-33 act on type 2 innate lymphoid cells (ILC2) to drive their more restricted secretion of IL-5 and IL-13. *DC*, Dendritic cell; *IL*, interleukin; *Th*, T helper.

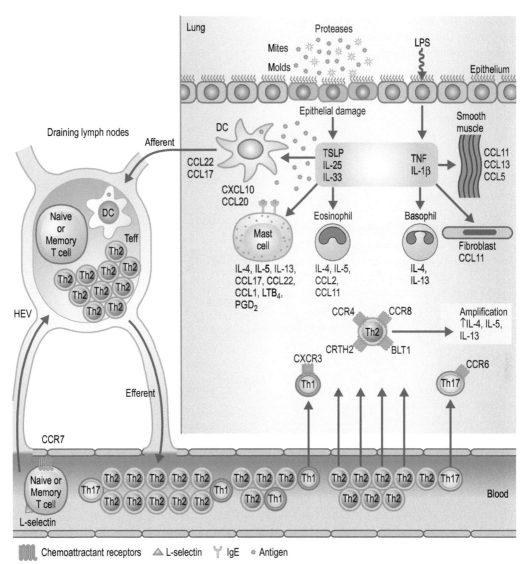

Fig. 1.8 Chemokines and asthma. Asthma is characterized by the infiltration of lung tissue with T helper type 2 *(Th2)* cells producing IL-4, IL-5, and IL-13. Allergen proteases disrupt airway epithelial integrity and induce thymic stromal lymphopoietin *(TSLP)*, IL-25, and IL-33, while epithelial toll-like receptor activation leads to IL-1β and tumor necrosis factor *(TNF)* production. These cytokines upregulate CC chemokine and Th2 cytokine production and release by smooth muscle cells, fibroblasts, mast cells, eosinophils, and basophils. Activated antigen-presenting cells travel to the draining lymph nodes and promote the generation of Th2 cells, which enter the lung and release more Th2 cytokines, thus amplifying the allergic response in the lung. *CCL,* C–C chemokine ligand; *CCR,* C–C chemokine receptor; *DC,* dendritic cell; *HEV,* high endothelial venules; *IgE,* immunoglobulin E; *IL,* interleukin; *LPS,* lipopolysaccharide.

for leukotriene B$_4$ (LTB$_4$). These receptors enable Th2 cells to move down the concentration gradient in response to CCL17, CCL22, CCL1, prostaglandin D$_2$ (PGD$_2$), and LTB$_4$, mediators released by DCs and activated mast cells. IL-4 and IL-13 induce lung-residing macrophages, DCs, epithelial cells, and endothelial cells to produce CCL11, CCL24, CCL26, CCL1, CCL17, and CCL22, thus amplifying the allergic inflammatory response by attracting more eosinophils and Th2 cells.

Atopic Dermatitis

AD is a pruritic chronic inflammatory disease of the skin in which CD4$^+$ memory T lymphocytes, DC subsets, eosinophils, and mast cells infiltrate the perivascular, subepidermal, and intraepidermal areas. A number of chemokines are aberrantly expressed in the skin of patients with AD and help recruit the

inflammatory infiltrate in this disorder. These include CCR2 and CCR3 ligands (CCL13, CCL11, and CCL26) for eosinophil and mast cell recruitment, CCR4 and CCR8 ligands (CCL22 and CCL1) for Th2 cell recruitment, CCR10 ligand (CCL27) for T cell entry into the epidermis, and CCL18.

The pathophysiology of AD begins with intense pruritus and the mechanical injury that results from chronic scratching (Fig. 1.9). Mechanical trauma can directly activate mast cells, which release histamine, neuropeptides, proteases, kinins, and cytokines, many of which further exacerbate pruritus. Furthermore, TSLP levels increase acutely in the skin after mechanical trauma. TSLP induces DC activation and DC production of CCL17 and CCL22.

The trafficking of memory T cells into the skin requires cutaneous lymphocyte antigen (CLA), which interacts with E-selectin on inflamed endothelium, and initiates rolling. The

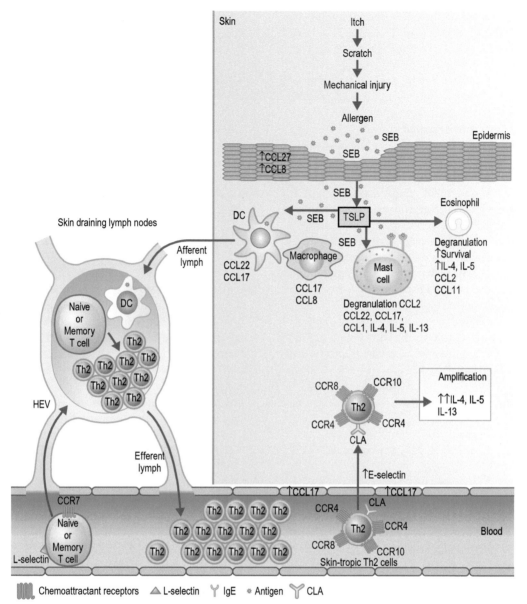

Fig. 1.9 Chemokines and atopic dermatitis. Atopic dermatitis begins with intense pruritus, chronic scratching, and mechanical injury to the skin. Mechanical trauma leads to mast cell release of Th2 cytokines and CC chemokines and upregulates local TSLP production, while loss of normal barrier function increases exposure to allergens and SEB. TSLP-activated dendritic cells travel to the draining lymph nodes and promote Th2 cell differentiation. Th2 cells enter the skin and release Th2 cytokines, thus amplifying the allergic response in the skin. *CCL,* C–C chemokine ligand; *CCR,* C–C chemokine receptor; *CLA,* cutaneous lymphocyte antigen; *DC,* dendritic cell; *IgE,* immunoglobulin E; *IL,* interleukin; *SEB,* staphylococcal enterotoxin B; *Th2,* T helper type 2; *TSLP,* thymic stromal lymphopoietin.

trafficking molecules most highly expressed by T cells isolated from healthy skin are CLA, CCR4, CCR6 (>80%–90%), and, to a lesser extent, CCR8 (50%). Whereas the ligands for CCR6 and CCR8 are upregulated in inflammation, skin endothelial cells and keratinocytes constitutively express CCL17 (one of the ligands for CCR4) and CCL27 (only known ligand for CCR10), respectively.

Eczema lesions as the hallmark of AD and allergic contact dermatitis lesions are induced by keratinocyte apoptosis, related to IFN-γ, Fas-Fas–ligand interaction, TNF-α, TNF-related weak inducer of apoptosis (TWEAK), and IL-32.[33,34]

BIOLOGY OF IMMUNE CELLS

T Lymphocytes

Two classes of α/β T lymphocytes that bear the co-receptors CD4 or CD8 are involved in adaptive immune responses. CD4+ T cells are traditionally called Th cells because they activate and direct other immune cells. There are also populations of CD4+ Treg cells that modulate immune responses. CD4+ T cells recognize antigen presented by class II MHC molecules on APCs, including DCs, B cells, and macrophages. Exogenous protein antigens are taken up by APCs and processed into peptides in endocytic vesicles, which are presented on the cell surface bound to class II MHC molecules. The CD8+ cytotoxic T cells (CTLs) recognize antigen presented on MHC class I molecules. Class I MHC molecules are present on the surface of all nucleated cells. Their cytotoxic functions are carried out by release of preformed effector molecules and by interactions of cell surface molecules.

Antigen-activated CD4+ T cells have the potential to differentiate into effector cells, each with distinct functional properties conferred by the pattern of cytokines they secrete (Fig. 1.10).[35] Th1 cells are a subset of CD4+ T cells that secrete IFN-γ, whereas Th2 cells produce IL-4, IL-5, IL-9, IL-10, and IL-13. Th17 cells produce IL-17A, IL-17F, and IL-22. Treg cells produce IL-10 and TGF-β1, are naturally occurring and induced, suppress T cell differentiation and APC activation, and are not considered effector cells. Th1 cells stimulate strong cell-mediated immune responses, particularly against intracellular pathogens. Th2 cells are elicited in immune responses that require a strong humoral component and in antiparasitic responses. Th17 serve critical host defense functions at mucosal surfaces.

Cytokines are the primary factors that influence the CD4+ Th cell generation and are considered the third signal in CD4+ T cell differentiation.[20] IFN-γ and IL-12 stimulate the induction of Th1 cells. IL-4 drives Th2 cell generation by direct action on CD4+ T cells. IL-13 is involved in the induction of Th2 cells by an unknown mechanism, although not through direct effects on

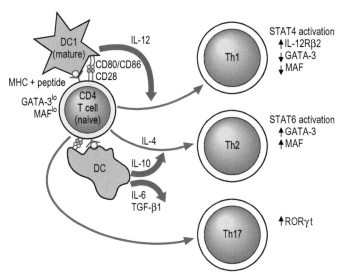

Fig. 1.10 Generation of helper T cell types 1, 2, and 17 (*Th1, Th2,* and *Th17*) from a naive CD4+ T cell. A naive CD4+ T cell does not secrete cytokines and has low expression levels of transcription factors GATA-3 and MAF. Differentiation along the Th1, Th2, or Th17 pathway is triggered by stimulation by antigen presented to the T cell receptor in the context of the major histocompatibility complex *(MHC)* by the appropriate antigen-presenting cell (APC) and a second signal imparted by ligation of costimulatory molecules CD80/CD86 and CD28. Dendritic cells *(DCs)* represent the key APCs for naive T cells. Those that produce interleukin-10 *(IL-10)* favor Th2 differentiation, and those that produce interleukin-12 *(IL-12)* stimulate Th1 differentiation. Th17 cells can be generated in the presence of interleukin-6 *(IL-6)* and transforming growth factor-β1 *(TGF-β1)*, presumably produced by DCs.

CD4+ T cells. IL-6, IL-1β, TGF-β1, and in some situations, IL-23 promote Th17 development.

In the secondary lymphoid tissue, a naive T cell differentiates into an effector cell. Compared with naive T cells, effector cells do not require costimulation to be activated, allowing these cells to respond to antigen with hair-trigger rapidity to produce high levels of cytokines and chemokines, which then direct the immune response. Most activated effector CD4+ T cells die subsequent to an immune response through the process of activation-induced cell death, but a subset of CD4+ T cells will persist as memory cells for the life of the host. CD4+ memory T cells persist in lymphoid organs as central memory cells and in nonlymphoid tissues as effector memory cells. The effector memory T cells respond rapidly to repeat exposures to antigen, whereas central memory T cells are slower to be mobilized.

B Lymphocytes

The humoral immune response is generated by B cells. Mature B cells express immunoglobulin on its cell surface, which constitutes the antigen-specific BCR. BCR is a molecular complex made up of antigen-binding or variable (V) regions. This region of the protein varies among immunoglobulins, allowing each antibody to bind to any foreign structure that the individual may encounter. To generate this diverse immunoglobulin repertoire, during development in the bone marrow, B cells undergo somatic deoxyribonucleic acid (DNA) recombination of the variability (V), diversity (D), and joining (J) regions of the immunoglobulin heavy and light chains. The invariant or constant region of the antibody is specialized for different effector functions in the immune system after antibody is secreted. There are five main constant-region forms: IgM, IgD, IgG, IgE, and IgA. The BCR in the membrane-bound form recognizes and binds antigen and transmits activation signals into the cell.

Naive B cells recirculate through peripheral lymphoid tissues until it binds specific antigen through surface immunoglobulin and is activated (i.e., signal 1). Most antibody responses, including antibody responses to protein antigens, require antigen-specific T cell help. Antigen bound to surface immunoglobulin is internalized, processed, complexed with MHC class II molecules, and displayed on the cell surface. Previously primed CD4+ T cells that recognize the peptide-MHC class II complex on the B cell provide the second signal for activation. The cytokines secreted by CD4+ Th cells during B cell activation regulate which immunoglobulin heavy-chain constant regions will be selected during class-switch recombination to best serve the functions of the specific immune response. Th2 responses to allergens stimulate B cell activation and result in elevated levels of allergen-specific IgE.

Innate Lymphoid Cells

Populations of lymphoid cells that lack rearranged antigen receptors, which were called ILCs, have been recently identified. These ILC populations can be divided into three groups, based on shared phenotypic and functional properties like T cells. Type 1 ILC (ILC1) constitutively express T-bet and are able to produce IFN-γ upon activation. Type 2 ILC (ILC2) constitutively express GATA-3 and in response to IL-25, IL-33, and

TSLP stimulation produce IL-5 and IL-13. Type 3 ILC (ILC3) constitutively express ROR-γ and in response to IL-1β and IL-23 produce IL-17, IL-22, and IFN-γ.[36]

ILC type 2 seems to be important in allergic responses. The ILC2/ILC1 ratio is high in patients with perennial AR sensitized to house dust mite; however, it turns to normal levels following a successful AIT. In the presence of retinoic acid, ILC2 cells transformed into regulatory ILCs (ILCregs) which produce IL-10. These cells can suppress Th2 cell and ILC2 activation. DCs that have the capability of retinoic acid production also induce peripheral Treg cell differentiation. Putting these together, one may suggest that ILCregs may participate in tolerance induction in the mechanisms of AIT.[13,19] ILC2s take place in many functions during the inflammatory process in asthma and AD (Fig. 1.11).

Another type of ILC, ILC type 3, may have essential roles in immune tolerance induction. CD40L-expressing ILC3s locate in close contact with B cells in tonsils. Both cells work interdependently, as ILC3s induce IL-15 production in B cells and IL-15 which is a potent growth factor for ILC3s increases CD40L expression on ILC3s. CD40L+ ILC3s induce IL-10–secreting Breg cells through the CD40L and BAFF-receptor–dependent pathway. ILC3-induced Breg cells are characterized by CD27– IgD+IgM+CD24highCD38highCD1d+ immature transitional (itBreg) phenotype. This interaction is important for the maintenance of immune tolerance against innocuous antigens and is inadequate in allergic diseases. In tonsils, generation of functional allergen-specific Treg cells takes place. ILC3s, Breg cells, and Treg cells localize side by side in the interfollicular regions of palatine tonsils. CD40L+ ILC3s may be essential in the maintenance of immune tolerance in tonsils through induction of

functional itBreg cells. These cells can contribute to immune tolerance induction and suppression of T cell responses both by a cell-to-cell contact through programmed cell death-ligand 1 and by secretion of IL-10.[13]

Dendritic Cells

DCs are the most important APCs found throughout the body and are mainly recognized for their exceptional potential to generate a primary immune response and sensitization to allergens. DCs determine the T cell polarization process that produces Th1 cells (generating mainly IFN-γ), Th2 cells (generating mainly IL-4, IL-5, and IL-13), Th17 cells (generating mainly IL-17), and Treg cells (generating mainly IL-10 and TGF-β). These cells are also recognized for their ability to produce ongoing effector responses that are crucial in maintaining allergic inflammation. In humans, circulating DCs can be broadly divided into two groups: (1) mDCs and (2) pDCs. Both subsets express a different repertoire of TLRs and display a diverse cytokine signature after microbial stimulation. mDCs selectively express TLR2–6 and TLR8 and respond to bacterial and viral infections by producing large amounts of IL-12. In contrast, pDCs constitutively express the endosome-associated TLR7 and TLR9, and they are the main producers of type 1 IFNs in humans.[6]

Mast Cells

Mast cells are present throughout connective tissues and mucosal surfaces and are especially prominent at the interface with the external environment, such as the skin, respiratory tract, conjunctiva, and gastrointestinal tract. Mast cells contribute to the maintenance of tissue homeostasis, with important roles in

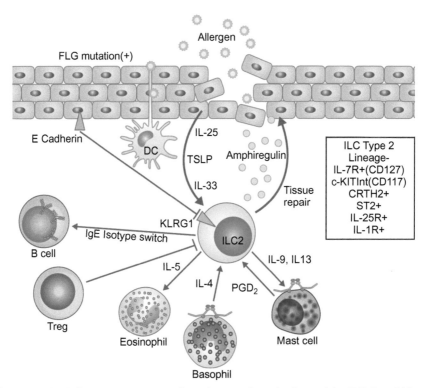

Fig. 1.11 The role of ILC2 during the inflammatory process in asthma and atopic dermatitis. *DC*, Dendritic cell; *IgE*, immunoglobulin E; *IL*, interleukin; *ILC*, innate lymphoid cell; *PGD₂*, prostaglandin D₂; *Treg*, regulatory T.

wound repair, revascularization, and protective responses to bacterial infection and envenomation. Their "misguided" activation by allergens contributes to the development of allergic symptoms.

The best-studied mechanism of mast cell activation, and the one considered most relevant to allergic disease, is activation mediated through the high-affinity IgE receptor FcεRI. IgE-dependent signaling in vivo is initiated when multivalent allergen binds to allergen-specific IgE bound to the FcεRIα chain. IgE-dependent activation of the mast cell induces granule swelling, crystal dissolution, and granule fusion. This sequence is followed by exocytosis with release of mediators into the extracellular space—a process termed *anaphylactic degranulation*. In addition to the stored granule-derived mediators, newly formed metabolites of arachidonic acid also are released from mast cells after IgE-dependent activation (Table 1.5).

Basophils

Basophil granulocytes develop in the bone marrow and are released into the circulation as mature end-stage cells representing less than 1% of blood leukocytes. Basophils play a critical role in allergic disease by infiltrating sites of allergic inflammation and releasing mediators and cytokines that perpetuate type I (immediate) hypersensitivity reactions. Degranulation events resulting in the release of these mediators are preceded by the interaction of allergen with specific IgE molecules bound to the high-affinity IgE receptors on the surface of these cells. This IgE-dependent activation also leads to the production of immunomodulatory cytokines. In particular, basophils are a significant source of IL-4 and IL-13, two Th2 cytokines, whose expression is characteristic of allergic lesions and which are now considered critical components in the pathogenesis of allergic disease.

Eosinophils

Eosinophils are bone marrow–derived granulocytes that play an important pathophysiologic role in a wide range of conditions, including asthma and related allergic diseases and parasitic helminth infections. Eosinophils are unique among circulating leukocytes in their prodigious capacity to produce a variety of mediators, including granule proteins, cytokines, lipids, oxidative products, and enzymes (Table 1.6). Eosinophils express receptors recognizing the Fc portion of various immunoglobulins (FcR). Beads coated with IgA or secretory IgA (sIgA) induce degranulation of eosinophils, and eosinophils from allergic individuals display enhanced FcαR expression. However, most reports suggest that ligation of FcεRI does not result in measurable eosinophil degranulation. Exposure of eosinophils ex vivo to various cytokines mimics in vivo primed eosinophils. IL-5 activates LTC_4 and O2− generation, phagocytosis, and helminthotoxic activity, as well as Ig-induced degranulation. Both TSLP and IL-33 activate eosinophil effector functions, such as adhesion to matrix proteins, cytokine production, and degranulation.

TABLE 1.5 Classical Preformed and Newly Generated Human Mast Cell Autacoid Mediators and Proteases With Examples of Their Biologic Effects

Mediator	Activity
Histamine (stored)	Bronchoconstriction; tissue edema; ↑vascular permeability; ↑ mucus secretion; ↑ fibroblast proliferation; ↑ collagen synthesis; ↑ endothelial cell proliferation, dendritic cell differentiation and activation
Heparin (stored)	Anticoagulant; mediator storage matrix; sequesters growth factors; fibroblast activation; endothelial cell migration
Tryptase (stored)	Degrades respiratory allergens and cross-linked IgE; generates C3a and bradykinin; degrades neuropeptides; TGF-β activation; increases basal heart rate and ASM contractility; ↑ fibroblast proliferation and collagen synthesis; epithelial ICAM-1 expression and CXCL8 release; potentiation of mast cell histamine release; neutrophil recruitment
Chymase (stored)	↑ mucus secretion; ECM degradation, type I procollagen processing; converts angiotensin I to angiotensin II; ↓ T cell adhesion to airway smooth muscle; activates IL-1β, degrades IL-4, releases membrane-bound SCF
PGD_2 (synthesized)	Bronchoconstriction; tissue edema; ↑ mucus secretion; dendritic cell activation; chemotaxis of eosinophils, Th2 cells, and basophils via the CRTH2 (CD294) receptor
LTC_4/LTD_4 (synthesized)	Bronchoconstriction; tissue edema; ↑ mucus secretion; enhances IL-13–dependent airway smooth muscle proliferation; dendritic cell maturation and recruitment; eosinophil IL-4 secretion; mast cell IL-5, IL-8, and TNF-α secretion; tissue fibrosis

ASM, Airway smooth muscle; *CRTH2*, chemoattractant receptor of Th2 cells; *ECM*, extracellular matrix; *ICAM-1*, intercellular adhesion molecule 1; *IgE*, immunoglobulin E; *IL*, interleukin; LTC_4, leukotriene C_4; LTD_4, leukotriene D_4; PGD_2, prostaglandin D_2; *SCF*, stem cell factor; *TGF-β*, transforming growth factor-β; *TNF-α*, tumor necrosis factor-α.

TABLE 1.6 Eosinophil Mediators

Granule proteins
Major basic protein (MBP)
MBP homolog (MBP2)
Eosinophil cationic protein (ECP)
Eosinophil-derived neurotoxin (EDN)
Eosinophil peroxidase (EPX)
Charcot–Leyden crystal (CLC) protein
Secretory phospholipase A_2 (sPLA_2)
Bactericidal/permeability-inducing protein (BPI)
Acid phosphatase
Arylsulfatase
β-Glucuronidase

Lipid mediators
Leukotriene B_4 (negligible)
Leukotriene C_4
5-HETE
5,15- and 8,15-diHETE
5-oxo-15-hydroxy-6,8,11,13-ETE
Platelet-activating factor (PAF)
Prostaglandin E_1 and E_2
Thromboxane B_2

(Continued)

TABLE 1.6 Eosinophil Mediators—cont'd

Oxidative products

Superoxide radical anion (OH⁻)

Hydrogen peroxide (H_2O_2)

Hypohalous acids

Enzymes

Collagenase

Metalloproteinase-9

Indoleamine 2,3-dioxygenase (IDO)

Cytokines[a]

IL-1α

IL-2

IL-3

IL-4

IL-5

IL-6

IL-9

IL-10

IL-11

IL-12

IL-13

IL-16

Leukemia inhibitory factor (LIF)

Interferon-γ (IFN-γ)

Tumor necrosis factor-α (TNF-α)

GM-CSF

APRIL

Chemokines

CXCL8 (IL-8)

CCL2 (MCP-1)

CCL3 (MIP-1α)

CCL5 (RANTES)

CCL7 (MCP-3)

CCL11 (eotaxin)

CCL13 (ECP-4)

Growth factors

Nerve growth factor (NGF)

Platelet-derived growth factor (PDGF)

Stem cell factor (SCF)

Transforming growth factor (TGF-α, TGF-β)

APRIL, A proliferation-inducing ligand; *ETE*, eicosatetraenoic acid; *GM-CSF*, granulocyte-macrophage colony-stimulating factor; *HETE*, hydroxyeicosatetraenoic acid; *IL*, interleukin.
[a]Physiologic significance of these cytokines needs to be confirmed.

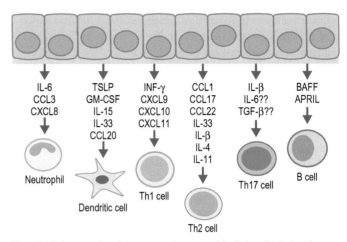

Fig. 1.12 Interaction between airway epithelial cell–derived cytokines and inflammatory cells. *APRIL*, A proliferation-inducing ligand; *BAFF*, B cell–activating factor of the TNF family; *CCL*, C–C chemokine ligand; *GM-CSF*, granulocyte-macrophage colony-stimulating factor; *IFN-γ*, interferon-γ; *IL*, interleukin; *TGF-β*, transforming growth factor-β; *Th*, helper T cell subset; *TSLP*, thymic stromal lymphopoietin.

response to inflammation. Accordingly, these structural cells play crucial roles in the pathogenesis and symptoms of allergic disease and asthma in concert with immune cells.

Airway Epithelial Cells

The epithelium constitutes the interface between the external environment and the internal milieu of the lung. It is the site of first contact with inhaled particles, pollutants, respiratory viruses, and airborne allergens. Consequently, the epithelium plays an important role as a physical and immune barrier. The epithelium senses PAMPs on inhaled foreign substances via their PRRs and regulates airway homeostasis through the production of a multitude of mediators, such as GM-CSF, TSLP, IL-25, and IL-33, which promote a Th2 bias in DC precursor (Fig. 1.12). In other words, epithelial cells bridge the innate and adaptive immune responses by translating environmental exposures into disease phenotypes.

Epithelial cell structure and function are abnormal in patients with asthma. At a gross level, the composition of the asthmatic airway epithelium is different from that of the non-asthmatic population. For example, goblet cell hyperplasia and excessive mucus production are common features of asthma that contribute significantly to morbidity and mortality. Moreover, epithelial cells isolated from patients who have asthma have a deficient innate immune response from type I antiviral IFNs, particularly of IFN-β release during rhinovirus infection. Changes of epithelial cell structure and function occur early in disease pathogenesis. These findings place the epithelium at the forefront of asthma pathogenesis, and understanding the mechanisms that underlie these abnormalities will have short- and long-term clinical significance for the treatment of this disease.

When the epithelial cells are exposed to an external insult, such as allergens, pollutants, viruses, fungi, and bacterial toxins, epithelial barrier is damaged, epithelial cytokines (TSLP, IL-25, and IL-33) called alarmins are released. IL-25 and IL-33

CONTRIBUTION OF STRUCTURAL CELLS TO ALLERGIC INFLAMMATION

While structural cells, such as epithelial, bone, smooth muscle cells, or fibroblast, have their proper function, they produce cytokines, chemokines, lipid mediators, and growth factors which control mobility of immune cells and local inflammatory milieu. Symptoms of allergic airway disease, such as sneezing, rhinorrhea, unproductive coughing, episodic bronchospasm, and sensations of breathlessness, are neuronally mediated in activate ILC2s to produce IL-4, IL-5, and IL-13. Rhinovirus can also induce IL-33 and promote type 2 inflammation. The epithelial barrier is disrupted by Th2 cells, type 2 ILCs, and their cytokines IL-4 and IL-13 in human bronchial epithelium. Meanwhile, CPG-DNA administration strengthens the tight junction (TJ) integrity of the bronchial epithelial barrier. In addition, TSLP-stimulated CD11c⁺ DCs can activate CRTH2⁺ Th2 effector memory cells and undergo further Th2 polarization to magnify their role in allergic inflammation. Periostin is secreted by stimulated airway epithelial cells. It is an ECM protein and is considered a biomarker of type 2 inflammation. Periostin gene expression is increased by IL-13 and IL-4 in bronchial epithelial cells. Periostin functions on fibroblasts to promote airway remodeling, increase mucus secretion, and recruit eosinophils.[37]

Epithelial TJs seal the epithelia and form an essential part of the barrier between the inner tissues and the external environment. They control the paracellular flux and epithelial permeability and prevent the entrance of foreign particles, such as allergens and toxins to subepithelial tissues. They form complexes with members of the claudin family, the marvel family, and the junctional adhesion molecule (JAM) family spanning the membrane and forming homo- and heterodimeric connections between adjacent cells. Scaffold proteins, such as the zonula occludens (ZO) family, link the TJ complex to the actin cytoskeleton. Epithelial barrier TJ defects are reported in several allergic and inflammatory disorders, such as AD, asthma, and chronic rhinosinusitis, and a role for TJ in smooth muscle cells is described in asthma pathogenesis.[38-45]

Epithelial TJs are very sensitive to environmental factors. A recent study with laundry detergents demonstrated the devastating effects on TJ barrier integrity and cellular toxicity of human bronchial epithelial cells, even at very high dilution, without affecting epigenome and TJ gene expression.[46]

Airway Smooth Muscle Cells

In asthma, the ASM contracts in response to multiple stimuli, but it also produces ECM proteins, proteases that modulate these proteins, and myriad growth factors and cytokines. These collectively lead to airway remodeling—the pathology that characterizes asthma and consists of thickening of the airway wall, increased angiogenesis, mucous cell hyperplasia, thickening of the basement membrane, and increased bulk of muscle. It was previously thought that remodeling was a response to chronic airway inflammation, but it seems more likely that inflammation and remodeling develop along separate pathways. This is consistent with the finding that bronchoconstriction alone in the absence of an inflammatory or allergic stimulus can lead to airway remodeling.

ASM is a functional part of the innate immune system. It expresses messenger RNAs (mRNAs) for TLR1 through TLR10 and functional TLR2 and TLR3, indicating ASM can respond to bacterial and viral infections. ASM modulates leukocyte trafficking and function in asthma by activating cell adhesion molecules and secretion of chemokines and cytokines. When the response from cells obtained from people with asthma and people without asthma were compared, higher levels of cytokines and profibrotic factors were observed in the asthma-derived cells.

Neuronal Control of Airway Function

Both the immune system and the nervous system are critical to host defense within the airways. The immune system uses cellular and humoral mechanisms to protect the peripheral air spaces from invasion and colonization by microorganisms. The nervous system protects the airways by orchestrating reflexes, such as sneezing, coughing, mucus secretion, and bronchospasm in response to inflammation. Therefore the nervous system serves as the principal transducer between immunologic aspects of allergic inflammation and the symptomatology of immediate hypersensitivity.

Nerve–immune interactions can be inappropriate and deleterious, as with allergy; the immune response triggered by allergen exposure can recruit the nervous system in a way that is not beneficial to the host and causes or exacerbates the symptoms of allergic disease: irritation, pruritus, sneezing, coughing, hypersecretion, reversible bronchospasm, and dyspnea. Relatively little is known about the specific pharmacology of allergen–immune–nerve interactions, but the mediators likely include histamine, arachidonic acid metabolites, tryptase, neurotrophins, chemokines, and cytokines. In addition, the allergic reaction in the respiratory tract is associated with overt activation, increases in electrical excitability, as well as phenotypic changes in sensory, central, and autonomic neurons. Future research into the mediators and mechanisms of allergen-induced neuromodulation will not only increase our basic understanding of the pathophysiology of allergic disease but also suggest novel therapeutic strategies.[47]

CYTOKINE NETWORKS IN ALLERGIC INFLAMMATION

Cytokines play a key role in the orchestration and perpetuation of allergic inflammation and are now targeted in therapy (Fig. 1.13).[48] Allergic inflammation is characterized by the secretion of Th2 cytokines, including IL-4, IL-5, IL-9, and IL-13, which are secreted mainly by Th2 cells. The use of biologic immune response modifiers that target and neutralize cytokines is beginning to shed new light on the role of individual Th2 cytokines. IL-4 and IL-13 play a key role in IgE synthesis through isotype switching of B cells and appear to play a critical role in animal models of asthma. Thus far, blocking IL-4 and IL-13 or their common receptor IL-4Rα has not yet been shown to be of clinical benefit in asthma, but many clinical trials are currently under way. IL-5 is of critical importance in the differentiation, survival, and priming of eosinophils. A humanized monoclonal IL-5 neutralizing antibody, mepolizumab, induced a profound decrease in eosinophils in the blood and in induced sputum in patients with mild asthma but had no effect on the response to inhaled allergen. Clinical trials of anti–IL-5 in unselected symptomatic asthmatic patients showed no overall clinical improvement. Yet in highly selected patients with severe asthma and sputum eosinophilia, despite high doses of inhaled or oral corticosteroids, mepolizumab decreased the frequency of exacerbations and reduced requirements for oral corticosteroids, although it did not lessen symptoms or AHR.

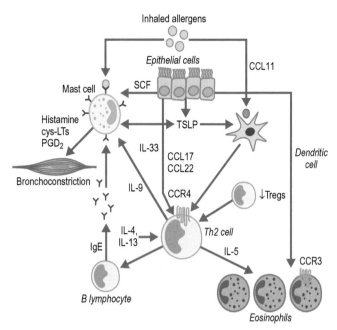

Fig. 1.13 Inflammation in allergy. Inhaled allergens activate sensitized mast cells by cross-linking surface-bound immunoglobulin E *(IgE)* molecules to release several bronchoconstrictor mediators, including cysteinyl leukotrienes *(cys-LTs)* and prostaglandin D_2 *(PGD$_2$)*. Epithelial cells release stem cell factor *(SCF)* (i.e., Kit ligand), which is important for maintaining mucosal mast cells at the airway or skin surface. Allergens are processed by myeloid dendritic cells, which are conditioned by thymic stromal lymphopoietin *(TSLP)* secreted by epithelial cells and mast cells to release the chemokines CCL17 and CCL22, which act on CCR4 to attract T helper 2 *(Th2)* cells. Th2 cells have a central role in orchestrating the inflammatory response in allergy through the release of interleukin *(IL)*-4 and IL-13 (which stimulate B cells to synthesize IgE), IL-5 (which is necessary for eosinophilic inflammation), and IL-9 (which stimulates mast cell proliferation). Epithelial cells release CCL11, which recruits eosinophils via CCR3. Patients with allergic disease may have a defect in regulatory T cells *(Tregs)*, which may favor further Th2 cell activation. *CCL*, C–C chemokine ligand; *CCR*, C–C chemokine receptor.

This observation suggests that blockade of individual cytokines may provide clinical benefit only in carefully selected patients.

Several proinflammatory cytokines have been implicated in allergic diseases, including IL-1β, IL-6, TNF-α, and GM-CSF, which are released from a variety of cells, including macrophages and epithelial cells, and may be important in amplifying the allergic inflammatory response. Although available evidence is persuasive that TNF-α may be important in patients with severe asthma, and earlier small clinical studies with anti–TNF-α therapies were promising, a large placebo-controlled trial of an anti-TNF antibody (golimumab) in severe asthma showed no overall benefit. Some of the subjects may have been responders, however, and patients with greater bronchodilator reversibility showed an apparent reduction in exacerbations. IL-17 also is increased in severe asthma, but anti–IL-17 antibodies have not yet been tested in asthma patients.

Interest has now focused on upstream regulatory cytokines in the pathogenesis of asthma because it is thought that they may

have greater therapeutic potential. TSLP is an upstream IL-7–like cytokine that may initiate and propagate allergic immune responses and plays an important role in immune responses to helminths. TSLP is produced predominantly by airways and nasal epithelial cells and by skin keratinocytes and also stimulates immature mDCs, which express the heterodimeric TSLP receptor to differentiate into mature DCs. TSLP-activated DCs promote naive CD4$^+$ T cells to differentiate into a Th2 phenotype and promote the expansion of Th2 memory cells through the release of Th2 chemotactic cytokines CCL17 and CCL22 and expression of the costimulatory molecule OX40 ligand. In addition, TSLP suppresses the IL-12 p40 receptor in DCs and, by suppressing Th1 responses, further enhances Th2 responses. TSLP also promotes allergic inflammation by activating the differentiation IL-4 gene transcription in Th2 cells and the production of IL-13 from mast cells, by recruiting eosinophils and by amplifying responses of basophils. TSLP may therefore play a pivotal role in the initiation of allergic asthma, rhinitis, and AD. It is highly expressed in the airways of asthmatic patients, and its expression is correlated with disease severity and the expression of CCL17. TSLP is also expressed in epithelial cells of patients with AR and AD. Overexpression of TSLP in skin keratinocytes of mice amplifies the inflammatory response of inhaled allergen in sensitized animals, thus providing a mechanism for the "allergic march" whereby AD commonly precedes the development of asthma in children.

IL-25 (IL-17E) is a member of the IL-17 family of cytokines and induces allergic inflammation through increased production of Th2 cytokines. Although originally shown to be produced by Th2 cells, it is now known to be released from many different cells, including mast cells, basophils, eosinophils, macrophages, and epithelial cells. Blockade of IL-25 is effective in animal models of allergic disease, and blocking antibodies are now in clinical development. IL-33 is another upstream cytokine and a member of the IL-1 family of cytokines, which is unusual in its localization within the nucleus, where it may regulate chromatin structure and gene expression. It appears to be released only on damage to epithelial or endothelial cells, presumably acting as an alarmin, and is constitutively expressed at mucosal surfaces such as the airways. It signals through a receptor, ST2, that activates NF-κB and MAPK pathways. Its relevance to allergic inflammation is that it enhances ILC2 and Th2 cell function, leading to eosinophilia, mast cell activation, and mucus hypersecretion, potentially acting as a bridge between innate and adaptive immunity in allergic inflammation. It also directly activates eosinophils, mast cells, epithelial cells, and DCs. It appears to switch alveolar macrophages to the alternatively activated form (M2) that has been found in animal models of asthma with increased secretion of CCL17, although whether this association is relevant to human allergic disease is uncertain. IL-33 shows increased expression in airway epithelium of asthmatic patients, and level of expression is related to disease severity. IL-33 is increased in the skin of patients with AD and is released into the circulation during as well as mediating anaphylactic shock. IL-33 also is expressed in mast cells after activation through IgE receptors and also activates mast cells, providing a means of maintaining mast cell activation. Antibodies that block IL-33 or ST2 are now in clinical development.

MICROBIOME AND IMMUNE SYSTEM

Bacteria can stimulate or suppress inflammatory events in many ways. Both bacterial cell wall components and some metabolites of the microbiome have been associated with immunoregulatory effects. *Bifidobacterium*, *Lactobacillus*, and *Clostridium* species have been shown to increase the proportion of Treg cells in animal models. Moreover, *Clostridia* stimulates ILC3s to produce IL-22, which results in a strengthening of the epithelial barrier in the gastrointestinal tract. Bifidobacteria and Lactobacilli increase the induction of Treg cells by promoting metabolic processes such as vitamin A metabolism and tryptophan metabolism in DCs. An exopolysaccharide from *Bifidobacterium longum* has been shown to suppress Th17 responses in the gut and lung. Ingestion of *B. longum* by healthy human volunteers stimulated Foxp3+ Treg cells in peripheral blood. Administration of this bacterial strain to patients with chronic inflammatory diseases resulted in decreased levels of serum proinflammatory biomarkers. Bacteria-derived metabolites also have some effects on immunoregulatory processes. Short-chain fatty acids (SCFAs) produced by the gut microbiota have been shown to affect DC and T cell functions by epigenetic mechanisms which are inhibition of histone deacetylases. Biogenic amines produced by bacteria in the human gut can change immune and inflammatory responses. In recent studies, microbiota-originated taurine and histamine have been shown to influence host–microbiome interactions in different ways such as co-modulating NLRP6 inflammatory signaling, production of epithelial IL-18, and suppressing the AMP production.[49]

FOOD ALLERGY AS A MODEL FOR ALLERGIC DISEASES

Food allergy frequently develops during infancy and this is explained by the immaturity of the gastrointestinal mucosa.[50] For this reason, exposure to food allergens early in life may be protective towards the development of allergy, establishing oral tolerance before sensitization to the allergen. LEAP study showed that early introduction of peanuts decreased the probability of peanut allergy development among children at high risk and resulted in the induction of oral tolerance to peanuts.[51] Although GUT mucosa are continuously exposed to allergens and commensal microorganisms, the immune system are mostly capable of tolerating these antigens. Induced Treg cells (iTregs) and Tr1 lymphocytes play an important role in this immune tolerance. Tolerogenic CD103+ DCs present the luminal antigens and induce Foxp3+ Tregs in a TGF-β–dependent and retinoic acid–dependent pathway.[52,53] In children who outgrow or become tolerant towards cow's milk allergy, the level of Tregs has been found to be higher than those with active allergies.[54] Genetic and environmental factors shape the immune responses in the skin when an exposure to food allergens occurs. In two epidemiologic studies, AD and the filaggrin gene mutation have been identified as potential risk factors for the development of food allergy.[55,56] In experimental food allergy models, exposure of the skin to food allergens resulted in the promotion of intestinal food allergy development in a Th2-dependent manner before the establishment of immune tolerance.[57,58] Despite the advancement in studies, the mechanism to which allergic sensitization in the skin is able to disrupt oral tolerance and how it leads to the development of food allergy in the gut remains unclear. It is proposed that the triggering effect of food allergens stimulates TSLP, IL-33, and IL-25 production in the skin keratinocytes and these alarmins in turn results in the activation of ILC2s and DCs.[52,53,58–62] The migration of DCs to the lymph nodes triggers the proliferation of Th2 effector and memory cells.[32] Following the ingestion of sensitized food, these Th2 cells are likely to migrate into the intestine and communicate with ILC2s leading to the production of IL-13. Intestinal epithelial cells also produce IL-33 and IL-25, further stimulating ILC2s. As a result of this, an allergic immune response develops towards the sensitized food.[63,64]

Tregs regulate the functions of ILC2s and suppress their type 2 cytokine production. Reciprocally, ILC2s secrete IL-4, which downregulates the Treg functions and increases the mast cell activation.[65] In the steady state, this network functions towards the food tolerance side. However, some genetic and environmental factors like microbiota dysregulation may stimulate alarmin production from the intestinal epithelial cells, which results in ILC2 activation.[66] Additionally, peanut allergens have been shown to increase alarmin production leading to food allergy development.[67] ILC2s produce many Th2 cytokines like IL-4, IL-5, IL-9, IL-13. IL-4, and IL-9 that amplifies the mast cells response.[68] As a result, iTregs are inhibited by the effect of IL-4.[65] After re-exposure to food allergens, activated mast cells can stimulate IL-33 production and ILC2 activation. This forms a positive feedback loop on mast cell activation and a negative feedback loop on iTregs, promoting the persistence of food allergy.[69,70]

Commensal bacteria also have some indirect effects on host immune responses towards food antigens. Some *Clostridia* strains induce the accumulation of Tregs in the colon.[71,72] *Clostridia* also trigger ILC3s to produce IL-22, strengthening the epithelial barrier. In mice, it was shown that *Clostridia*-containing microbiota suppresses the response to food allergy.[73] In response to the microbial signals, macrophages secrete IL-1β which mediates GM-CSF release from ILC3s. GM-CSF induces IL-10 and retinoic acid production by DCs and macrophages and subsequently promotes the induction of Tregs. Any interference with this crosstalk results in loss of oral tolerance to food allergens.[74]

RESOLUTION OF ALLERGIC INFLAMMATION AND MAJOR PATHWAYS

Inflammation resolution is a tightly regulated and active process essential for the restoration of tissue homeostasis after an inflammatory insult. Dysregulated resolution results in chronic inflammation, tissue remodeling, and fibrosis. Granulocyte apoptosis–mediated caspase family proteins are essential for the clearance of these infiltrating inflammatory cells; cell survival is increased during inflammation, and apoptosis is accelerated during the resolution phase.

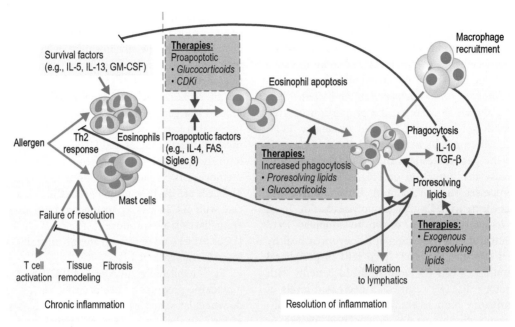

Fig. 1.14 Inflammation resolution and therapeutic opportunities. After the initial Th2-mediated proinflammatory events that occur in allergic inflammation and that are characterized by increased eosinophil recruitment, activation, and survival along with mast cell degranulation, progression to the resolution phase of inflammation allows return of normal tissue structure and function. Increasing proapoptotic factors drive eosinophil apoptosis for their timely clearance by macrophages, a process that is controlled by and increases the production of proresolving lipids. Apoptosis can be enhanced through the use of glucocorticoids, which can also increase the phagocytic capacity of macrophages and a variety of proresolving lipids. IL-10 released from a variety of cell types, including macrophages, can indirectly attenuate eosinophil survival and promote resolution. *CDKi*, Cyclin-dependent kinase inhibitor; *GM-CSF*, granulocyte-macrophage colony-stimulating factor; *IL*, interleukin; *Siglec*, sialic acid–binding immunoglobulin-like lectin; *TGF-β*, transforming growth factor-β; *Th2*, T helper type 2 cell.

Phagocytosis of apoptotic cells by macrophages ensures the safe disposal of dead and dying cells without release of toxic intracellular mediators. Engulfment of apoptotic cells signals to the phagocytosing macrophage that inflammation is coming to an end and alters macrophage mediator production from predominantly proinflammatory to proresolution, with enhanced production of cytokines with antiinflammatory properties, including IL-10 and TGF-β. This pattern contrasts with macrophage phagocytosis of necrotic eosinophils, which leads to enhanced proinflammatory mediator production such as GM-CSF.

Several proresolving lipids promote and control the resolution phenotype. The delivery of exogenous protectins, lipoxins, and resolvins has increased inflammation resolution and improved clinical outcomes in a variety of allergic murine models. Advances in our understanding of proresolving lipids, granulocyte apoptosis, and phagocytic clearance of dead and dying cells are creating new avenues for generation of novel proresolving agents with which to tackle allergic inflammation (Fig. 1.14).

REFERENCES

1. Castillo EF, Zheng H, Yang XO. Orchestration of epithelial-derived cytokines and innate immune cells in allergic airway inflammation. Cytokine Growth Factor Rev. 2018;39:19–25.
2. Lambrecht BN, Hammad H. The airway epithelium in asthma. Nat Med. 2012;18(5):684–692.
3. Maeda K, Caldez MJ, Akira S. Innate immunity in allergy. Allergy. 2019;74(9):1660–1674.
4. Joiner KA, Brown EJ, Frank MM. Complement and bacteria: chemistry and biology in host defense. Annu Rev Immunol. 1984;2:461–491.
5. Liu J, Cao X. Cellular and molecular regulation of innate inflammatory responses. Cell Mol Immunol. 2016;13(6):711–721.
6. Palomares O, Ruckert B, Jartti T, et al. Induction and maintenance of allergen-specific FOXP3+ Treg cells in human tonsils as potential first-line organs of oral tolerance. J Allergy Clin Immunol. 2012;129(2):510–520, 520. e511–519.
7. Kaur BP, Secord E. Innate immunity. Pediatr Clin North Am. 2019;66(5):905–911.
8. Kubelkova K, Macela A. Innate immune recognition: an issue more complex than expected. Front Cell Infect Microbiol. 2019;9:241.
9. Mellor AL, Munn DH. Physiologic control of the functional status of Foxp3+ regulatory T cells. J Immunol. 2011;186(8):4535–4540.
10. Pierce SK, Liu W. The tipping points in the initiation of B cell signalling: how small changes make big differences. Nat Rev Immunol. 2010;10(11):767–777.
11. Macaubas C, DeKruyff RH, Umetsu DT. Respiratory tolerance in the protection against asthma. Curr Drug Targets Inflamm Allergy. 2003;2(2):175–186.
12. Metzger TC, Anderson MS. Control of central and peripheral tolerance by Aire. Immunol Rev. 2011;241(1):89–103.
13. Komlosi ZI, Kovacs N, Sokolowska M, van de Veen W, Akdis M, Akdis CA. Mechanisms of subcutaneous and sublingual

aeroallergen immunotherapy: what is new? Immunol Allergy Clin North Am. 2020;40(1):1–14.

14. Globinska A, Boonpiyathad T, Satitsuksanoa P, et al. Mechanisms of allergen-specific immunotherapy: Diverse mechanisms of immune tolerance to allergens. Ann Allergy Asthma Immunol. 2018;121(3):306–312.

15. Sindher SB, Long A, Acharya S, Sampath V, Nadeau KC. The use of biomarkers to predict aero-allergen and food immunotherapy responses. Clin Rev Allergy Immunol. 2018;55(2):190–204.

16. Penagos M, Durham SR. Duration of allergen immunotherapy for inhalant allergy. Curr Opin Allergy Clin Immunol. 2019;19(6):594–605.

17. Wang M, Yang IV, Davidson EJ, et al. Forkhead box protein 3 demethylation is associated with tolerance induction in peanut-induced intestinal allergy. J Allergy Clin Immunol. 2018;141(2):659–670. e652.

18. Stanic B, van de Veen W, Wirz OF, et al. IL-10-overexpressing B cells regulate innate and adaptive immune responses. J Allergy Clin Immunol. 2015;135(3):771–780. e778.

19. Shamji MH, Durham SR. Mechanisms of allergen immunotherapy for inhaled allergens and predictive biomarkers. J Allergy Clin Immunol. 2017;140(6):1485–1498.

20. Akdis M, Akdis CA. Mechanisms of allergen-specific immunotherapy: multiple suppressor factors at work in immune tolerance to allergens. J Allergy Clin Immunol. 2014;133(3):621–631.

21. Buchbinder EI, Desai A. CTLA-4 and PD-1 pathways: similarities, differences, and implications of their inhibition. Am J Clin Oncol. 2016;39(1):98–106.

22. Fort MM, Cheung J, Yen D, et al. IL-25 induces IL-4, IL-5, and IL-13 and Th2-associated pathologies in vivo. Immunity. 2001;15(6):985–995.

23. Schmitz J, Owyang A, Oldham E, et al. IL-33, an interleukin-1-like cytokine that signals via the IL-1 receptor-related protein ST2 and induces T helper type 2-associated cytokines. Immunity. 2005;23(5):479–490.

24. Khodoun MV, Tomar S, Tocker JE, Wang YH, Finkelman FD. Prevention of food allergy development and suppression of established food allergy by neutralization of thymic stromal lymphopoietin, IL-25, and IL-33. J Allergy Clin Immunol. 2018;141(1):171–179. e171.

25. Chen CC, Kobayashi T, Iijima K, Hsu FC, Kita H. IL-33 dysregulates regulatory T cells and impairs established immunologic tolerance in the lungs. J Allergy Clin Immunol. 2017;140(5):1351–1363. e1357.

26. Shen P, Roch T, Lampropoulou V, et al. IL-35-producing B cells are critical regulators of immunity during autoimmune and infectious diseases. Nature. 2014;507(7492):366–370.

27. Wang RX, Yu CR, Dambuza IM, et al. Interleukin-35 induces regulatory B cells that suppress autoimmune disease. Nat Med. 2014;20(6):633–641.

28. Collison LW, Chaturvedi V, Henderson AL, et al. IL-35-mediated induction of a potent regulatory T cell population. Nat Immunol. 2010;11(12):1093–1101.

29. Wirtz S, Billmeier U, McHedlidze T, Blumberg RS, Neurath MF. Interleukin-35 mediates mucosal immune responses that protect against T-cell-dependent colitis. Gastroenterology. 2011;141(5):1875–1886.

30. Vignali DA, Kuchroo VK. IL-12 family cytokines: immunological playmakers. Nat Immunol. 2012;13(8):722–728.

31. Layhadi JA, Eguiluz-Gracia I, Shamji MH. Role of IL-35 in sublingual allergen immunotherapy. Curr Opin Allergy Clin Immunol. 2019;19(1):12–17.

32. Wang YH, Ito T, Wang YH, et al. Maintenance and polarization of human TH2 central memory T cells by thymic stromal lymphopoietin-activated dendritic cells. Immunity. 2006;24(6):827–838.

33. Klunker S, Trautmann A, Akdis M, et al. A second step of chemotaxis after transendothelial migration: keratinocytes undergoing apoptosis release IFN-gamma-inducible protein 10, monokine induced by IFN-gamma, and IFN-gamma-inducible alpha-chemoattractant for T cell chemotaxis toward epidermis in atopic dermatitis. J Immunol. 2003;171(2):1078–1084.

34. Rebane A, Zimmermann M, Aab A, et al. Mechanisms of IFN-gamma-induced apoptosis of human skin keratinocytes in patients with atopic dermatitis. J Allergy Clin Immunol. 2012;129(5):1297–1306.

35. Zhu J, Yamane H, Paul WE. Differentiation of effector CD4 T cell populations (*). Annu Rev Immunol. 2010;28:445–489.

36. Sonnenberg GF, Mjosberg J, Spits H, Artis D. SnapShot: innate lymphoid cells. Immunity. 2013;39(3) 622-622. e621.

37. Boonpiyathad T, Sozener ZC, Satitsuksanoa P, Akdis CA. Immunologic mechanisms in asthma. Semin Immunol. 2019;46:101333.

38. Schulzke JD, Gunzel D, John LJ, Fromm M. Perspectives on tight junction research. Ann N Y Acad Sci. 2012;1257:1–19.

39. Matter K, Balda MS. SnapShot: epithelial tight junctions. Cell. 2014;157(4) 992-992. e991.

40. De Benedetto A, Rafaels NM, McGirt LY, et al. Tight junction defects in patients with atopic dermatitis. J Allergy Clin Immunol. 2011;127(3):773–786. e771-777.

41. de Boer WI, Sharma HS, Baelemans SM, Hoogsteden HC, Lambrecht BN, Braunstahl GJ. Altered expression of epithelial junctional proteins in atopic asthma: possible role in inflammation. Can J Physiol Pharmacol. 2008;86(3):105–112.

42. Fujita H, Chalubinski M, Rhyner C, et al. Claudin-1 expression in airway smooth muscle exacerbates airway remodeling in asthmatic subjects. J Allergy Clin Immunol. 2011;127(6):1612–1621. e1618.

43. Holgate ST. Epithelium dysfunction in asthma. J Allergy Clin Immunol. 2007;120(6):1233–1244, quiz 1245–1236.

44. Soyka MB, Wawrzyniak P, Eiwegger T, et al. Defective epithelial barrier in chronic rhinosinusitis: the regulation of tight junctions by IFN-gamma and IL-4. J Allergy Clin Immunol. 2012;130(5):1087–1096. e1010.

45. Xiao C, Puddicombe SM, Field S, et al. Defective epithelial barrier function in asthma. J Allergy Clin Immunol. 2011;128(3):549–556. e541-512.

46. Wang M, Tan G, Eljaszewicz A, et al. Laundry detergents and detergent residue after rinsing directly disrupt tight junction barrier integrity in human bronchial epithelial cells. J Allergy Clin Immunol. 2019;143(5):1892–1903.

47. Kipnis J. Multifaceted interactions between adaptive immunity and the central nervous system. Science. 2016;353(6301):766–771.

48. Barnes PJ. The cytokine network in asthma and chronic obstructive pulmonary disease. J Clin Invest. 2008;118(11):3546–3556.

49. Sokolowska M, Frei R, Lunjani N, Akdis CA, O'Mahony L. Microbiome and asthma. Asthma Res Pract. 2018;4:1.

50. Sampson HA. Food allergy. Part 1: immunopathogenesis and clinical disorders. J Allergy Clin Immunol. 1999;103(5 Pt 1):717–728.

51. Du Toit G, Roberts G, Sayre PH, et al. Randomized trial of peanut consumption in infants at risk for peanut allergy. N Engl J Med. 2015;372(9):803–813.

52. Schulz O, Jaensson E, Persson EK, et al. Intestinal CD103+, but not CX3CR1+, antigen sampling cells migrate in lymph and serve classical dendritic cell functions. J Exp Med. 2009;206(13): 3101–3114.

53. Coombes JL, Siddiqui KR, Arancibia-Carcamo CV, et al. A functionally specialized population of mucosal CD103+ DCs induces Foxp3+ regulatory T cells via a TGF-beta and retinoic acid-dependent mechanism. J Exp Med. 2007;204(8): 1757–1764.

54. Karlsson MR, Rugtveit J, Brandtzaeg P. Allergen-responsive CD4+CD25+ regulatory T cells in children who have outgrown cow's milk allergy. J Exp Med. 2004;199(12):1679–1688.

55. Hill DJ, Hosking CS, de Benedictis FM, et al. Confirmation of the association between high levels of immunoglobulin E food sensitization and eczema in infancy: an international study. Clin Exp Allergy. 2008;38(1):161–168.

56. Lack G, Fox D, Northstone K, Golding J. Avon Longitudinal Study of Parents and Children Study Team. Factors associated with the development of peanut allergy in childhood. N Engl J Med. 2003;348(11):977–985.

57. Noti M, Kim BS, Siracusa MC, et al. Exposure to food allergens through inflamed skin promotes intestinal food allergy through the thymic stromal lymphopoietin-basophil axis. J Allergy Clin Immunol. 2014;133(5):1390–1399. 1399. e1391–1396.

58. Tordesillas L, Goswami R, Benede S, et al. Skin exposure promotes a Th2-dependent sensitization to peanut allergens. J Clin Invest. 2014;124(11):4965–4975.

59. Reese TA, Liang HE, Tager AM, et al. Chitin induces accumulation in tissue of innate immune cells associated with allergy. Nature. 2007;447(7140):92–96.

60. Roediger B, Kyle R, Yip KH, et al. Cutaneous immunosurveillance and regulation of inflammation by group 2 innate lymphoid cells. Nat Immunol. 2013;14(6):564–573.

61. Salimi M, Barlow JL, Saunders SP, et al. A role for IL-25 and IL-33-driven type-2 innate lymphoid cells in atopic dermatitis. J Exp Med. 2013;210(13):2939–2950.

62. Kim BS, Siracusa MC, Saenz SA, et al. TSLP elicits IL-33-independent innate lymphoid cell responses to promote skin inflammation. Sci Transl Med. 2013;5(170): 170ra116.

63. Shik D, Tomar S, Lee JB, Chen CY, Smith A, Wang YH.IL-9-producing cells in the development of IgE-mediated food allergy. Semin Immunopathol. 2017;39(1):69–77.

64. Lee JB.Regulation of IgE-mediated food allergy by IL-9 producing mucosal mast cells and type 2 innate lymphoid cells. Immune Netw. 2016;16(4):211–218.

65. Noval Rivas M, Burton OT, Oettgen HC, Chatila T. IL-4 production by group 2 innate lymphoid cells promotes food allergy by blocking regulatory T-cell function. J Allergy Clin Immunol. 2016;138(3):801–811. e809.

66. Palmer G, Gabay C.Interleukin-33 biology with potential insights into human diseases. Nat Rev Rheumatol. 2011;7(6):321–329.

67. Li J, Wang Y, Tang L, et al. Dietary medium-chain triglycerides promote oral allergic sensitization and orally induced anaphylaxis to peanut protein in mice. J Allergy Clin Immunol. 2013;131(2):442–450.

68. Osterfeld H, Ahrens R, Strait R, Finkelman FD, Renauld JC, Hogan SP.Differential roles for the IL-9/IL-9 receptor alpha-chain pathway in systemic and oral antigen-induced anaphylaxis. J Allergy Clin Immunol. 2010;125(2):469–476. e462.

69. Lefrancais E, Duval A, Mirey E, et al. Central domain of IL-33 is cleaved by mast cell proteases for potent activation of group-2 innate lymphoid cells. Proc Natl Acad Sci U S A. 2014;111(43):15502–15507.

70. Hsu CL, Neilsen CV, Bryce PJ.IL-33 is produced by mast cells and regulates IgE-dependent inflammation. PLoS One. 2010;5(8):e11944.

71. Atarashi K, Tanoue T, Shima T, et al. Induction of colonic regulatory T cells by indigenous Clostridium species. Science. 2011;331(6015):337–341.

72. Atarashi K, Tanoue T, Oshima K, et al. Treg induction by a rationally selected mixture of Clostridia strains from the human microbiota. Nature. 2013;500(7461):232–236.

73. Stefka AT, Feehley T, Tripathi P, et al. Commensal bacteria protect against food allergen sensitization. Proc Natl Acad Sci U S A. 2014;111(36):13145–13150.

74. Mortha A, Chudnovskiy A, Hashimoto D, et al. Microbiota-dependent crosstalk between macrophages and ILC3 promotes intestinal homeostasis. Science. 2014;343(6178):1249288.

2

Precision Medicine

Gurjit K. Khurana Hershey, Michael G. Sherenian, and Tesfaye B. Mersha

PRECISION MEDICINE: A BRIEF HISTORY AND DEFINITION

Starting in the 19th century, developments in the basic and clinical sciences allowed scientists to start understanding the underlying causes and treatments of disease.[1] In recent years, the concept of personalized medicine has become part of the everyday language. However, medical practice has always been about treating each patient based on personal characteristics. Clinicians understand that patients respond differently to specific therapies, and this makes it challenging to identify what management strategy is appropriate for a given patient. Precision medicine (PM) offers the promise of improving prognostication and diagnostic accuracy and enhancing individualization therapy based on a patient's genetics, environmental exposures, and lifestyle choices. The terms *PM, personalized medicine, genomic medicine, stratified medicine, individualized medicine,* and *P4 medicine* (personalized, predictive, preventive, and participatory) are often used interchangeably.[2–4] Although the term *PM* was first coined in 2008, it was not until 2011 that it became widely used following a report from the

U.S. National Research Council (US NRC) entitled *Toward Precision Medicine: Building a Knowledge Network for Biomedical Research and a New Taxonomy of Disease.*[5,6] What all of these terms have in common is that they recognize that a "one-size-fits-all" approach to medicine is not sufficient.

In January 2015, President Obama launched the Precision Medicine Initiative (PMI). PMI "is a long-term research endeavor, involving the National Institutes of Health (NIH) and multiple other research centers, which aims to understand how a person's genetics, environment, and lifestyle can help determine the best approach to prevent or treat disease."[5] The overarching goal of PM, despite its varied definitions,[1,6–8] is to provide each patient with the most accurate therapy management based on genetics/genomics, environmental exposures, and lifestyle choices.[9] This is being achieved through the national research program called *All of Us*, which is currently recruiting at least one million volunteers from populations of diverse ancestry to help build a database of genetic information, biological samples, and other health data that will be used to predict disease risk, understand how diseases occur, and improve the diagnosis and treatment of medical conditions.[10] The Trans-Omics for

TABLE 2.1	Potential Benefits of Precision Medicine
Drug developers	A national knowledge repository (with high-quality genotype–phenotype data) would allow for the repurposing of existing drugs and the development of novel therapeutics for specific subsets of populations within allergic disorders.
Researchers	Increasingly large integrated datasets of individual clinical and molecular data over time are becoming available for interrogation. This will allow for increased characterization of populations within allergic disorders.
Medical insurers	Extensive information to identify specific subsets of patients with allergic disorders will allow for the optimization of management algorithms that mutually benefit the insurer and the patient. A novel, potentially more expensive treatment might be made available to patients who will more likely respond to that specific treatment. This would allow for increased cost-effectiveness of allergic disorder management by (1) advocating use in patients who are most likely to respond to the therapy and (2) avoiding use in patients who are more likely to have serious adverse effects.
Healthcare providers	New algorithms that tailor the development or use of medical therapies to the key characteristics of population subsets will improve efficacy and satisfaction while decreasing treatment failures that result in healthcare utilization.

Precision Medicine (TOPMed) Program is gathering omics data across diverse populations, including those that have been traditionally underrepresented in research.[11] The potential impact of PM to improve the diagnosis of and alleviate the suffering from allergic diseases is significant. This initiative and PM on the whole is centered on four core values: predictive, preventive, personalized, and participatory, which together are called P4 Medicine.[12] Some of the important potential short- and long-term benefits of PM are presented in Table 2.1.

While the initial goals of the PMI have focused primarily on applying PM to cancer, its long-term goals include applying PM to all areas of health and healthcare, including allergic diseases. Allergic disorders have significant potential to benefit from implementing PM practices. Its use in oncology and cancer management provides a clear example of the successful use of the practice.[13-16] For example, HER2-positive breast cancer patients are being targeted with specific therapies that reduce treatment time and speed recovery.[14] Moreover, a meta-analysis of phase II clinical trials of different cancers suggests that the use of a precision approach to select participants, based on subset characteristics, for specific trials resulted in increased therapeutic response rates when compared with randomly selected participants ($p<0.001$).[16] The development of new precision management strategies is made possible by integrating clinical, research, environmental, and lifestyle information—collectively known as information commons.[17] By incorporating this framework into allergic disorders, we allow for the potential to generate similar outcomes as the cancer field. In this chapter, we will briefly discuss the key components of the PMI. We will then focus on recent advancements made in PM for allergic disorders, including biologic therapies as a recent example of using PM approaches within allergic disorders.

EVIDENCE-BASED VERSUS PRECISION MEDICINE

Published practice parameters provide evidence-based medicine (EBM) guidelines for the diagnosis and management of allergic disorders. For decades, the allergy community has collected demographic, immunologic, genomic, biomarker, and clinical data to generate disease phenotypes and endotypes. Recently, novel technological advances enabled the rapid generation of increasing amounts of tissue- and cell-level molecular data. These data allow individuals with a given allergic disorder to be placed into subgroups that define disease subsets based on biologic pathways and pathogenic mechanisms. The synthesis of this information allows PM to account for individual variability and then to apply the EBM principles to each allergic disorder and its subtype. Expanding on an EBM approach, whereby the best disease management strategy is determined for a heterogeneous group of individuals with a given disorder, PM aims to determine the best management strategy for each subset of individuals stratified based on their molecular data (Fig. 2.1). In contrast, by using the PM approach, clinical management and prevention strategies can target the pathogenic mechanisms rather than applying one type of treatment across heterogeneous patients with different endotypes, but similar phenotypes, as is done using traditional EBM.[18]

COMPONENTS OF PRECISION MEDICINE IN ALLERGIC DISORDERS

Patients with allergic diseases present and respond to treatments differently, which can create a major dilemma in providing optimal management. Patients with asthma often share similar clinical symptoms, yet these similar presentations may optimally respond to different treatments.[19,20] Indeed, 40%–70% of asthma treatments are considered to have absent or incomplete efficacy,[21] including responses to corticosteroids.[21,22] This is due to underlying -omic (genetic, genomic, epigenomic, metabolomic, etc.), immune, environmental, and microbiome differences among patients. Thus PM in allergy extends beyond genetic sequence analysis. Assays that measure multiple biomarkers can now be used to interrogate several key steps in the transcription (transcriptome), translation (proteome), regulation of gene expression (epigenome), host–microbial interactions (immunome and microbiome), exposures and their metabolites (metabolome), and their combined synergies (multi-omics).

Endotypes/Biomarkers in Allergic Disorders

Endotypes are characterized by the immunological, inflammatory, metabolic, and remodeling pathways that explain the

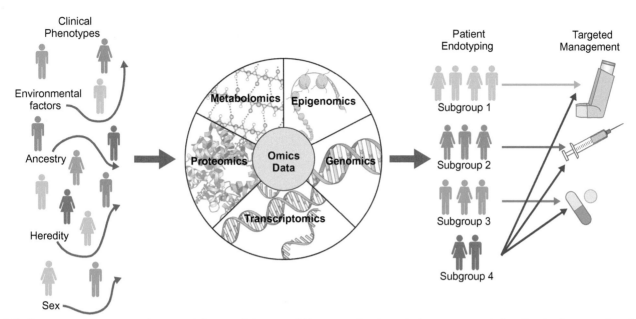

Fig. 2.1 Conceptual diagram on how precision medicine can aid in generating targeted managements for allergic diseases. A patient's clinical phenotype will be integrated with -omics level data to identify their disease-specific endotype category and subgroup. This endotype will then be used to identify which targeted management recommendations would lead to the best outcome(s) for a given patient.

mechanisms underlying a clinical presentation (phenotype) of a disease.[23–26] In allergic disorders, endotypes are an important tool for disease management. As part of determining endotypes, biologic markers (i.e., biomarkers) are biological compounds used to define different aspects of a disease such as severity or the likelihood of a response to a given treatment.[24,27,28] Ideal biomarkers share three important characteristics. First, they are stable over time. Second, they link disease endotypes and phenotypes to appropriately discern management strategies. Third, they are detectable among populations with genetically distinct backgrounds.[29] Several potential biomarkers have been identified for allergic disorders (Table 2.2).[28]

Immune Profiling of Allergic Disorders

The immune response is affected by several factors including an individual's immune predisposition based on underlying genetic characteristics, personal immune history, infection history, age, sex, and season. New technologies allow for the detailed study of the immune response in allergic disorders. These technologies can provide a means to determine "immune fingerprints" associated with the development of a given allergic disease throughout an individual's life spectrum.

For example, the functional heterogeneity, and thus specific subpopulations, of T helper type 2 (Th2) cells drive specific Th2-based pathologies.[55] However, allergic disorders are increasingly recognized as having additional T cell subtypes involved in their pathogenesis. Allergic asthma is often characterized by a Th2 phenotype, with increased eosinophils and Th2 cytokine (e.g., interleukin [IL]-4, IL-5, and IL-13) levels. Yet, severe corticosteroid-resistant asthma is often characterized by mixed Th2/Th17 responses.[56] Moreover, like Th2 cells, Th17 cells also show considerable heterogeneity. Th17 cells that are polarized in vitro with IL-1β, IL-6, and IL-23 adopt a more pathogenic state, whereas

Th17 cells polarized with transforming growth factor-β (TGF-β) and IL-6 are nonpathogenic.[57,58] Also, single-cell transcriptomic sequencing has recently been shown to identify unique subsets of T cells associated with clinical disease.[59,60] These findings highlight the importance of accurate immune profiling in allergic disorders. Characterizing patients by T cell phenotype will likely become an important part of PM in allergic disorders.

Role of -omics

Through technological advances such as the use of high-throughput assays that allow for hundreds of thousands of experimental samples to be processed simultaneously, next-generation sequencing, computational biology, clinical bioinformatics, and genome-wide assay sequencing, these advances are coming together in multi-omics form to increase the predictive accuracy of disease classification.[61] The pathogenesis of complex diseases such as allergy involves several cascades of events at various levels of -omics as including transcriptomics of gene expression, epigenomics of gene regulation, proteomics, and metabolomics, which may have direct effects on disease endotypes. These methods are now being applied at the level of the single cell, which is extremely powerful and reveals the considerable heterogeneity within cell types.[59]

Genomics

Genomic studies in allergy can be subdivided into different approaches: whole-genome sequencing (WGS), whole-exome sequencing, genome-wide association studies (GWAS), or candidate gene association studies. GWAS focus mainly on detecting nucleotide polymorphisms (single-nucleotide polymorphisms) across the whole genome. WGS is being increasingly applied to allergic disorders and yielding promising results for application as a key part of PM. The International HapMap Project,[62] the

TABLE 2.2 Established and Emerging Biomarkers for Major Allergic Disorders

Disease	Source	Marker	Phenotype/Outcome	Reference (s)
Asthma	Blood, serum	Serum IgE		30
		Blood eosinophils	T2-high asthma, lung function	31
		Serum periostin	T2-high asthma	32
	Urine	LTE4	Asthma severity, aspirin-sensitive asthma, susceptibility to leukotriene receptor antagonists	33
		Metabolomic profile	Asthma severity, corticosteroid-resistant asthma, early-onset asthma	34–36
	Exhaled breath	Volatile organic compounds	Eosinophilic asthma, neutrophilic asthma, persistent asthma	37,38
		Fractional exhaled nitric oxide	Eosinophilic airway inflammation, response to treatment	39
	Sputum	Eosinophils	T2-high asthma, asthma severity, lung function, predictor of exacerbations, response to treatment	31,40,41
AD	Blood, serum	Serum TARC/CCL17	AD severity	42
	DNA	Filaggrin genotype	Screening and prognostic biomarker for AD risk, AD severity, early-onset AD	43
	Skin	Transcriptome profile	Treatment response	44
		Microbiome profile	AD severity	45
Allergic rhinitis	Skin prick test	Allergen sensitization	Diagnosis, distinguishes allergic from non-allergic rhinitis	46
	Nasal secretions	TARC/CCL17, endothelin-1	Distinguishes allergic from non-allergic rhinitis	47
	Nasal lavage following nasal allergen challenge	Eosinophils, IL-5, IL-6, macrophage inflammatory protein	Diagnosis, monitoring of treatment	48
Food allergy	Skin prick test	Allergen sensitization	Diagnosis	49
	Blood, serum	Allergen-specific IgE levels	Diagnosis	49
	Blood	Basophil activation test	Diagnosis	50
	Plasma	Mast cell activation	Diagnosis	51,52
	Blood	FOXP3 methylation in antigen-induced Treg cells	Predictive of response to oral immunotherapy	53
	Tissue, serum	Eotaxins	Disease activity	54
Eosinophilic esophagitis	Tissue, serum	IL-5, IL-13	Disease activity	
	Tissue, serum	Eosinophil-derived neurotoxin	Disease activity	
	Tissue, serum	Transcriptomics	Disease activity, remission	
	Tissue	Mast cell quantification	Disease activity	

AD, Atopic dermatitis; *IgE,* immunoglobulin E; *IL,* interleukin; *LTE4,* leukotriene E4; *TARC/CCL17,* thymus- and activation-regulated chemokine/CC chemokine ligand 17.

1000 Genomes Project,[63] and the Exome Sequencing Project[64] along with publicly available databanks, including PubMed, EBI/Ensembl, University of California, Santa Cruz, Genome Browser, the National Human Genome and Research Institute, among others, have helped shape a new era of research for many diseases and disorders, including allergic disorders. A catalog of almost all published GWAS can be accessed at https://www.ebi.ac.uk/gwas.[65] According to the GWAS catalog, 85 studies and more than 600 associations are related to asthma alone.[66] Recently, an increasing number of GWAS involve other allergic disorders.[67,68] One drawback of GWAS results is that they generally fail to take into account gene–gene and gene–environment interactions.[68] In the future, integrating molecular biomarkers that help characterize patients into groups according to pathogenic mechanisms of disease and more cost-efficient next-generation sequencing approaches will ultimately enable genome-wide studies with the ability to yield more genetic causality.

Transcriptomics

Transcriptomic approaches in allergy encompass two main techniques: gene expression microarrays and RNA-sequencing

(RNA-seq). The study of how genes are expressed during specific conditions (e.g., health status, exposures, and disease state) in different tissues and/or cells is known as transcriptomics. The transcriptome varies from cell to cell, and to precisely analyze how the disease affects gene expression it is necessary to select tissues/cells directly affected from disease to be studied. In the case of allergic disorders, transcriptomes from whole blood, neutrophils, CD4+ T cells, lung and airway tissues, airway smooth muscle cells, induced sputum, and nasal lavage fluids have been studied.[69] For example, genome-wide profiling of bronchial epithelial brushings in individuals revealed two different asthma phenotypes: "Th2-High" and "Th2-Low" based on microarray expression of IL-5 and IL-13.[22] These findings have been replicated in nasal epithelial brushings,[70] opening the possibility of using nasal airway gene profiles as biological markers for asthma diagnostics and treatment,[70] which is very attractive, as this sample can be easily obtained without anesthesia at a clinical point of care. Recent approaches utilizing single-cell RNA-seq enable the characterization of all cell subpopulations. For example, a recent study of asthmatic patients found that suboptimal asthma control was associated with signatures of eosinophilic and granulocytic inflammatory signals, while optimal asthma control signatures were associated with immature lymphocytic patterns.[71] This study highlights the existence of specific, reproducible transcriptomic components in the blood that vary with the degree of asthma control.[71] Thus transcriptomic signatures from easily accessible tissue (nasal cells, blood, skin) could potentially be utilized to monitor disease control and determine responsiveness to treatments including corticosteroids.

Epigenomics

Epigenetics study the changes in genetic functions that are not related to genetic alterations. Epigenetic variations are dynamic and affected by environmental factors such as diet, chemical compounds (including the use of medication), air pollution, smoking, and others. Epigenetic studies in allergy often focus on changes in DNA methylation patterns, which can be examined by epigenome-wide association studies. Other epigenetic studies may include the investigation of patterns of histone modifications or noncoding RNAs. Together, these epigenetic mechanisms regulate the gene expression program of a cell by being responsive to changes in the environment of a cell. A compelling hypothesis is that environmental cues associated with diseases might initiate or influence the epigenetic processes of host cells, leading to epigenetic reprogramming of host cells to favor their pathogenic function and contributing to the development of the disease.[24,25]

Proteomics

Proteins play a significant role in cellular processes, and their levels reflect the momentary state of tissues/cells at the time of the investigation. Analytical proteomic techniques allow the characterization, identification, and quantification of proteins and their associated functions. Different methods of proteomics are available, which can roughly be subdivided into immunoassay-based methods (e.g., enzyme-linked immunosorbent assay [ELISA], immunohistochemistry, and Western blot), mass spectrometry

(MS)-based methods (e.g., tandem MS, electron capture, or electron-transfer dissociations), and protein microarray methods. Like transcriptomics and epigenomics, it is important to note that proteome collected from a single body compartment/site or at a certain moment (e.g., exacerbation, stable, etc.) will not provide the information on the complete dynamic proteome linked to the disease process. Thus comparative evaluation of the information collected from different sample sites and in different disease conditions and/or times may be needed to get more comprehensive information about the asthma–proteome link.

Metabolomics

Metabolomics concerns the study of low molecular weight organic compounds (50–1500 Da) that originate from human-/microorganism-related metabolism and are involved in biological processes.[69,72] The techniques used in metabolomics belong mainly to gas or liquid chromatography coupled with MS. Another method is nuclear magnetic resonance (NMR) spectroscopy, which has lower sensitivity and specificity compared to MS-based techniques and therefore requires higher analyte concentrations.

Microbiome

The human body comprises at least 10 times more bacteria in numbers than human cells. Microbiome investigations are divided into two main approaches: 16S ribosomal RNA sequencing and shotgun metagenomics. The former is less costly and less computationally intensive compared to metagenomics, and therefore used more frequently. However, it has a lower potential to detect microbial taxa up to species level. Data strongly support that dysbiosis contributes to the mechanistic underpinnings of the hygiene hypothesis that was first described in the 1980s.[73] Indeed, site-specific dysbiosis has been shown to affect all allergic disorders.[74] For example, skin bacteria dysbiosis is associated with atopic dermatitis (AD) pathogenesis and outcomes.[45,75–78] In addition, airway dysbiosis has been associated with both asthma[79] and allergic rhinitis.[80] This dysbiosis can extend beyond the primary affected organ of an allergic disease as well. Several studies have shown that intestinal dysbiosis can lead to detrimental immune-mediated outcomes including asthma and allergies.[81,82]

Exposomics

Environmental exposure factors, which might influence asthma risk, are numerous, ranging from lifestyle-related factors such as diet, smoking, exercise, and stress to environmental exposures related to pollution, allergens, occupational factors, as well as many others. Linking the exposome to other-omics layers is now a focus of allergy research. An example is the EXPOsOMICS consortium that investigates short- and long-term exposures to air and water contaminants and their biological effects on chronic diseases (including asthma) using a multi-omics approach.[83]

Comprehensive Integrative Omics

Integrative omics (multi-omics) in allergy is the process of combining the information of multiple-omics layers, to get more insight into the disease process. Each omics data type typically provides a list of differential factors potentially associated with the disease. These data can be useful as disease markers while providing insight as to which biological pathways or processes are different between the disease and control groups. However, analysis of only one-omic(s) data type is limited to correlations and provides a partial view of the biological system. Integrating different-omics data types is often used to elucidate the potential causative changes that lead to disease or can be used to identify potential therapeutic targets for further molecular studies. A large number of publicly available tools have been developed for omics data integration.[84]

Pharmacogenomics and Drug Dosing

Pharmacogenomics is the study and application of genetic factors relating to the body's response to drugs. By predicting the drug response of an individual, the goal is to increase the success of therapies and reduce the incidence of adverse side effects. Currently, there are more than 130 medications that have labels from the Food and Drug Administration (FDA) with warnings about possible serious implications based on genotypes for drug response.[85] There are at least 35 companies offering pharmacogenetics (PGx) testing panels on different genes associated with the metabolism of drugs for various diseases (e.g., cardiovascular, diabetes, neurological, psychiatry).[86,87] While no PGx testing exists for allergic disorders currently, pharmacogenomic studies targeting drugs used for the treatment of asthma are being conducted and were summarized in a recent review.[88] One reason that pharmacogenomics has not already been successful in allergic disorders is because it is difficult to interpret differential drug responses by "groups" when the "group" definition is imprecise, fluid, and time-dependent, such as the case with asthma and other allergic disorders.

PRECISION MEDICINE IN THE MANAGEMENT OF ALLERGIC DISORDERS

Nutrition

Nutrition is a key area that can enhance PM in allergic disorders. Vitamin D and omega-3 polyunsaturated fatty acids (PUFAs) are two examples of where PM can influence allergic disorders. The following discussion is not meant to be a complete survey of the effects of nutrition on allergic disease, but rather to highlight key findings and convey where PM can make an impact on patient care.

Vitamin D

One of the most studied nutrition factors within allergic disease has been vitamin D. Vitamin D3 is the most common nutritional source of vitamin D and is determined by measuring serum 25-hydroxyvitamin D (25OH-D3) levels.[89] However, the most biologically active form of vitamin D is that of 1,25-dihydroxyvitamin D (1,25[OH]$_2$-D3) obtained through several mechanisms including sun exposure. Sufficient vitamin D levels depend on several factors including age and race.[90,91] Serum levels less than 30 ng/mL are considered insufficient.[91] Vitamin D affects several aspects of the immune system including both innate[92,93] and adaptive immune function.[94–96] For example, vitamin D is also known to enhance skin barrier function,[97] antimicrobial peptide expression,[98] and IL-10 production by regulatory T (Treg) cells.[94,95]

Importantly for the clinician, multiple studies have investigated the influence of vitamin D (25OH-D3) levels on allergic disorders. As a result, insufficient vitamin D levels have been attributed to a variety of outcomes and pathogenic mechanisms in allergic diseases. In subjects with AD, seasonal low levels of vitamin D have been associated with worse disease severity.[99] Moreover, AD severity has been associated with vitamin D levels, whereby mild AD has higher levels than moderate or severe AD.[100] Indeed, correcting vitamin D insufficiency among individuals with AD has been shown to improve disease severity.[101] In children, insufficient vitamin D levels have been correlated with asthma,[102] including an inverse association between the level of vitamin D and inhaled corticosteroid dose.[103] Vitamin D supplementation in children with asthma has also been shown to reduce the frequency of seasonal asthma exacerbations[101,104] and the risk for respiratory tract infections.[105] Studies have also reported a prenatal role for vitamin D in allergic disease development as decreased maternal vitamin D levels are correlated with an increased risk of childhood wheezing.[106,107] Yet, other studies have shown the inverse correlation,[108] suggesting a potential dynamic relationship between vitamin D and prenatal asthma risk. Similarly, both increased and decreased levels of vitamin D have been associated with increased immunoglobulin E (IgE) levels,[109] although levels may vary with vitamin D supplementation.[108] Vitamin D sufficiency in children is associated with decreased odds of having allergen-specific sensitizations.[110] However, several studies have also shown that vitamin D supplementation leads to an increased risk of allergic disease development.[111,112] With the increasing amount and complexity of data, PM has the potential to guide management based on a patient's vitamin D level in the context of other individual factors.

Fatty Acids

PUFAs have also been shown to impact allergic disease. Omega-6 (n-6) PUFAs and omega-3 (n-3) PUFAs have been shown to have differential effects on the immune system.[113,114] In general, n-6 PUFAs contribute to a proinflammatory state[113,114] and come from sources such as corn, soybean, and sunflower oils—including products made from these oils,[115] whereas n-3 PUFAs are considered antiinflammatory,[113,114] with the major source coming from oily fish.[115] Indeed, n-3 PUFAs have direct immunoregulatory effects[113,114,116] and have been shown to downregulate both Th1 and Th2 responses.[117] n-3 PUFAs can also decrease antigen-presenting cell production of cytokines.[118]

PUFAs have been studied on their impact on allergic disorders, particularly during childhood. For example, children who regularly eat oily fish are significantly less likely to develop asthma compared with their peers.[118] Conversely, increased consumption of n-6 PUFAs is associated with an increased risk of allergic disease.[119] A diet high in n-6 PUFAs has been linked with increased risk of allergic diseases including asthma,[120–122] AD,[121] and allergic rhinitis[120,121,123] prevalence. While these data have been compelling, there is uncertainty around the true benefit of n-3 PUFA supplementation, as others have shown an increased risk of allergic disease with increased n-3 PUFA intake.[122,124] Several studies have shown that dietary supplementation with fish oil decreases inflammatory mediators[125,126] and leukocyte chemotaxis.[126–128] In children, fish oil supplementation has been associated with improved asthma symptom scores and reduced need for rescue medication.[128,129] Furthermore, dietary n-3 PUFA supplementation has been associated with improvement in peak expiratory flow measurements.[129] Despite data suggesting that n-3 PUFA intake may reduce the risk of or improve outcomes related to allergic disease, current opinion on best practice related to management remains unclear as other studies show no long-term benefit.[120,130,131] Moreover, a meta-analysis has shown no association between n-3 PUFA supplementation on allergic disease pathogenesis.[132] PM can help provide the tools to appropriately make management decisions regarding those patients who will benefit the most from n-3 PUFA supplementation.

There is also evidence that n-3 PUFA supplementation may act in disease prevention and that the immunomodulatory benefits are relevant before disease onset. Children who receive fish oil supplementation have shown a decrease in wheezing incidence.[133] Also, fish oil supplementation in pregnant women has been shown to decrease IL-13 levels in umbilical cord plasma[134] as well as IL-5, IL-10, and interferon-γ.[135] Conversely, increases in dietary n-6 PUFA have been associated with increases in the above cytokines from umbilical cord blood.[134] Infants with AD whose mothers received fish oil supplementation have also been shown to have less severe disease and less egg sensitization than those whose mothers did not have supplementation.[134] PM could provide clearer insight into those populations who would benefit most from increased n-3 PUFA maternal dietary supplementation to help reduce the risk of allergic disease development in infants and children.

Respiratory Pathogens and Allergic Disease

Early life wheezing due to viruses and other respiratory pathogens is associated with later onset of asthma and allergic sensitization.[136–138] Indeed, preschool children who develop wheezing during either viral or bacterial respiratory illnesses have an increased asthma risk. Respiratory syncytial virus (RSV) and rhinovirus are two of the largest contributors to viral wheezing illnesses in children.[139] Treatment using RSV-specific monoclonal antibodies (mAbs) in preterm infants who have RSV infection has also been shown to reduce the incidence of later wheezing.[140,141] Rhinovirus management presents a key opportunity for PM using patient genotyping. Cadherin-related family member 3 (CDHR3) is an entry factor for airway epithelial cells for rhinovirus C,[142] one of the main types of serious rhinoviral infections in infants.[140] A *CDHR3* polymorphism increases the amount of CDHR3 present on cell surfaces and is thus associated with an increased risk of childhood asthma.[142] Therefore using PM techniques could identify these individuals as high risk for asthma development before disease onset and potentially alter management. Moreover, while no current preventative measures exist to ameliorate the risk of later wheeze after rhinovirus

infection, one could anticipate the utility of PM in a situation where this is possible, whereby PM identifies those individuals with the highest risk of viral-induced wheeze based on genetic risk factors and identifies appropriate strategies to mitigate the risk of future asthma and allergic disease development.

BIOLOGICS AND PRECISION MEDICINE

Biologics are discussed briefly here in the context of PM. Briefly, a biologic is a targeted therapy manufactured using living organisms rather than via chemical synthesis. Biologics are large, complex molecules consisting of proteins, peptides, nucleic acids, sugars, other cellular structures, or a combination of these, produced within living cells or microorganisms. Biologics represent an increasingly important means to use PM in allergic disorders (Fig. 2.2). Both small- and large-molecule drugs interact with a patient's biology; however, small-molecule drugs work as inhibitors disrupting the process through penetrating cells, whereas large biologic drugs are designed to bind to specific targets with extreme precision. Biologics target inflammatory modulators that are important within a given allergic disease. Thus far asthma has the most available biologic therapies. A key area where PM could be useful in the rapidly developing landscape of biologic therapy for allergic diseases is to identify which patients would benefit most from a given biologic by using key patient biomarkers and other characteristics. The discussion below presents a brief overview of biologics in several allergic diseases and what biomarkers could be used in a PM approach to patient management.

Asthma
Anti-IgE

Omalizumab was the first biologic used to treat allergic disease by targeting circulating IgE and preventing binding to its receptor.[143] Omalizumab significantly improves asthma outcomes[143,144]; however, these effects are stronger in certain individuals based on their underlying characteristics. For example, patients with high fractional exhaled nitric oxide (FeNO >19.5–25 ppb) are more likely to have a positive response to omalizumab.[145] Also, patients with asthma and a baseline peripheral absolute eosinophil counts of at least 300 cells/μL are more likely to have reduced asthma exacerbations by 67% relative to placebo and those with 400 cells/μL had reductions of 74%.[146] In contrast, an observational study compared omalizumab treatment with placebo and found that blood eosinophils, as well as FeNO and total IgE levels, did not predict the more likely response to omalizumab.[145] This lack of evidence for eosinophil levels was also observed in a second observational study.[147] In situations with conflicting results like this, PM could serve as a means to determine and then identify those individuals who would benefit from eosinophil-guided omalizumab therapy.

Anti–IL-5 or Anti–IL-5 Receptor

Anti–IL-5 antibodies such as mepolizumab, reslizumab, and benralizumab have also shown efficacy in treating asthma.[148–150] These antibodies act by either binding and depleting IL-5 (mepolizumab, reslizumab)[151] or blocking the IL-5 receptor alpha chain

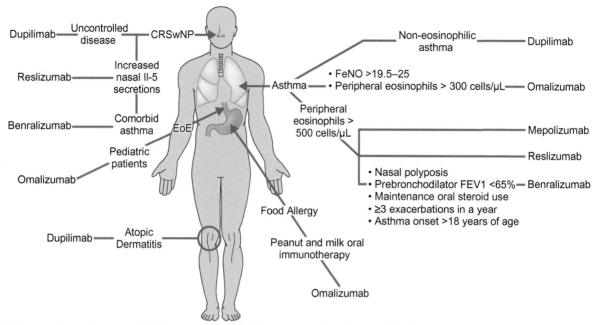

Fig. 2.2 Phenotypic and endotypic influences on biologic therapies in patients with allergic disease. This figure illustrates select examples of different endotypes and phenotypes and their associations with improved outcomes using a given biologic for several allergic diseases. *CRSwNP*, Chronic rhinosinusitis with nasal polyposis; *EoE*, eosinophilic esophagitis.

(benralizumab).[152] Either mechanism leads to a decrease in eosinophil count. Importantly, the patient biomarker that best predicts response to any of these agents is blood eosinophilia, rather than sputum eosinophilia.[153] Moreover, patients with eosinophil counts of 500 cells/µL or more show better improvement in both pre- and post-bronchodilator FEV1 compared with lower eosinophil counts.[154] Also, in patients with high blood eosinophils, several other markers were predictive of benralizumab responsiveness: nasal polyposis, prebronchodilator FEV1 <65% predicted, maintenance oral corticosteroid use, three or more exacerbations in the last year, and age of asthma onset of 18 years or older.[155] Therefore when considering a PM approach to biologics, the provider would likely find more benefit from using blood eosinophil counts over those from patient sputum.

Anti–IL-4/IL-13

Dupilumab binds to the IL-4 receptor alpha chain, which leads to both IL-4 and IL-13 receptor signaling blockade[156] and has shown to be effective in treating asthma.[157]

Other

Anti–IL-33 mAbs have shown promising results for the improvement of asthma outcomes.[158] Similarly, anti–thymic stromal lymphopoietin mAbs have shown promise in reducing asthma exacerbations, particularly in individuals with noneosinophilic asthma.[159,160] Thus mAbs top the list when compared to other biological drug types, such as proteins, enzymes, and vaccines.

Atopic Dermatitis

The only currently approved biologic therapy for AD is dupilumab, an IL-4 receptor alpha-antagonist. IL-4 and IL-13 are two key cytokines involved with AD pathogenesis.[161] Studies have found that dupilumab improves AD outcomes.[162] Dupilumab has also been shown to alter the AD transcriptome by upregulating structural proteins, lipid metabolism proteins, and epidermal barrier proteins as well as downregulating inflammatory mediators, and markers of epidermal proliferation.[44]

Chronic Rhinosinusitis With Nasal Polyposis

While not yet standard-of-care in clinical practice, several biologic therapies have been developed for chronic rhinosinusitis with nasal polyposis (CRSwNP). Dupilumab has been shown to improve outcomes in patients with uncontrolled CRSwNP.[163] After treatment with dupilumab, individuals have been shown to have an improvement in sinonasal symptom scores, sense of smell, sinonasal imaging, nasal polyp size, and a decreased need for systemic corticosteroids or sinus surgery.[163,164] Omalizumab has also been shown to be an effective biologic therapy for CRSwNP and can lead to improvements in nasal congestion, rhinorrhea, and a sense of smell.[165] These findings were increased in subjects without atopic disease.[166] Anti–IL-5 mAb therapies have also shown efficacy in treating CRSwNP.[167] Mepolizumab has shown particular promise and has been found to decrease nasal polyp size, decrease in need for sinus surgery, and improved congestion, postnasal drip, and sense of smell.[167] Reslizumab has also been shown to reduce total nasal polyp scores, particularly among those individuals with increased IL-5 nasal secretions.[168] Benralizumab is most effective in patients with both CRSwNP and asthma, with improvements in both diseases over patients who only have either asthma or CRSwNP.[169]

Each of these therapies has the potential to be a part of PM management. PM approaches could use patient biomarkers and medical history to determine the medicine most likely to produce beneficial results.

Eosinophilic Esophagitis (EoE)

Mepolizumab has been trialed for use within EoE and is an effective treatment for decreasing overall eosinophilia and improving symptoms in adults with disease resistance to other therapies.[170,171] However, while esophageal eosinophils decreased in children, mepolizumab appears to not have a significant effect on decreasing clinical symptoms in children.[172] Similarly, reslizumab therapy in EoE was shown to decrease esophageal eosinophil counts but did not affect patient symptom scores.[173] While one study showed no benefit of omalizumab therapy in EoE,[174] a second showed potential benefit, particularly in children.[175] These results, whereby a greater benefit is seen using omalizumab in children, highlight the potential role for a PM approach using biologics within EoE.

Food Allergy

The most promising biologic at this time for use within food allergy is omalizumab. Omalizumab has been shown to increase the tolerability of cow's milk[176,177] and peanut oral immunotherapy.[178] Further investigation is needed on relevant biomarkers within these populations to help guide PM approaches.

CHALLENGES IN PRECISION MEDICINE

PM has significant potential for providing improved management in allergic disorders, but it is in its infancy. Notably, many challenges exist facing the progress and implementation of PM in everyday healthcare. Incredibly large amounts of data are being accumulated creating a vast knowledge network, but considerable work remains in mining and understanding the data and finally interpreting it for the benefit of the healthcare practitioner and patients and families. Although great progress has been made to technologies and platforms for use in the clinic, there are still diagnostic, technical, and therapeutic challenges that need to be taken into account and resolved.[179] One of the major selling points of PM is that it is participatory, meaning that the patient will play a big role in the decision-making process. Thus additional tools are needed to discuss with patients the individual-level data clearly and effectively. This presents a challenge in the sense that doctors will need to develop sufficient skills and knowledge in genomics, pharmacogenomics, and related fields.[180] There is also the challenge of economic feasibility; while the costs are decreasing, they remain high. Many people are opting to pay out of pocket to companies that sell genomic and other tests directly to the consumer. Moreover, other patients discard the possibility of testing completely because they are afraid they will be discriminated against based on their genetic predispositions.[181] Lastly, many ethical aspects including individual privacy issues have to be taken into consideration when applying PM to practice.

SUMMARY

Biologics are becoming the primary focus for a growing number of therapeutic developers in the era of PM. Although they are both challenging (produced in living cells) and expensive to develop,

they have applications for a wide range of diseases that are not being adequately addressed with existing medicines. The concept of clinical care practice to fit specific treatment to the individual patient in PM paradigm is an evolving concept becoming a reality.

REFERENCES

1. US Food and Drug Administration. Paving the Way for Personalized Medicine: FDA's Role in a New Era of Medical Product Development. Silver Spring, MD: US Food and Drug Administration; 2013.
2. Khoury MJ, Gwinn ML, Glasgow RE, Kramer BS. A population approach to precision medicine. Am J Prev Med. 2012;42:639–645.
3. Hood L, Flores M. A personal view on systems medicine and the emergence of proactive P4 medicine: predictive, preventive, personalized and participatory. N Biotechnol. 2012;29:613–624.
4. Roden DM, Tyndale RF. Genomic medicine, precision medicine, personalized medicine: what's in a name? Clin Pharmacol Ther. 2013;94:169–172. https://doi.org/10.1038/clpt.2013.101.
5. Genetics Home Reference. https://ghr.nlm.nih.gov/. Accessed September 10, 2020.
6. Redekop WK, Mladsi D. The faces of personalized medicine: a framework for understanding its meaning and scope. Value Health. 2013;16:S4–S9.
7. Ginsburg GS, Willard HF. Genomic and personalized medicine: foundations and applications. Transl Res. 2009;154:277–287.
8. Abrahams E, Silver M. The history of personalized medicine. Integr Neurosci Personal Med. 2010:3–16.
9. Juengst E, McGowan ML, Fishman JR, Settersten Jr. RA. From "Personalized" to "Precision" medicine: the ethical and social implications of rhetorical reform in genomic medicine. Hastings Cent Rep. 2016;46:21–33. https://doi.org/10.1002/hast.614.
10. Denny JC, Rutter JL, Goldstein DB, et al. The "All of Us" Research Program. N Engl J Med. 2019;381:668–676. https://doi.org/10.1056/NEJMsr1809937.
11. Kowalski MH, Qian H, Hou Z, et al. Use of >100,000 NHLBI Trans-Omics for Precision Medicine (TOPMed) Consortium whole genome sequences improves imputation quality and detection of rare variant associations in admixed African and Hispanic/Latino populations. PLoS Genet. 2019;15:e1008500. https://doi.org/10.1371/journal.pgen.1008500.
12. Hood L, Friend SH. Predictive, personalized, preventive, participatory (P4) cancer medicine. Nat Rev Clin Oncol. 2011;8:184–187.
13. Hoberg-Vetti H, Bjorvatn C, Fiane BE, et al. BRCA1/2 testing in newly diagnosed breast and ovarian cancer patients without prior genetic counselling: the DNA-BONus study. Eur J Hum Genet. 2016;24:881–888. https://doi.org/10.1038/ejhg.2015.196.
14. Incorvati JA, Shah S, Mu Y, Lu J. Targeted therapy for HER2 positive breast cancer. J Hematol Oncol. 2013;6:38.
15. Druker BJ, Guilhot F, O'Brien SG, et al. Five-year follow-up of patients receiving imatinib for chronic myeloid leukemia. N Engl J Med. 2006;355:2408–2417.
16. Schwaederle M, Zhao M, Lee JJ, et al. Impact of precision medicine in diverse cancers: a meta-analysis of phase II clinical trials. J Clin Oncol. 2015;33:3817–3825. https://doi.org/10.1200/JCO.2015.61.5997.
17. Council NR. Toward Precision Medicine: Building a Knowledge Network for Biomedical Research and a New Taxonomy of Disease. Washington, DC: National Academies Press; 2011.
18. Muraro A, Lemanske Jr RF, Hellings PW, et al. Precision medicine in patients with allergic diseases: airway diseases and atopic

dermatitis-PRACTALL document of the European Academy of Allergy and Clinical Immunology and the American Academy of Allergy, Asthma & Immunology. J Allergy Clin Immunol. 2016;137:1347–1358. https://doi.org/10.1016/j.jaci.2016.03.010.

19. Fassl BA, Nkoy FL, Stone BL, et al. The Joint Commission Children's Asthma Care quality measures and asthma readmissions. Pediatrics. 2012;130:482–491. https://doi.org/10.1542/peds.2011-3318.

20. Akinbami L, Centers for Disease Control and Prevention National Center for Health Statistics. The state of childhood asthma, United States, 1980-2005. Adv Data. 2006;381:1–24.

21. Woodruff PG, Boushey HA, Dolganov GM, et al. Genome-wide profiling identifies epithelial cell genes associated with asthma and with treatment response to corticosteroids. Proc Natl Acad Sci U S A. 2007;104:15858–15863. https://doi.org/10.1073/pnas.0707413104.

22. Woodruff PG, Modrek B, Choy DF, et al. T-helper type 2-driven inflammation defines major subphenotypes of asthma. Am J Respir Crit Care Med. 2009;180:388–395. https://doi.org/10.1164/rccm.200903-0392OC.

23. Lotvall J, Akdis CA, Bacharier LB, et al. Asthma endotypes: a new approach to classification of disease entities within the asthma syndrome. J Allergy Clin Immunol. 2011;127:355–360. https://doi.org/10.1016/j.jaci.2010.11.037.

24. Agache I, Akdis CA. Endotypes of allergic diseases and asthma: an important step in building blocks for the future of precision medicine. Allergol Int. 2016;65:243–252. https://doi.org/10.1016/j.alit.2016.04.011.

25. Desai M, Oppenheimer J. Elucidating asthma phenotypes and endotypes: progress towards personalized medicine. Ann Allergy Asthma Immunol. 2016;116:394–401. https://doi.org/10.1016/j.anai.2015.12.024.

26. Anderson GP. Endotyping asthma: new insights into key pathogenic mechanisms in a complex, heterogeneous disease. Lancet. 2008;372:1107–1119. https://doi.org/10.1016/s0140-6736(08)61452-x.

27. Akdis CA, Ballas ZK. Precision medicine and precision health: building blocks to foster a revolutionary health care model. J Allergy Clin Immunol. 2016;137:1359–1361. https://doi.org/10.1016/j.jaci.2016.03.020.

28. Berry A, Busse WW. Biomarkers in asthmatic patients: has their time come to direct treatment? J Allergy Clin Immunol. 2016;137:1317–1324. https://doi.org/10.1016/j.jaci.2016.03.009.

29. Agache I, Rogozea L. Asthma biomarkers: do they bring precision medicine closer to the clinic? Allergy Asthma Immunol Res. 2017;9:466–476. https://doi.org/10.4168/aair.2017.9.6.466.

30. Sonntag H-J, Filippi S, Pipis S, Custovic A. Blood biomarkers of sensitization and asthma. Front Pediatr. 2019;7:251. https://doi.org/10.3389/fped.2019.00251. https://europepmc.org/articles/PMC6593482, https://europepmc.org/articles/PMC6593482?pdf=render.

31. Tiotiu A. Biomarkers in asthma: state of the art. Asthma Res Pract. 2018;4:10. https://doi.org/10.1186/s40733-018-0047-4.

32. van Rensen EL, Straathof KC, Veselic-Charvat MA, et al. Effect of inhaled steroids on airway hyperresponsiveness, sputum eosinophils, and exhaled nitric oxide levels in patients with asthma. Thorax. 1999;54:403–408. https://doi.org/10.1136/thx.54.5.403.

33. Hoffman BC, Rabinovitch N. Urinary leukotriene E(4) as a biomarker of exposure, susceptibility, and risk in asthma: an update. Immunol

Allergy Clin North Am. 2018;38:599–610. https://doi.org/10.1016/j.iac.2018.06.011.

34. Carraro S, Bozzetto S, Giordano G, et al. Wheezing preschool children with early-onset asthma reveal a specific metabolomic profile. Pediatr Allergy Immunol. 2018;29:375–382. https://doi.org/10.1111/pai.12879.

35. Park YH, Fitzpatrick AM, Medriano CA, Jones DP. High-resolution metabolomics to identify urine biomarkers in corticosteroid-resistant asthmatic children. J Allergy Clin Immunol. 2017;139:1518–1524.e1514. https://doi.org/10.1016/j.jaci.2016.08.018.

36. Papamichael MM, Katsardis C, Erbas B, Itsiopoulos C, Tsoukalas D. Urinary organic acids as biomarkers in the assessment of pulmonary function in children with asthma. Nutr Res. 2019;61:31–40. https://doi.org/10.1016/j.nutres.2018.10.004.

37. Cavaleiro Rufo J, Paciência I, Mendes FC, et al. Exhaled breath condensate volatilome allows sensitive diagnosis of persistent asthma. Allergy. 2019;74:527–534. https://doi.org/10.1111/all.13596.

38. Schleich FN, Zanella D, Stefanuto P-H, et al. Exhaled volatile organic compounds are able to discriminate between neutrophilic and eosinophilic asthma. Am J Respir Crit Care Med. 2019;200:444–453. https://doi.org/10.1164/rccm.201811-2210OC.

39. Menzies-Gow A, Mansur AH, Brightling CE. Clinical utility of fractional exhaled nitric oxide (FeNO) in severe asthma management. Eur Respirat J. 2020;1901633. https://doi.org/10.1183/13993003.01633-2019.

40. Hastie AT, Moore WC, Meyers DA, et al. Analyses of asthma severity phenotypes and inflammatory proteins in subjects stratified by sputum granulocytes. J Allergy Clin Immunol. 2010;125:1028–1036. e1013. https://doi.org/10.1016/j.jaci.2010.02.008.

41. Licari A, Castagnoli R, Brambilla I, et al. Asthma endotyping and biomarkers in childhood asthma. Pediatr Allergy Immunol Pulmonol. 2018;31:44–55. https://doi.org/10.1089/ped.2018.0886\\192.168.60.5\Public\Hari

42. Thijs J, Krastev T, Weidinger S, et al. Biomarkers for atopic dermatitis: a systematic review and meta-analysis. Curr Opin Allergy Clin Immunol. 2015;15:453–460. https://doi.org/10.1097/ACI.0000000000000198.

43. Carpagnano GE, Scioscia G, Lacedonia D, et al. Looking for airways periostin in severe asthma: could it be useful for clustering type 2 endotype? Chest. 2018;154:1083–1090. https://doi.org/10.1016/j.chest.2018.08.1032.

44. Hamilton JD, Suárez-Fariñas M, Dhingra N, et al. Dupilumab improves the molecular signature in skin of patients with moderate-to-severe atopic dermatitis. J Allergy Clin Immunol. 2014;134:1293–1300.

45. Kong HH, Oh J, Deming C, et al. Temporal shifts in the skin microbiome associated with disease flares and treatment in children with atopic dermatitis. Genome Res. 2012;22:850–859. https://doi.org/10.1101/gr.131029.111.

46. Fornadley JA. Skin testing for inhalant allergy. Int Forum Allergy Rhinol. 2014;4(Suppl 2):S41–S45. https://doi.org/10.1002/alr.21393.

47. Tsybikov NN, Egorova EV, Kuznik BI, Fefelova EV, Magen E. Biomarker assessment in chronic rhinitis and chronic rhinosinusitis: endothelin-1, TARC/CCL17, neopterin, and α-defensins. Allergy Asthma Proc. 2016;37:35–42.

48. Badorrek P, Müller M, Koch W, Hohlfeld JM, Krug N. Specificity and reproducibility of nasal biomarkers in patients with allergic rhinitis after allergen challenge chamber exposure. Ann Allergy Asthma Immunol. 2017;118:290–297. https://doi.org/10.1016/j.anai.2017.01.018\\192.168.60.5\Public\Hari.

49. Oriel RC, Wang J. Diagnosis and management of food allergy. Pediatr Clin North Am. 2019;66:941–954. https://doi.org/10.1016/j.pcl.2019.06.002.

50. Hemmings O, Kwok M, McKendry R, Santos AF. Basophil activation test: old and new applications in allergy. Curr Allergy Asthma Rep. 2018;18:77. https://doi.org/10.1007/s11882-018-0831-5.

51. Bahri R, Custovic A, Korosec P, et al. Mast cell activation test in the diagnosis of allergic disease and anaphylaxis. J Allergy Clin Immunol. 2018;142:485–496.e416. https://doi.org/10.1016/j.jaci.2018.01.043.

52. Santos AF, Couto-Francisco N, Bécares N, Kwok M, Bahnson HT, Lack G. A novel human mast cell activation test for peanut allergy. J Allergy Clin Immunol. 2018;142:689–691.e689. https://doi.org/10.1016/j.jaci.2018.03.011.

53. Syed A, Garcia MA, Lyu S-C, et al. Peanut oral immunotherapy results in increased antigen-induced regulatory T-cell function and hypomethylation of forkhead box protein 3 (FOXP3). J Allergy Clin Immunol. 2014;133:500–510. https://doi.org/10.1016/j.jaci.2013.12.1037.

54. Bhardwaj N, Ghaffari G. Biomarkers for eosinophilic esophagitis: a review. Ann Allergy Asthma Immunol. 2012;109:155–159. https://doi.org/10.1016/j.anai.2012.06.014.

55. Wambre E, Bajzik V, DeLong JH, et al. A phenotypically and functionally distinct human TH2 cell subpopulation is associated with allergic disorders. Sci Transl Med. 2017;9. https://doi.org/10.1126/scitranslmed.aam9171.

56. Lloyd CM, Hessel EM. Functions of T cells in asthma: more than just T(H)2 cells. Nat Rev. 2010;10:838–848. https://doi.org/10.1038/nri2870.

57. Gaublomme JT, Yosef N, Lee Y, et al. Single-cell genomics unveils critical regulators of Th17 cell pathogenicity. Cell. 2015;163:1400–1412. https://doi.org/10.1016/j.cell.2015.11.009.

58. Wang C, Yosef N, Gaublomme J, et al. CD5L/AIM regulates lipid biosynthesis and restrains Th17 cell pathogenicity. Cell. 2015;163:1413–1427. https://doi.org/10.1016/j.cell.2015.10.068.

59. Papalexi E, Satija R. Single-cell RNA sequencing to explore immune cell heterogeneity. Nat Rev Immunol. 2018;18:35–45. https://doi.org/10.1038/nri.2017.76.

60. Seumois G, Ramírez-Suástegui C, Schmiedel BJ, et al. Single-cell transcriptomic analysis of allergen-specific T cells in allergy and asthma. Sci Immunol. 2020;5:eaba6087. https://doi.org/10.1126/sciimmunol.aba6087.

61. Li CX, Wheelock CE, Sköld CM, Wheelock Å. M. Integration of multi-omics datasets enables molecular classification of COPD. Eur Respir J. 2018;51. https://doi.org/10.1183/13993003.01930-2017.

62. Gibbs RA, et al. The international HapMap project. Nature. 2003;426:789–796.

63. Siva, N. Nature Publishing Group, 2008.

64. Auer PL, Johnsen JM, Johnson AD, et al. Imputation of exome sequence variants into population-based samples and blood-cell-trait-associated loci in African Americans: NHLBI GO Exome Sequencing Project. Am J Hum Genet. 2012;91:794–808.

65. Hindorff L, Junkins H, Mehta J, Manolio T. A catalog of published genome-wide association studies 2010. Ref Type: Generic. 2011

66. Welter D, MacArthur J, Morales J, et al. The NHGRI GWAS Catalog, a curated resource of SNP-trait associations. Nucleic Acids Res. 2014;42:D1001–D1006.

67. Paternoster L, Standl M, Waage J, et al. Multi-ancestry genome-wide association study of 21,000 cases and 95,000 controls identifies new risk loci for atopic dermatitis. Nat Genet. 2015;47:1449–1456. https://doi.org/10.1038/ng.3424.

68. Meyers DA, Bleecker ER, Holloway JW, Holgate ST. Asthma genetics and personalised medicine. Lancet Respir Med. 2014;2:405–415.

69. Kan M, Shumyatcher M, Himes BE. Using omics approaches to understand pulmonary diseases. Respir Res. 2017;18:149.

70. Poole A, Urbanek C, Eng C, et al. Dissecting childhood asthma with nasal transcriptomics distinguishes subphenotypes of disease. J Allergy Clin Immunol. 2014;133:670–8.e612.

71. Croteau-Chonka DC, Qiu W, Martinez FD, et al. Gene expression profiling in blood provides reproducible molecular insights into asthma control. Am J Respir Crit Care Med. 2017;195:179–188.

72. Turi KN, Romick-Rosendale L, Ryckman KK, Hartert TV. A review of metabolomics approaches and their application in identifying causal pathways of childhood asthma. J Allergy Clin Immunol. 2017;141:1191–1201.

73. Strachan DP. Hay fever, hygiene, and household size. BMJ: Br Med J. 1989;299:1259–1260.

74. Huang YJ, Marsland BJ, Bunyavanich S, et al. The microbiome in allergic disease: current understanding and future opportunities-2017 PRACTALL document of the American Academy of Allergy, Asthma & Immunology and the European Academy of Allergy and Clinical Immunology. J Allergy Clin Immunol. 2017;139:1099–1110. https://doi.org/10.1016/j.jaci.2017.02.007.

75. Kennedy EA, Connolly J, O'B Hourihane J, et al. Skin microbiome before development of atopic dermatitis: early colonization with commensal staphylococci at 2 months is associated with a lower risk of atopic dermatitis at 1 year. J Allergy Clin Immunol. 2017;139:166–172. https://doi.org/10.1016/j.jaci.2016.07.029.

76. Baurecht H, Rühlemann MC, Rodríguez E, et al. Epidermal lipid composition, barrier integrity, and eczematous inflammation are associated with skin microbiome configuration. J Allergy Clin Immunol. 2018;141:1668–676.e1616. https://doi.org/10.1016/j.jaci.2018.01.019.

77. Nakatsuji T, Chen TH, Narala S, et al. Antimicrobials from human skin commensal bacteria protect against Staphylococcus aureus and are deficient in atopic dermatitis. Sci Transl Med. 2017;9:eaah4680. https://doi.org/10.1126/scitranslmed.aah4680.

78. Meylan P, Lang C, Mermoud S, et al. Skin colonization by Staphylococcus aureus precedes the clinical diagnosis of atopic dermatitis in infancy. J Invest Dermatol. 2017;137:2497–2504. https://doi.org/10.1016/j.jid.2017.07.834.

79. Chung KF. Airway microbial dysbiosis in asthmatic patients: a target for prevention and treatment? J Allergy Clin Immunol. 2017;139:1071–1081. https://doi.org/10.1016/j.jaci.2017.02.004.

80. Chiu C-Y, Chan Y-L, Tsai Yu-S, et al. Airway microbial diversity is inversely associated with mite-sensitized rhinitis and asthma in early childhood. Scientific Rep. 2017;7:1820. https://doi.org/10.1038/s41598-017-02067-7.

81. Arrieta MC, Stiemsma LT, Dimitriu PA, et al. Early infancy microbial and metabolic alterations affect risk of childhood asthma. Sci Transl Med. 2015;7:307ra152. https://doi.org/10.1126/scitranslmed.aab2271.

82. Fujimura KE, Sitarik AR, Havstad S, et al. Neonatal gut microbiota associates with childhood multisensitized atopy and T cell differentiation. Nat Med. 2016;22:1187–1191. https://doi.org/10.1038/nm.4176.

83. Vineis P, Chadeau-Hyam M, Gmuender H, et al. The exposome in practice: design of the EXPOsOMICS project. Int J Hyg Environ Health. 2017;220:142–151. https://doi.org/10.1016/j.ijheh.2016.08.001.

84. Wanichthanarak K, Fahrmann JF, Grapov D. Genomic, proteomic, and metabolomic data integration strategies. Biomark Insights. 2015;10:1–6. https://doi.org/10.4137/BMI.S29511.

85. Cavallari L, Beitelshees AL, Blake KV, et al. The IGNITE Pharmacogenetics Working Group: an opportunity for building evidence with pharmacogenetic implementation in a real-world setting. Clin Trans Sci. 2017;10:143–146.

86. Haga SB, Mills R. A review of consent practices and perspectives for pharmacogenetic testing. Pharmacogenomics. 2016;17:1595–1605.

87. Mills R, Voora D, Peyser B, Haga SB. Delivering pharmacogenetic testing in a primary care setting. Pharmacogen Personal Med. 2013;6:105–112. https://doi.org/10.2147/PGPM.S50598.

88. Kersten ET, Koppelman GH. Pharmacogenetics of asthma: toward precision medicine. Curr Opin Pulm Med. 2017;23:12–20. https://doi.org/10.1097/MCP.0000000000000335.

89. Muehleisen B, Gallo RL. Vitamin D in allergic disease: shedding light on a complex problem. J Allergy Clin Immunol. 2013;131:324–329. https://doi.org/10.1016/j.jaci.2012.12.1562.

90. Tsiaras WG, Weinstock MA. Factors influencing vitamin D status. Acta Derm Venereol. 2011;91:115–124. https://doi.org/10.2340/00015555-0980.

91. Holick MF, Binkley NC, Bischoff-Ferrari HA, et al. Evaluation, treatment, and prevention of vitamin D deficiency: An Endocrine Society Clinical Practice Guideline. J Clin Endocrinol Metabol. 2011;96:1911–1930. https://doi.org/10.1210/jc.2011-0385.

92. Bikle DD, Teichert A, Arnold LA, Uchida Y, Elias PM, Oda Y. Differential regulation of epidermal function by VDR coactivators. J Steroid Biochem Mol Biol. 2010;121:308–313. https://doi.org/10.1016/j.jsbmb.2010.03.027.

93. Hawker NP, Pennypacker SD, Chang SM, Bikle DD. Regulation of human epidermal keratinocyte differentiation by the vitamin D receptor and its coactivators DRIP205, SRC2, and SRC3. J Invest Dermatol. 2007;127:874–880. https://doi.org/10.1038/sj.jid.5700624.

94. Khoo AL, Chai LYA, Koenen HJPM, et al. Regulation of cytokine responses by seasonality of vitamin D status in healthy individuals. Clin Exp Immunol. 2011;164:72–79. https://doi.org/10.1111/j.1365-2249.2010.04315.x.

95. Biggs L, Yu C, Fedoric B, Lopez AF, Galli SJ, Grimbaldeston MA. Evidence that vitamin D3 promotes mast cell–dependent reduction of chronic UVB-induced skin pathology in mice. J Experiment Med. 2010;207:455–463. https://doi.org/10.1084/jem.20091725.

96. Hewison M. Vitamin D and innate and adaptive immunity. Vitam Horm. 2011;86:23–62. https://doi.org/10.1016/b978-0-12-386960-9.00002-2.

97. Hong SP, Kim MJ, Jung M-Y, et al. Biopositive effects of low-dose UVB on epidermis: coordinate upregulation of antimicrobial peptides and permeability barrier reinforcement. J Invest Dermatol. 2008;128:2880–2887. https://doi.org/10.1038/jid.2008.169.

98. Gorman S, Judge MA, Hart PH. Immune-modifying properties of topical vitamin D: focus on dendritic cells and T cells. J Steroid Biochem Mol Biol. 2010;121:247–249. https://doi.org/10.1016/j.jsbmb.2010.02.034.

99. Vähävihu K, Ala-Houhala M, Peric M, et al. Narrowband ultraviolet B treatment improves vitamin D balance and alters antimicrobial peptide expression in skin lesions of psoriasis and atopic dermatitis. Br J Dermatol. 2010;163:321–328. https://doi.org/10.1111/j.1365-2133.2010.09767.x.

100. Peroni DG, Piacentini GL, Cametti E, Chinellato I, Boner AL. Correlation between serum 25-hydroxyvitamin D levels and severity of atopic dermatitis in children. Br J Dermatol. 2011;164:1078–1082. https://doi.org/10.1111/j.1365-2133.2010.10147.x.

101. Sidbury R, Sullivan AF, Thadhani RI, Camargo Jr CA. Randomized controlled trial of vitamin D supplementation for winter-related atopic dermatitis in Boston: a pilot study. Br J Dermatol. 2008;159:245–247. https://doi.org/10.1111/j.1365-2133.2008.08601.x.

102. Brehm JM, Celedón JC, Soto-Quiros ME, et al. Serum vitamin D levels and markers of severity of childhood asthma in Costa Rica. Am J Respir Crit Care Med. 2009;179:765–771. https://doi.org/10.1164/rccm.200808-1361OC.

103. Goleva E, Searing DA, Jackson LP, Richers BN, Leung DYM. Steroid requirements and immune associations with vitamin D are stronger in children than adults with asthma. J Allergy Clin Immunol. 2012;129:1243–1251. https://doi.org/10.1016/j.jaci.2012.01.044.

104. Urashima M, Segawa T, Okazaki M, Kurihara M, Wada Y, Ida H. Randomized trial of vitamin D supplementation to prevent seasonal influenza A in schoolchildren. Am J Clin Nutr. 2010;91:1255–1260. https://doi.org/10.3945/ajcn.2009.29094.

105. Majak P, Olszowiec-Chlebna M, Smejda K, Stelmach I. Vitamin D supplementation in children may prevent asthma exacerbation triggered by acute respiratory infection. J Allergy Clin Immunol. 2011;127:1294–1296. https://doi.org/10.1016/j.jaci.2010.12.016.

106. Camargo Jr CA, Clark S, Kaplan MS, Lieberman P, Wood RA. Regional differences in EpiPen prescriptions in the United States: the potential role of vitamin D. J Allergy Clin Immunol. 2007;120:131–136. https://doi.org/10.1016/j.jaci.2007.03.049.

107. Nurmatov U, Devereux G, Sheikh A. Nutrients and foods for the primary prevention of asthma and allergy: systematic review and meta-analysis. J Allergy Clin Immunol. 2011;127:724–733.e730. https://doi.org/10.1016/j.jaci.2010.11.001.

108. Gale CR, Robinson SM, Harvey NC, et al. Maternal vitamin D status during pregnancy and child outcomes. Eur J Clin Nutr. 2008;62:68–77. https://doi.org/10.1038/sj.ejcn.1602680.

109. Hyppönen E, Berry DJ, Wjst M, Power C. Serum 25-hydroxyvitamin D and IgE - a significant but nonlinear relationship. Allergy: Euro J Allergy Clin Immunol. 2009;64:613–620. https://doi.org/10.1111/j.1398-9995.2008.01865.x.

110. Sharief S, Jariwala S, Kumar J, Muntner P, Melamed ML. Vitamin D levels and food and environmental allergies in the United States: results from the National Health and Nutrition Examination Survey 2005-2006. J Allergy Clin Immunol. 2011;127:1195–1202. https://doi.org/10.1016/j.jaci.2011.01.017.

111. Bäck O, Blomquist HK, Hernell O, Stenberg B. Does vitamin D intake during infancy promote the development of atopic allergy? Acta Derm Venereol. 2009;89:28–32. https://doi.org/10.2340/00015555-0541.

112. Hyppönen E, et al. Ann N Y Acad Sci. 2004;1037:84–95.

113. Calder PC, Grimble RF. Polyunsaturated fatty acids, inflammation and immunity. Eur J Clin Nutr. 2002;56 (Suppl 3):S14–S19. https://doi.org/10.1038/sj.ejcn.1601478.

114. Calder PC. N-3 polyunsaturated fatty acids and inflammation: from molecular biology to the clinic. Lipids. 2003;38:343–352. https://doi.org/10.1007/s11745-003-1068-y.

115. Prescott SL, Calder PC. N-3 polyunsaturated fatty acids and allergic disease. Curr Opin Clin Nutr Metab Care. 2004;7:123–129. https://doi.org/10.1097/00075197-200403000-00004.

116. Harizi H, Juzan M, Moreau JF, Gualde N. Prostaglandins inhibit 5-lipoxygenase-activating protein expression and leukotriene B4 production from dendritic cells via an IL-10-dependent mechanism. J Immunol. 2003;170:139–146. https://doi.org/10.4049/jimmunol.170.1.139.

117. Calder PC, Yaqoob P, Thies F, Wallace FA, Miles EA. Fatty acids and lymphocyte functions. Br J Nutr. 2002;87(Suppl 1)S31–S48. https://doi.org/10.1079/bjn2001455.

118. Hughes DA, Pinder AC. N-3 polyunsaturated fatty acids modulate the expression of functionally associated molecules on human monocytes and inhibit antigen-presentation in vitro. Clin Exp Immunol. 1997;110:516–523. https://doi.org/10.1046/j.1365-2249.1997.4351455.x.

119. Dunder T, Kuikka L, Turtinen J, Räsänen L, Uhari M. Diet, serum fatty acids, and atopic diseases in childhood. Allergy. 2001;56:425–428. https://doi.org/10.1034/j.1398-9995.2001.056005425.x.

120. von Mutius E, Martinez FD, Fritzsch C, Nicolai T, Roell G, Thiemann H. Prevalence of asthma and atopy in two areas of West and East Germany. Am J Respir Crit Care Med. 1994;149:358–364. https://doi.org/10.1164/ajrccm.149.2.8306030.

121. Pöysä L, Korppi M, Pietikäinen M, Remes K, Juntunen-Backman K. Asthma, allergic rhinitis and atopic eczema in Finnish children and adolescents. Allergy. 1991;46:161–165. https://doi.org/10.1111/j.1398-9995.1991.tb00564.x.

122. Haby MM, Peat JK, Marks GB, Woolcock AJ, Leeder SR. Asthma in preschool children: prevalence and risk factors. Thorax. 2001;56:589–595. https://doi.org/10.1136/thorax.56.8.589.

123. von Mutius E, Weiland SK, Fritzsch C, Duhme H, Keil U. Increasing prevalence of hay fever and atopy among children in Leipzig, East Germany. Lancet. 1998;351:862–866. https://doi.org/10.1016/s0140-6736(97)10100-3.

124. Takemura Y, Sakurai Y, Honjo S, et al. The relationship between fish intake and the prevalence of asthma: the Tokorozawa childhood asthma and pollinosis study. Prev Med. 2002;34:221–225. https://doi.org/10.1006/pmed.2001.0978.

125. Arm JP, Horton CE, Mencia-Huerta JM, et al. Effect of dietary supplementation with fish oil lipids on mild asthma. Thorax. 1988;43:84–92. https://doi.org/10.1136/thx.43.2.84.

126. Okamoto M, Mitsunobu F, Ashida K, et al. Effects of dietary supplementation with n-3 fatty acids compared with n-6 fatty acids on bronchial asthma. Intern Med. 2000;39:107–111. https://doi.org/10.2169/internalmedicine.39.107.

127. Broughton KS, Johnson CS, Pace BK, Liebman M, Kleppinger KM. Reduced asthma symptoms with n-3 fatty acid ingestion are related to 5-series leukotriene production. Am J Clin Nutr. 1997;65:1011–1017. https://doi.org/10.1093/ajcn/65.4.1011.

128. Nagakura T, Matsuda S, Shichijyo K, Sugimoto H, Hata K. Dietary supplementation with fish oil rich in omega-3 polyunsaturated fatty acids in children with bronchial asthma. Eur Respir J. 2000;16:861–865. https://doi.org/10.1183/09031936.00.16586100.

129. Hodge L, Salome CM, Hughes JM, et al. Effect of dietary intake of omega-3 and omega-6 fatty acids on severity of asthma in children. Eur Respir J. 1998;11:361–365. https://doi.org/10.1183/09031936.98.11020361.

130. Marks GB, Mihrshahi S, Kemp AS, et al. Prevention of asthma during the first 5 years of life: a randomized controlled trial. J Allergy Clin Immunol. 2006;118:53–61. https://doi.org/10.1016/j.jaci.2006.04.004.

131. Almqvist C, Garden F, Xuan W, et al. Omega-3 and omega-6 fatty acid exposure from early life does not affect atopy and asthma at age 5 years. J Allergy Clin Immunol. 2007;119:1438–1444. https://doi.org/10.1016/j.jaci.2007.01.046.

132. Anandan C, Nurmatov U, Sheikh A. Omega 3 and 6 oils for primary prevention of allergic disease: systematic review and meta-analysis. Allergy. 2009;64:840–848. https://doi.org/10.1111/j.1398-9995.2009.02042.x.

133. Mihrshahi S, Peat JK, Marks GB, et al. Eighteen-month outcomes of house dust mite avoidance and dietary fatty acid modification in the Childhood Asthma Prevention Study (CAPS). J Allergy Clin Immunol. 2003;111:162–168. https://doi.org/10.1067/mai.2003.36.

134. Dunstan JA, Mori TA, Barden A, et al. Maternal fish oil supplementation in pregnancy reduces interleukin-13 levels in cord blood of infants at high risk of atopy. Clin Exp Allergy. 2003;33:442–448. https://doi.org/10.1046/j.1365-2222.2003.01590.x.

135. Dunstan JA, Mori Trevor A, Barden A, et al. Fish oil supplementation in pregnancy modifies neonatal allergen-specific immune responses and clinical outcomes in infants at high risk of atopy: a randomized, controlled trial. J Allergy Clin Immunol. 2003;112:1178–1184. https://doi.org/10.1016/j.jaci.2003.09.009.

136. Turunen R, Koistinen A, Vuorinen T, et al. The first wheezing episode: respiratory virus etiology, atopic characteristics, and illness severity. Pediatr Allergy Immunol. 2014;25:796–803.

137. Jackson DJ, Gangnon RE, Evans MD, et al. Wheezing rhinovirus illnesses in early life predict asthma development in high-risk children. Am J Respir Crit Care Med. 2008;178:667–672.

138. Lukkarinen M, Koistinen A, Turunen R, Lehtinen P, Vuorinen T, Jartti T. Rhinovirus-induced first wheezing episode predicts atopic but not nonatopic asthma at school age. J Allergy Clin Immunol. 2017;140:988–995.

139. Jackson DJ, Gern JE, Lemanske Jr. RF. The contributions of allergic sensitization and respiratory pathogens to asthma inception. J Allergy Clin Immunol. 2016;137:659–665, quiz 666. https://doi.org/10.1016/j.jaci.2016.01.002.

140. Cox DW, Bizzintino J, Ferrar G, et al. Human rhinovirus species C infection in young children with acute wheeze is associated with increased acute respiratory hospital admissions. Am J Respir Crit Care Med. 2013;188:1358–1364.

141. Lee W-M, Lemanske Jr RF, Evans MD, et al. Human rhinovirus species and season of infection determine illness severity. Am J Respir Crit Care Med. 2012;186:886–891.

142. Bochkov YA, Watters K, Ashraf S, et al. Cadherin-related family member 3, a childhood asthma susceptibility gene product, mediates rhinovirus C binding and replication. Proc Natl Acad Sci. 2015;112:5485–5490.

143. Walker S, Monteil M, Phelan K, Lasserson TJ, Walters EH. Anti-IgE for chronic asthma in adults and children. Cochrane Database Syst Rev. 2006

144. Busse W, Corren J, Lanier BQ, et al. Omalizumab, anti-IgE recombinant humanized monoclonal antibody, for the treatment of severe allergic asthma. J Allergy Clin Immunol. 2001;108:184–190. https://doi.org/10.1067/mai.2001.117880.

145. Casale TB, Luskin AT, Busse W, et al. Omalizumab effectiveness by biomarker status in patients with asthma: evidence from PROSPERO, a prospective real-world study. J Allergy Clin Immunol Pract. 2019;7:156–164.e151. https://doi.org/10.1016/j.jaip.2018.04.043.

146. Casale TB, Chipps BE, Rosén K, et al. Response to omalizumab using patient enrichment criteria from trials of novel biologics in asthma. Allergy. 2018;73:490–497. https://doi.org/10.1111/all.13302.

147. Humbert M, Taillé C, Mala L, et al. Omalizumab effectiveness in patients with severe allergic asthma according to blood eosinophil count: the STELLAIR study. Eur Respir J. 2018;51:1702523.

148. Pavord ID, Korn S, Howarth P, et al. Mepolizumab for severe eosinophilic asthma (DREAM): a multicentre, double-blind, placebo-controlled trial. Lancet. 2012;380:651–659. https://doi.org/10.1016/s0140-6736(12)60988-x.

149. Castro M, Zangrilli J, Wechsler ME, et al. Reslizumab for inadequately controlled asthma with elevated blood eosinophil counts: results from two multicentre, parallel, double-blind, randomised, placebo-controlled, phase 3 trials. Lancet Respir Med. 2015;3:355–366. https://doi.org/10.1016/s2213-2600(15)00042-9.

150. Castro M, Wenzel SE, Bleecker ER, et al. Benralizumab, an anti-interleukin 5 receptor alpha monoclonal antibody, versus placebo for uncontrolled eosinophilic asthma: a phase 2b randomised dose-ranging study. Lancet Respir Med. 2014;2:879–890. https://doi.org/10.1016/s2213-2600(14)70201-2.

151. Tan LD, Bratt JM, Godor D, Louie S, Kenyon NJ. Benralizumab: a unique IL-5 inhibitor for severe asthma. J Asthma Allergy. 2016;9:71–81. https://doi.org/10.2147/jaa.S78049.

152. Kolbeck R, Kozhich A, Koike M, et al. MEDI-563, a humanized anti-IL-5 receptor alpha mAb with enhanced antibody-dependent cell-mediated cytotoxicity function. J Allergy Clin Immunol. 2010;125:1344–53.e1342. https://doi.org/10.1016/j.jaci.2010.04.004.

153. Rothenberg ME. Eosinophilia. N Engl J Med. 1998;338:1592–1600. https://doi.org/10.1056/nejm199805283382206.

154. Ortega HG, Liu MC, Pavord ID, et al. Mepolizumab treatment in patients with severe eosinophilic asthma. N Engl J Med. 2014;371:1198–1207. https://doi.org/10.1056/NEJMoa1403290.

155. FitzGerald JM, Bleecker ER, Menzies-Gow A, et al. Predictors of enhanced response with benralizumab for patients with severe asthma: pooled analysis of the SIROCCO and CALIMA studies. Lancet Respir Med. 2018;6:51–64. https://doi.org/10.1016/s2213-2600(17)30344-2.

156. Kau AL, Korenblat PE. Anti-interleukin 4 and 13 for asthma treatment in the era of endotypes. Curr Opin Allergy Clin Immunol. 2014;14:570–575. https://doi.org/10.1097/aci.0000000000000108.

157. Wenzel S, Ford L, Pearlman D, et al. Dupilumab in persistent asthma with elevated eosinophil levels. N Engl J Med. 2013;368:2455–2466. https://doi.org/10.1056/NEJMoa1304048.

158. Donovan C, Hansbro PM. IL-33 in chronic respiratory disease: from pre-clinical to clinical studies. ACS Pharmacol Transl Sci. 2019;3:56–62.

159. Corren J, Parnes JR, Wang L, et al. Tezepelumab in adults with uncontrolled asthma. N Engl J Med. 2017;377:936–946.

160. Gauvreau GM, O'Byrne PM, Boulet L-P, et al. Effects of an anti-TSLP antibody on allergen-induced asthmatic responses. N Engl J Med. 2014;370:2102–2110.

161. Gandhi NA, Pirozzi G, Graham NM. Commonality of the IL-4/IL-13 pathway in atopic diseases. Exp Rev Clin Immunol. 2017;13:425–437.

162. Beck LA, Thaçi D, Hamilton JD, et al. Dupilumab treatment in adults with moderate-to-severe atopic dermatitis. N Engl J Med. 2014;371:130–139.

163. Bachert C, Mannent L, Naclerio RM, et al. Effect of subcutaneous dupilumab on nasal polyp burden in patients with chronic sinusitis and nasal polyposis: a randomized clinical trial. JAMA. 2016;315:469–479.

164. Bachert C, Han JK, Desrosiers M, et al. Efficacy and safety of dupilumab in patients with severe chronic rhinosinusitis with nasal polyps (LIBERTY NP SINUS-24 and LIBERTY NP SINUS-52): results from two multicentre, randomised, double-blind, placebo-controlled, parallel-group phase 3 trials. Lancet. 2019;394:1638–1650.

165. del Carmen Vennera M, Picado C, Mullol J, Alobid I, Bernal-Sprekelsen M. Efficacy of omalizumab in the treatment of nasal polyps. Thorax. 2011;66:824–825.

166. Gevaert P, Calus L, Van Zele T, et al. Omalizumab is effective in allergic and nonallergic patients with nasal polyps and asthma. J Allergy Clin Immunol. 2013;131:110–116.e111.

167. Gevaert P, Van Bruaene N, Cattaert T, et al. Mepolizumab, a humanized anti-IL-5 mAb, as a treatment option for severe nasal polyposis. J Allergy Clin Immunol. 2011;128:989–995.e988.

168. Gevaert P, Lang-Loidolt D, Lackner A, et al. Nasal IL-5 levels determine the response to anti–IL-5 treatment in patients with nasal polyps. J Allergy Clin Immunol. 2006;118:1133–1141.

169. Zangrilli J, Maspero J, Harrison T, Werkstrom V, Wu Y. Clinical efficacy of benralizumab in patients with severe, uncontrolled eosinophilic asthma and nasal polyposis: pooled analysis of the SIROCCO and CALIMA trials. Pneumologie. 2019;73:P254.

170. Stein ML, Collins MH, Villanueva JM, et al. Anti-IL-5 (mepolizumab) therapy for eosinophilic esophagitis. J Allergy Clin Immunol. 2006;118:1312–1319. https://doi.org/10.1016/j.jaci.2006.09.007.

171. Straumann A, Conus S, Grzonka P, et al. Anti-interleukin-5 antibody treatment (mepolizumab) in active eosinophilic oesophagitis: a randomised, placebo-controlled, double-blind trial. Gut. 2010;59:21–30. https://doi.org/10.1136/gut.2009.178558.

172. Assa'ad AH, Gupta SK, Collins MH, et al. An antibody against IL-5 reduces numbers of esophageal intraepithelial eosinophils in children with eosinophilic esophagitis. Gastroenterology. 2011;141:1593–1604. https://doi.org/10.1053/j.gastro.2011.07.044.

173. Spergel JM, Rothenberg ME, Collins MH, et al. Reslizumab in children and adolescents with eosinophilic esophagitis: results of a double-blind, randomized, placebo-controlled trial. J Allergy Clin Immunol. 2012;129:456–463, 463.e451–453. https://doi.org/10.1016/j.jaci.2011.11.044.

174. Clayton F, Fang JC, Gleich GJ, et al. Eosinophilic esophagitis in adults is associated with IgG4 and not mediated by IgE. Gastroenterology. 2014;147:602–609. https://doi.org/10.1053/j.gastro.2014.05.036.

175. Loizou D, Enav B, Komlodi-Pasztor E, et al. A pilot study of omalizumab in eosinophilic esophagitis. PLoS One. 2015;10:e0113483. https://doi.org/10.1371/journal.pone.0113483.

176. Wood RA, Kim JS, Lindblad R, et al. A randomized, double-blind, placebo-controlled study of omalizumab combined with oral immunotherapy for the treatment of cow's milk allergy. J Allergy Clin Immunol. 2016;137:1103–1110.e1111. https://doi.org/10.1016/j.jaci.2015.10.005.

177. Nadeau KC, Schneider LC, Hoyte L, Borras I, Umetsu DT. Rapid oral desensitization in combination with omalizumab therapy in patients with cow's milk allergy. J Allergy Clin Immunol. 2011;127:1622–1624. https://doi.org/10.1016/j.jaci.2011.04.009.

178. Schneider LC, Rachid R, LeBovidge J, Blood E, Mittal M, Umetsu DT. A pilot study of omalizumab to facilitate rapid oral desensitization in high-risk peanut-allergic patients. J Allergy

Clin Immunol. 2013;132:1368–1374. https://doi.org/10.1016/j.jaci.2013.09.046.

179. Goldfeder RL, Wall DP, Khoury MJ, Ioannidis JP, Ashley EA. Human genome sequencing at population scale: a primer on high throughput DNA sequencing and analysis. Am J Epidemiol. 2017;186:1000–1009.

180. Rothstein, M.A. *Structural Challenges of Precision Medicine*. 2017.

181. U.S. National Library of Medicine. Help me understand genetics. 2017. https://ghr.nlm.nih.gov/primer.

3

Epidemiology of Allergic Diseases

Adnan Custovic

CHAPTER OUTLINE

SUMMARY OF IMPORTANT CONCEPTS

- Epidemiology is the study of the distribution of disease and, by extension, its causes and consequences, mostly in general populations.
- The rates of allergic sensitization and allergic diseases have been increasing, although the increase in prevalence of asthma may have slowed among children in some parts of the developed world.
  - The atopic march model of a linear progression from atopic dermatitis (AD) in infancy to asthma and then allergic rhinitis in later childhood is not, in most cases, an accurate descriptor of the natural history of atopic diseases in individual patients and does not capture the heterogeneity of allergic phenotypes.
  - Allergic diseases coexist in a multimorbidity framework in which no single condition holds priority over any of the co-occurring conditions.
- Allergic diseases are generally less common in low-income countries and in populations with traditional farming lifestyles, and the great changes observed in prevalence and distribution strongly suggest a major role for the environment.
- Allergies are affected by environmental factors, including diet; exposure to a normal, diverse microflora; infections; exposure to air pollutants; and occupational exposures.

- Factors that initiate allergy and allergic diseases should be differentiated from factors that exacerbate them after they have been established.

INTRODUCTION

Epidemiology studies the distribution of diseases in populations and addresses the issues related to the definition of the outcome (disease) of interest, the overall morbidity and mortality in a given community, factors that may cause or predispose to the development of disease(s), and the effects of interventions. Therefore, the focus of epidemiological studies is on populations rather than individual patients. At the simplest level, this involves surveys that measure disease frequency at a single time point within a given population. Such studies may also identify factors that are associated with disease and that can be quantified in terms of risk.

A large number of cross-sectional studies have been carried out, both in adults and in children, to ascertain the prevalence of allergic disease and explore their associated risk factors. Some of these crucially important studies, such as the International Study of Asthma and Allergies in Childhood (ISAAC; http://isaac.auckland.ac.nz/) and the European Community Respiratory Health Survey (ECRHS; http://www.ecrhs.org/), will be reviewed in this chapter. The chapter will not offer a complete overview of the epidemiology of allergic diseases but will focus on examining the definitions of the relevant clinical outcomes, the estimates of prevalence (including changes in prevalence over time and the differences by geographical area/place), and the association between allergic (immunoglobulin E [IgE]-mediated) sensitization and symptomatic allergic diseases (asthma, atopic dermatitis [AD], allergic rhinitis, and IgE-mediated food allergy). Some of the major risk factors will be examined.

EPIDEMIOLOGICAL DEFINITIONS OF ALLERGIC DISEASES: PART OF THE CHALLENGE

Precise definitions of the primary disease outcomes are key to our understanding of the epidemiology, pathophysiology, and etiology of human diseases, and one of the challenges in the area of allergic diseases is the lack of consensus in defining these conditions. We will use "asthma" as an exemplar but will also discuss briefly the definitions of allergic rhinitis, AD allergic sensitization, anaphylaxis, and food allergy.

Asthma

Despite many attempts to reach a consensus definition of asthma for clinical practice and research studies (Table 3.1), to date, no single definition or validated diagnostic standard has gained universal acceptance.[1] As a result, at least 60 different definitions were used in studies investigating the risk factors associated with childhood asthma.[2] Although there are only subtle differences between many of these definitions and some of them may appear almost identical, the overall impact of the heterogeneity in the definition of the primary outcome on the reported prevalence and associated risk factors may be considerable. For example, when the four of the most commonly used definitions were applied to a high-risk population of children, the overall agreement was relatively low (61%), suggesting that over a third of the study participants could move from being considered as having asthma to being assigned as non-asthmatic controls depending on a definition used.[2]

Since 2010, there has been a fundamental change in the approach to asthma, with a gradual emergence of a consensus that asthma is not a single disease but an umbrella term for a collection of several diseases with similar symptoms and clinical manifestations, which are underpinned by different underlying pathophysiological mechanisms[3] and which are usually referred to as asthma endotypes.[4] The heterogeneity of asthma may result in difficulties in the interpretation of findings across different populations and in discrepancies between studies investigating asthma epidemiology.

Despite ongoing efforts to disaggregate asthma, the reductionist view of asthma as a single disease remains the norm in clinical practice and most epidemiological studies and underpins most asthma management guidelines. This is one of the key barriers preventing genuine advances toward personalized treatment,[5,6] as the focus is on treating the diagnosis (or "asthma disease") rather than addressing the pathological mechanism that causes symptoms in an individual patient.[7] A consequence of such an approach is that patients with different asthma subtypes are forced into a single group for empirical treatment.[5] Furthermore,

regulatory approvals for asthma therapies are mostly based on randomized controlled trials focused on relatively short-term improvements in clinical indices, and group mean data are used to compare the effects of investigational medicinal products. The results of such trials, and systematic reviews thereof, are currently the backbone of evidence-based medicine. However, a prerequisite to fully understand epidemiology of asthma-related diseases and deliver a genuinely personalized approach is to understand disease heterogeneity and pathophysiological mechanism(s), which give rise to symptoms in specific endotypes, and to use this knowledge to deploy mechanism-based treatment(s)/prevention strategies[8]—that is, to move away from diagnosis-based or symptom-based toward mechanism-based treatments.[7] Similarly, unless epidemiologic studies find better ways to distinguish between different endotypes at a population level, it will be difficult to discover their underlying genetic risk factors, pathophysiological processes, or identify novel therapeutic targets for stratified treatment, as any signal will be diluted by phenotypic heterogeneity.[9] Further problems for asthma epidemiology arise from the difficulties in distinguishing the disease state (i.e., the presence or absence) from triggers of acute asthma attacks. Since "asthma" encompasses a range of linked conditions, until the time comes when we have genuinely understood different endotypes, one possible approach would be to consider categorizing it as a spectrum and use the term "Asthma spectrum disorder," which is likely better suited to the current state of knowledge than the term "Asthma."[7] It is of note that at the time of writing this chapter, the framework of asthma endotypes remains primarily a hypothetical construct, and not a single "asthma endotype" has been identified with absolute certainty.[5]

Allergic Rhinitis

Epidemiologic studies of rhinitis have been undertaken less frequently than those of asthma but are arguably as difficult to interpret. It is likely that phenotypic heterogeneity in rhinitis mirrors that of asthma, with the existence of several different but as yet poorly defined endotypes of rhinitis.[10] Most studies rely only on reported symptoms, and most questionnaires collect self-reports of responders confirming that they have "allergic rhinitis" or "hay fever." Symptoms suggestive of rhinitis include nasal blockage and/or itching, runny nose (rhinorrhea) and sneezing, which may be seasonal (e.g., related to pollen exposure in hay fever) or perennial. In the case of rhinoconjunctivitis, symptoms also include ocular involvement such as conjunctival irritation and lachrymation. However, these symptoms are relatively nonspecific, and when using only questionnaire surveys, they may be confused with viral upper respiratory tract infections. Acknowledging all the aforementioned potential pitfalls, epidemiological studies reported to date show that allergic rhinitis is among the most common chronic diseases, particularly among school-age children and young adults in developed countries.

Atopic Dermatitis/Eczema

AD is one of the most common skin diseases but, similar to asthma and rhinitis, there is no universally accepted definition for epidemiological studies,[11] and there is no objective

TABLE 3.1 Asthma Definitions

Source	Year	Definition
CIBA Foundation[6]	1959	Condition of subjects with widespread narrowing of the bronchial airways, which changes its severity over short periods spontaneously or during treatment.
American Thoracic Society[8]	1962	Disease characterized by increased responsiveness of the trachea and bronchi to various stimuli and manifested by widespread narrowing of the airways that changes in severity spontaneously or as a result of therapy.
World Health Organization (WHO)[9]	1975	Chronic condition characterized by recurrent bronchospasm resulting from a tendency to develop reversible narrowing of the airway lumina in response to stimuli of a level or intensity not inducing such narrowing in most individuals.
American Thoracic Society[10]	1987	Clinical syndrome is characterized by increased responsiveness of the tracheobronchial tree to a variety of stimuli. Major symptoms are paroxysms of dyspnea, wheezing, and cough, which may vary from mild and almost undetectable to severe and unremitting (i.e., status asthmaticus). Primary physiologic manifestation of this hyperresponsiveness is variable airway obstruction, occurring in the form of fluctuations in the severity of obstruction after bronchodilator or corticosteroid use, or increased obstruction caused by drugs or other stimuli, as well as evidence of mucosal edema of bronchi, infiltration of bronchial mucosa or submucosa with inflammatory cells (especially eosinophils), shedding of epithelium, and obstruction of peripheral airways with mucus.
NHLBI/NIH[11]	1991	Lung disease with the following characteristics: (1) airway obstruction that is reversible (but not completely in some patients) spontaneously or with treatment, (2) airway inflammation, and (3) increased airway responsiveness to a variety of stimuli.
NHLBI/NIH[12,13]	1993 1995 1997	Chronic inflammatory disorder of the airways in which many cells play a role, particularly mast cells, eosinophils, and T lymphocytes. In susceptible individuals, this inflammation causes recurrent episodes of wheezing, breathlessness, chest tightness, and cough in early morning. Symptoms are usually associated with widespread but variable airflow limitation that is at least partly reversible spontaneously or with treatment. Inflammation also causes an increase in airway responsiveness that is associated with a variety of stimuli.
NIH/NHLBI[14]	2002	Chronic inflammatory disorder of the airways in which many cells and cellular elements play a role. The chronic inflammation causes an increase in airway hyperresponsiveness that leads to recurrent episodes of wheezing, breathlessness, chest tightness, and coughing, particularly at night or in the early morning. These episodes are usually associated with widespread but variable airflow obstruction that is often reversible spontaneously or with treatment.

NHLBI/NIH, National Heart, Lung, and Blood Institute/National Institutes of Health.

test that can confirm the diagnosis.[12] Despite efforts to reach a consensus on nomenclature, two terms (AD and eczema) currently coexist to describe a clinically defined, pruritic, inflammatory skin condition, characterized by chronic and relapsing dermatitis in specific anatomical sites.[13] These terms are usually used interchangeably,[14] and further denominations such as atopic eczema/dermatitis syndrome (AEDS) have also been proposed.[15] Currently, AD remains the most commonly used term, but it is of note that the nomenclature differs between publications in different languages and specialties.[14] Even when the same term (e.g., AD) is used in epidemiological studies,[16] similar to the situation in asthma described earlier, individuals are assigned as "Cases" and "Controls" using numerous different definitions,[16–19] which hinders the generalizability and comparisons across different studies and geographical areas. It has been shown that the use of different definitions of AD results in a substantial difference in prevalence estimates, the performance of prediction models, and association with risk factors.[20]

Atopic March, Comorbidity or Multimorbidity of AD, Asthma, and Allergic Rhinitis

As outlined in previous sections, AD, asthma, and allergic rhinitis encompass a range of linked complex and multifactorial conditions that are caused by a variety of different mechanisms and

that result in multiple heterogeneous clinical phenotypes. For example, some patients have symptoms affecting a single organ, while others may have symptoms involving multiple organs (e.g., skin, upper, and lower airways). The pattern of expression of symptoms in different organs/systems (such as skin, lungs, and nose) may provide clues about the underlying pathophysiology, but the age of onset, progression, and resolution of symptoms differ considerably between different individuals. The term "atopic march" (or "allergic march") is usually interpreted as a sequential development of symptoms (or diseases) from AD in infancy to asthma, and then allergic rhinitis in later childhood.[21,22] The use of the term "march" emphasizes that there is an exclusive sequence of events, and the origins are observations from epidemiological studies that the point prevalence of AD is the highest in early life, which is followed by the high period prevalence of asthma in mid-school age and then an increase in allergic rhinitis in late childhood. Such population-level observations could reflect the progression of symptoms within individual patients, and this assumption has been used to suggest that clinicians in primary care "should inform parents that children with eczema may later develop asthma,"[23] that "effective eczema treatment may decrease the risk of asthma,"[24] and that "effective atopic eczema control … may also prevent the atopic march."[23] However, some studies suggested that there is considerable heterogeneity between patients in the pattern of symptom development, thus questioning the existence of the atopic march.[25]

Artificial intelligence and machine learning provide new ways to discern the heterogeneity in patterns of different symptoms within individual patients, where conventional epidemiological approaches might over-aggregate the underlying complexity. For example, a Bayesian machine learning modeling has been used to model the development of AD, wheeze, and rhinitis during childhood in ~10,000 children from two UK birth cohorts with a specific focus on longitudinal changes within individual children.[26] Overall, ~50% of children had at least one of these allergic diseases, but only ~6% of those with such symptoms followed trajectory profile resembling the "atopic march." A further six disease classes (Fig. 3.1) were characterized by the presence of only one or two of the three symptoms, indicating that well over 90% of

children with symptoms commonly associated with atopy in childhood do not follow the trajectory of the atopic march.[26] Among >2500 children with AD, ~60% had only AD, but not any other allergic disease, revealing that the atopic march model of a linear progression from one symptom to another is not, in most cases, an accurate descriptor of the natural history of allergic diseases in individual patients and does not capture the heterogeneity of allergic phenotypes. A subsequent study has confirmed differential genetic associations across different disease classes ($p = 3.3 \times 10^{-13}$),[27] suggesting that genetic architecture differs between different combinations of symptoms (e.g., the filaggrin locus that is traditionally considered to be a genetic marker of AD was associated with all profiles that included AD, but more strongly for those with co-occurrent wheeze and rhinitis).[27] The available evidence to date suggests that rather than following a specific sequential development of symptoms, allergic diseases likely coexist in

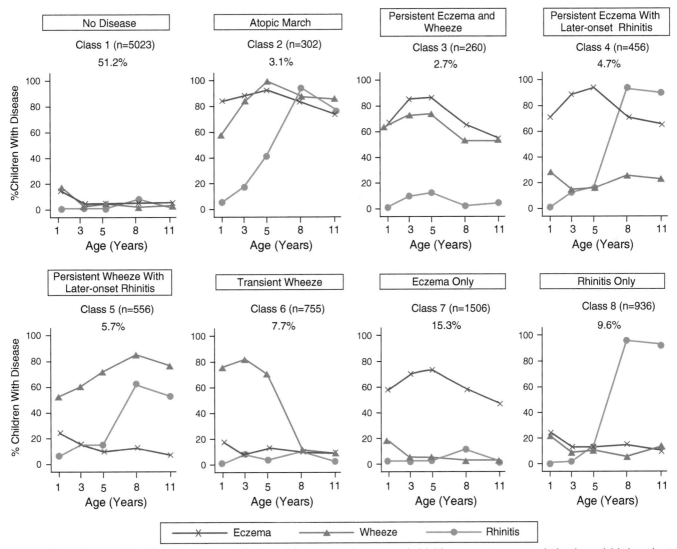

Fig. 3.1 Bayesian machine learning joint modeling of eczema, wheeze, and rhinitis across two population-based birth cohorts revealed eight distinct disease profiles—latent classes of allergic diseases (LCADs). The number of children and the proportion of the study population are indicated for each class. Plots indicate longitudinal trajectories of wheeze, eczema, and rhinitis within each class. (From Belgrave DC, Granell R, Simpson A, Guiver J, Bishop C, Buchan I, et al. Developmental profiles of eczema, wheeze, and rhinitis: two population-based birth cohort studies. PLoS Med 2014;11:e1001748.)

a multimorbidity framework in which no single condition holds priority over any of the co-occurring conditions.[28]

Allergic Sensitization

A large number of epidemiologic studies have indicated that allergic sensitization is a strong risk factor for asthma, rhinitis, and AD/eczema,[29] and the US National Institutes of Health expert group recommended a multiallergen sensitization screening as the principal biomarker for asthma.[30] However, in different areas, there is a considerable variability in the strength of the association between sensitization and asthma,[31] and at a population level, a sizeable proportion of sensitized subjects (i.e., those producing IgE antibodies toward common inhalant and food allergens) have no evidence of allergic disease.[32] One of the reasons for the inconsistencies of findings on the association between sensitization and asthma may be due to phenotypic heterogeneity of the primary disease outcomes, which is outlined above. However, similar concerns can be raised about the current definitions of allergic sensitization used in epidemiology and clinical practice. Most epidemiologic studies define sensitization as a positive allergen-specific serum IgE (most commonly $>0.35\,kU_A/L$) or a positive skin prick test (usually, but not exclusively, a wheal diameter $>3\,mm$) to at least one common food or inhalant allergen. However, positive "allergy" tests indicate only the presence of allergen-specific IgE (either in serum or bound to the membrane of mast cells in the skin) and are not necessarily related to the development of clinical symptoms upon allergen exposure. A number of studies have shown that the level of specific IgE antibodies and the size of the skin test wheal diameter predict much better the presence and severity of allergic diseases (both respiratory and food allergies) than the mere presence of a positive allergy test.[32–34] A stratification of sensitization into several subtypes was achieved by data-driven machine learning approaches with Bayesian inference applied to "allergy tests" (skin prick tests and allergen-specific IgE antibody measurements), which were longitudinally collected in two population-based birth cohorts from birth to school age.[35,36] These analyses took into account the timing of the onset of sensitization, its progression and/or remission, and the type of allergens causing sensitization. Most of the children who would be considered "sensitized" using conventional epidemiological definitions clustered into four distinct subtypes. Based on their characteristics, these atopy subtypes were named "Multiple Early," "Multiple Late," "Predominantly Dust Mite," and "Non-Dust Mite" atopic vulnerabilities.[35] The relevance of this to the epidemiological studies can be highlighted using the relationship between sensitization and asthma as an example. The data-driven approach described above uncovered an unexpected but very strong risk factor for asthma; although less than one-third of the children defined as "sensitized" using conventional definitions clustered to the Multiple Early class, the risk of asthma was markedly increased among the children in this class (with the odds ratio of 29.3) but not among those in other atopy subtype (Fig. 3.2). In addition, children in the "Multiple Early" atopy subtype had significantly lower lung function and were at high risk

of severe asthma exacerbations compared to all other classes (subtypes).[35,36] However, these sensitization classes can only be identified by modeling large amounts of data collected longitudinally in a large number of subjects, and cannot as yet be differentiated or confirmed in a clinical situation or in cross-sectional studies. A recent approach utilized machine learning to demonstrate that the pattern of interaction between allergen component-specific IgEs on component-resolved diagnostic (CRD) arrays, but not IgE to any individual allergen(s), predicted asthma.[37] A further study in the U-BIOPRED severe asthma cohort has shown that asthma severity can be predicted by interaction patterns between IgE and multiple allergenic proteins,[38] suggesting that it may be possible to develop interpretation algorithms for CRD arrays to help disaggregate allergic sensitization and facilitate asthma diagnosis[37] and prediction of future risk among sensitized individuals.[39]

Given the aforementioned evidence, in this chapter, allergic sensitization will not be referred to as a simple yes/no phenomenon, but rather a sum of several atopic vulnerabilities that differ in their relationship with clinical allergy.

Food Allergy

The focus of this chapter is on IgE-mediated food allergy. Diagnosis of food allergy is based on clinical history and diagnostic test results, and the gold standard test to confirm or refute the diagnosis is a double-blind, placebo-controlled oral food challenge.[40] However, many reported food allergies are not confirmed using such a thorough diagnostic evaluation. As a result, conducting large epidemiologic surveys that rely only on questionnaires may not provide accurate data on true prevalence, and estimates of prevalence obtained from questionnaires are likely to be inflated. It is therefore not surprising that systematic reviews of the literature on the prevalence of food allergies have reported considerable heterogeneity between different studies and confirmed that the prevalence estimates based on self-reported symptoms tend to be higher than those based on objective assessments.[41]

To facilitate the conduct of future studies, it would be useful to develop simpler tests that discriminate accurately food-allergic from food-tolerant subjects, without the need to perform placebo-controlled oral food challenges.[41]

ESTIMATES OF WORLDWIDE PREVALENCE OF ASTHMA, RHINITIS, AD, AND FOOD ALLERGY

Most studies collected the data using standardized questionnaires enquiring about the symptoms, usually assessing point prevalence (the proportion of individuals in a population with a disease at a particular time point) of allergic diseases or their lifetime prevalence (the proportion of individuals in a population who have had a disease at some point in their life up to the time of assessment). For children, the most widely used questionnaire was developed for the ISAAC.[42–44] For studies in adults, the questionnaire developed for the International Union against Tuberculosis and Lung Disease (IUATLD)[45] was adapted for use in the ECRHS[46] and the World Health Survey.[47] Studies using these tools have reported that across the

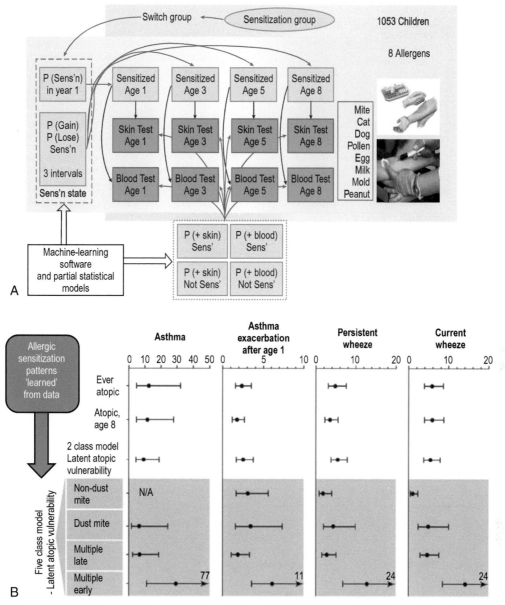

Fig. 3.2 Hypothesizing with data (A) revealed a stratification of atopy (B): an unexpected risk factors for asthma discovered. (Adapted from Simpson A, Tan VY, Winn J, Svensen M, Bishop CM, Heckerman DE, et al. Beyond atopy: multiple patterns of sensitization in relation to asthma in a birth cohort study. Am J Respir Crit Care Med 2010;181(11):1200–1206.)

world, there is a large variability in the prevalence of asthma (Figs. 3.3–3.5), upper airway allergic disease (such as allergic rhinitis), allergic sensitization, and food allergy.[48,49] Generally, low rates have been reported from developing countries, with much higher prevalence in the developed "western" countries.[50] Furthermore, within the same ethnic group, there is considerable variation in the prevalence over time and across different geographical areas.[31,51–55] In general, allergic sensitization and allergic diseases increase with affluence, both at a country and the individual level.[51] Today, high socio-economic status as assessed by parental education remains a risk factor, even in affluent countries. In contrast, in inner city areas of the US, increased rates of allergic sensitization and asthma are related to poverty.[56] These observations are a further proof that there is a strong environmental component to the causation of

these conditions, and that the recent epidemic of allergic diseases in developed countries is predominantly caused by the changes in environment. On the other hand, genetic studies have demonstrated a clear familial aggregation, and numerous genetic loci have been reproducibly linked to asthma, atopy, and total IgE in genome-wide association studies and linkage analyses,[57–59] suggesting an additional and important genetic component.

Asthma

Asthma is one of the most common chronic diseases globally, and individuals of all ages throughout the world are affected by this disorder, which can be severe and sometimes fatal. It is estimated that approximately 300 million people worldwide have asthma, and by 2025, a further 100 million will likely be

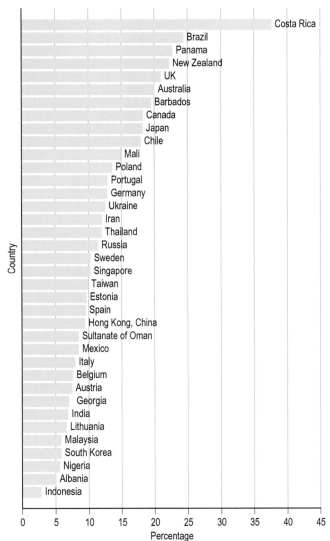

Fig. 3.3 Prevalence of asthma symptoms by country among children 6 to 7 years of age according to the 1999–2004 International Study of Asthma and Allergies in Childhood (ISAAC) III study. (From Asher MI, Montefort S, Bjorksten B, et al. Worldwide time trends in the prevalence of symptoms of asthma, allergic rhinoconjunctivitis, and eczema in childhood: ISAAC Phases One and Three repeat multicountry cross-sectional surveys. Lancet 2006;368:733–743.)

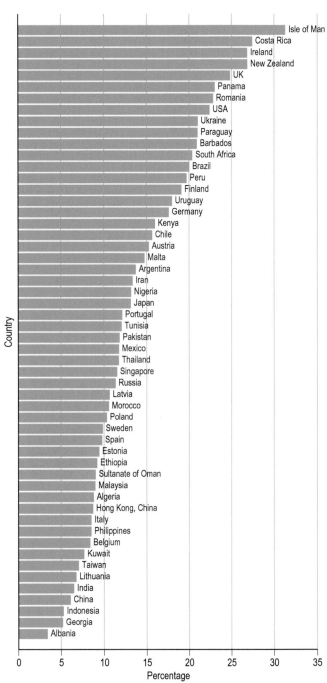

Fig. 3.4 Prevalence of asthma symptoms by country among children 13 to 14 years of age according to the 1999–2004 International Study of Asthma and Allergies in Childhood (ISAAC) III study. (From Asher MI, Montefort S, Bjorksten B, et al. Worldwide time trends in the prevalence of symptoms of asthma, allergic rhinoconjunctivitis, and eczema in childhood: ISAAC Phases One and Three repeat multicountry cross-sectional surveys. Lancet 2006;368:733–743.)

affected. The direct cost of uncontrolled asthma in in the US over the next two decades is likely to be a staggering $1.5 trillion,[60] highlighting the importance of devising and implementing effective strategies for long-term control.[61] Deaths from asthma are relatively rare and do not correlate well with prevalence; the annual worldwide mortality from asthma has been estimated to be 250,000. While the overall asthma-related mortality has declined in the US from 1999 to 2015, the mortality rate among children aged 1–14 years has not changed.[62] Mortality continues to be higher in women (particularly Black women),[62] and we need to better understand these disparities to develop accurate risk-prediction tools. One of the risk factors for asthma death identified by the UK National Review of Asthma Deaths is the recent severe acute

asthma attack—approximately 10% of patients who died had hospitalization with severe exacerbation within a month prior to death and 20% had emergency departments attendance in the 12-month period before death.[63] Furthermore, the overuse of reliever medication (more than one inhaler per month) was an indicator of risk.

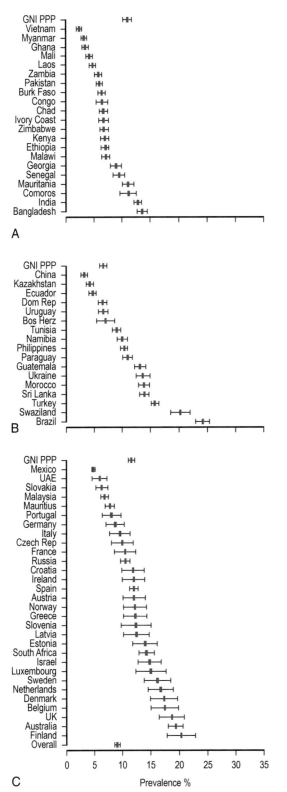

Fig. 3.5 (A–C) Estimates of adult asthma prevalence from the World Health Survey by country and gross national income. *Bos Herz*, Bosnia Herzegovina; *Burk Faso*, Burkina Faso; *Dom Rep*, Dominican Republic; *GNI PPP*, gross national income per capita at purchasing power parity rates; *Rep*, Republic; and *UAE*, United Arab Emirates; *UK*, United Kingdom. (From Sembajwe G, Cifuentes M, Tak SW, et al. National income, self-reported wheezing and asthma diagnosis from the World Health Survey. Eur Respir J 2010;35:279–286.)

Geographical Variations in the Prevalence of Asthma

Data from standardized, multicenter international studies have shown striking geographical variations in the prevalence of asthma symptoms throughout the world, with the highest prevalence rates observed in English-speaking countries (the UK, Australia, New Zealand, Ireland, and the US) and Latin America and the lowest in the Mediterranean, Eastern Europe, and rural areas of Africa and China.[43,45,48,54,64] These patterns appear comparable between children and adults, and the global asthma prevalence seems to range from 1% to 18%.

Childhood Asthma

The ISAAC[42–44,48] was established in 1991 and used a global and standardized approach to address the perceived increase in prevalence of asthma and allergies worldwide and the paucity of reliable and comparable data to measure the scale of the problem. ISAAC Phase One was conducted between 1992 and 1998 and used a simple validated questionnaire to measure worldwide prevalence of asthma, rhinitis, and hay fever in 56 countries in a study involving ~700,000 children aged 6–7 years and 13–14 years.[44] Asthma was defined as a positive answer to the question "Have you (has your child) had wheezing or whistling in the chest in the last 12 months?". There was a staggering 20-fold variation worldwide in the prevalence, with the highest rates reported in the UK, Australia, New Zealand, and Ireland, and the lowest in Eastern Europe, Indonesia, Greece, China, Taiwan, India, and Ethiopia. Wide variations in asthma prevalence were observed in populations that appeared genetically similar, leading to a series of follow-up studies in "ISAAC Phase Two," which investigated a range of environmental factors that could contribute to disease risk (including diet, infection, indoor and outdoor environment, climate, and allergens).[43] These studies investigated variations in prevalence, which emerged from Phase One, among children aged 10–12 years. Comparisons between populations in different centers have been undertaken using objective measures and assessment of environment, lifestyle, and clinical management. However, no single unifying factor has emerged to account for the observed differences.

Adult Asthma

The ECRHS is a multicenter study designed to estimate geographical variation in the prevalence, management, and determinants of asthma and allergy among 140,000 adults aged 22–44 years from 22 countries, using standardized instruments and definitions.[46] This study used a validated questionnaire to assess the prevalence of asthma and allergic diseases and collect information on possible risk factors. "Diagnosed current asthma" was defined as a positive answer to either having had an attack of asthma in the previous 12 months or being on current medication for asthma. This study also aimed to assess the prevalence of airway hyperresponsiveness, estimate variations in exposures to known or suspected risk factors for asthma, and assess their contribution in explaining the variations in the prevalence of disease.

A smaller random sample of participants from multiple centers was selected for more detailed questionnaires, skin prick testing, blood tests for the measurement of total and specific IgE, spirometry and methacholine challenge during Stage II, which took place from 1991 to 1993. ECRHS II was conducted subsequently, directed toward assessment of the incidence and risk factors for the development of allergic disease, atopy, and rapid loss of lung function in middle-aged adults (with collection of dust samples and air pollution data). ECRHS III is a follow-up survey of more than 10,000 adults who were first recruited in 1992–1994, aiming (among other things) to describe the change in the prevalence of respiratory symptom and IgE sensitization in adults as they age.

The ECRHS reported a six-fold variation in the prevalence of current asthma between different countries.[46] There was a large variation in self-reported asthma symptoms, for example, from 4.1% (95% CI 3.1–5.2) in India to 32.0% (95% CI 30.1–33.9) in Dublin for recent wheeze. The prevalence of respiratory symptoms and asthma tended to be low in Western Europe (Belgium, France, Germany, Switzerland, Austria, and Iceland); in Mediterranean countries (Greece, Italy, Spain Portugal, and Algeria); and in India. In Australia, New Zealand, Ireland, the UK, and the single center in the US, prevalence rates of asthma symptoms were high. The geographical distribution of airway hyperresponsiveness fitted well with that for symptoms. A high prevalence of allergic sensitization was found in English-speaking countries (Australia, New Zealand, the US, and the UK), while it was low in Iceland, Greece, Norway, and parts of Spain.

Allergic Rhinitis

In ISAAC, allergic rhino-conjunctivitis was defined based on questionnaire responses as sneezing or a runny or a blocked nose without a cold or flu, accompanied by itchy, watery eyes. There was a 30-fold variation in the prevalence rate among children aged 13–14 years between different sites from 56 countries (from 1.4% to 39.7%). Estimates for adults obtained in the ECRHS suggested median prevalence of nasal allergies of approximately 21%, with a range from 9.5% (95% CI 8.5–10.6) in Algeria to 40.9% (95% CI 39.2–42.7) in Australia. Countries with high prevalence rates included the Netherlands, Belgium, France, Switzerland, the UK, New Zealand, Australia, and the US.

Atopic Dermatitis

In contrast to high-income countries (HICs) where AD is very common,[65] it is a rare disease in low- and middle-income countries (e.g., rural areas of Africa). According to the ISAAC, the lifetime prevalence by age 13 years was reported to be >20% in HICs, 16% in Cape Town, and 6% in Addis Ababa.[66] A questionnaire-based population survey in Ethiopia reported the lifetime prevalence of AD to be as low as 0.3% in the rural areas.[67] A population-based South African study of rural, peri-urban, and urban Xhosa children aged 3–11 years reported a prevalence of visible flexural eczema according to the UK diagnostic criteria of 1.8% and a point prevalence of AD according to a dermatologist of 1.0%.[68]

Food Allergy

IgE-mediated food allergy is estimated to affect up to 8% of children in HICs such as the US,[69] and similar to other allergic diseases, the prevalence seems to be increasing in low-and middle-income countries such as Vietnam and South Africa,[70,71] as well as in other parts of Asia and Africa (particularly in urban areas).[72]

Most of the estimates about the prevalence of food allergy to date are based on data from telephone surveys and cross-sectional surveys. A telephone survey in the US reported that 2.3% of the general population reported allergy to fish or shellfish.[73] Another telephone survey estimated the prevalence rate of peanut or tree nut allergy to be ~1.4% among adults and ~2.1% among children.[74] A school-based survey in Singapore and the Philippines estimated a prevalence rate of peanut and tree nut allergy to be less than 1%.[75] In Australia, the prevalence of peanut allergy may be higher than that observed in the US or the UK and the prevalence of peanut allergy among 1-year-old children was estimated to be ~3%.[76]

In contrast to the aforementioned data, a report from the UK, which interrogated a large health database on almost three million patients registered with 422 general practices, suggested a much lower prevalence rate of peanut allergy of 0.05%.[77] This reported prevalence rate was markedly lower than the estimates derived from other reports from England, such as findings from unselected birth cohorts from Southampton and Manchester, which corroborated questionnaire data with objective assessment such as skin tests, peanut-specific IgE measurement, and oral peanut challenges, and estimated the prevalence of peanut allergy among school-age children to be ~2%.[32,41] These data suggest a worrying possibility that in the UK (and probably in many other countries), a considerable proportion of children with peanut allergy are not diagnosed by their primary care physicians and consequently are not appropriately managed. A metaanalysis of studies that used objective measures (such as peanut sensitization or food challenge) reported little heterogeneity between different studies in children aged 0–4 years and 5–16 years, with the estimates of prevalence of peanut allergy based on oral peanut challenge ranging from 0.2% to 1.6% in different countries.[78] A pressing need to address this issue is further emphasized by the evidence, which suggests that the prevalence of IgE-mediated food allergy among children may be increasing at an alarming rate.

TRENDS IN PREVALENCE OVER TIME

There has been a steep rise in the prevalence of asthma and allergic diseases in the last century, which has been documented in a number of repeated cross-sectional surveys over time[79] (Fig. 3.6). This increasing prevalence of symptomatic allergic diseases has been accompanied by the rising trends in allergic sensitization.[52] It appears that since the 1990s, the prevalence of some allergic diseases (e.g., asthma) may have peaked in regions with previously documented high prevalence, whereas an increase was recorded in several centers with presumed lower prevalence, mostly in low- and mid-income countries.[48] It is of note that the increases in different allergic diseases may

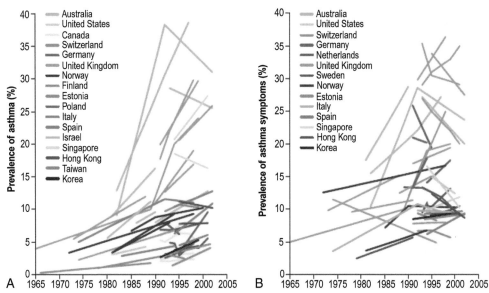

Fig. 3.6 Changes in the prevalence of diagnosed asthma (A) and asthma symptoms (B) over time in children and young adults. (From Eder W, Ege MJ, von Mutius E. The asthma epidemic. N Engl J Med 2006; 355(21):2226–2235.)

not have occurred contemporaneously; there are some data to suggest that hay fever has increased in the US as early as the mid-20th century, followed by an increase in asthma between the 1960s and 1990s, whilst the rise in food allergies may be a phenomenon that started in the late 20th century, with this trend continuing into the first decades of the current century.

Asthma, Allergic Rhinitis, and Sensitization

ISAAC Phase Three (conducted 1999–2004) was broadly a repetition of Phase One, with an approximately 7-year interval to investigate the differences in time trends internationally.[48] When all results are pooled together, there has been an overall increase in the prevalence of asthma and rhinitis in both age groups from 13.2% to 13.7% in the 13–14 years age group and from 11.1% to 11.6% in the 6 to 7 years age group.[48] However, wide variations were observed between centers, and different patterns were noted in different regions. For example, increases were seen in Asia Pacific, India, North America, Eastern Mediterranean, and Western Europe in the younger age group and Africa, Asia Pacific, India, Latin America, and Northern and Eastern Europe amongst children in the older age group. The most marked reduction in asthma symptoms was observed in English-speaking countries (0.5% reduction at age 13–14 years and 0.1% reduction at age 6 to 7 years). A similar effect was seen for severe asthma. Overall, the global burden of allergic airway diseases and atopic sensitization has likely increased, and the geographical differences in prevalence globally appear to have decreased.

Other investigators have studied the variation in asthma prevalence in different communities who live within the same country. For example, in Ghana, the prevalence of exercise-induced bronchospasm (objective marker of airway hyperreactivity and asthma) was found to be significantly higher among urban affluent children (4.7%) compared to urban poor children (2.2%) and children living in rural communities (3.8%).[51]

Similar differences were observed for atopy (determined objectively using skin prick tests). A subsequent study using identical methodology has demonstrated that the prevalence of both atopy and exercise-induced bronchospasm doubled over a 10-year period between 1993 and 2003.[52]

The proportion of patients consulting their primary care physicians for asthma has also changed with time, with an eight-fold increase for children aged up to 14 years between 1960 and 1990 and a three- to four-fold increase amongst adults (but notably with fewer consultations per patient). Asthma prevalence recorded by the general practice research databases increased from 3% to 5% from 1990 to 1998 in all age groups; however, the rates of incident asthma recorded in the same database fell during the same period of time.

Rates of hospital admissions have possibly shown the most dramatic trends, with a steady and significant increase in all age groups between 1960 and 1985 (especially for children under the age of 4 years),[80] after which a steady fall has occurred during the 1990s and early 2000s (possibly due to the better provision of medical care). The analysis of asthma mortality across 46 countries (36 were high-income and 10 middle-income countries) estimated the global asthma mortality rate to be 0.44 deaths per 100,000 (90% CI 0.39–0.48) in 1993 and 0.19 deaths per 100,000 (0.18–0.21) in 2006.[81] However, there was no further reduction from 2006 to 2012 when the estimate remained at 0–19 deaths per 100,000 people (0.16–0.21) (Fig. 3.7).

Asthma attacks (exacerbation) remain one of the most troublesome aspects of asthma for patients and families and a major burden on healthcare resources. In a study of >50,000 asthmatics in England, one-third had at least one confirmed exacerbation over an 8-year period between 2007 and 2015, but <1% had yearly exacerbations.[82] Although exacerbation frequency increased with asthma severity, they occurred across all severity levels, and more than half of patients with frequent exacerbations had mild/moderate disease, suggesting that rather than being driven only by severity, the exacerbation risk reflects specific susceptibility, which may characterize an exacerbation-prone asthma endotype.[83]

Food Allergy

In the US, three nationwide telephone surveys suggested that the prevalence of self-reported peanut allergy in children in 2008 was 1.4%, compared with 0.8% in 2002 and 0.4% in 1997. In the UK, reported rates of peanut allergy in three cohorts of children aged 3–5 years born in 1989, 1994–1996, and 2001–2002 in the same geographical area were 0.5%, 1.4%, and 1.2%. These increasing trends have been indirectly confirmed in a report from the ECRHS on the prevalence of sensitization to foods in a sample of young adults from Western Europe, the US, and Australia, which reported that prevalence of sensitization to peanut was the highest in the US center in Portland.[84]

Unfortunately, the data to provide accurate estimates on time trends of food allergies are lacking.

To summarize, the prevalence rates of asthma, other allergic diseases, and allergic sensitization vary considerably throughout the world and are the highest in the English-speaking nations, higher in western than eastern parts of Europe, and higher in urban than rural parts of Africa. Overall, the evidence suggests that there has been a marked increase (two- to three-fold) in the prevalence of asthma in the latter part of the last century, seen across all grades of severity of symptoms and all ages. Evidence collected more recently suggests that the increase in asthma may have flattened off, and that at least in some age groups, asthma prevalence may be decreasing. However, ISAAC Phase III suggests that in many parts of the world, asthma prevalence continues to increase, and that the global differences may be shrinking in magnitude.

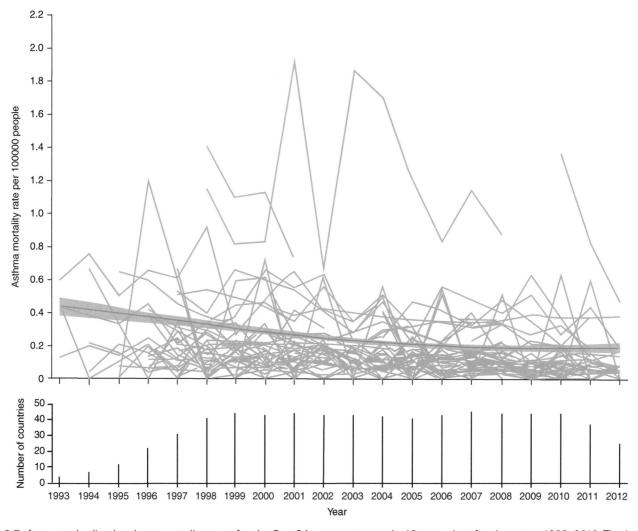

Fig. 3.7 Age-standardized asthma mortality rates for the 5 to 34-year age group in 46 countries, for the years 1993–2012. The locally weighted scatterplot smoother (LOESS) rates with 90% confidence limits, weighted by country population, are shown in *red*. The countries included are Australia, Austria, Belgium, Bulgaria, Canada, Croatia, Czech Republic, Denmark, Egypt, Estonia, Finland, France, Georgia, Germany, Greece, Hong Kong, Hungary, Iceland, Israel, Italy, Japan, Kuwait, Kyrgyzstan, Latvia, Lithuania, Luxembourg, Macedonia, Malta, Mauritius, Moldova, Netherlands, New Zealand, Norway, Poland, Portugal, Romania, Serbia, Singapore, Slovakia, Slovenia, South Korea, Spain, Sweden, UK: England and Wales, UK: Scotland, and US. (From Ebmeier S, Thayabaran D, Braithwaite I, Benamara C, Weatherall M, Beasley R. Trends in international asthma mortality: analysis of data from the WHO Mortality Database from 46 countries (1993–2012). Lancet 2017;390(10098):935–945.)

The sharp increase in the prevalence of asthma and allergic diseases observed since the mid-20th century has occurred in a time frame that is too short for the increase to be attributable to genetic factors alone. The explanation for the increasing trends therefore must lie in the influences brought about by environmental exposures and associated lifestyle, both of which have undergone rapid and profound changes in the last half of the century. Numerous environmental changes have occurred in parallel during this period, including changes in diet and exercise, patterns of microbial exposure in early life, family size and childcare arrangements, changes to housing design, and environmental exposure to a number of pollutants. It is important to emphasize that the increase in the prevalence of asthma and allergic diseases is likely a consequence of environmental factors increasing the risk in genetically susceptible individuals mediated through gene–environment interactions, and that the effect of environmental exposures is usually context-dependent.

RISK FACTORS FOR ASTHMA AND ALLERGIC DISEASES

In general, risk factors for asthma and allergic diseases can be divided into those that cause their development and those that trigger symptoms amongst patients with established disease (although some do both, and the mechanisms by which this happens are complex and interactive). For example, multiple genes interact with each other and with the environment in determining individual susceptibility. In addition to gene–environment interactions, environmental factors may also interact with each other (e.g., some air pollutants may increase the allergenicity of pollen grains). There is a wealth of information about the putative risk factors for asthma development in children, coming mainly from a number of birth cohort studies; however, there is a relative paucity of data for adult-onset disease. Numerous environmental exposures, such as exposure to indoor and outdoor allergens, tobacco smoke, air pollution, viral and bacterial infections, and diet (especially obesity) are important in the etiology and severity of asthma, and we will briefly discuss some of them.

In the developed world where the prevalence of allergic diseases is high, the general trend is to have smaller family size, cleaner living conditions, and highly processed and often sterilized food, with additives and altered nutrient content. A proportion of the population in the developing countries (particularly in the urban areas) is following this pattern and adopting certain aspects of the "westernized" lifestyle, and this may be associated with an increase in allergic disease. Similarly, migration from developing to developed countries may result in an increased risk for allergies amongst migrants.

Protective Environments

Epidemiological studies have shown markedly reduced prevalence of asthma and sensitization among children in traditional farming families compared to control rural populations, highlighting the key role of specific protective environmental exposures.[85,86] Similar observations have been reported from studies

in adults (e.g., the prevalence of allergic rhinitis in subjects aged 20–44 years in the ECRHS was 20.7%, with a considerably lower rate of 14.0% found among animal farmers of the same age).[87] The strongest protection was consistently demonstrated for the contact with farm animals and intake of unprocessed farm milk,[88] with the effect being stronger among genetically susceptible individuals.[89] Both of these protective features are associated with high microbial exposures.

Further studies capitalized on "natural experiments," which enabled comparisons of genetically similar populations with different lifestyles and/or living conditions. Examples include marked differences in asthma prevalence between Amish and Hutterite schoolchildren[90] or populations living in Finnish and Russian Karelia.[91] These studies offer insights into potential mechanisms of protection, such as the finding that exposure to household dust from Amish environment protects against asthma by engaging and modulating innate immunity.[90] Mechanistic studies in the murine model have shown that intranasal exposure of pregnant mice to extracts of one of the main microbial constituents of farm dust (*Acinetobacter lwoffii*) protected against asthma development in offspring.[92] The evidence to date indicates that microbial diversity is a hallmark of farm homes and associated with reduced risk of asthma, but importantly a farm-like microbial compositional structure in nonfarm homes is also associated with protection.[93] Driven by these findings, a focus of current research is on therapeutic strategies to enhance the resistance of infants and preschool children by immune modulation to reduce the community burden of persistent asthma.[94]

Air Pollution

In addition to microbial exposures, other environmental exposures may also be associated with urban living (e.g., air pollution and sedentary lifestyle). It is well established that outdoor air pollution contributes to worsening asthma control and increased risk of asthma attacks. Recent new data linked air pollution to adverse outcomes across the life-course, from increased risk of asthma deaths[95] and impaired lung function,[96] but also higher risk of asthma development.[97] A study in China investigated the association between short-term exposure to air pollution and asthma mortality, using information on >7000 asthma deaths between 2013 and 2018.[95] Short-term exposures to fine particulate matter <2.5 μm in diameter ($PM_{2.5}$), NO_2, and O_3 were all significantly associated with asthma mortality.[95] Similarly, in Peruvian children, ambient air pollution (including $PM_{2.5}$, black carbon, and NO_2) negatively affected asthma control and quality of life.[98] These findings raise a possibility that reducing air pollution may decrease asthma prevalence and mortality worldwide[99] and highlight the need for enacting effective policy measures in low- and middle-income countries affected by rising pollution.

CONCLUDING REMARKS

The prevalence rates of allergic sensitization, asthma, and other allergic diseases vary throughout the world, and are the highest in English-speaking nations, higher in western than eastern parts of Europe, and higher in urban than rural parts of Africa. In the last several decades, there has been a marked increase in the prevalence of these disorders across all ages and ranges of disease severity. More recent evidence suggests that this increase may have reversed for some of the outcomes (such as asthma) in some developed countries and in certain age groups. However, in developing parts of the world, the prevalence continues to increase, and global differences may be getting smaller. The fundamental role of the environment in allergy epidemic is suggested by the relatively short time frame within which the increase in allergies and asthma has occurred. Numerous environmental changes have occurred at the same time as the increase in allergies, and among many factors, these include changes in the family size and childcare arrangements, pattern of microbial exposures, housing design, exposure to a number of pollutants, exercise, diet, etc. It is likely that the increase in allergic diseases is a consequence of numerous different environmental factors increasing the risk in genetically susceptible individuals, mediated through gene–environment interactions. However, all this effort has as yet failed to identify a single intervention that could be used to prevent the development of asthma, and at present time, we cannot give any meaningful advice on primary prevention. The exception is findings that early introduction of peanuts significantly decreases the frequency of the development of peanut allergy in high-risk children with severe eczema, egg allergy, or both in early life.[100]

Epidemiology of asthma and allergic diseases has made major contributions to our understanding of the worldwide prevalence and environmental risk and protective factors, and has informed numerous basic science studies aiming to discover the underlying pathophysiological mechanisms of these disorders. However, due to many factors discussed earlier, which include residual confounding, heterogeneity in the definition of primary outcomes, multiple influences of modest effect size, and lack of statistical power to detect interactions between numerous factors, traditional epidemiology may be reaching the limit of what can be achieved through conventional hypothesis-driven research. Different manifestations of asthma symptom profiles over time may be a reflection of distinct causes and underlying biological mechanisms and may help identification of different asthma subtypes. However, the proposed subtypes (or endotypes) of asthma remain as yet ill-defined hypothetical constructs, and unless epidemiology finds better ways of distinguishing between different diseases under this umbrella diagnosis, it will be difficult to identify their unique risk and protective factors and discover their underlying pathophysiological processes, as any signal is likely to be diluted by phenotypic heterogeneity.

The ability to generate new data in research studies has increased exponentially over a short period of time, resulting in a vast amount of collected data. We seek to use this information to predict disease outcomes and understand their causes, so that we can design personalized prevention strategies and targeted treatments. To map a way forward in the areas of asthma and allergic diseases, the enormous body of evidence that has been generated on these topics need to be harnessed in an iterative way to inform next steps. The major challenges facing epidemiology in the 21st century are how best to utilize a vast amount of available data and how to integrate different scales of data (spanning from molecular-level, genetic and epigenetic, to population-level variables, including symptoms and objective measures of lung function and atopy); and different levels of directness of the measurement of the many variables of interest (including multiple environmental exposures). Instead of using a "black box" or "data-mining" approach, this process should be informed by and capitalize on the current and future biological and clinical knowledge about asthma and allergies. To do this effectively, it is essential to integrate the data with models/methods that can be tailored in full to the problem space of asthma, and the human expertise to make sense of the results. This can be achieved through pooling resources and multidisciplinary expertise from different disciplines and centers of excellence to maximize the potential of existing and newly collected data. The future of research in asthma and allergic diseases should be a genuine iterative interdisciplinary dialogue between epidemiologists, clinicians, statisticians, computer scientists, mathematicians, geneticists, and basic scientists, all working on a common problem—to solve the puzzle of asthma and allergies.[5]

REFERENCES

1. Guilbert TW, Bacharier LB, Fitzpatrick AM. Severe asthma in children. J Allergy Clin Immunol Pract. 2014;2(5):489–500.
2. Van Wonderen KE, Van Der Mark LB, Mohrs J, et al. Different definitions in childhood asthma: how dependable is the dependent variable? Eur Respir J. 2010;36(1):48–56.
3. Pavord ID, Beasley R, Agusti A, et al. After asthma: redefining airways diseases. Lancet. 2018;391(10118):350–400.
4. Lotvall J, Akdis CA, Bacharier LB, et al. Asthma endotypes: a new approach to classification of disease entities within the asthma syndrome. J Allergy and Clin Immunol. 2011;127(2):355–360.
5. Custovic A, Henderson J, Simpson A. Does understanding endotypes translate to better asthma management options for all? J Allergy Clin Immunol. 2019;144(1):25–33.
6. Belgrave D, Henderson J, Simpson A, Buchan I, Bishop C, Custovic A. Disaggregating asthma: Big investigation versus big data. J Allergy Clin Immunol. 2017;139(2):400–407.
7. Custovic A. "Asthma" or "asthma spectrum disorder"? J Allergy Clin Immunol Pract. 2020;8(8):2628–2629.
8. Saglani S, Custovic A. Childhood asthma: advances using machine learning and mechanistic studies. Am J Respir Criti Care Med. 2019;199(4):414–422.
9. Belgrave DC, Custovic A, Simpson A. Characterizing wheeze phenotypes to identify endotypes of childhood asthma, and the implications for future management. Expert Rev Clin Immunol. 2013;9(10):921–936.
10. Papadopoulos NG, Bernstein JA, Demoly P, et al. Phenotypes and endotypes of rhinitis and their impact on management: a PRACTALL report. Allergy. 2015;70(5):474–494.
11. Bieber T. Why we need a harmonized name for atopic dermatitis/atopic eczema/eczema! Allergy. 2016;71(10):1379–1380.
12. Bieber T, D'Erme AM, Akdis CA, et al. Clinical phenotypes and endophenotypes of atopic dermatitis: where are we, and where should we go? J Allergy Clin Immunol. 2017;139(4):S58–S64.
13. Silverberg JI, Thyssen JP, Paller AS, et al. What's in a name? Atopic dermatitis or atopic eczema, but not eczema alone. Allergy. 2017;72(12):2026–2030.

14. Kantor R, Thyssen JP, Paller AS, Silverberg JI. Atopic dermatitis, atopic eczema, or eczema? A systematic review, meta-analysis, and recommendation for uniform use of 'atopic dermatitis'. Allergy. 2016;71(10):1480–1485.

15. Johansson SG, Hourihane JO, Bousquet J, et al. A revised nomenclature for allergy. An EAACI position statement from the EAACI nomenclature task force. Allergy. 2001;56(9):813–824.

16. Kim JP, Chao LX, Simpson EL, Silverberg JI. Persistence of atopic dermatitis (AD): a systematic review and meta-analysis. J Am Acad Dermatol. 2016;75(4):681–687. e11.

17. Simpson EL, Keck LE, Chalmers JR, Williams HC. How should an incident case of atopic dermatitis be defined? A systematic review of primary prevention studies. J Allergy Clin Immunol. 2012;130(1):137–144.

18. Vakharia PP, Chopra R, Silverberg JI. Systematic review of diagnostic criteria used in atopic dermatitis randomized controlled trials. Am J Clin Dermatol. 2017;19(1):15–22.

19. Paternoster L, Standl M, Chen C-M, et al. Meta-analysis of genome-wide association studies identifies three new risk loci for atopic dermatitis. Nat Genet. 2011;44(2):187–192.

20. Nakamura T, Haider S, Custovic A. Understanding the heterogeneity of atopic dermatitis in childhood. Curr Allergy Clin Immunol. 2018;31(3):124–130.

21. Spergel JM. From atopic dermatitis to asthma: the atopic march. Ann Allergy Asthma Immunol. 2010;105(2):99–106. quiz 7–9, 17.

22. Bantz SK, Zhu Z, Zheng T. The atopic march: progression from atopic dermatitis to allergic rhinitis and asthma. J Clin Cell Immunol. 2014;5(2):202.

23. Munidasa D, Lloyd-Lavery A, Burge S, McPherson T. What should general practice trainees learn about atopic eczema? J Clin Med. 2015;4(2):360–368.

24. Galli E, Gianni S, Auricchio G, Brunetti E, Mancino G, Rossi P. Atopic dermatitis and asthma. Allergy Asthma Proc. 2007;28(5):540–543.

25. Hopper JL, Bui QM, Erbas B, et al. Does eczema in infancy cause hay fever, asthma, or both in childhood? Insights from a novel regression model of sibling data. J Allergy Clin Immunol. 2012;130(5):1117–1122.

26. Belgrave DC, Granell R, Simpson A, et al. Developmental profiles of eczema, wheeze, and rhinitis: two population-based birth cohort studies. PLoS Med. 2014;11(10):e1001748.

27. Clark H, Granell R, Curtin JA, et al. Differential associations of allergic disease genetic variants with developmental profiles of eczema, wheeze and rhinitis. Clin Exp Allergy. 2019;49(11):1475–1486.

28. Custovic A, Custovic D, Kljaic Bukvic B, Fontanella S, Haider S. Atopic phenotypes and their implication in the atopic march. Expert Rev Clin Immunol. 2020;16(9):873–881.

29. Custovic A, Lazic N, Simpson A. Pediatric asthma and development of atopy. Curr Opin Allergy Clin Immunol. 2013;13(2):173–180.

30. Szefler SJ, Wenzel S, Brown R, et al. Asthma outcomes: biomarkers. J Allergy Clin Immunol. 2012;129(3):S9–S23.

31. Pekkarinen PT, von Hertzen L, Laatikainen T, et al. A disparity in the association of asthma, rhinitis, and eczema with allergen-specific IgE between Finnish and Russian Karelia. Allergy. 2007;62(3):281–287.

32. Nicolaou N, Poorafshar M, Murray C, et al. Allergy or tolerance in children sensitized to peanut: prevalence and differentiation using component-resolved diagnostics. J Allergy Clin Immunol. 2010;125(1):191–197. e1–13.

33. Simpson A, Soderstrom L, Ahlstedt S, Murray CS, Woodcock A, Custovic A. IgE antibody quantification and the probability of wheeze in preschool children. J Allergy Clin Immunol. 2005;116(4):744–749.

34. Yunginger JW, Ahlstedt S, Eggleston PA, et al. Quantitative IgE antibody assays in allergic diseases. J Allergy Clin Immunol. 2000;105(6 Pt 1):1077–1084.

35. Simpson A, Tan VY, Winn J, et al. Beyond atopy: multiple patterns of sensitization in relation to asthma in a birth cohort study. Am J Respir Crit Care Med. 2010;181(11):1200–1206.

36. Lazic N, Roberts G, Custovic A, et al. Multiple atopy phenotypes and their associations with asthma: similar findings from two birth cohorts. Allergy. 2013;68(6):764–770.

37. Fontanella S, Frainay C, Murray CS, Simpson A, Custovic A. Machine learning to identify pairwise interactions between specific IgE antibodies and their association with asthma: a cross-sectional analysis within a population-based birth cohort. PLoS Med. 2018;15(11):e1002691.

38. Roberts G, Fontanella S, Selby A, et al. Connectivity patterns between multiple allergen specific IgE antibodies and their association with severe asthma. J Allergy Clin Immunol. 2020;146(4):821–830.

39. Howard R, Belgrave D, Papastamoulis P, Simpson A, Rattray M, Custovic A. Evolution of IgE responses to multiple allergen components throughout childhood. J Allergy Clin Immunol. 2018;142(4):1322–1330.

40. Sicherer SH, Sampson HA. Food allergy: epidemiology, pathogenesis, diagnosis, and treatment. J Allergy Clin Immunol. 2014;133(2):291–307. quiz 8.

41. Custovic A, Nicolaou N. Peanut allergy: overestimated in epidemiology or underdiagnosed in primary care? J Allergy Clin Immunol. 2011;127(3):631–632.

42. Ellwood P, Asher MI, Beasley R, Clayton TO, Stewart AW. ISAAC Steering Committee. The International Study of Asthma and Allergies in Childhood (ISAAC): phase three rationale and methods. Int J Tuberc Lung Dis. 2005;9(1):10–16.

43. Weiland SK, Bjorksten B, Brunekreef B, et al. Phase II of the International Study of Asthma and Allergies in Childhood (ISAAC II): rationale and methods. Eur Respir J. 2004;24(3): 406–412.

44. Asher MI, Keil U, Anderson HR, et al. International Study of Asthma and Allergies in Childhood (ISAAC): rationale and methods. Eur Respir J. 1995;8(3):483–491.

45. Burney PG, Chinn S, Britton JR, Tattersfield AE, Papacosta AO. What symptoms predict the bronchial response to histamine? Evaluation in a community survey of the bronchial symptoms questionnaire (1984) of the International Union Against Tuberculosis and Lung Disease. Int J Epidemiol. 1989;18(1): 165–173.

46. Variations in the prevalence of respiratory symptoms, self-reported asthma attacks, and use of asthma medication in the European Community Respiratory Health Survey (ECRHS). Eur Respir J 1996;9(4):687–695.

47. Sembajwe G, Cifuentes M, Tak SW, Kriebel D, Gore R, Punnett L. National income, self-reported wheezing and asthma diagnosis from the World Health Survey. Eur Respir J. 2010;35(2): 279–286.

48. Asher MI, Montefort S, Bjorksten B, et al. Worldwide time trends in the prevalence of symptoms of asthma, allergic rhinoconjunctivitis, and eczema in childhood: ISAAC Phases One and Three repeat multicountry cross-sectional surveys. Lancet. 2006;368(9537):733–743.

49. Upton MN, McConnachie A, McSharry C, et al. Intergenerational 20 year trends in the prevalence of asthma and hay fever in adults: the Midspan family study surveys of parents and offspring. BMJ. 2000;321(7253):88–92.

50. Dharmage SC, Perret JL, Custovic A. Epidemiology of asthma in children and adults. Front Pediatr. 2019;7:246.

51. Addo Yobo EO, Custovic A, Taggart SC, Asafo-Agyei AP, Woodcock A. Exercise induced bronchospasm in Ghana: differences in prevalence between urban and rural schoolchildren. Thorax. 1997;52(2):161–165.

52. Addo-Yobo EO, Woodcock A, Allotey A, Baffoe-Bonnie B, Strachan D, Custovic A. Exercise-induced bronchospasm and atopy in Ghana: two surveys ten years apart. PLoS Med. 2007;4(2):e70.

53. von Mutius E, Martinez FD, Fritzsch C, Nicolai T, Roell G, Thiemann HH. Prevalence of asthma and atopy in two areas of West and East Germany. Am J Respir Crit Care Med. 1994;149(2 Pt 1):358–364.

54. Wong GW, Ko FW, Hui DS, et al. Factors associated with difference in prevalence of asthma in children from three cities in China: multicentre epidemiological survey. BMJ. 2004;329(7464):486.

55. Vartiainen E, Petays T, Haahtela T, Jousilahti P, Pekkanen J. Allergic diseases, skin prick test responses, and IgE levels in North Karelia, Finland, and the Republic of Karelia, Russia. J Allergy Clin Immunol. 2002;109(4):643–648.

56. Lewis SA, Weiss ST, Platts-Mills TA, Syring M, Gold DR. Association of specific allergen sensitization with socioeconomic factors and allergic disease in a population of Boston women. J Allergy Clin Immunol. 2001;107(4):615–622.

57. Demenais F, Margaritte-Jeannin P, Barnes KC, et al. Multiancestry association study identifies new asthma risk loci that colocalize with immune-cell enhancer marks. Nat Genet. 2018;50(1):42–53.

58. Kim KW, Ober C. Lessons learned from GWAS of asthma. Allergy Asthma Immun. 2019;11(2):170–187.

59. Ober C. Asthma genetics in the post-GWAS era. Ann Am Thorac Soc. 2016;13:S85–S90.

60. Yaghoubi M, Adibi A, Safari A, FitzGerald JM, Sadatsafavi M. The projected economic and health burden of uncontrolled asthma in the United States. Am J Respir Crit Care Med. 2019;200(9):1102–1112.

61. Nurmagambetov TA, Krishnan JA. What will uncontrolled asthma cost in the United States? Am J Respir Crit Care Med. 2019;200(9):1077–1078.

62. Pennington E, Yaqoob ZJ, Al-Kindi SG, Zein J. Trends in asthma mortality in the United States: 1999 to 2015. Am J Respir Crit Care Med. 2019;199(12):1575–1577.

63. Levy ML, Winter R. Asthma deaths: what now? Thorax. 2015;70(3):209–210.

64. Weinmayr G, Weiland SK, Bjorksten B, et al. Atopic sensitization and the international variation of asthma symptom prevalence in children. Am J Respir Crit Care Med. 2007;176(6):565–574.

65. Shaw TE, Currie GP, Koudelka CW, Simpson EL. Eczema prevalence in the United States: data from the 2003 National Survey of Children's Health. J Investigative Dermatology. 2011;131(1):67–73.

66. Williams H, Stewart A, von Mutius E, Cookson W, Anderson HR. Is eczema really on the increase worldwide? J Allergy Clin Immunol. 2008;121(4):947–954. e15.

67. Yemaneberhan H, Flohr C, Lewis SA, et al. Prevalence and associated factors of atopic dermatitis symptoms in rural and urban Ethiopia. Clin Exp Allergy: J (BSACI). 2004;34(5):779–785.

68. Chalmers DA, Todd G, Saxe N, et al. Validation of the U.K. Working Party diagnostic criteria for atopic eczema in a Xhosa-speaking African population. Br J Dermatol. 2007;156(1):111–116.

69. Gupta RS, Warren CM, Smith BM, et al. The public health impact of parent-reported childhood food allergies in the United States. Pediatrics. 2018;142(6):e20181235.

70. Le TTK, Nguyen DH, Vu ATL, Ruethers T, Taki AC, Lopata AL. A cross-sectional, population-based study on the prevalence of food allergies among children in two different socio-economic regions of Vietnam. Pediatr Allergy Immunol. 2019;30(3):348–355.

71. Botha M, Basera W, Facey-Thomas HE, et al. Rural and urban food allergy prevalence from the South African Food Allergy (SAFFA) study. J Allergy Clin Immunol. 2019;143(2):662–668. e2.

72. Peters RL, Krawiec M, Koplin JJ, Santos AF. Update on food allergy. Pediatr Allergy Immunol. 2021;32(4):647–657.

73. Sicherer SH, Munoz-Furlong A, Sampson HA. Prevalence of seafood allergy in the United States determined by a random telephone survey. J Allergy Clin Immunol. 2004;114(1):159–165.

74. Sicherer SH, Munoz-Furlong A, Sampson HA. Prevalence of peanut and tree nut allergy in the United States determined by means of a random digit dial telephone survey: a 5-year follow-up study. J Allergy Clin Immunol. 2003;112(6):1203–1207.

75. Shek LP, Cabrera-Morales EA, Soh SE, et al. A population-based questionnaire survey on the prevalence of peanut, tree nut, and shellfish allergy in 2 Asian populations. J Allergy Clin Immunol. 2010;126(2):324–331. e1–7.

76. Osborne NJ, Koplin JJ, Martin PE, et al. Prevalence of challenge-proven IgE-mediated food allergy using population-based sampling and predetermined challenge criteria in infants. J Allergy Clin Immunol. 2011;127(3):668–676. e1–2.

77. Kotz D, Simpson CR, Sheikh A. Incidence, prevalence, and trends of general practitioner-recorded diagnosis of peanut allergy in England, 2001 to 2005. J Allergy Clin Immunol. 2011;127(3):623–630. e1.

78. Rona RJ, Keil T, Summers C, et al. The prevalence of food allergy: a meta-analysis. J Allergy Clin Immunol. 2007;120(3):638–646.

79. Eder W, Ege MJ, von Mutius E. The asthma epidemic. N Engl J Med. 2006;355(21):2226–2235.

80. Mitchell EA. International trends in hospital admission rates for asthma. Arch Dis Child. 1985;60(4):376–378.

81. Ebmeier S, Thayabaran D, Braithwaite I, Benamara C, Weatherall M, Beasley R. Trends in international asthma mortality: analysis of data from the WHO Mortality Database from 46 countries (1993–2012). Lancet. 2017;390(10098):935–945.

82. Bloom CI, Palmer T, Feary J, Quint JK, Cullinan P. Exacerbation patterns in adults with asthma in England. A population-based study. Am J Respir Crit Care Med. 2019;199(4):446–453.

83. Sears MR. Can we predict exacerbations of asthma? Am J Respir Crit Care Med. 2019;199(4):399–400.

84. Woods RK, Abramson M, Bailey M, Walters EH. International prevalences of reported food allergies and intolerances. Comparisons arising from the European Community Respiratory Health Survey (ECRHS) 1991–1994. Eur J Clin Nutr. 2001;55(4):298–304.

85. Braun-Fahrlander C, Riedler J, Herz U, et al. Environmental exposure to endotoxin and its relation to asthma in school-age children. N Engl J Med. 2002;347(12):869–877.

86. Ege MJ, Mayer M, Normand AC, et al. Exposure to environmental microorganisms and childhood asthma. N Engl J Med. 2011;364(8):701–709.

87. Radon K, Danuser B, Iversen M, et al. Respiratory symptoms in European animal farmers. Eur Respir J. 2001;17(4):747–754.
88. Illi S, Depner M, Genuneit J, et al. Protection from childhood asthma and allergy in Alpine farm environments-the GABRIEL advanced studies. J Allergy Clin Immunol. 2012;129(6):1470–1477. e6.
89. Loss GJ, Depner M, Hose AJ, et al. The early development of wheeze. Environmental determinants and genetic susceptibility at 17q21. Am J Respir Crit Care Med. 2016;193(8):889–897.
90. Stein MM, Hrusch CL, Gozdz J, et al. Innate immunity and asthma risk in Amish and Hutterite farm children. N Engl J Med. 2016;375(5):411–421.
91. Haahtela T, Laatikainen T, Alenius H, et al. Hunt for the origin of allergy-comparing the Finnish and Russian Karelia. Clin Exp Allergy. 2015;45(5):891–901.
92. Conrad ML, Ferstl R, Teich R, et al. Maternal TLR signaling is required for prenatal asthma protection by the nonpathogenic microbe Acinetobacter lwoffii F78. J Exp Med. 2009;206(13):2869–2877.
93. Kirjavainen PV, Karvonen AM, Adams RI, et al. Farm-like indoor microbiota in non-farm homes protects children from asthma development. Nat Med. 2019;25(7):1089–1095.
94. Holt PG, Strickland DH, Custovic A. Targeting maternal immune function during pregnancy for asthma prevention in offspring: Harnessing the "farm effect"? J Allergy Clin Immunol. 2020;146(2):270–272.
95. Liu Y, Pan J, Zhang H, et al. Short-term exposure to ambient air pollution and asthma mortality. Am J Respir Crit Care Med. 2019;200(1):24–32.
96. Wooding DJ, Ryu MH, Huls A, et al. Particle depletion does not remediate acute effects of traffic-related air pollution and allergen. A randomized, double-blind crossover study. Am J Respir Crit Care Med. 2019;200(5):565–574.
97. Lavigne E, Donelle J, Hatzopoulou M, et al. Spatiotemporal variations in ambient ultrafine particles and the incidence of childhood asthma. Am J Respir Crit Care Med. 2019;199(12):1487–1495.
98. Hansel NN, Romero KM, Pollard SL, et al. Ambient air pollution and variation in multiple domains of asthma morbidity among Peruvian children. Ann Am Thorac Soc. 2019;16(3):348–355.
99. Beamer PI. Air pollution contributes to asthma deaths. Am J Respir Crit Care Med. 2019;200(1):1–2.
100. Du Toit G, Roberts G, Sayre PH, et al. Randomized trial of peanut consumption in infants at risk for peanut allergy. N Engl J Med. 2015;372(9):803–813.

4

Indoor and Outdoor Allergens and Pollutants

Geoffrey A. Stewart and Clive Robinson

CHAPTER OUTLINE

SUMMARY OF IMPORTANT CONCEPTS

- Allergens in and outside the home are primarily proteins, capable of stimulating immunoglobulin E (IgE) synthesis in genetically susceptible people.
- Subsequent exposures to allergen may precipitate diseases such as allergic rhinitis, asthma, conjunctivitis, and urticaria.
- The major route of exposure, both inside and outside the home, is by inhalation, and the size of allergen-containing particles will influence both sensitization and symptoms, with submicronic particles likely to be associated with asthma rather than allergic rhinitis.
- The main sources of outdoor allergen exposure are pollens and fungi, but stinging and biting insects are also important.

- In the home, the most important allergen sources are house-dust mites, cockroaches, and furry animals such as cats and dogs.
- Methods exist to monitor allergen exposure, and sensitization thresholds for clinically important allergen sources have been established.
- Allergic symptoms may occur in patients due to cross-reactivity between aeroallergens and certain foods, giving rise to oral allergy or pollen food allergy syndromes.
- That indoor and outdoor air pollution exacerbates asthma symptoms is established but, with the exception of tropospheric ozone, evidence that pollution causes new asthma is hard to assess.
- Pollutant exposure can induce allergic and/or nonallergic inflammation in people with asthma.

- Air pollution can modify the allergome and thus allergen exposure in allergic individuals.
- Rising carbon dioxide levels and increasing surface temperatures affect plant pollination in ways that might affect pollination and pollen potency.

INTRODUCTION

Individuals are exposed to a range of potentially allergenic sources in both domestic and work settings, and each source will contain a variety of proteins, some of which may stimulate specific immunoglobulin E (IgE) production in genetically predisposed individuals. Such proteins are referred to as allergens, and a protein with such a propensity is described as being allergenic and allergenicity is the property of being allergenic (Table 4.1). The route by which an allergen enters a susceptible individual will influence the types of allergic symptoms ensuing, with exposure to aerosolized allergens (aeroallergen) giving rise to respiratory symptoms, in contrast with those resulting from ingestion, injection, or absorption. However, the most clinically significant route involves the respiratory tract (Fig. 4.1). There has been much interest in characterizing the clinically relevant allergens within a source, stimulated

by the desire to produce better diagnostic reagents, develop more effective immunotherapies, and establish exposure thresholds. In addition, the characterization of allergens has enabled researchers to determine whether allergen biochemistry influences immunogenicity. This chapter is devoted to describing indoor and outdoor aeroallergens, and, in so doing, posit how inherent biochemical characteristics contribute to allergenicity. We also include a brief discussion of allergens produced by biting and stinging insects as they represent an important and potentially life-threatening outdoor source of allergen, and as an adjunct to the chapter on the clinical aspects of insect allergy described elsewhere in this edition (see Chapter 15). We conclude by reviewing the qualitative and quantitative effects of climate change and air pollution on allergens in the environment as well as on the role of pollution in facilitating or exacerbating allergic diseases.

ALLERGENS AND ALLERGENICITY

The terms *allergen* and *allergy* were introduced into our lexicon in 1906 by Clemens von Pirquet (1874–1929) to describe a body's hyperreactivity to a foreign substance. Today, they are synonymous with immediate hypersensitivity. Although the term

TABLE 4.1 Glossary of Allergen and Allergy Terms

Allergy/Allergen	Term	Definition
Allergy-related	Atopy	The genetic tendency to produce specific immunoglobulin E (IgE) to common environmental allergens
	Monosensitization	Sensitization to one allergenic source
	Polysensitization	Sensitization to two or more allergenic sources
	Polyallergy	Both sensitization and symptoms associated with two or more allergen sources
Allergen-related	Allergen	A molecule shown to induce IgE in a susceptible person
	Allergenic	Adjective for allergen
	Allergenicity	The capacity of a molecule to become an allergen
	Major/immunodominant allergen	One that is recognized by more than 50% of a sensitized population (see Box 4.2 for other parameters)
	Isoallergen	An allergen sharing approximately 67% or more sequence identity with another allergen
	Isoform/variant	An allelic allergen
	Cross-reactive allergen	Allergens that react with antibodies produced to a (unrelated or related) primary sensitizing allergen because of the presence of significant sequence homology and hence common epitopes
	Risk allergen(s)	An allergen or a group of allergens stimulating IgE production in early childhood that predict asthma and/or rhinitis in the teenage years
	Initiator allergen	An allergen that, because of some biochemical characteristic, appears to lead, over time, to the production of IgE to associated proteins in the same source
	Pan-allergen	A minor cross-reacting allergen found in a wide variety of evolutionary unrelated sources
	Marker allergen	An allergen that clearly identifies the primary sensitizing source
	Epitope	A region of an antigen that binds to a B cell receptor or antibody combining site (B cell epitope) or to the T cell receptor (T cell epitope)
	Immunodominant epitope	An epitope present on an allergen which fits most favorably into the groove of MHC Class I or II molecules, thus stimulating a dominant T cell or B cell response
	Hapten	A chemical that is capable of modifying a host antigen (or other carrier protein) to render it immunogenic/allergenic
	Cross-reacting carbohydrate determinant (CCD)	An immunogenic glycan structure on a glycoprotein that stimulates the production of specific IgE which will then bind to similar moieties found on a diverse array of other glycoproteins

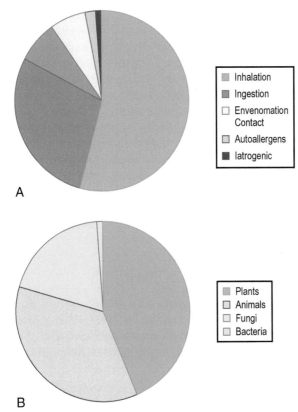

A

B

Fig. 4.1 Percent distribution of allergens present in the Allergome database, based on route of exposure (A) and origin (B). (Data from Radauer C, Bublin M, Wagner S, Mari A, Breiteneder H. Allergens are distributed into few protein families and possess a restricted number of biochemical functions. J Allergy Clin Immunol 2008;121:847–852, e7; Stewart GA, Robinson C. The structure and function of allergens. In: Burks AW, Holgate S, O'Hehir R, Bacharier L, Broide D, Hershey GK, et al., editors. Middleton's Allergy: Principles and Practice. 9th ed. London: Elsevier; 2019. p. 387–427.)

allergenic (Table 4.1) is used to describe the IgE-inducing property of an allergen, allergens may also stimulate the induction of other immunoglobulin isotypes in susceptible individuals, particularly IgG and IgG4. The clinical significance of such responses is unclear, but there are data to suggest that an IgG response precedes the appearance of an IgE one. A potentially allergenic source may contain several allergens, and each allergen may possess a number of potential epitopes, that is, areas of a protein that interact with the B and T cell receptors on lymphocytes, which stimulate their own specific IgE. Thus, serum IgE is polyclonal, reflecting that produced to different allergens as well as that to different parts of an individual allergen. The use of the term *marker allergen*, defined as an allergen (Table 4.1) that unambiguously identifies an initiating allergen source rather than a cross-reacting one, has arisen due to our ability to produce multiple purified single allergens for use in component-resolved diagnosis of allergy.

Allergens may also be described as *cross-reactive* allergens (Table 4.1), which means that a patient may produce IgE to an allergen, which not only reacts with the sensitizing allergen but, because of significant sequence identity and, hence, common epitopes, will also react with phylogenetically related proteins. Because of this, it is sometimes difficult to identify the initiating

allergenic stimulus. *Cross-reactivity* may also be evident between phylogenetically dissimilar species such as the tropomyosin allergens in mites, snails, cockroaches, and shellfish in which sequence identity may be >80%. It can also occur with allergens in physiologically dissimilar tissues such as pollen and distantly related fruits and vegetables. Such allergens are known as *pan-allergens* and respiratory sensitization can give rise to *oral allergy syndrome* (OAS), sometimes known as *pollen food allergy syndrome* (PFAS), in pollen-sensitized patients.

INDOOR AND OUTDOOR ALLERGEN SOURCES

The majority of these allergens are derived from plant, fungal, and animal sources. Outdoor sources (other than those from arthropod stings and bites) are associated with structures evolved for the dispersal of genetic material, such as pollen and spores. In contrast, mammalian indoor allergens are often secretions/excretions such as urine and saliva that are deposited onto danders, whereas indoor arthropod–derived allergens are usually derived from fecal pellets. Thus, most individuals are exposed to particulate or sub-particulate allergen–containing material. Such particulates contain mixtures of (glyco)proteins and other components that play essential roles in the physiology of the source, with the most complex being the pollens, fungal spores, and fecal pellets from arthropods.

Susceptible patients usually produce IgE to more than one protein present within a source, and a spectrum of reactivities in an individual serum will exist. In addition, individuals can be monosensitized, that is, they are sensitized to a single allergen source (e.g., house-dust mites [HDMs]) or polysensitized to multiple allergen sources (Table 4.1) such as pollen, HDMs, and danders, although sensitization to more than five sources is uncommon. Polysensitization is, however, common in asthma and atopic dermatitis,[1] and such patients manifest more severe clinical symptoms.[2] Within a single source, some constituent allergens will be recognized by a greater percentage of the members of an exposed population than others, and some will stimulate significantly more IgE than others. These and other criteria (Box 4.1) are used to define them as *major (or immunodominant/serodominant) allergens* in contrast to *minor* or *intermediate* allergens. However, some allergens considered to be *minor* on a population basis may be clinically significant for a particular individual. Similarly, some allergens considered to be *major* within a particular allergic population in a specific geographical location may not be so dominant in another location, indicating that local environmental, cultivar, or genetic factors may influence specific allergen production.

AEROBIOLOGY OF INDOOR AND OUTDOOR ALLERGEN SOURCES

Sensitization is dependent upon inhalation which, in turn, will require allergen aerosolization. Outdoors, the process will be influenced by climate, humidity, seasonality, and other ecological factors. Indoors, aerosolization will depend on anthropogenic factors such as bed-making, vacuuming, and pest and pet

BOX 4.1 IUIS Allergen Nomenclature Criteria and Criteria for Defining a Major Allergen

Physicochemical requirements	It is of proven homogeneity. Its molecular weight, isoelectric point (pI), and carbohydrate composition have been determined. Its nucleotide sequence and/or amino acid sequence has been determined. Specific antisera (mono- or polyclonal) are available.
Allergenicity requirements	Allergenicity can be demonstrated using both immunochemical and biologic assays such as enzyme-linked immunosorbent assay (ELISA), skin testing, or basophil histamine release. The allergenic activity of a recombinant protein is comparable to that of the native allergen.
Major allergen designation requirements	It sensitizes ≥50% of a predisposed and exposed population. A significant proportion of total serum IgE is directed to the allergen (>10%). Removal of the allergen from the source material greatly reduces the biologic and immunochemical (IgE) activity of the extract. The allergen represents a significant proportion of the total extractable protein in the extract. The allergen may be used as a marker of environmental exposure. The allergen, its cDNA, or its constituent peptides can be shown to be effective in an allergy vaccine. Both humoral (IgE) and cellular (T cell/basophil) responses to the allergen can be measured in a high proportion of a sensitized population.

Modified from Chapman MD. Allergen nomenclature. In: Lockey RF, Ledford DK, editors. Allergens and allergen immunotherapy. Boca Raton: CRC Press; 2008:47–58.

mitigation. The aerodynamic size of the aerosolized particles generated is also significant, as it will influence the site of deposition in the respiratory tree and, therefore, symptoms. Large particles (>10 μm) will be trapped in the nose, giving rise to nasal symptoms, whereas smaller particles enter the bronchi giving rise to lower airways inflammation resulting in asthma rather than rhinitis. Size will also influence the length of time particles remain suspended in the atmosphere and, therefore, exposure, because smaller-sized allergenic particles remain airborne for extended periods.

ALLERGEN MONITORING—WHOLE SPORES, POLLENS, AND MITES

Quantifying allergen sources or individual allergens provides a means of determining whether they are likely to precipitate symptoms of allergic rhinitis and conjunctivitis, predicting when increased emergency room visits for asthma are likely, and establishing allergen concentration thresholds for sensitization and how reductions might be achieved in the home and workplace. Various methods for quantifying morphologically distinct allergen sources are available. For example, spore

and pollen concentrations are measured using gravimetric, impaction, and trapping devices (Fig. 4.2) in combination with microscopy. The resulting counts can be expressed either as the number of grains or spores per m^3 of air per 24 hours or as an index representing the potential risk (pollen index) of developing symptoms, taking into consideration the known allergy provoking potential of the pollen or fungal species identified. The public dissemination of pollen data is often supported by national allergy organizations, and public and commercial broadcasting organizations, via the Internet (e.g., https://www.aaaai.org/global/nab-pollen-counts?ipb=1&desktop=1 and http://www.weatherzone.com.au/pollen-index/). In contrast, HDMs present in carpet or mattress dust are isolated by floatation over saturated sodium chloride and then counted using a stereo microscope, and data expressed as HDMs per g of dust per m^2 per unit time of vacuuming.

MEASURING SPECIFIC ALLERGENS

Quantification of a specific allergen in air or reservoir dusts is achieved by immunoassay using allergen-specific antisera and reference standards, making it possible to correlate allergen exposure with sensitization. A number of threshold concentrations have now been described, above which sensitization and/or provocation of symptoms may occur in susceptible individuals (Table 4.2). In establishing these, a linear relationship between exposure, sensitization, and induction of symptoms is assumed. However, data indicate that the concentration of allergen required to cause sensitization will often be lower than that for induction of symptoms, and that dose–response relationships may be bell-shaped, with very high exposure inducing tolerance (see the later section). Similarly, the ability to measure specific allergen enables allergen extract manufacturers to provide standardized preparations for use in both diagnosis and immunotherapy. Because the availability of specific standards has been limited, an Allergen Standardization Committee, through the auspices of the World Health Organization (WHO) and the International Union of Immunological Societies (IUIS), has facilitated the development of a universal allergen standard (UAS) containing purified natural and recombinant proteins, including Der p 1, Der f 1, Der p 2, Fel d 1, Can f 1, Rat n 1, Mus m 1, and Bla g 2, for robust standardization purposes.[5]

THE CHEMICAL NATURE OF ALLERGENS

Most allergens (and antigens) are proteins of varying sizes, but certain low molecular weight chemically reactive compounds may be allergenic (*haptens*, Table 4.1) only when they have modified host proteins. The most common haptens are the beta-lactam antibiotics such as the benzyl penicillins. Every protein allergen contains a number of potential *epitopes* (Table 4.1), which may comprise linear amino acid sequences or adjacent but distal sections of a sequence (conformational) that engage with either the B cell receptor or its soluble antibody form or the T cell receptor of a lymphocyte. The number of amino acid residues comprising a B cell or T cell epitope is about 5 and 13 to 17 amino acid residues, respectively (Fig. 4.3). Some epitopes

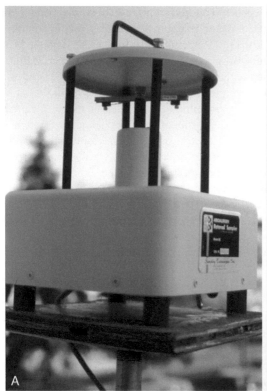
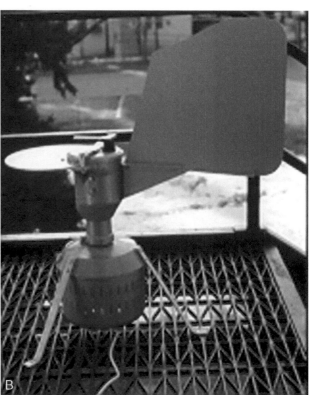
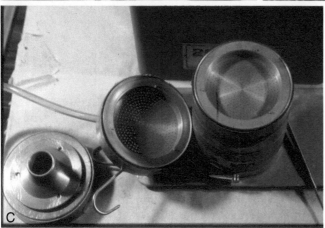

Fig. 4.2 Examples of equipment used in monitoring outdoor pollen and fungal spore concentrations, and allergen-bearing aerodynamic particle size. (A) Rotorod intermittent rotary impactor sampler; (B) Burkard suction drum Hirst-type spore trap, with rain guard and large weather vane; and (C) disassembled Andersen multistage cascade impactor. (Photographs from Davies JM, Weber RW. Aerobiology of outdoor allergens. In: Burks AW, Holgate S, O'Hehir R, Bacharier L, Broide D, Hershey GK, et al., editors. Middleton's allergy: principles and practice. 1. 9th ed. London: Elsevier; 2019:428–450.) Middletons 9e, Figures 24.4–24.6 as a composite.

stimulate a stronger immune response than others for a variety of reasons, for example, such as being better able to fit into the groove of the major histocompatibility complex (MHC) Class I or II binding cleft. In addition, the type of antigen presenting cell, the endosomal proteases present within it, and the susceptibility of the acquired antigen/allergen to them will likely play a role. In this regard, it has been demonstrated that the presence of the phytoprostane E_1 ligand bound to the Bet v 1 allergen confers resistance to proteolysis by inhibiting lysosomal cathepsin S activity which, in turn, enhances Th2 responses.[6] An individual may also recognize epitopes that are different to those recognized by other individuals because of differences in their MHC haplotype.

Lipids do not appear to be allergenic, but IgE may be produced against glycan structures on some glycoprotein allergens and approximately 15% to 30% of allergic patients, particularly teenagers, may produce IgE to these. Whether the IgE is specific for a particular glycoprotein allergen is unclear because glycoproteins from diverse sources possess immunochemically similar glycan moieties and are referred to as *cross-reacting carbohydrate determinants* (CCDs). A number of CCDs have been described and, in general, they do not appear to be particularly important. However, the Galα1-3Galβ1-4GlcNAc-R (α-Gal) epitope is immunogenic and IgE to α-Gal on animal serum immunoglobulins, red meat proteins, and therapeutic murine monoclonal antibody (Cetuximab) may cause immediate anaphylaxis in certain patients given Cetuximab and delayed anaphylaxis (3–6 h) in some patients after ingesting red meat. This IgE is thought to be stimulated by prior exposure to tick bite salivary proteins and its presence in these individuals may give rise to false positive results when using certain allergen extracts in skin testing, for example, cat extracts.

TABLE 4.2 **Proposed Pollen/Allergen Threshold Concentrations for Sensitization and Symptom Manifestation**

Allergen	Sensitization Threshold Concentration in Reservoir Dust (µg Allergen/g Dust/sq m) or Grains per Cubic Meter	Percent Homes in the US with Allergen Concentration Exceeding that Required for Sensitization	Concentrations which will Elicit Symptoms of Asthma or Rhinitis (for Pollen) in Sensitized patients	Percent Homes in the US with Allergen Concentrations Exceeding that Required for Asthma Symptoms in Sensitized Patients
Fel d 1[a]	1 (0.29)	66	8 (2.32)	35
Bla g 1	2 units/g	Living room, 11 Kitchen, 3	8 units/g	Living room, 13 Kitchen, 10
Bla g 2	0.8 (0.45)	-	8	-
Can f 1[a]	2 (0.34)	56	10 (1.7)	35
Der p 1	2 (1.18)	46	10 (5.9)	24
Der f 1	2 (0.16)	-	10 (0.8)	-
Mus m 1	1.6	82	1.6	-
Grass pollen[b]	?	-	5	-
Weed pollen	?	-	15	-
Tree pollen	?	-	10	-

[a]Cat and dog allergens detected in most homes irrespective of pet ownership;[3] mite allergen detectable in most homes (National Survey of Lead and Allergens in Housing publications). Figures in parentheses indicate the threshold values converted on the basis of the availability of the Universal Allergen Standard.[4]
[b]Pollen data from National Allergy Bureau. 2017. Retrieved from American Academy of Allergy Asthma and Immunology: http://www.aaaai.org/global/nab-pollen-counts?ipb=1

ALLERGEN NOMENCLATURE AND ALLERGEN DATABASES

Through the auspices of the WHO and IUIS, an Allergen Nomenclature Subcommittee was established in 1984 to bring order to the previously ad hoc way in which allergens were described. This Committee introduced a systematic nomenclature system based on a set of specific criteria using the first three letters of the genus (e.g., _Dermatophagoides_) combined with the first one or two letters of the species name (e.g., _pteronyssinus_) and an Arabic numeral reflecting either the order in which the allergen was isolated or its clinical importance, or both, are used.[7] To avoid confusion where such abbreviations of the genus are identical, four letters rather than three may be used (e.g., Cand and Can for _Candida_ and _Canis_, respectively). With the development of molecular biological techniques in the 1980s, the determination of the primary amino acid sequence of allergens and thus their biochemical identification was made easier, as was the capacity to produce recombinant proteins. As a result, the denomination process was modified to differentiate the recombinant from the natural form, using the prefixes r and n, respectively (e.g., rDer p 1, nDer p 1).

Similar allergens from related species use the same nomenclature. For example, HDM cysteine protease allergens from the species _Dermatophagoides pteronyssinus, D. farinae, Euroglyphus maynei,_ and _Blomia tropicalis_ are individually referred to as Der p 1, Der f 1, Eur m 1, and Blo t 1, respectively, with sequence identity ranging from 40% to 88%. Collectively, they are referred to as the Group 1 mite allergens or as the mite cysteine proteases, and a similar approach is routinely used to describe allergens

of similar function and sequence identity, for example, grass, weed, and tree pollen allergen groups. As a source may produce allergens that are clearly related by size, function, and sequence identity, the terms _isoallergen, isoform/variant_ were introduced to describe closely related allergens (Table 4.1). An arbitrary definition for an isoallergen within a source is that it should have at least 67% sequence identity (arising from gene duplication or alternate splicing) and be denominated using a suffix (e.g., Amb a 1.01, Amb a 1.02). Similarly, isoforms/variants (polymorphisms) of an allergen/isoallergen in the same source differing by only a few residues are denominated using an additional two digits (e.g., Amb a 1.0101).

The Subcommittee also created the first official allergen database but other allergen databases have followed, each with different emphases (Table 4.3). Of particular relevance to the denomination of allergens are the databases Pfam[8] and the derivative AllFam.[9] Pfam is a database of all known proteins curated into families based on sequence identity within a functional domain—for example, binding or enzymatic domains. Proteins with similar domains and functions are assumed to be evolutionarily related and are assigned to a specific family and/or clan (a large collection of evolutionary related families). As allergens are proteins, they will have been curated into Pfam families together with every other known protein (Table 4.3). The advantage of this is that the evolutionary relatedness of similar allergens, but with little sequence homology outside of the domain portion, will be clearly identified (e.g., Asp f 11 and Asp f 27, both of which are cyclophilins). AllFam uses the Pfam database to specifically group allergens into one of 151 allergen families

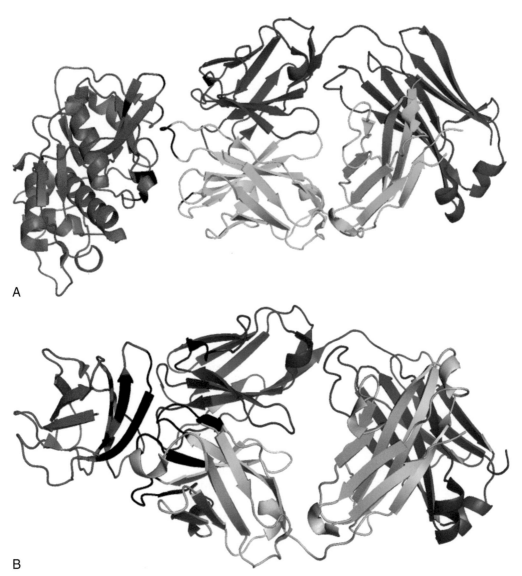

Fig. 4.3 Three-dimensional structure of allergenic B cell epitopes on a mite (Der p 1) and grass pollen allergen (Phl p 2). (A) Binding of the Fab fragment of a genetically engineered IgE antibody molecule to a conformational B cell epitope on the timothy grass pollen allergen Phl p 2; (B) binding of the Fab fragment of a mouse IgG monoclonal antibody to Der p 1. Both allergens are shown in *red*, whereas the light and heavy chains of the Fab portions are shown in *blue* and *green*, respectively. The actual amino acid residues comprising each of the two epitopes binding to the hypervariable regions of the Fab fragments are shown in *black*, as are the interacting amino acid residues of the hypervariable regions of the antibody combining sites in the Fab fragments (the paratope). *IgE*, Immunoglobulin E; *IgG*, immunoglobulin G. The images were constructed with the PyMOL molecular graphics system using Worldwide Protein Data Bank (PDB) entries 2VXQ and 3RVX. (Figure from Stewart GA, Robinson C. The structure and function of allergens. In: Burks AW, Holgate S, O'Hehir R, Bacharier L, Broide D, Hershey GK, et al., editors. Middleton's Allergy: Principles and Practice. 9th ed. London: Elsevier; 2019:387–427.)

(Table 4.4) but does not take into account whether an allergen contains more than one type of Pfam domain.

OUTDOOR ALLERGENS

Outdoor aeroallergens, typically derived from pollens and fungal spores, constitute the most common cause of allergic disease. All pollen types are >2.5 μm in diameter (e.g., grass pollen 25–45 μm and tree [e.g., birch], 15–27 μm) and each pollen grain will contain picograms of allergen. A high proportion of pollen aeroallergen-exposed individuals become sensitized (30%–40%) depending on the community. Allergy is typically seasonal, and is influenced by conditions, including temperature, wind, rain, and thunderstorm activity. Symptoms generally correlate with atmospheric concentrations or, in their absence, submicronic allergenic particles (fragmented pollen or fungal spores or released starch granules). Similarly, the age of the pollen will also influence symptoms, as immature and aging pollens are less potent than mature pollen.

Fungal spores (undifferentiated) are also present in the atmosphere at varying concentrations, ranging from a few hundred to >100,000 per m³, depending on humidity,[11] but the percentage of known allergenic species ranges from 3% to 11%. Spores are generally smaller than pollen with many in the range of 5 to 15 μm. The sensitization rate in the general population is about 15% depending on age of the individual and season. Fungal

TABLE 4.3 Various Databases Containing Information on Allergen Structure and Function, and Available Allergen Prediction Software

Database/Software	Content	Web Address
Non–Allergen Specific[a]		
European Nucleotide Archive (ENA)	Nucleotide sequences	ebi.ac.uk/ena/browser/home
GenBank	Nucleotide sequences	ncbi.nlm.nih.gov/genbank/
MEROPS	Peptidases and peptidase inhibitors	ebi.ac.uk/merops/
Protein family (Pfam)	Protein structures and domain architectures	pfam.xfam.org
Universal Protein Knowledge Base (UniProtKB)	Protein sequences and function	uniprot.org
Worldwide Protein Data Bank (wwPDB)	Three-dimensional protein structures	wwpdb.org/
Allergen-specific		
Allergome	Similar to the IUIS database but contains other information, as well as data on allergens yet to be denominated by the IUIS Subcommittee	allergome.org
AllFam	A database of allergens curated on basis of information contained in Allergome and Pfam	meduniwien.ac.at/allfam/
Immune Epitope Database and Analysis Resource	A database of epitopes of both antigens and allergens	IEDB.org
InFormAll	A database of allergens relevant to the food industry	research.bmh.manchester.ac.uk/informall/allergenic-foods/
International Union of Immunological Societies (IUIS) Allergen Nomenclature Subcommittee	A curated database of all officially recognized allergens	allergen.org
Structural Database of Allergenic Proteins (SDAP)	An allergen database, including epitope data, together with a collection of bioinformatics tools for their analysis	fermi.utmb.edu/SDAP/index.html
Allergenicity/Cross-Reactivity Prediction Servers		
AlgPred	In silico prediction of allergenicity and epitopes	crdd.osdd.net/raghava/algpred/
AllerTOP	In silico prediction of allergenicity and route of exposure	ddg-pharmfac.net/AllerTOP/
Cross-React	In silico prediction of allergen cross-reactivity	curie.utmb.edu
Food Allergy Research and Resource Program Allergen Database	A database of allergens relevant to the food industry	allergenonline.com

[a]Although not allergen-focused *per se*, these databases may cross-reference structure and sequence data with allergenicity data.

allergens are found in both mycelia and spores but expression may be growth phase dependent. Thus, some of the spore-derived allergens may be absent in mycelial extracts, and vice versa. In addition to outdoor exposure to pollens and fungal spores, individuals may be exposed to allergens associated with stinging and biting insects.

Outdoor Aeroallergens—Pollen

Pollen from allergenic plants arises predominantly from wind-pollinated (anemophilous) angiosperms and gymnosperms, including trees, herbaceous dicotyledons (weeds), and grasses (Fig. 4.4) (Table 4.5). Exposure usually reflects the types of plants growing in a particular location since most pollen settle close to their origin. However, pollen-specific physical characteristics mean that pollens may travel many hundreds of kilometers from their original source and reach heights of several hundred meters. A concentration of 20 to 100 pollen grains per m³ is sufficient to provoke disease, but the concentrations of specific pollen-derived allergens required to initiate symptoms are unknown.

Pollen Structure

Pollens are structures containing a cytoplasm within which may be found the male gametophyte and a range of components essential for ensuring the successful fertilization of the plant ovum, some of which will be allergenic or immunomodulatory. This is then surrounded by an internal (intine) layer made up of cellulose and pectin, and a rigid, external (exine) layer made up of sporopollenin. On top of the exine may be found the pollenkitt, a sticky adhesive layer that contains a variety of proteins, lipids, and pigments, which have important functions in pollen–stigma interactions as well as pollen tube growth. In addition, the pollen surface may be covered with anther-derived orbicles (Ubisch bodies) of some but not all grass, weed, and tree species. Similarly, the pollen surface may harbor a microbiome of bacteria and fungi.[12]

In angiosperms, pollen produced by anthers, lands on the stigma (dry), and a pollen tube develops, which then enters the ovum via the micropyle at a relatively fast rate. In stigma-less gymnosperms, in particular, Cupressaceae species associated with allergy, the predominant method involves whole pollen,

TABLE 4.4   The Pfam and AllFam Codes for Common Outdoor, Indoor, and Stinging and Biting Insect Allergens

Pfam Code	Domain Description	Aeroallergen Example(s)	AllFam Code
Hydrolytic Enzymes			
PF00082	Subtilisin-like proteases	Asp f 13, Pen ch 18, Cuc m 1	AF021
PF00089	Trypsin	Mite Group 3, Api m 7	AF024
PF00112	Papain family cysteine protease	Mite Group 1, Act d 1, Ana c 2	AF030
PF00151	Lipase	Vespid Group 1	AF037
PF00295	Polygalacturonase	Cry j 2, Phl p 13, Jun a 2	AF057
PF00314	Thaumatin family	Act d 2, Cup a 3, Jun a 3	AF060
PF01620	Ribonuclease (pollen allergen)	Grass Groups 5/6	AF102
PF01630	Hyaluronidase	Vespid Group 2, Tab y 2	AF103
Nonhydrolytic Enzymes			
PF00113	Enolase, C-terminal riose phosphate isomerase (TIM) barrel domain	Cla h 6, Alt a 6	AF031
PF03952	Enolase, N-terminal domain	Cla h 6, Alt a 6	AF031
PF00544	Pectate lyase	Amb a 1, Amb a 3, Cha o 1, Cry j 1, Jun v 1, Cup a 1	AF073
Enzyme Inhibitors			
PF00234	Protease inhibitor/seed storagelipid transfer protein family	Amb a 6, Art v 3	AF050
PF01190	Pollen proteins Ole e 1 family	Ole e1, Phl p 11, Pla a 1	AF087
Lipid-binding Proteins			
PF00061	Lipocalin/cytosolic fatty acid–binding protein family	Blo t 13, Bos d 5, Can f 2	AF015
PF02221	MD-2 related lipid recognition (ML) domain	Mite Group 2, Der p 22, Der p 35	AF111
PF00407	Pathogenesis-related protein Bet v 1 family	Group 1 Fagales, Pru av 1, Gly m 4	AF069
PF00273	Serum albumin family	Bos d 6, Can f 3, Fel d 2	AF056
Calcium-binding Proteins			
PF00036	EF hand	Bos d 3, Bet v 3, grass Group 7	AF007
Actin-associated Proteins			
PF00235	Profilin	Phl p 12, Ole e 2, Ara h 5	AF051
PF00261	Tropomyosin	Der p 10, Per a 7, Pen a 1	AF054
Transport and Nonlipid Ligand–binding Proteins			
PF00012	HSP70	Alt a 3, Cla h 5, Mala s 10	AF002
PF00042	Globin	Chi t 1–9	AF009
Other			
PF00188	Cysteine-rich secretory protein family (CAP)	Group 5 vespid, Sol r 3, Art v 2, Cyn d 4	AF044
PF00428	Acid ribosomal P1 protein	Alt a 12, Asp f 8, Cla h 10	AF070
PF00578	AhpC/thiol-specific antioxidant (TSA) family	Asp f 3, Mala f 3, Cand b 2	AF131
PF01357	Expansin and expansin-like	Grass pollen Groups 1, 2, 3	AF093
PF06757	Insect allergen-related repeat, nitrile-specifier detoxification	Per a 1, Bla g 1	AF127
PF01099	Uteroglobin	Fel d 1, Ory c 3	AF134

The standard IUIS nomenclature is used throughout this chapter, although allergens yet to receive the IUIS imprimatur, but reported either in the literature or denominated in the Allergome database, are described using the first three (or four) letters of genus name and the first letter of the species name followed by some abbreviation of the biochemical identity, for example, Lol p CYP for the cyclophilin allergen from rye grass pollen. *HSP*, heat shock protein.

Data taken from the Pfam data base[8] and the AllFam database.[9,10]

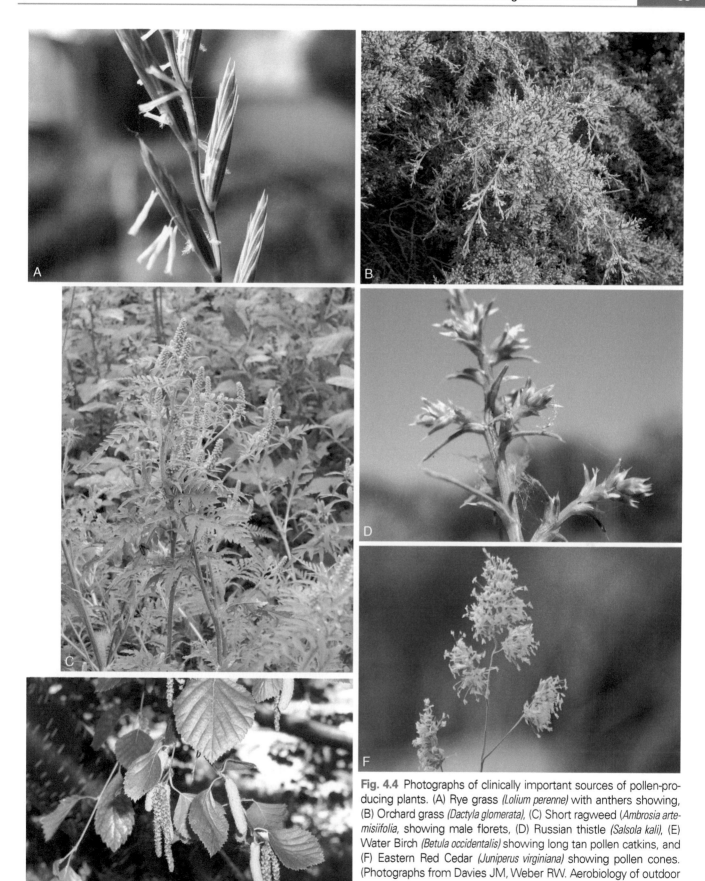

Fig. 4.4 Photographs of clinically important sources of pollen-producing plants. (A) Rye grass *(Lolium perenne)* with anthers showing, (B) Orchard grass *(Dactyla glomerata)*, (C) Short ragweed (*Ambrosia artemisiifolia*, showing male florets, (D) Russian thistle *(Salsola kali)*, (E) Water Birch *(Betula occidentalis)* showing long tan pollen catkins, and (F) Eastern Red Cedar *(Juniperus virginiana)* showing pollen cones. (Photographs from Davies JM, Weber RW. Aerobiology of outdoor allergens. In: Burks AW, Holgate S, O'Hehir R, Bacharier L, Broide D, Hershey GK, et al., editors. Middleton's allergy: principles and practice. 1. 9th ed. London: Elsevier; 2019:428–450. Middletons 9e, Figures 27.11 (a), 27.10 (b), 27.35 (c), 27.15 (d), 27.32 (e), 27.7 (f).)

TABLE 4.5 Common Sources of Allergenic Pollens

Cross-reacting Groups	Representative Genera[a]
Grasses	
Pooideae	*Poa* (bluegrass), *Dactylis* (orchard), *Festuca* (fescue), *Lolium* (perennial rye), *Agrostis* (redtop), *Anthoxanthum* (vernal), *Phleum* (timothy)
Chloridoideae	*Cynodon* (Bermuda)
Panicoideae	*Paspalum* (Bahia), *Sorghum* (Johnson)
Herbaceous dicotyledons	
Chenopodiaceae	*Atriplex* (scales, saltbush), *Chenopodium* (lamb's quarter), *Salsola* (Russian thistle), *Kochia* (firebush)
Asteraceae	*Artemisia* (mugworts, wormwood, sages), *Ambrosia* (ragweeds), *Xanthium* (cocklebur)
Amaranthaceae	*Amaranthus* (careless weed, pigweeds), *Acnida* (Western water hemp)
Plantaginaceae	*Plantago* (plantain)
Polygonaceae	*Rumex* (dock, sorrel)
Trees	
Aceraceae	*Acer* (maples, box elder)
Betulaceae	*Alnus* (alder), *Betula* (birches), *Corylus* (hazelnut)
Cupressaceae	*Cupressus* (cypress), *Juniperus* (junipers, cedars), *Taxodium* (bald cypress)
Fabaceae	*Acacia* (mimosa), *Robinia* (locust), *Prosopis* (mesquite)
Fagaceae	*Quercus* (oaks), *Fagus* (beech)
Juglandaceae	*Carya* (hickory, pecan), *Juglans* (walnut)
Moraceae	*Morus* (mulberry)
Oleaceae	*Olea* (olive), *Fraxinus* (ash), *Ligustrum* (privet)
Pinaceae	*Pinus* (pines)
Platanaceae	*Platanus* (sycamore)
Salicaceae	*Populus* (cottonwood, poplars), *Salix* (willows)
Ulmaceae	*Ulmus* (elms)

[a]Representative genera are members of the same botanical family or subfamily. Manufacturers currently offer allergen products derived from one or more species of each listed genus.
Adapted from Davies JM, Weber RW. Aerobiology of outdoor allergens. In: Burks AW, Holgate S, O'Hehir R, Bacharier L, Broide D, Hershey GK, et al., editors. Middleton's allergy: principles and practice. 1. 9th ed. London: Elsevier; 2019:428–50.

pollenkitt, cytoplasm, and the intine and exine walls. In grass and ragweed pollens, cytoplasmic contents such as allergen-containing starch granules may be rapidly discharged through the germination pore. However, in tree pollens (e.g., birch), the expulsion of granules arises through the rupturing of the tips of emerging, abortive pollen tube growth.[13]

Allergenic Pollen

Grasses belong to a single family (Poaceae), and the majority of allergenic grasses (temperate and tropical) belong to the subfamilies Pooideae, Chloridoideae, and Panicoideae. Many allergens have been described with most, but not all, represented in the various grass subfamilies (Table 4.6). The allergens from different species and families have been grouped together, based on sequence identity. Pollens from herbaceous dicotyledon species, often referred to as *weeds*, may also be allergenic, particularly in species of the Amaranthaceae, Asteraceae, Euphorbiaceae, Plantaginaceae, and Urticaceae families (Table 4.7) but, unlike the unifamiliar grasses, the immunodominant groups vary both within and between families. However, allergenic cross-reactivity is high between biochemically identical allergens from different families, but marker allergens for some species (e.g., timothy grass) have been identified. With regard to tree pollens, allergens from both angiosperms and gymnosperms are clinically important (Table 4.8). The most clinically relevant angiosperm and families include the Fagales, the Lamiales and the Proteales, within each order, different allergen groups appear immunodominant (some of which are restricted to specific families). Allergens from the clinically important gymnosperm species, namely, cedar, juniper, and cypress have been described.

Pollen Allergens

Allergens from pollens are biochemically active and facilitate the pollination process, particularly pollen tube development (Tables 4.6–4.8). They include plant cell wall modifying enzymes, proteins associated with abiotic and biotic stressors, actin cytoskeleton–associated proteins, and calcium-binding proteins. Pollens from all plant types produce proteins that facilitate the emergence of the pollen tube, which may be achieved in different ways and involving biochemically different proteins/enzymes. These reflect cell wall carbohydrate polymer composition, but there are some similarities across the three pollen types. Many of these proteins are immunodominant allergens, although some may be minor. For example, the Group 1 β-expansins in grass pollen are prominent, whereas in weed and tree pollen, the pectin degrading polygalacturonases (e.g., Phl p 13, Pla a 2, Cry j 2), pectin lyases (e.g., Amb a 1, Art v 6, Cry j 1), and pectin methylesterases (e.g., Sal k 1, Cry j 1) dominate. Interestingly, analogous polymer-degrading enzymes have yet to be described in Fagales pollen and, similarly, the gymnosperm Group 1 pectate lyase allergens are absent from angiosperm tree pollen. All pollens contain allergenic proteases (e.g., Cyn d CP), which may also play a role in pollen tube growth by degrading the pellicle that covers the stigma.

Pollens have also been shown to contain proteins that are likely to play a role in protection against pathogens, given they

produced by pollen cones, entering the ovum via a pollen capture process. Here, pollen lands on a drop of fluid sitting atop the micropyle and then sinks into the ovum and only then does the pollen tube start to grow, a process that can take from weeks to months. When pollens land on the dry stigma or nasal membranes or water bodies, they hydrate through the microchannels in the pollen cell wall resulting in their expansion and activation. During this process, proteins (allergens) together with several pro-inflammatory molecules such as pollen-associated lipid mediators and adenosine may be released from orbicles,

TABLE 4.6 Physicochemical and Biochemical Characteristics of Grass Pollen Aeroallergens

Allergen	Frequency of Reactivity (%)[a]	Mol. Size (kDa)[b]	Function
Order Poales, Subfamily Poaceae: *Phleum pratense, Lolium perenne, Holcus lanatus, Dactylis glomerata, Agrostis longata, Oryza sativa, Secale cereale, Triticum aestivum, Poa pratensis*			
Subfamily Panicoideae: *Cynodon dactylon, Sorghum halepense, Paspalum notatum, Zea mays*			
Group 1 (e.g., Lol p 1)	>90	30	β-Expansin; involved in cell wall loosening; shows C-terminal sequence similarity with Group 2 and 3 allergens and the mite Group 2 allergen; C-terminal domain demonstrates oxidized cellulose binding activity, present in all Poaceae subfamilies
Group 2 (e.g., Lol p 2)	>60	11	Shows sequence similarity with the C-terminal half of Group 1 allergens; shows sequence similarity with Group 3 allergens
Group 3 (e.g., Lol p 3)	70	11	Shows sequence similarity with Group 1 and Group 2 allergens
Group 4 (e.g., Phl p 4)	22–92	57	Berberine bridge enzyme, member of flavoprotein oxidoreductase superfamily
Group 5 (e.g., Lol p 5)	62–80	29–31	Single-stranded nuclease with topoisomerase-like activity; shows sequence similarity with the Group 6 allergens; present in Pooideae subfamily only
Group 6 (e.g., Phl p 6)	14–64	11	Shows sequence similarity with Group 5 allergens; associated with P-particles, may be restricted to timothy grass pollen
Group 7 (e.g., Phl p 7)	>10	6	Polcalcin, 2EF-hand calcium-binding protein; shows sequence similarity with Bet v 4, Ole e 3, Aln g 4, Jun o 2
Group 10 (e.g., Lol p 10)	?	12	Cytochrome c
Group 11 (e.g., Lol p 11)	66	16	Function unknown; shows sequence similarity with tree allergen Ole e 1, lamb's quarters allergen Che a 1, and soybean trypsin inhibitor
Group 12 (e.g., Phl p 12)	20–36	14	Profilin
Group 13 (e.g., Phl p 13)	40–100	55–60	Polygalacturonase; degrades pectin, a major plant cell wall polymer of α-linked galacturonic acid
Group 15 (e.g., Cyn d 15)	?	9	β-Expansin, shows sequence similarity with other grass groups 1, 2, and 3
Group 22 (e.g., Cyn d 22)	?	48	Enolase, may be restricted to Bermuda grass pollen
Group 23 (e.g., Cyn d 23)	?	9	Function unknown
Group 24 (e.g., Cyn d 24)	66	21	Pathogenesis-related protein; PR-1
Cyn d CP	63	23	Cysteine protease; shows sequence similarity with enzymes from maize and rice, enzyme also found in timothy and Johnson grass pollen
Phl p CP	?	23	Cysteine protease
Cyn d EXY	75	30	Endoxylanase; shows sequence similarity with enzymes from maize and rice
Lol p Cyp	42	26	Cytophilin
Lol p FT	16	71.3	Fructosyltransferase
Lol p Legumin	21	38	11 S globulin

Data obtained from http://www.allergen.org and http://www.allergome.org or from original references.

Tables of allergens taken from Stewart GA, Robinson C. The structure and function of allergens. In: Burks AW, Holgate S, O'Hehir R, Bacharier L, Broide D, Hershey GK, et al., editors. Middleton's allergy: principles and practice. 1. 9th ed. London: Elsevier; 2019:387–427.

[a]Frequency data presented in these tables are indications only, because they will vary with the population studied, geographic location and the number of allergic individuals in a cohort. In addition, the data presented may reflect immediate hypersensitivity diseases, including atopic dermatitis and ABPA, as well as delayed-type hypersensitivity disease although this will be specifically indicated. "?" Indicates lack of data at the time of the publication although there is evidence of allergenicity. When frequency data are shown for allergens described in groups, the data refer to the example in parentheses. Classification of species throughout tables is derived from the Catalogue of Life (www.catalogueoflife.org).

share sequence similarity with 6 of the known 17 pathogenesis-related protein (PR) families (Table 4.9) found in nonpollen plant tissue.[14] Generally, they are minor allergens but some are immunodominant, including, for example, the PR-1 allergens, for example, Cyn d 24 and Art v 2; the PR-10 allergens, for example, the Group 1 Fagales allergens; the PR-12 allergens, for example, Par h 1; and the PR-14 allergens. The PR-14 related allergens are also involved in OAS or PFAS, in particular, the Group 1

TABLE 4.7   Physicochemical and Biochemical Characteristics of Pollen-Derived Aeroallergens From Herbaceous Dicotyledon (Weed) Species

Allergen	Frequency of Reactivity (%)	Mol. Size (kDa)	Function
Order Asterales, Asteraceae family: Short Ragweed (*A. artemisiifolia, A. elatior, A. psilostachya, A. trifida*)			
Group 1 (e.g., Amb a 1)[a]	>90	38	Pectate lyase, cleaved into two chains by pollen trypsin-like protease; shows sequence similarity with Art v 6; several isoforms exist; cleave pectin by eliminative cleavage rather than by hydrolysis
Group 3 (e.g., Amb a 3)	51	11	Plastocyanin, a copper-containing protein
Group 4 (e.g., Amb a 4)	20–39	30	Defensin-like protein with a proline-rich C-terminal domain; shows sequence similarity with Art v 1
Group 5 (e.g., Amb a 5)	10–15	5	Secreted basic protein
Group 6 (e.g., Amb a 6)	21	10	Nonspecific lipid transfer protein type 1
Group 7 (e.g., Amb a 7)	15–20	12	Plastocyanin, possible isoallergen of Amb a 3
Group 8 (e.g., Amb a 8)	25–56	14	Profilin
Group 9 (e.g., Amb a 9)	10–15	9	Polcalcin, 2EF-hand calcium-binding protein
Group 10 (e.g., Amb a 10)	9–26	17	Polcalcin, 3EF-hand binding protein
Group 11 (e.g., Amb a 11)	53	37	Cysteine protease
Group 12 (e.g., Amb a 12)	66	48	Enolase
Order Asterales, Asteraceae family: Mugwort (*Artemisia vulgaris, A. annua, A. absinthium, A. argyi, A. californica, A. ludoviciana, A. tridenta*)			
Art v 1	95	28	Plant defensin-like domain and a proline-rich domain (PR-12); the defensin-like domain shows sequence similarity with Amb a 4, Par h 1
Art v 2	58–63	20	Pathogenesis-related protein PR-1 like
Art v 3	25–56	12	Nonspecific lipid transfer protein type 1, recognition is a consequence of peach ingestion and sensitization
Art v 4	47–46	14	Profilin
Art v 5	0–28	10	Polcalcin, 2EF-hand calcium-binding protein
Art v 6	89	44	Pectate lyase; shows sequence similarity with Amb a 1
Art an 7	94	62	Galactose oxidase, may involve recognition due to presence of CCD
Order Asterales, Asteraceae family: Feverfew (*Parthenium hysterophorus*)			
Par h 1	>90	31	Defensin-like protein; contains a defensin-like domain fused to a proline-rich region (PR-12); the defensin-like domain shows sequence similarity with Amb a 4 and Art v 1
Order Asterales, Asteraceae family: Sunflower (*Helianthus annuus*)			
Hel a 1	57	34	Function unknown
Hel a 2	31	15	Profilin
Hel a 6	37	42	Pectate lyase
Order Rosales, Urticaceae Family: Wall Pellitory (*Parietaria judaica/officinalis*)			
Group 1 (e.g., Par o 1)	95	15	Nonspecific lipid transfer protein type 1, Par j 1.0101 isoform with a 37 amino acid extension possess LPS binding activity
Group 2 (e.g., Par o 2)	82	10–14	Nonspecific lipid transfer protein type 1
Group 3 (e.g., Par j 3)	6.5	14	Profilin
Group 4 (e.g., Par j 4)	6	9	Polcalcin, 2EF-hand calcium-binding protein

(Continued)

TABLE 4.7   Physicochemical and Biochemical Characteristics of Pollen-Derived Aeroallergens From Herbaceous Dicotyledon (Weed) Species—cont'd

Allergen	Frequency of Reactivity (%)	Mol. Size (kDa)	Function
Order Malpighiales, Euphorbiaceae Family: Annual Mercury (Mercurialis annua)			
Mer a 1	16	14	Profilin
Caryophyllales, Amaranthaceae Family			
Lamb's Quarters or Goosefoot (Chenopodium album)			
Che a 1	77	17	Ole e 1-related protein
Che a 2	50–60	14	Profilin
Che a 3	46	10	Polcalcin, 2EF-hand calcium-binding protein
Russian Thistle (S. kali)			
Sal k 1	67	43	Pectin methylesterase
Sal k 2	?	36	Protein kinase homolog
Sal k 3	67	45	Methionine synthase
Sal k 4	47	14	Profilin
Sal k 5	34–64	18	Ole e 1-like protein
Sal k 6	32	47	Polygalacturonase
Sal k 7	40	9	Polycalcin
Order Lamiales, Plantaginaceae Family: English Plantain (Plantago lanceolata)			
Pla l 1	86	18	Ole e 1-related protein
Pla l 2	71–86	15	Profilin

Both taxonomic Order and Family are indicated.

[a]Amb a 2 is now considered to be an isoallergen of Amb a 1 and is designated Amb a 1.05.

TABLE 4.8   Physicochemical and Biochemical Characteristics of Tree Pollen Aeroallergens

Allergen	Frequency of Reactivity (%)	Mol. Size (kDa)	Function
Angiosperms (Flowering Plants with Seeds Enclosed Within Fruit)			
Order Fagales, Fagaceae Family: Birch (Betula verrucosa), Alder (Alnus glutinosa), Hazel (Corylus avellana), Hornbeam (Carpinus betulus), Oak (Quercus alba), Chestnut (Castanea sativa)			
Group 1 (e.g., Bet v1)	>95	17	Plant steroid carrier; shows sequence similarity with pathogenesis-related proteins (e.g., PR-10)
Group 2 (e.g., Bet v 2)	5–37	15	Profilin
Group 3 (e.g., Bet v 3)	10	24	Polcalcin, 3EF-hand calcium-binding protein
Group 4 (e.g., Bet v 4)	20	7–8	Polcalcin, 2EF-hand calcium-binding protein; shows sequence similarity with Aln g 4, Ole e 3, Syr v 3
Group 6 (e.g., Bet v 6)	32	35	Isoflavone reductase, shows homology with Ole e 12
Group 7 (e.g., Bet v 7)	21	18	Peptidyl-prolyl cis-trans isomerase (cyclophilin)
Group 8 (e.g., Bet v 8)	13	27	Glutathione S-transferase
Bet v TLP	3–7[a]	25	Thaumatin-like protein
Order Lamiales, Oleaceae Family: Olive (Olea europaea), Lilac (Syringa vulgaris), Privet (Ligustrum vulgare), Ash (Fraxinus excelsior)			
Group 1 (e.g., Ole e 1)	>90	16	Shows limited sequence similarity with soybean trypsin inhibitor and Lol p 11
Group 2 (e.g., Ole e 2)	16–70	15	Profilin
Group 3 (e.g., Ole e 3)	20–>50	9	Polcalcin, 2EF-hand calcium-binding protein
Group 4 (e.g., Ole e 4)	80	32	Glucanase

(Continued)

TABLE 4.8 Physicochemical and Biochemical Characteristics of Tree Pollen Aeroallergens—cont'd

Allergen	Frequency of Reactivity (%)	Mol. Size (kDa)	Function
Group 5 (e.g., Ole e 5)	35	16	Cu/Zn superoxide dismutase
Group 6 (e.g., Ole e 6)	5–20	10	Cysteine-rich protein
Group 7 (e.g., Ole e 7)	47–100	10	Nonspecific lipid transfer protein type 1
Group 8 (e.g., Ole e 8)	13	21	Polcalcin, 4EF-hand calcium-binding protein
Group 9 (e.g., Ole e 9)	65	46	β-1,3-Glucanase (Family 17), contains a carbohydrate-binding domain; shows sequence similarity with peptide originally designated Ole e 10
Group 10 (e.g., Ole e 10)	55	11	Shows sequence similarity with the C-terminal domain of Ole e 9, carbohydrate-binding module CBM-43
Group 11 (e.g., Ole e 11)	62–65	37	Pectate methylesterase
Group 12 (e.g., Ole e 12)	35	37	Isoflavone reductase, shows homology with Bet v 6
Group 13	2–7[a]	23	Thaumatin-like protein
Group 14 (e.g., Ole e 14)	13	47	Polygalacturonase
Group 15 (e.g., Ole e 15)	22	19	Cyclophilin
Order Proteales, Platanaceae Family: London Plane Tree (Platanus acerifolia) *and American Sycamore* (P. orientalis)			
Pla a 1	87	18	Invertase/pectin methylesterase inhibitor
Pla a 2	83	43	Polygalacturonase
Pla a 3	61	10	Nonspecific lipid transfer protein type 1
Pla a TLP	7–21[a]	25	Thaumatin-like protein
Gymnosperms (Conifers: Fruitless, Flowerless Plants Where Seeds are on Surface of Scales or Leaves) *Order Cupressales, Cupressaceae Family: Juniper Species (e.g.,* **Juniperus ashei, J. rigida, J. virginiana, J. oxycedrus, J. sabinoides),** *Cypress (e.g.,* **Cupressus sempervirens, C. arizonica),** *Japanese Cypress* **(Chamaecyparis obtusa),** *Japanese Cedar* **(Cryptomeria japonica)**			
Group 1 (e.g., Jun a 1)	71	43	Pectate lyase
Group 2 (e.g., Jun a 2)	100	43	Polygalacturonase
Group 3 (e.g., Jun a 3)	33	30	Thaumatin-like protein, osmotin, and amylase/trypsin inhibitor; PR-5–related
Group 4 (e.g., Jun o 4)	15	29	Polcalcin, 4EF-hand calcium-binding protein
Group 7 (e.g., Jun a 7)	100[b]	7	Gibberellin-regulated protein, Cypmaclein; member of a cysteine-rich antimicrobial protein family. Homologous allergen associated with peach allergy
Cha o 3	88	63	Cellulase (glycosyl hydrolase)

[a]Higher value associated with patients with food allergy.
[b]Frequency determined in patients with both pollinosis and peach allergy.

Lamiales allergens, for example, Bet v 1. Initial sensitization to the pollen results in the production of IgE which, due to cross-reactivity with similar allergens, causes oral symptoms in uncooked fruit and vegetables. Similar reactions may occur with pollen-derived lipid transfer proteins (e.g., Amb a 6) and the profilin allergens (e.g., Bet v 2). The function of some immunodominant allergens remains unclear, for example, the Lamiales Group 1 allergens but immunodominant homologs are found in both grasses and weeds (e.g., Lol p 11 and Che a 1). Other immunodominant pollen allergens (e.g., the grass pollen Group 4 berberine bridge enzymes) may also play a defense function because of their role in the production of secondary metabolites such as phytoalexin and alkaloids.

Outdoor Allergens—Fungi

Fungi are significant sources of allergens, and the incidence of fungal allergy within people with atopy and asthma may be high (up to 44% and 80%, respectively). A large number of species have been shown to be allergenic and many allergens characterized but the clinically relevant species belong to Ascomycota and Basidiomycota (Table 4.10).[11,15] All use airborne conidia (spores) dispersal for reproduction, and the spores comprise cytoplasm surrounded by a wall made up of three layers (mannoproteins, glucans, and chitin). They are often produced in concentrations exceeding those seen with pollens by orders of magnitude. Meteorological conditions play an important role in spore release. For example, dry and windy conditions are important for species belonging to the Ascomycota whereas humidity plays an important role in species from the Basidiomycota. The most important indoor fungal allergens are derived from Ascomycota species (Fig. 4.5). Many of the important species are saprophytic and have evolved to live in soil and on decaying organic matter using extracellular digestion. This is achieved by

TABLE 4.9 Relationship Between Plant Pathogenesis-Related Proteins and Allergens

Family	Description or Characteristics	Typical Size (kDa)	Grass/Weed Pollen Allergen	Tree Pollen Allergen
PR-1	Antifungal, mechanism unknown	15	Art v 2, Cyn d 24	
PR-2	Endo-β-1,3-glucanases	30		Ole e 4/9
PR-5	Thaumatin-like proteins; antifungal; may have endo-β-1,3-glucanase activity	25		Cry j 3, Jun a 3 Cup a 3
PR-10[a]	Plant steroid carrier (ribonuclease-like)	17		Bet v 1, Cor a 1, Aln g 1
PR-12	Defensins	5	Art v 1, Amb a 4	
PR-14	Non-specific lipid transfer proteins	9	Art v 3, Amb a 6, Par j 1, 2, Amb a 6, Art v 3	Ole e 7

[a]Members of this PR family are involved in OAS/PFAS.
Modified from Stewart GA, Robinson C. The structure and function of allergens. In: Burks AW, Holgate S, O'Hehir R, Bacharier L, Broide D, Hershey GK, et al., editors. Middleton's allergy: principles and practice. 1. 9th ed. London: Elsevier; 2019:387–427.

TABLE 4.10 Physicochemical and Biochemical Characteristics of Indoor and Outdoor Fungi-Derived Aeroallergens

Allergen	Frequency of Reactivity (%)	Mol. Size (kDa)	Function
Phylum Ascomycota			
Alternaria alternata			
Alt a 1	>80	16	Secreted protein homologous with the fungal cytotoxin mitogillin from *Aspergillus restrictus* and α-sarcin from *Aspergillus giganteus*
Alt a 2	0–61	25	Shows very high homology (>98%) with bacterial adenosine triphosphate (ATP) binding proteins
Alt a 3	5	70	Heat shock protein 70
Alt a 4	42	57	Protein disulfide isomerase
Alt a 5	8	11	Ribosomal P_2 protein; shows sequence similarity with Cla h 5
Alt a 6	22	45	Enolase
Alt a 7	7	22	Flavodoxin, electron transfer protein; shows sequence similarity Cla h 7
Alt a 8	41	29	Mannitol dehydrogenase
Alt a 10	2	53	Aldehyde dehydrogenase; shows sequence similarity with Cla h 10
Alt a 12	?	11	Acid ribosomal P1 protein
Alt a 13	?	26	Glutathione *S*-transferase
Alt a 14	?	24	Manganese superoxide dismutase, shows homology with Asp f 6
Alt a 15	6	58	Subtilisin-like serine protease
Cladosporium herbarum			
Cla h 2	43	23	Function unknown
Cla h 5	22	11	Acidic ribosomal protein P2 (previously Cla h 4)
Cla h 6	20	46	Enolase
Cla h 7	22	22	Flavodoxin, electron transfer protein; shows sequence similarity Alt a 7
Cla h 8	57	28	Mannitol dehydrogenase
Cla h 9	16	45	Subtilisin-like protease
Cla h 10	36	53	Aldehyde dehydrogenase
Cla h 12	?	11	Acidic ribosomal P1 protein
Cla h HSP70	38	70	Heat shock protein 70
Cla h TCTP	50	19	Histamine-releasing factor, shows sequence similarity with human translationally controlled tumor protein (TCTP)
Aspergillus fumigatus			
Asp f 1	85	17	Ribonuclease; ribotoxin shows sequence similarity with mitogillin
Asp f 2	96[a]	37	Shows sequence similarity with *Candida albicans* fibrinogen-binding protein

(Continued)

TABLE 4.10 Physicochemical and Biochemical Characteristics of Indoor and Outdoor Fungi-Derived Aeroallergens—cont'd

Allergen	Frequency of Reactivity (%)	Mol. Size (kDa)	Function
Asp f 3	72	19	Peroxisomal membrane protein; belongs to the peroxiredoxin family; thiol-dependent peroxidase
Asp f 4	0–83[a]	30	Shows sequence similarity with bacterial ATP-binding cassette (ABC) transporter–binding protein; associated with peroxisome
Asp f 5	74–93[a]	40	Metalloprotease
Asp f 6	0–56[a]	27	Manganese superoxide dismutase; shows sequence similarity with Alt a 14, Mal s 11
Asp f 7	7–46[a]	12	Shows sequence similarity with fungal riboflavin, aldehyde-forming enzyme
Asp f 8	8–15[a]	11	Ribosomal P_2 protein
Asp f 9	31–89[a]	34	Shows sequence similarity with plant and bacterial endo-β1,3;1,4-glucanases
Asp f 10	3–28[a]	34	Aspartic protease
Asp f 11	90	24	Peptidyl-prolyl cis-trans isomerase (cyclophilin)
Asp f 12	?	90	Heat shock protein P90
Asp f 13	?[a]	34	Subtilisin-like protease
Asp f 15	?	16	Cerato-platanin, only found in fungi and thought to function as cell wall loosening agents akin to the expansins in plant pollen
Asp f 16	0–70[a]	43	Glycosyl hydrolase, shows homology with Asp f 9
Asp f 17	?	27	Galactomannoprotein
Asp f 18	79	34	Subtilisin-like protease
Asp f 22	30	46	Enolase, shows sequence similarity with Pen c 22
Asp f 23	27	44	L3 ribosomal protein
Asp f 27	75	18	Peptidyl-prolyl cis-trans isomerase (cyclophilin)
Asp f 28	30	13	Thioredoxin
Asp f 29	50	13	Thioredoxin
Asp f 34	93	20	Phi A cell wall protein
Penicillium brevicompactum			
Pen b 13	91	33	Alkaline serine protease
Pen b 26	73	11	Acidic ribosomal protein P1
Penicillium chrysogenum (Formally notatum)			
Pen ch 13	>80	34	Subtilisin-like protease
Pen ch 18	77–100	32	Subtilisin-like protease
Pen ch 20	56	68	β-N-acetylglucosaminidase from *Candida albicans*
Pen ch 31	?	?	Calreticulin, a calcium-binding protein
Pen ch 33	?	16	Hypothetical protein
Pen ch 35	?	37	Transaldolase
Penicillium citrinum			
Pen c 3	46	18	Peroxisomal membrane protein; belongs to the peroxiredoxin family; thiol-dependent peroxidase
Pen c 13	?	33	Subtilisin-like protease
Pen c 19	41	70	Heat shock protein P70
Pen c 22	30	46	Enolase
Pen c 24	8	25	Elongation factor 1β
Pen c 30	48	97	Catalase
Pen c 32	100[c]	40	Pectate lyase
Penicillium oxalicum			
Pen o 18	89	34	Subtilisin-like protease

(Continued)

TABLE 4.10 Physicochemical and Biochemical Characteristics of Indoor and Outdoor Fungi-Derived Aeroallergens—cont'd

Allergen	Frequency of Reactivity (%)	Mol. Size (kDa)	Function
Candida albicans/boidinii			
Cand a 1	77	40	Alcohol dehydrogenase
Cand b 2	100	20	Peroxisomal membrane protein A
Cand a 3	56	29	Function unknown
Trichophyton rubrum			
Tri r 2	43	29	Subtilisin-like protease
Tri r 4	?	85	Dipeptidyl peptidase
Curvularia lunata			
Cur l 1	80	31	Subtilisin-like protease
Cur l 2	75	48	Enolase
Cur l 3	60	12	Cytochrome c
Cur l 4	81	54	Subtilisin-like protease
Phylum Basidiomycota			
Malassezia furfur			
Mala f 2	72	21	Peroxisomal membrane protein; belongs to the peroxiredoxin family, thiol-dependent peroxidase; shows sequence similarity with Asp f 3
Mala f 3	70	20	Peroxisomal membrane protein; belongs to the peroxiredoxin family, thiol-dependent peroxidase; shows sequence similarity with Asp f 3, Mala f 2
Mala f 4	83	35	Mitochondrial malate dehydrogenase
Malassezia sympodialis			
Mala s 1	61	37	Function unknown; cell wall protein
Mala s 5	19–35	18	Oxidoreductase
Mala s 6	21–92	17	Peptidyl-prolyl cis-trans isomerase (cyclophilin)
Mala s 7	60	16	Function unknown
Mala s 8	72	19	Function unknown
Mala s 9	36	37	Function unknown
Mala s 10	69	86	Heat shock protein P70
Mala s 11	75	23	Manganese superoxide dismutase; shows sequence similarity with Asp f 6
Mala s 12	62[b]	67	Glucose–methanol–choline (GMC) oxidoreductase
Mala s 13	50	13	Thioredoxin
Coprinus comatus			
Cop c 1	34	11	Leucine zipper protein
Cop c 2	?	12	Thioredoxin
Cop c 3	?	37	Nucleotide binding protein
Cop c 5	?	16	Function unknown
Cop c 7	?	16	Function unknown
Psilocybe cubensis			
Psi c 1	?	46	Function unknown
Psi c 2	82	16	Peptidyl-prolyl cis-trans isomerase (cyclophilin)

HSP, Heat shock protein; NaDP, nicotinamide-adenine dinucleotide phosphate.
[a]Higher frequency determined in patients with ABPA.
[b]Tested using M. sympodialis-sensitized atopic asthmatic patients.
[c]Based on three patients.

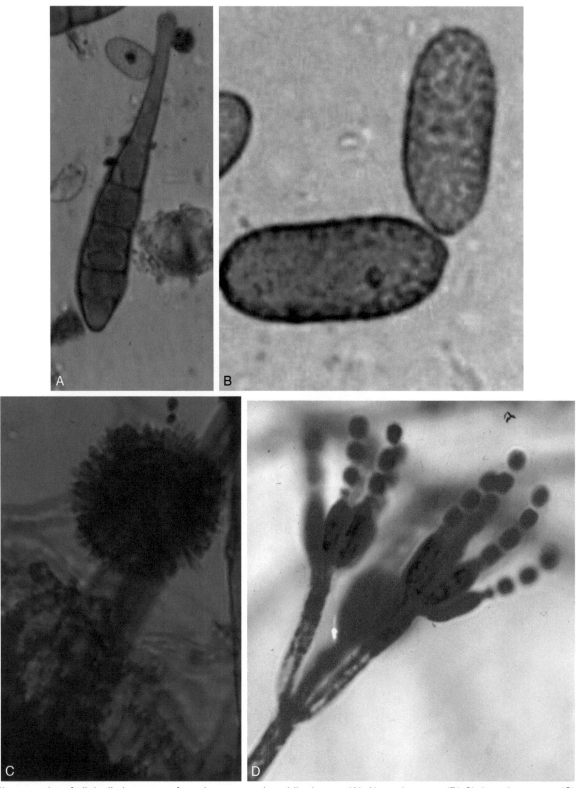

Fig. 4.5 Photographs of clinically important fungal spores and conidiophores. (A) *Alternaria* spore, (B) *Cladosporium* spore, (C) *Aspergillus* conidiophore and (D) *Penicillium* conidiophore. (Figure from Stewart GA, Robinson C. The structure and function of allergens. In: Burks AW, Holgate S, O'Hehir R, Bacharier L, Broide D, Hershey GK, et al., editors. Middleton's Allergy: Principles and Practice. 9th ed. London: Elsevier; 2019:387–427.)

secreting a variety of hydrolases (e.g., proteases, amylases, carbohydrases such as pectinases and cellulases, and lipases) that break down complex organic molecules in plant cell walls and passively absorbing catabolites. Similarly, fungal proteases play a role in spore release.

The Ascomycetes of aeroallergenic importance include the saprophytes *Alternaria*, *Cladosporium*, *Penicillium*, *Curvularia*, and *Candida* species. While the number of immunodominant allergens in these species varies with regard to biochemical identity, it is likely that they are all secreted rather than cytoplasmic proteins

(Fig. 4.5) (Table 4.10). They include a cytotoxic mitogillin, mannitol dehydrogenase, and serine proteases. However, they demonstrate varying similarities with regard to the presence of minor allergens, most of which are derived from the cytoplasm such as enolases, heat shock proteins (HSPs), aldehyde dehydrogenases, thioredoxins, and cyclophilins (peptidyl-prolyl isomerase) (Table 4.10).

The other clinically important Ascomycete aeroallergen source is *Aspergillus*, which also plays a role in a number of other clinical conditions in which IgE production is stimulated, notably, allergic bronchopulmonary aspergillosis (ABPA). At least 33 allergens have been described with several (secreted) being established as immunodominant using sera from rhinitis and asthma patients (e.g., Asp f 1, ribonuclease) and some of cytoplasmic origin using sera from patients with ABPA (e.g., Asp f 5, metalloprotease). The clinically minor Ascomycetes such as *Candida* and *Curvularia* also produce serine proteases, dipeptidyl peptidases, aspartic proteases, enolases, and peroxisomal membrane proteins or are of unknown

function (Table 4.10). The dermatophyte species *Trichophyton* also produces allergens such as serine proteases that play a role in asthma. Basidiomycetes also produce allergens, in particular, those species involved in atopic dermatitis such as *Malassezia* species. The immunodominant allergens include peroxisomal membrane proteins (Mala f 2, 3) and malate dehydrogenase (Mala f 4).

Outdoor Allergens—Stinging and Biting Arthropods

Venoms of bees, wasps, ants, and hornets contain various components, including, for example, enzymes, vasoactive compounds, neurotoxins, and phospholipids, several of which are allergenic, with the potential to cause local and systemic (anaphylaxis) reactions in sensitized patients. It is estimated that the prevalence of insect allergy is about 5% to 7.5% of a population, although several-fold higher in beekeepers. At least 12 allergen groups have been delineated for honeybee, including various enzymes and melittin (Table 4.11). Melittin accounts

TABLE 4.11 Physicochemical and Biochemical Characteristics of Outdoor Arthropod-Derived Allergens

Allergen	Frequency of Reactivity (%)	Mol. Size (kDa)	Function
Envenomating Insects			
Apidae			
Honey Bee *(Apis mellifera, A. cerana, A. dorsata, A. florea)*			
Group 1 (e.g., Api m 1)	12–91	16	Phospholipase A$_2$
Group 2 (e.g., Api m 2)	48–100	39	Hyaluronidase; shows sequence similarity with yellow jacket wasp allergen Ves v 2
Group 3 (e.g., Api m 3)	38–50	43	Acid phosphatase
Group 4 (e.g., Api m 4)	23	3	Melittin
Group 5 (e.g., Api m 5)	58	100	Dipeptidyl peptidase IV; shows sequence similarity with Ves v 3
Group 6 (e.g., Api m 6)	42–88	8	Serine protease inhibitor
Group 7 (e.g., Api m 7)	?	39	CUB (Complement C1r/C1s, Uegf, Bmp1) serine protease
Group 8 (e.g., Api m 8)	46	70	Carboxylesterase
Group 9 (e.g., Api m 9)	80	60	Serine carboxypeptidase
Group 10 (e.g., Api m 10)	52–75	50–55	Icarapin variant 2
Group 11 (e.g., Api m 11)	15–34	50	Major jelly protein
Group 12 (e.g., Api m 12)	47	200	Vitellogenin; shows sequence similarity with Ves v 6
Bumble Bee **(Bombus pensylvanicus/terrestris)**			
Group 1 (e.g., Bom p 1)	82	16	Phospholipase A$_2$
Group 2 (e.g., Bom p 2)	82	39	Hyaluronidase
Group 3 (e.g., Bom p 3)	82	49	Acid phosphatase
Group 4 (e.g., Bom p 4)	82	27	Protease
Vespidae			
White-Faced and Yellow Hornets *(Dolichovespula Species)*, Paper Wasps *(Polistes species)*, and Yellow Jackets *(Vespula species)*			
Group 1 (e.g., Pol a 1)	46	34	Phospholipase A$_1$
Group 2 (e.g., Ves v 2)	50–76	39	Hyaluronidase
Group 3 (e.g., Ves v 3)	50	100	Dipeptidyl peptidase IV
Group 4 (e.g., Pol d 4)	?	32–34	Serine protease
Group 5 (e.g., Ves v 5)	51–90	23	Belongs to the cysteine-rich secretory (SCP) family of proteins (includes PR-1 plant proteins); shows sequence similarity with group 3 allergens from fire ant
Group 6 (e.g., Ves v 6)	39	200	Vitellogenin

(Continued)

TABLE 4.11   Physicochemical and Biochemical Characteristics of Outdoor Arthropod-Derived Allergens—cont'd

Allergen	Frequency of Reactivity (%)	Mol. Size (kDa)	Function
Formicidae			
Fire Ant *(Solenopsis invicta, S. geminata, S. richteri, S. saevissima)*			
Group 1 (e.g., Sol i 1)	87	18	Phospholipase A$_1$
Group 2 (e.g., Sol i 2)	61	14	Function unknown
Group 3 (e.g., Sol i 3)	61	26	SCP domain containing family of proteins. Shows sequence similarity with the vespid group 5 allergens
Group 4 (e.g., Sol i 4)	74	12	Shows sequence similarity with Sol i 2
Australian Jumper Ant (Myrmecia pilosula)			
Myr p 1	52	9	Pilosulin 1, histamine-releasing protein
Myr p 2	35	5	Pilosulin 3
Myr p 3	?	9	Pilosulin 4.1
Hematophagous Insects			
Culicidae			
Mosquito *(Aedes aegypti, A. albopictus, Anopheles darlingi, Culex aegypti)*			
Aed a 1	29–65	68	Apyrase
Aed a 2	11–32	37	Female specific protein D7
Aed a 3	32	30	Function unknown
Aed a 4	47	67	α-Glucosidase
Aed a 5	67	22	Sarcoplasmic calcium-binding protein
Aed a 6	33	31	Porin 3
Aed a 7	50	24	Function unknown
Aed a 8	83	70	Heat shock protein 70
Aed a 10	60	32	Tropomyosin
Aed a 11	50	42	Lysosomal aspartate protease
Pulicidae			
Cat Flea *(Ctenocephalides felis)*			
Cte f 1	80[a]	18	Function unknown
Cte f 2	?	27	Salivary protein; shows sequence similarity with ant Sol i 3 allergen and vespid group 5 allergens
Cte f 3	40[a]	25	Function unknown
Tabaninae			
Horse Fly *(Tabanus yao)*			
Tab y 1	81–100	70	Apyrase
Tab y 2	91	35	Hyaluronidase
Tab y 5	86	26	Shows sequence similarity with wasp venom antigen 5
Argasidae			
Pigeon Tick *(Argasidae reflexus)*			
Arg r 1	100	17	Lipocalin
Reduviidae			
Kissing Bug *(Triatoma protracta)*			
Tria p 1	89	20	Procalin, a member of the lipocalin family; shows sequence similarity with triabin, a thrombin inhibitor
Chinese Red-Headed Centipede (Scolopendra mutilans)			
Sco m 5	83	20	Venom allergen 5

for approximately 50% of the injected venom in this species (although absent from wasps and ants) and causes pain by activation of transient receptor potential channels and nociceptive sodium channels.

Allergenic enzymes present in bees include phospholipase A_2, the Group 2 hyaluronidases, the Group 3 acid phosphatases, and various peptidases (Table 4.11). Some enzymes are common to wasps, such as the hyaluronidases and acid phosphatases, but the phospholipase present in wasp venom is type A_1, which cleaves phospholipid differently to type A_2. The Group 5 allergens are major allergens in wasps, but absent from bee venom. They belong to a family of cysteine-rich secretory proteins (CAP) homologous with PR-1 proteins and those associated with mammalian reproduction. Additionally, other venom enzymes show sequence similarity with sperm hyaluronidases and prostatic-like acid phosphatases, suggesting they probably evolved from proteins associated with insect reproduction. Attempts have been made to determine venom-associated marker allergens, but cross-reactivity between certain groups of allergens is high.

Several venom allergens have also been described in the fire and jumper ants, some of which correspond to those in wasp or bee venoms such as the vespid Group 5 allergen and phospholipase A_1, although minor (Table 4.11). The major but not immunodominant allergen in the jumper ant is pilosulin, a basic, low molecular weight peptide, whereas the major fire ant allergen has unknown function. The major ant venom allergens are the Group 2 proteins of unknown function. Saliva from hematophagous insects such as fleas, mosquitos, and horse flies contains several minor and major allergens (Table 4.6). Most extensively studied is the mosquito, in which at least 15 allergen groups have been delineated. Compared with other allergen sources, no allergen dominates, but a mixture of Aed a 6, Aed a 8, and Aed a 10 identifies more than 80% of mosquito-allergic individuals.

INDOOR ALLERGENS

When describing indoor allergens in the context of respiratory allergy, we are principally referring to those present in reservoir house-dust (floor and bedding) and to fungal allergens released from contaminated walls and fixture (see the previous section). In this regard, the significance of house-dust as a cause of allergic disease was first recognized by Kern in 1921, who observed that many patients with rhinitis or asthma had positive skin responses to an extract of dust from their own homes. It is a compositionally diverse matrix comprising components from HDMs, mammals, insects, fungal spores, and pollen grains, as well as materials introduced from the outside world (Box 4.2). However, a major advance in our understanding of house-dust allergenicity was the discovery, in 1967, by Voorhorst et al. that the HDM, D. pteronyssinus, was an important source of indoor allergens.[16] In humid temperate climates, HDMs trigger the development of high allergen-specific IgE titers in susceptible individuals and they form the single most important allergen source associated with asthma. Given the largely sedentary, indoor lifestyle in affluent countries coupled with the creation

BOX 4.2	Sources of Allergens in House-Dust	
Source and origin	Form	Examples
Acarids—house-dust mites, indoors	Fecal pellets and body debris	*Dermatophagoides pteronyssinus* *Dermatophagoides farinae* *Euroglyphus maynei* *Blomia tropicalis* Storage mites
Arachnids—spiders, indoors		
Mammals, indoors	Danders	Pets Cats *(Felis domesticus)* Dogs *(Canis familiaris)* Rabbits Ferrets Rodents—pets such as mice, gerbils, guinea pigs, chinchilla, and others Rodents—pests such as mice *(Mus musculus)* and rats *(Rattus norvegicus)*
Insects, indoors	Fecal pellets and body debris	Cockroaches: *Blattella germanica* (German cockroach) *Periplaneta americana* (American cockroach) *Blatta orientalis* (Oriental cockroach) Others: *Harmonia axyridis* (Asian lady beetle) Crickets Flies Fleas Moths Midges Silverfish *(Lepisma saccharina)*
Fungi, indoors	Spores and mycelium	*Penicillium* *Aspergillus* *Cladosporium* (growing on surfaces of rotting wood) Other species
Fungi, outdoors	Spores	Multiple species from entry with incoming air
Pollens, outdoors	Whole pollen and aerosolized contents	Multiple species from entry with incoming air
Miscellaneous, indoors		Horse hair from furniture Kapk (insulation, fillings, silky fibers from ceiba tree) Food remnants

Adapted from Matsui E, Thomas AE, Platts-Mills TAE. Indoor allergens. In: Burks AW, Holgate S, O'Hehir R, Bacharier L, Broide D, Hershey GK, et al., editors. Middleton's allergy: principles and practice. 1. 9th ed. London: Elsevier; 2019:451–466.

of warm, draught-free, and increasingly humid living and working conditions, human exposure to HDMs is extreme—up to 23 h/day—with important consequences for allergic disease.

Population-based, cross-sectional and prospective studies show that individuals with specific IgE to one or more major allergens derived from house-dust, particularly HDMs, are significantly more likely to have asthma than nonsensitized individuals.[17–21] Historically, chronic rhinitis, asthma, atopic dermatitis, conjunctivitis, and urticaria, but rarely anaphylaxis, have been associated with exposure to HDM or other indoor allergens. In the case of atopic dermatitis, the epidemiologic evidence is mainly from HDM sensitization, with high IgE (>30 IU/mL) strongly associated with the condition. A common finding in surveys of allergic sensitization is that up to 15% of asymptomatic individuals are sensitized to an indoor allergen. This raises questions about why and how individuals become sensitized and why only some develop clinical symptoms.

Mammalian allergens may also be a prominent feature of domestic or occupational dusts and are encountered in the form of cat, dog, rat, and mouse proteins from pets, from domestic rodent infestations or in animal rearing institutions. The aerodynamics of the particles carrying cat and dog allergens differ from those associated with mite and cockroach allergens and confer them with greater airborne persistence. This results in cat and dog allergens becoming widely distributed by passive carriage on people.[22] Dogs, especially, may bring significant lipopolysaccharide (LPS) from Gram-negative bacteria as well as bacteriologic diversity into the home, and there are reasons to believe this may further influence the development of allergy.

In addition to the above, fungi can be detected in reservoir house-dust, and several studies link their presence with allergic diseases, including asthma, for example, high fungal contamination of homes with infants, determined using the environmental relative moldiness index (ERMI), was a predictor of asthma at age 7.[23] In other studies, remediation of dampness in homes with a high ERMI resulted in reduced hospitalization of asthmatic children. The main species in house-dust are *Cladosporium*, *Penicillium*, and *Aspergillus*. However, a link between fungal allergen-specific IgE and specific fungal allergen concentrations in dust and allergic disease, as shown for arthropod and mammalian allergens, has not been clearly determined. Despite this, it should be noted that fungi not only stimulate IgE production but may have non–IgE-mediated detrimental effects on lung health due to proteases and cell wall constituents such as chitin and β-glucan that activate pattern recognition receptors (PRRs),[24] which will be discussed in a later section.

Indoor Allergen Sources—Nonmammalian

Arthropods, particularly from the Insecta and Arachnida classes, are the main nonmammalian sources of indoor allergens. Of these, HDMs and cockroaches are clinically important, with their allergens being derived from whole bodies, salivary secretions, and fecal pellets accumulating in house-dust.

Acaridae

Mites are eight-legged, sightless creatures living on a diet of skin and other debris such as bacteria shed from human bodies. The clinically important species belong to the Pyroglyphidae, Acaridae, Glycyphagidae, and Echimyopodidae families. While

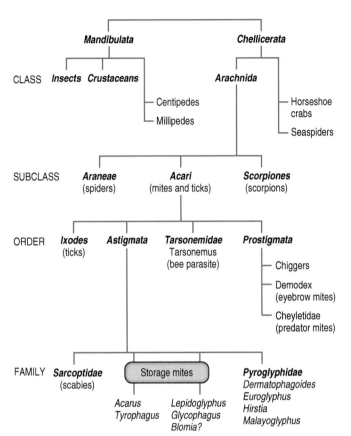

Fig. 4.6 Phylogenetic relationships between different arthropods, showing the clinically important mite genera. (From Matsui E, Thomas AE, Platts-Mills TAE. Indoor allergens. In: Burks AW, Holgate S, O'Hehir R, Bacharier L, Broide D, Hershey GK, et al., editors. Middleton's allergy: principles and practice. 1. London: Elsevier; 2019:451–466.) (Middletons 9e, Figure 28.2.)

many mite species are found in house-dust, in most parts of the world, the pyroglyphid family (e.g., *D. pteronyssinus*, *D. farinae*, and *E. maynei*), dominates (Fig. 4.6). In tropical or semi-tropical climates, allergy to *B. tropicalis* may also be prevalent. Domestic dwellings can also contain mites usually associated with stored agricultural products such as grains (e.g., *Lepidoglyphus destructor*, *Tyrophagus putrescentior*) and large predator mites of the family Cheyletidae or the smaller *Tarsonemus* spp.

HDMs thrive in a warm, moist environment and, accordingly, mite abundance is seasonal (Fig. 4.7). The optimum growth temperature for mites is 65 to 80°F (18 to 27°C), and there is a requirement for atmospheric moisture (75% relative humidity, RH), which is absorbed through their leg joints or produced through metabolism since they are unable to drink. Domestic environments often show significant microclimatic variation such that when free air is relatively dry, HDMs are able to withdraw into the pockets of humidity within carpets, soft furnishings, and clothing so that even with dehumidification (<50% RH) it may take months for mites to die, and longer for allergen levels to decline.

HDMs excrete digested food mixed with their digestive enzymes, other proteins, and endosymbiotic bacteria as fecal pellets surrounded by a chitinous peritrophic membrane.[25] Although indoor allergens are carried on particles that are amorphous compared to pollen or fungal spores found outdoors,

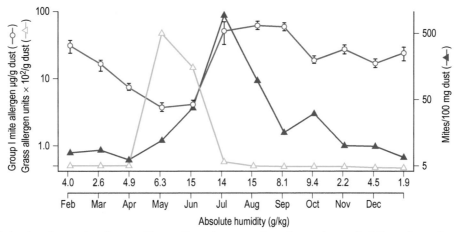

Fig. 4.7 Seasonal variation in mites, mite allergen (Group 1), and grass pollen allergen in a sofa followed over 1 year in central Virginia. A sharp rise in mite numbers (▲-▲) follows the rise in outdoor absolute humidity. Mite allergen levels rise during the summer but remain high until after Christmas (○-○). Allergen from ryegrass pollen (△-△) was detected only in May, June, and July. (Adapted from Platts-Mills TA, Hayden ML, Chapman MD, et al. Seasonal variation in dust mite and grass pollen allergens in dust from the houses of patients with asthma. J Allergy Clin Immunol 1987;79:781; Matsui E, Thomas AE, Platts-Mills TAE. Indoor allergens. In: Burks AW, Holgate S, O'Hehir R, Bacharier L, Broide D, Hershey GK, et al., editors. Middleton's Allergy: Principles and Practice. 9th ed. London: Elsevier; 2019:451–466.)

HDM fecal pellets are similar in diameter to some pollen grains (10–35 μm), with a similar allergen load (~0.2 ng). As with pollens, the contents of the pellets are rapidly released after impacting upon the hydrating and reducing agent-rich environment of airway surface liquid, creating a high concentration of enzymatically active allergens (e.g., the Group 1 allergens) at the site of deposition.

Mite species produce numerous allergens, and the first mite allergens to be cloned were Der p 1, Der p 2, and Der p 5 in the late 1980s. Almost 40 groups of allergenic proteins are now denominated and they comprise digestive enzymes (e.g., cysteine proteases, trypsins, chymotrypsins, amylases, and chitinases), actin-associated proteins (e.g., tropomyosin, troponin C, and paramyosin), ligand-binding proteins, or proteins of unknown function (Table 4.12). According to immunodominance, the major HDM allergens have generally been considered to be those of Groups 1 and 2, followed by the intermediate allergen Groups 4, 5, and 6, and then a large group of minor allergens. However, more recently, other allergens such as the peritrophin-A related allergen involved in the formation of the chitin-containing peritrophic membrane (Der p 15) (Fig. 4.8), and ubiquinol-cytochrome c reductase binding protein-like protein (Der f 24)[26] have now been added to the immunodominant list.

Insecta

Insects such as cockroaches, moths, crickets, locusts, beetles, non-biting midges, lake flies, houseflies, and lady beetles are established allergy triggers, but of these, cockroaches form the most significant allergenic insect threat in the indoor environment, particularly in the inner-city areas of the US.[27]

TABLE 4.12 Physicochemical and Biochemical Characteristics of Arthropod-Derived Indoor Allergens

Allergen	Frequency of Reactivity (%)	Mol. Size (kDa)	Function
Class Insecta: Order Diptera			
Chironomidae* (non-biting midges), *Chironomus thummi, Cladotanytarsus lewisi, Polypedilum nubifer, Chironomus kiiensis			
Groups 1–9 (e.g., Chi t I to 9)	>50	15	Hemoglobin
Group 10 (e.g., Chi k 10)	81	33	Tropomyosin
Superorder: Dictyoptera, Order *Blattodea*, Family Ectobiidae: German Cockroach *(Blattella germanica)* and American Cockroach *(Periplaneta americana)*			
Group 1 (e.g., Bla g 1)	1–77	46	Function unknown, may be involved in lipid transport; contains three insect allergen–related repeat, nitrile-specifier detoxification domains, although such a detoxification role has not been demonstrated
Group 2 (e.g., Bla g 2)	7–62	36	Aspartate protease (pseudoprotease); shows sequence similarity with pepsin

(Continued)

TABLE 4.12   Physicochemical and Biochemical Characteristics of Arthropod-Derived Indoor Allergens—cont'd

Allergen	Frequency of Reactivity (%)	Mol. Size (kDa)	Function
Group 3 (e.g., Per a 3)	26–95	79	Arthropod hemocyanin; hexameric copper-containing proteins involved in oxygen transport in hemolymph
Group 4 (e.g., Bla g 4)	5–53	21	Lipocalin, found only in the male reproductive tract, binds tyramine and octopamine, involved in pheromone transport
Group 5 (e.g., Bla g 5)	7–72	23	Glutathione S-transferase (delta class); the equivalent allergen from American cockroach is a sigma class enzyme with low sequence similarity to Bla g 5
Group 6 (e.g., Bla g 6)	50	21	Troponin C; a muscle-associated calcium-binding protein
Group 7 (e.g., Bla g 7)	2–31	31	Tropomyosin
Group 8 (e.g., Bla g 8)	14	20	Myosin light chain
Group 9 (e.g., Per a 9)	34–100	43	Arginine kinase; shows sequence similarity with mite group 20 allergens, the meal moth allergen Plo i 1 and the shell B group 2 allergens such as Pen m 2
Group 10 (e.g., Per a 10)	82	28	Trypsin
Group 11 (e.g., Bla g 11)	41	57	Amylase
Group 12 (e.g., Per a 12)	45	60–64	Chitinase
Bla g Chymotrypsin	29	23	Chymotrypsin
Bla g Enolase	25	45	Enolase
Bla g Vitellogenin	47	50	Shows sequence similarity with Der p 14

Order Lepidoptera

***Family Pyralidae, Indianmeal Moth* (Plodia interpunctella)**

Allergen	Frequency of Reactivity (%)	Mol. Size (kDa)	Function
Plo i 1	25	40	Arginine kinase; shows sequence similarity with mite group 20 allergens and the cockroach group 9 allergens
Plo i 2	8	12	Thioredoxin

Family Bombycidae

***Silkworm Larvae* (Bombyx Mori)**

Allergen	Frequency of Reactivity (%)	Mol. Size (kDa)	Function
Bomb m 1	>90	42	Arginine kinase; shows sequence similarity with mite group 20 allergens and the cockroach group 9 allergens
Bomb m 7			Tropomyosin

Class Arachnida, Subclass Acari (mites)

***Families Pyroglyphidae/Glycyphagidae/Acaridae/Echimyopodidae*, Dermatophagoides pteronyssinus, D. farinae, Euroglyphus maynei, Blomia tropicalis, Tyrophagus putrescentiae, Lepidoglyphus destructor**

Allergen	Frequency of Reactivity (%)	Mol. Size (kDa)	Function
Group 1 (e.g., Der p 1)	>90	25	Cysteine protease
Group 2 (e.g., Der p 2)	>90	14	MD-2–related protein, lipid binding, binds LPS
Group 3 (e.g., Der p 3)	90	25	Trypsin
Group 4 (e.g., Der p 4)	25–46	60	Amylase
Group 5 (e.g., Der p 5)	9–70	14	Function unknown; possible ligand-binding protein
Group 6 (e.g., Der p 6)	39	25	Chymotrypsin
Group 7 (e.g., Der p 7)	24–53	26–31	Bactericidal permeability-increasing-like proteinFunction unknown; belongs to the juvenile hormone-binding family of proteins found in insects; may have lipid-binding properties; binds the lipopeptide polymyxin B
Group 8 (e.g., Der p 8)	40	27	Glutathione S-transferase
Group 9 (e.g., Der p 9)	>90	29	Collagenase-like serine protease
Group 10 (e.g., Der p 10)	81	36	Tropomyosin
Group 11 (e.g., Der f 11)	82	103	Paramyosin
Group 12 (e.g., Blo t 12)	50	16	May be a chitinase; shows sequence similarity with Der f 15 due to chitin-binding domain
Group 13 (e.g., Lep d 13)	11–23	15	Fatty acid–binding protein

(Continued)

TABLE 4.12 Physicochemical and Biochemical Characteristics of Arthropod-Derived Indoor Allergens—cont'd

Allergen	Frequency of Reactivity (%)	Mol. Size (kDa)	Function
Group 14 (e.g., Der f 14)	84	177	Vitellogenin or lipophorin
Group 15 (e.g., Der f 15)	95	98, 109[a]	Chitinase; shows sequence similarity with the cockroach group 12 allergen and mite group 18; contains a chitin-binding peritrophin-A domain (CBM-14) characteristic of peritrophic membranes of insects and belongs to the GH 18 chitinase family
Group 16 (e.g., Der f 16)	50–62	53	Gelsolin/villin
Group 17 (e.g., Der f 17)	35	30	Calcium-binding protein
Group 18 (e.g., Der f 18)	63	60	Chitinase; shows sequence similarity with the cockroach group 12 allergen and mite group 15; contains a chitin-binding peritrophin-A domain (CBM-14) characteristic of peritrophic membranes of insects and a glyco 18 chitinase domain; is a GH 18 chitinase superfamily member
Group 19 (e.g., Blo t 19)	10	7	Function unknown; shows high sequence similarity with putative antibacterial peptides from helminthic worms
Group 20 (e.g., Der p 20)	0–44	40	Arginine kinase
Group 21 (e.g., Der p 21)	26	15	Function unknown; shows sequence similarity with group 5 allergens
Group 22 (e.g., Der f 22)	?	17	Shows sequence similarity with group 2 mite allergen; belongs to MD-2-related lipid recognition (ML) domain family; implicated in lipid binding
Group 23 (e.g., Der p 23)	74	14	Unknown function; shows sequence similarity with peritrophin-A domain and contains a chitin-binding domain
Group 24 (e.g., Der f 24)	100	13	Ubiquinol-cytochrome c reductase binding protein-like protein
Group 25 (e.g., Der f 25)	76	34	Triosephosphate isomerase
Group 26 (e.g., Der f 26)	62	14	Myosin alkali light chain
Group 27 (e.g., Der f 27)	35–100	48	Serpin-trypsin inhibitor
Group 28 (e.g., Der f 28)	68	70	Heat shock protein
Group 29 (e.g., Der f 29)	70–86	16	Peptidyl-prolyl cis-trans isomerase (cyclophilin)
Group 30 (e.g., Der f 30)	63	16	Ferritin
Group 31 (e.g., Der f 30)	31–100	15	Cofilin, actin-binding protein
Group 32 (e.g., Der f 32)	15–100	35	Secreted inorganic pyrophosphatase
Group 33 (e.g., Der f 33)	25–100	52	Alpha tubulin
Group 34 (e.g., Der f 34)	68	16	Enamine/imine deaminase
Group 35 (e.g., Der f 35)	78	14	MD-2-related protein, shows sequence similarity with mite group 2 allergens
Group 36 (e.g., Der f 36)	42	23	Function unknown, contains a C-terminal C2 domain (pfam00168), which is associated with signal transduction enzymes
Group 37 (e.g., Der f 37)	21	29	Chitin-binding protein
Group 38 (e.g., Der p 38)	78	15	Bacteriolytic enzyme belonging to the NlpC/P60 family
Group 39 (e.g. Der f 39)	9	18	Troponin C; a muscle-associated calcium-binding protein

HSP, Heat shock protein; *MD-2*, myeloid differentiation factor-2.
[a]Glycosylated forms, DNA sequence indicates a nonglycosylated protein of 63 kDa. Frequency determined in dogs with atopic dermatitis.

Sensitization is associated with *Blattella germanica*, *Periplaneta americana*, and *P. fuliginosa* (Box 4.2), with the first of these common in urban settings where the climate is warm or domestic heating maintained. The allergenic components of cockroaches are associated with their feces, saliva, and the debris of dead insects, and substantial quantities of these aerodynamically large particulates can accumulate and persist even after the eradication of live insects.

In contrast to HDM, which predominate in the bedroom and living room, the greatest numbers of cockroaches and the highest concentrations of allergen are usually found in kitchens because of their proximity to food. However, cockroach allergen concentrations in bedrooms may correlate with the frequency of hospitalization. Cockroaches produce more than 10 groups of denominated allergens, of which several are recognized as immunodominant (Table 4.12). The first cockroach allergens to be cloned were shown to be homologous with aspartate proteases (Bla g 2), though catalytically inert, and a lipocalin (Bla g 4). Other allergens include the gut-associated Group 1 allergens, which are thought to play a detoxifying function, digestive enzymes (e.g., the Group 11 amylases and the Group 10 trypsins), and arginine kinases (Group 9 allergens).[28]

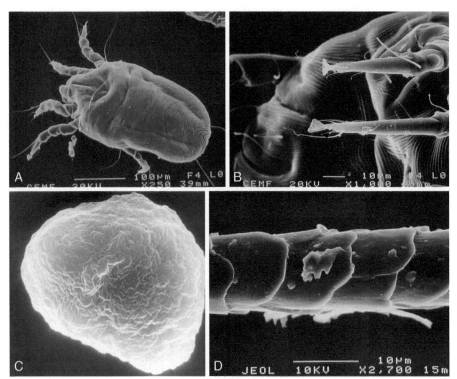

Fig. 4.8 Photomicrographs of clinically important indoor allergen sources. (A) *Dermatophagoides farinae*, showing legs and mouth parts. (B) Details of the legs of a dust mite, showing the pads on their ends allowing them to hold on to surfaces. (C) A mite fecal particle, with a chitinous, outer peritrophic membrane. (D) Cat hair showing adherent particles of dander/skin scales that carry antigen. (From scanning electron micrographs (A)–(C) courtesy John Vaughan; (D) courtesy Judith Woodfolk; Matsui E, Thomas AE, Platts-Mills TAE. Indoor allergens. In: Burks AW, Holgate S, O'Hehir R, Bacharier L, Broide D, Hershey GK, et al., editors. Middleton's Allergy: Principles and Practice. 9th ed. London: Elsevier; 2019:451–466.)

TABLE 4.13 Physicochemical and Biochemical Characterization of Animal-Derived Indoor Allergens

Allergen	Frequency of Reactivity (%)	Mol. Size (kDa)	Function
Cat (Felix domesticus)			
Fel d 1	95	33–39[a]	Secretoglobin family member, tetramer of two heterodimers (chains 1 and 2), a possible ligand-binding molecule; chain 1 shows sequence similarity with 10-kDa secretory protein from human Clara cells, mouse salivary androgen-binding protein subunit, rabbit uteroglobin, and a Syrian hamster protein
Fel d 2	20–35	69	Serum albumin: food allergen, cross reacts with pork, beef albumin
Fel d 3	10	11	Cystatin
Fel d 4	60	20	Lipocalin, shows sequence similarity with other mammalian lipocalin allergens
Fel d 5	38	400	Immunoglobulin A; food allergen, IgE is directed against the galactose β-1,3-galactose moiety, also found on the heavy chain of immunoglobulin M; present in pork, beef, and lamb
Fel d 6	?	900	Immunoglobulin M
Fel d 7	38	18	Von Ebner gland protein, cysteine protease inhibitor
Fel d 8	19	24	Latherin, surfactant protein
Dog (Canis familiaris)			
Can f 1	50	19–25	Lipocalin; shows sequence similarity with Von Ebner gland protein, which has cysteine protease inhibitory activity
Can f 2	20–22	27	Lipocalin; shows sequence similarity with Can f 1 and Fel d 4, and with other lipocalin allergens
Can f 3	16–40	69	Serum albumin
Can f 4	35	23	Lipocalin, shows sequence similarity with bovine odorant-binding protein
Can f 5	70	28	Prostatic kallikrein; shows sequence similarity with human prostate-specific antigen (PSA), which is also allergenic

(Continued)

TABLE 4.13 Physicochemical and Biochemical Characterization of Animal-Derived Indoor Allergens—cont'd

Allergen	Frequency of Reactivity (%)	Mol. Size (kDa)	Function
Can f 6	38	27, 29	Lipocalin
Can f 7	17	16	Epidydimal secretory protein, member of the NPC2 family
Can f Fel d 1-like	?	20	Shows high sequence similarity with Fel d 1
Horse (Equus caballus)			
Equ c 1	100	25	Lipocalin; shows sequence similarity with rodent urinary proteins
Equ c 2	100	17	Lipocalin; shows sequence similarity with rodent urinary proteins
Equ c 3	50	67	Serum albumin
Equ c 4	77	17, 20.5	Latherin, surfactant protein
Cow (Bos taurus)			
Bos d 2	97	20	Lipocalin
Bos d 3	?	11	S100 calcium-binding protein
Bos d OSCP	31	21	Oligomycin sensitivity-conferring protein of the mitochondrial adenosine triphosphate synthase complex
Guinea Pig (Cavia porcellus)			
Cav p 1	70	20	Lipocalin; shows sequence similarity with Cav p 2
Cav p 2	65	17	Lipocalin; shows sequence similarity with Bos d 2
Cav p 3	54	19	Lipocalin
Cav p 4	53	66	Serum albumin
Cav p 6	53	18	Lipocalin; shows sequence similarity with various other mammalian lipocalin allergens
Mouse (Mus musculus)			
Mus m 1	>80	17	Major urinary protein; shows sequence similarity with lipocalins such as β-lactoglobulin, odorant-binding proteins, Rat n 2 Rat (Rattus norvegicus)
Rat (Rattus norvegicus)			
Rat n 1	>90	17	Lipocalin; shows sequence similarity with lipocalins such as β-lactoglobulin Bos d 5, odorant-binding proteins, Mus m 1
Rat n 4	100	69	Serum albumin
Rat n 7	47	150	Immunoglobulin G
Rabbit (Oryctolagus cuniculus)			
Ory c 1	100	18	Lipocalin
Ory c 3	77–100	19–21	Lipophilin, glycosylated heterodimer and similar to Fel d 1
Ory c 4	46	24	Lipocalin
Ory c 6	6	69	Serum albumin

[a]Molecular size given represents dimer form, with two chains of approximately 18 kDa each. Note that for NAC (nascent polypeptide–associated complex alpha subunit) and keratin, deduced molecular masses are given.

Indoor Allergen Sources—Mammalian

The clinically important animals in either domestic or occupational settings are cats, dogs, cows, rats, mice, horses, rabbits, mice, gerbils, and guinea pigs often referred to collectively as *furry animals*.[29] Their associated allergens are derived from dander, epithelium, fur, urine, or saliva and, in most of these species, the allergens fall into two major groupings, namely, the lipocalins (e.g., Can f 1, 4, 6), comprising >50% of all furry animal allergens thus far described) and the secretoglobins (e.g., Fel d 1, Ory c 3) with a third minor group containing a small diversity of other proteins such as animal immunoglobulins (Fel d 5, Rat n 4) and albumins (e.g., Fel d 2, Can f 3) (Table 4.13).

Cats, Dogs, and Rabbits

Cat-allergic patients report symptoms on entering a house in which a cat is living, indicating that cat allergen can be airborne in undisturbed air. This is because 10% to 40% of cat allergens are carried on particles that sediment only slowly (aerodynamically equivalent to 1–7 μm spheres) such that free undisturbed air concentrations of cat allergen may be 10 to 50 times higher than those of HDM allergens.[30] Modern housing is relatively airtight when windows are closed (0.2–0.5 air changes per hour)[31] so the otherwise beneficial effect of ventilation to remove small airborne particulates such as pet allergens is lost. Compared with the HDM allergen, Der p 1, inhalational exposures to cat or dog allergens may be up to 100-fold (1 μg/day) greater in homes with pets. This situation results from the greater persistence of the pet allergens in air, and from the tendency of cat dander to be carried passively.[32] In communities where 20% or more of resident families have animals, these allergens will be measurable in dust from schools or in homes without a cat, and this can result in sensitization to animals occurring without direct exposure to the animals.

Although inhalant exposure to cat allergens may be greater than for HDM allergens, this does not readily translate to individuals having a greater prevalence of cat sensitization or higher titer IgE antibodies against cat allergens. Indeed, there is clear evidence of greater sensitization to HDM despite the imbalance in airborne concentrations. This paradox is complemented by studies reporting that cat (or dog) ownership is protective against developing cat allergy[33] and that the dose–response relationship is bell-shaped rather than linear. These, seemingly, counter-intuitive findings do not have proven explanations, but mechanisms have been proposed. In the case of cat allergens (Table 4.13), which certainly do have the potential to evoke IgE-dependent sensitization and cause disease, the protection phenomenon may be a function of the dose, with high levels of allergens inducing tolerance rather than sensitization, consistent with the apparently selective nature of the "protection" and the ability of cat allergens to remain airborne for extended periods. The more general protective effect evoked by cats and dogs may be related to increased LPS exposure on floors but not in beds.[34]

Rodents and Rodent Allergens

Rodents are a source of domestic indoor allergens and prominent sources in animal facilities where they are a well-recognized cause of occupational allergy. The National Cooperative Inner-City Asthma Study showed the presence of mouse allergens in dust was correlated with IgE antibodies to these allergens and with asthma. Sensitization is common; in laboratory animal workers, for example, allergy prevalence is ~40%, with most becoming sensitized within 3 years of exposure (approximately 60%) and the remainder becoming sensitized within 5 to 20 years. The rat and mouse urinary lipocalin proteins (Rat n 1, Mus m 1) (Table 4.13) induce IgE- and IgG-directed immune responses, with IgG and IgG_4 being seen in the absence of IgE in occupational cases. Like cat and dog allergens, rat and mouse allergens are formed on small particles and remain airborne for extended periods. When kept as pets, the quantity of allergen becoming and remaining airborne is dependent upon both disturbance and the condition of the animal litter; where dry, larger quantities will remain airborne for longer.

ALLERGENS AND ALLERGENICITY

Why do some proteins trigger allergic responses? Early attempts to grapple with this problem sought to determine whether a universal explanation could explain allergenicity. However, no simple description accounts for the phenomenon. One early idea was that the amino acid sequence of an allergenic protein encoded a signal for allergenicity and that this signal was shared amongst all allergens. In essence, this concept is akin to there being a universal linear epitope for allergenicity. While linear epitopes are crucial immune recognition features, there is no evidence of a universal signature for allergenicity. Epitopes are also formed three-dimensionally to create specific conformations, so a further evolution of thought was the possible existence of a universal structural feature. Although not all allergen structures have been solved, it is clear that this does not explain allergenicity *per se*, although it highlights similarities in structure between certain allergens and, importantly, provides an explanation of cross-reactivity syndromes such as OAS/PFAS.

Allergens and Functionalism

The molecular structure of allergens is of profound interest beyond the definition of three-dimensional epitopes because molecular structure determines both protein function and molecular recognition on the broadest level. These attributes are of relevance to allergenicity because they illuminate the immune mechanisms that may initiate and then sustain allergic sensitization. This concept has been dubbed the "functionalist" view of allergenicity[35] in which understanding the intrinsic bioactivity of an allergen provides a rationalization for why some allergens are clinically more important than others from the same source, and why some purified allergens alone are weak sensitizers, but become strikingly allergenic when other allergens or even nonallergenic materials are present. The functionalist view of allergenicity attempts to explain some of these phenomena in terms of the ability of different allergens to form an effective bridge between innate and adaptive immunity through their intrinsic bioactivity. Allergens most adept in this regard may be classified "risk" or "initiator" allergens.

In addition to intrinsic properties, allergen sources contain a variety of nonallergenic factors that contribute adjuvant-like properties to allergens sources or, as mentioned earlier for Bet v 1, are potentially capable of influencing epitope selection and biasing toward a Th2 response. For example, pollens absorb bacteria and pollutants onto their surfaces, and carry pollen-derived biologically active lipid molecules. In addition, allergen sources such as indoor dusts (or arthropods *per se*) may contain significant amounts of microbe-associated molecular pattern (MAMP) molecules such as LPS and peptidoglycan that can exert immunomodulatory effects. Recently, it has been demonstrated that MAMPs are responsible for eliciting *trained immunity* (TRIM), a process whereby the innate immune system is primed (memory) by epigenetic changes to produce an enhanced pro-inflammatory response on subsequent exposure. Both LPS, through toll-like receptor-4 (TLR4), and β-glucan, through CLEC7A (aka Dectin-1), have been shown to reprogram macrophages and monocytes, and differential (upregulated v nonresponsive) TLR-mediated gene expression may occur. Similarly, significant concentrations of MAMPs also occur in dusts within the home from a variety of sources. As indicated earlier for cat and dog allergy, as well as being observed in farming communities, susceptible individuals may be protected, particularly in environments rich in these MAMPs.

Allergens as Proteases

Allergens that are proteolytically active are well represented in the cadre of "risk" allergens and are present in the allergomes of most clinically important allergen sources, including arthropods, pollens and fungi, and in some occupational agents. They are preeminent examples because they possess a bioactivity profile that fosters both allergen delivery and the breaking of immune tolerance in a Th2-directed manner. For example, they possess the ability to enhance the probability of contacting antigen presenting cells directly by proteolysis of conserved cleavage sites within the intercellular tight junctions of epithelial barriers,[36] which enables them to breach epithelial barriers and, indirectly, through the generation of cytokines (e.g., IL-13) which impair barrier function.[37] The release of other cytokines and chemokines by the cleavage of protease-activated receptors (PARs) also facilitates polarization towards a Th2 immune response due to the triggering of intracellular signaling.[38] In the case of the Group 1 HDM allergens (Fig. 4.9), this is possible because they behave as prothrombinases, thus enabling the canonical activation of PAR1 and PAR4 by thrombin.[38] In the case of serine peptidase HDM allergens, cleavage of PAR2 is directly due to the allergens with tryptic or chymotryptic specificity.[38]

Allergens and Toll-like Receptors (TLRs)

Allergens can also interact directly or indirectly with a range of receptors other than PARs, such as the PRRs which detect MAMPS. When activated, they facilitate the release of damage-associated molecular pattern mediators (DAMPs, e.g., ATP, high-mobility box protein, HMGB1) that provide adjuvant-like effects that boost allergy. Notable PRRs orchestrating responses to allergens, in particular, HDM allergens, include members of the TLR family such as TLR 2, 4, and 6.[39] In this regard, studies indicate that TLR4, expressed by structural cells, plays a central role in the development of HDM sensitization, prompting questions about its activation, although evidence suggesting that Group 1 HDM allergens interact directly with TLR4 is lacking. However, they activate a signaling mechanism in airway epithelial cells, which stimulates TLR4 through the formation of endogenous ligands. The consequence of TLR4 activation is the generation of reactive oxidants and the redox-sensitive transcription of genes encoding inflammatory cytokines and chemokines. Reactive oxidants, in turn, are also involved in the release of IL-33, which is stored pre-formed in epithelial cells and which is cleaved to a super-active form by the proteolytic activity of Group 1 HDM allergens[38,39]

The endogenous ligands responsible for TLR4 activation are incompletely characterized, but evidence implicates fibrinogen fragments in a way which may be like that described for the activation of TLR4 by extracts of *A. oryzae*.[40] As already noted, Group 2 HDM allergens have functional homology with the MD-2 component of the TLR4 receptor complex and their interaction with TLR4 may facilitate its activation by a range of stimuli, including LPS. An MD-2 recognition domain has been identified in Der f 35 suggesting a similar mechanism, although it is currently unclear if the domain is functionally active.[39] The homology of several HDM allergens with molecules that have

lipid transport function (Groups 5, 7, 13, 14, 21, 35) suggests these might bind a variety of lipid cargoes, in addition to LPS and lipoteichoic acid from Gram-positive bacteria, and interact either with TLR4 or heterodimers of TLR2 with TLR1 or TLR6.

Allergens and C-type Lectin Receptors (CTLRs)

Many allergens are potentially capable of binding to CTLRs due to the presence of glycan structures on their surface, as are materials that might be associated with them. For example, chitins (polymeric β-(1-4)-poly-N-acetyl-D-glucosamine) are found in both the HDM exoskeleton and peritrophic membranes of their fecal pellets. Experimental evidence supports the notion that chitins might signal autonomously through TLR2 or in conjunction with allergens with putative chitin-binding domains (e.g., Der p 23).[39] In addition, polysaccharide signaling may also be mediated by CTLRs activated by glucans found within mite fecal pellets and fungal cell walls. As with chitins, understanding the significance of such mechanisms is hampered by the structural diversity of glucans, which determines their physicochemistry and bioactivity profile. While glucans have been associated with both pro-inflammatory and anti-inflammatory effects in allergy, a surprising finding is that one of the CTLR receptor family, namely, CLEC7A (expressed on epithelial cells) involved in glycan recognition, binds arthropod tropomyosin allergens such as the Group 10 HDM allergens rather than β-glucan.[41] Normally, CLEC7A is involved in the suppression of IL-33 release, but in allergic patients, CLEC7A expression in bronchial and sino-nasal epithelial cells is reduced, possibly due to a polymorphism associated with reduced lung function in children.[41]

ENVIRONMENTAL MODIFIERS OF ALLERGIC SENSITIZATION AND DISEASE

In addition to genetic factors, environmental components have significant roles in allergen aerobiology and allergic diseases. Some have been alluded to previously but, in this section, the effects of climate and pollution on allergenicity and allergic diseases will be discussed, as well as the potential therapeutic impact of deliberate environmental intervention.

Avoidance Measures for Indoor Allergens

Reducing exposure to obvious trigger factors is a standard component in the management of allergic diseases due to indoor allergens, and complete avoidance of allergens (sanatoria, clean rooms, and home modifications) can reduce the symptoms of asthma and bronchial hyper-reactivity.[42] However, maintaining the strict regimens required for optimal results is onerous and the procedures achieve only a static improvement, which does not follow the daily perambulations of patients into allergen-laden environments. A further limitation is that many patients receive inadequate advice and fail to see the association between allergen exposure and disease. For avoidance measures to work, it is essential that the inciting trigger(s) be clearly identified and that the countermeasures adopted achieve an effective reduction in allergen exposure. The former can be addressed by skin

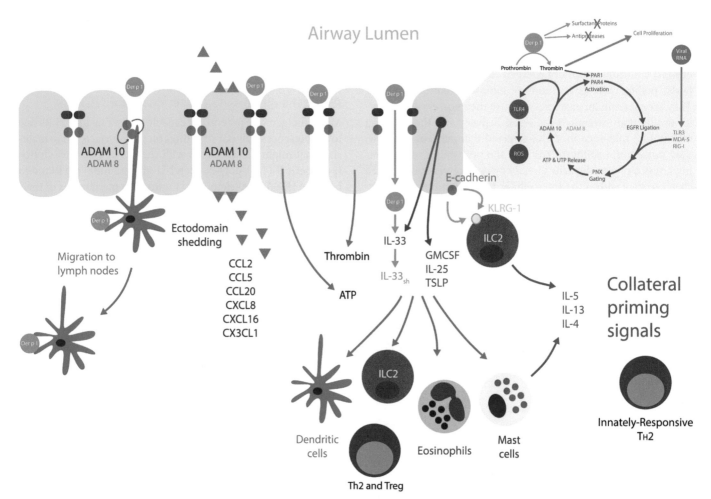

Fig. 4.9 Immunological effector pathways activated by Group 1 house-dust mite (HDM) allergens (e.g., Der p 1) in the airway epithelium. These pathways involve the cleavage of cell surface molecules which (A) facilitate the interaction of any allergen with dendritic antigen presenting cells, (B) increase the expression of inflammatory cytokines, (C) recruit migratory effector cells, and (D) liberate danger signals such as ATP and IL-33. Increased allergen contact with dendritic cells arises from cleavage of occludin and claudin adhesion proteins found in interepithelial tight junctions (shown in purple) which increases epithelial permeability nonspecifically. Inflammatory cytokine expression (e.g., granulocyte macrophage colony-stimulating factor (GM-CSF), IL-25, thymic stromal lymphopoietin (TSLP)) is upregulated in a TLR4- and reactive oxidant species (ROS)-dependent manner following canonical activation of PAR1 and PAR4 by the prothrombinase activity of Group 1 HDM allergens (see signaling cycle summarized in the cream shaded box). Migratory cells are recruited through ectodomain shedding of chemoattractant (CCL, CXCL) proteins triggered directly by Group 1 HDM allergens or, indirectly, through their activation of a disintegrin and metalloprotease 10 (ADAM 10). In addition to triggering ectodomain shedding of chemokines, ADAM 10 facilitates the untethering of dendritic cells from junctional E-cadherin, enabling their migration to lymph nodes. It also promotes the untethering of type 2 innate lymphoid cells from the epithelium by disrupting interaction between nonjunctional E-cadherin and killer cell lectin-like subfamily G member 1 (KLRG1). Danger signals such as ATP and IL-33 are stored constitutively in the airway epithelium and are released in response to ROS-dependent signaling. Acting in concert with upregulated cytokines, they recruit and activate effector cells in an IgE-independent manner to provide a population of innately responsive cells which prime the development and maintenance of allergic sensitization to HDM and other allergens. (Reproduced from Zhang J, Chen J, Robinson C. Cellular and molecular events in the airway epithelium defining the interaction between house dust mite group 1 allergens and innate defenses. Int J Mol Sci. 2018;19(11):3549. Licensed under CC BY 4.0.)

testing, which helps educate patients about exposure and disease as well as confirming a diagnosis; the latter can be addressed by measuring specific allergens in the environment (Table 4.2) before and after instituting the avoidance measures.

House-Dust Mites

Even with public awareness, it can be hard to convince patients of the association between HDM exposure and their allergic condition, as they and their allergens cannot be perceived in the same way as some outdoor pollutants, whose presence may be readily visible. This failure to appreciate the association can limit the acceptance of an allergen avoidance strategy. In addition, the perception of allergen avoidance has been affected by a widely misunderstood metaanalysis of controlled trials of HDM allergen avoidance in homes, which concluded that it was not an effective treatment for asthma (Gotzsche and Johansen, 2008).

In reality, this metaanalysis was more a test of the achievability of allergen reduction under different regimens because the survey included trials that were of insufficient duration to achieve a meaningful reduction in HDMs and their allergens and, unsurprisingly, returned no benefit for asthma symptoms.[43] In contrast, evidence from studies in sanatoria and in hospital clean rooms shows that a reduction in HDM allergen levels is dependably effective, provided sufficient allergen reduction can be achieved. Controlled trials in clean rooms, achieving a reduction for >6 months, have consistently reported a decrease in symptoms and/or bronchial hyper-reactivity and in atopic dermatitis patients.[44]

The necessary actions to reduce HDM exposure are divided into those for the bedroom and those for the remainder of the house[45,46] (Box 4.3). In the bedroom, the most effective long-term measure is the removal of carpets but covering mattresses and pillows with impermeable covers and washing bedding at 130 °F/55 °C weekly are also effective. These should be supplemented with vacuum cleaning to eliminate dust where mites proliferate but, elsewhere, the greatest problem is associated with carpets and sofas. On unventilated damp floors, carpets are a particular problem (e.g., in basements and on ground floors of concrete slab construction) because water can condense on cold surfaces, or because of leakage. Once the carpet is wet and the temperature rises, it provides an excellent growth environment for fungi and HDMs.

For mitigation, homes can be designed with uncarpeted floors and leather furniture to limit mite growth; ventilation and/or air conditioning can be used to control humidity and chemical treatments can be applied to carpets and furniture to control mite growth or to denature allergens. Acaricides kill mites with varying efficacy, but the challenge is to achieve a sufficient effect in a carpet. However, they do not tackle the allergen reservoir dispersed throughout the carpet or in furnishings. Tannic acid (1%–3% w/v) may be used to inactivate allergens, but its effect is temporary as it is not acaricidal.

Furry Animals

Avoiding allergens from furry animals provides a special challenge and requires tact because many are considered full members of the family. A number of environmental control measures have been proposed[45,47] but the effects of removing a cat are progressive, and several months may be required for levels to fall below 8 µg/g dust, the recognized sensitizing threshold concentration (Table 4.2). This, and the airborne persistence of their allergens, explains why many patients with cat allergy find that they experience symptoms when they move into a home in which a cat has previously been present. Keeping a cat outdoors is only a partially successful measure because of the ease with which cat allergens are subject to passive transfer. Removal of carpets, air filtration, and regular washing of the cat (twice weekly) are additionally helpful (Box 4.3). Avoidance measures for dogs are similar.

Cockroaches and Other Allergens

Measures to avoid cockroaches are effective when part of an overall strategy which includes baiting, careful housekeeping to

BOX 4.3 Avoidance Measures for Common Indoor Allergens

Allergen Source	Avoidance Measures
Mites	Bedrooms Cover mattresses and pillows with impermeable covers. For pillow cases or duvets, covers should be "fine woven"; for mattress covers, plastic or other impermeable fabric can be used together with a mattress pad. Bedding should be washed weekly regularly at 130 °F/55 °C. Remove carpets, stuffed animals, and clutter from bedroom. Vacuum weekly (wearing a mask) using vacuum cleaner with a double-thickness bag or a high-efficiency particulate air (HEPA) filter. Rest of house Minimize carpets, particularly on unventilated floors and upholstered furniture. Reduce humidity below 45% relative humidity (or 6 g H_2O/kg air).
Furry animals	Remove animals from the home, but may take 20–30 weeks for allergen levels to drop to levels seen in a non–cat dwelling house. Failing removal, reduce allergen exposure in situ by reducing cat allergen reservoirs (e.g., carpets, sofas) using vacuum cleaners with effective filtration systems. Increase ventilation or use high-efficiency particulate air (HEPA) filters to remove small airborne particles. Wash animals weekly, if feasible. Cover mattresses and pillows with impermeable covers, as above for mites. Do not allow animals to access bedrooms.
Fungi	Reduce humidity. Wash contaminated surfaces (if feasible) with detergent and/or vinegar/water (80:20 ratio). Use HEPA filter equipped air conditioning. Restrict entry of spores by keeping windows and doors closed.
Cockroaches	Use baits where cockroaches are present such as the kitchen. Maintain good hygiene standards and ensure prompt removal of food debris.
Rodents	Use traps and cats. Maintain good hygiene standards to restrict access to food and water.

Modified from Matsui E, Thomas AE, Platts-Mills TAE. Indoor allergens. In: Burks AW, Holgate S, O'Hehir R, Bacharier L, Broide D, Hershey GK, et al., editors. Middleton's allergy: principles and practice. 1. 9th ed. London: Elsevier; 2019:451–466.

enclose all food sources, cleaning to remove and prevent allergen accumulation, and the sealing of access points[45] (Box 4.3). Insecticidal sprays are generally ineffective and the volatile organic vehicles in which their active ingredients are dissolved can be problematic for people with asthma. For wild rodents, the measures required are obvious,[48] but it may be difficult to obtain consent to remove a domestic pet. In urban areas of the mid-west and northeast US, rodents are significant sources of allergens, and skin testing with rodent extracts should be routine in clinics that treat patients from cities in these regions. Current recommendations for the avoidance of fungal allergens include controlling humidity, removing growth sites, cleaning with fungicides, and the avoidance of damp living environments[49] (Box 4.3). Closing of windows will reduce fungal entry from outside, but as this may also reduce ventilation, it could create conditions, allowing other allergens to thrive or remain airborne.

The Indoor Microbiome

Bacterial proteins *per se* within dusts, as opposed to those associated with bacterial commensals on skin from atopic dermatitis patients such as the staphylococcal super-antigens, are generally discounted as a significant allergen source. However, their cell wall constituents such as LPS from Gram-negative bacteria significantly influence allergic disease. Exposure can both suppress and stimulate allergic responses, suggesting that the operative mechanisms are complex and multifactorial.[39] In farming villages, children who are exposed to cow barns in early life appear to be protected against allergic sensitization and asthma. In homes generally, other data suggest that there is an inverse relationship between concentrations of LPS and the prevalence of allergic sensitization. Paradoxically, other data suggest that LPS exposure in the homes of mite-allergic children predicts the severity of asthma better than mite exposure.[50]

ENVIRONMENTAL AIR POLLUTION, ALLERGIC SENSITIZATION, AND DISEASE

Interactions between genetic predispositions and allergens are crucial events in the development of allergic conditions, but environmental factors also have relevance to disease pathogenesis (Box 4.4).[51] For example, air pollution, a contamination of the indoor or outdoor atmosphere by chemical, physical, or biologic agents, is one among many that might potentiate respiratory allergies. Air pollution and poor air quality are global issues, which express themselves at the macro (transboundary, outdoor atmospheric pollution) and the micro (indoor air pollution) levels, although both are relevant to the health effects of indoor allergens. The WHO recognizes indoor air pollution as one of the top 10 preventable risk factors for global disease. Unsurprisingly, many ethnic minority populations are deemed to incur a higher risk of ill health because of the likelihood that they inhabit areas with higher indoor and outdoor pollution.

People with preexisting allergic disorders, especially those of the respiratory tract, are especially sensitive to airborne pollutants.[51] While air pollution has the potential to affect all, stratification exists through age (typically affecting the very young or the very old), co-morbidities, genetic susceptibility, and socioeconomic factors. In some instances, the young, fit, and active also form a vulnerable group because exposure of the respiratory tract to pollutants increases with physical activity. Collectively, these factors point to the mechanisms and medical consequences of air pollution being complex. While there are important associations with morbidities such as cardiovascular disease and cancer, there has, for obvious reasons, been considerable interest in understanding the primary medical effects of air pollution per se and addressing the issue of whether it has a significant role in the induction and/or exacerbation of asthma and related conditions of the airways.

Sources of Air Pollution

The contaminants commonly responsible for poor air quality (both indoor and outdoor) are carbon monoxide, lead, sulfur dioxide, oxides of nitrogen, ozone, polyaromatic hydrocarbons (PAH), particulates, and miscellaneous biologics such as LPS. Permissible levels of pollutants are declared in air quality standards and air quality indices issued by nation states and by the WHO (Tables 4.14 and 4.15). Of the contaminants listed above, all except carbon monoxide and lead are potentially relevant to the pathogenesis and exacerbation of asthma through actions that directly affect airway tone or which promote inflammation directly or indirectly.

Regardless of whether the inciting pollutant is an oxidizing agent per se, oxidative stress is a component of the cellular mechanisms activated by these pollutants and responses will, therefore, be exaggerated in individuals with loss of function polymorphisms in antioxidant defense enzymes. Outdoor pollution ranges from discharges at point sources, such as industrial plant and machinery, to mobile sources, such as motor vehicles, aircraft, and marine craft. The spectrum of outdoor pollutants is wide, but the main sources of indoor air pollution include biomass combustion (wood, crop, dung, grass, and coal), nitrogen oxides (NO_x), tobacco smoke, and LPS.[51]

TABLE 4.14 **Interactions Between Pollutant and Allergen Exposures**			
Effect of Airway Pollutant Challenge in Allergic Volunteers	**Ozone**	**Diesel Exhaust Particles**	**Lipopolysaccharide**
Response to recall eosinophilic response to nasal allergen challenge	Increased	Increased	Increased
Immediate phase response to inhaled allergen (PD_{20})	Increased	Unknown	Increased
Effect on development of IgE response to a neoantigen	Unknown	Increased	Unknown
Effect on local (airway) IgE levels	Unknown	Increased	Unknown

PD_{20}, provocative dose causing a 20% drop in forced expiratory volume in 1 s.
Table from Hernandez ML, Peden DB. Air pollution: indoor and outdoor. In: Burks AW, Holgate S, O'Hehir R, Bacharier L, Broide D, Hershey GK, et al., editors. Middleton's allergy: principles and practice. 1. London: Elsevier; 2019:479–499.[51] and Peden DB. The epidemiology and genetics of asthma risk associated with air pollution. J Allergy Clin Immunol 2005;115:213–219.[52]

TABLE 4.15	National Ambient Air Quality Standards of the United States of America (NAAQS)			
Pollutant	**Primary or Secondary Standards[a]**	**Average Sampling Time**	**Level**	**Form**
Carbon monoxide	Primary	8 h	9 ppm	Not to be exceeded more than once per year
		1 h	35 ppm	
Lead	Primary and secondary	Rolling 3-month average	0.15 µg/m³	Not to be exceeded
Nitrogen dioxide	Primary	1 h	100 ppb	98th percentile of 1 h daily maximum concentrations, averaged over 3 years
	Primary and secondary	1 year	53 ppb	Annual mean
Ozone	Primary and secondary	8 h	0.070 ppm	Annual fourth-highest daily maximum 8-h concentration, averaged over 3 years
Particulate matter pollution (PM)	$PM_{2.5}$	Primary 1 year	12 µg/m³	Annual mean, averaged over 3 years
		Secondary 1 year	15 µg/m³	Annual mean, averaged over 3 years
		Primary and secondary 24 h	35 µg/m³	98th percentile, averaged over 3 years
	PM_{10}	Primary and secondary 24 h	150 µg/m³	Not to be exceeded more than once per year on average over 3 years
Sulfur dioxide		Primary 1 h	75 ppb	99th percentile of 1-h daily maximum concentrations, averaged over 3 years
		Secondary 3 h	0.5 ppm	Not to be exceeded more than once per year

PM_{10}, Particulate matter of 10 µm or less in diameter; $PM_{2.5}$, particulate matter of 2.5 µm or less in diameter. The above NAAQS standards reflect the six main air pollutants.
Modified from the U.S. Environmental Protection Agency (EPA), Air and Radiation, National Ambient Air Quality Standards (NAAQS). Table based on the US Environmental Protection agency table at http://www.epa.gov/air/criteria.html (accessed August 2020).
[a]Primary standards provide public health protection, including protecting the health of sensitive populations, such as asthmatics, children, and the elderly. Secondary standards provide public welfare protection, including protection against decreased visibility and damage to animals, crops, vegetation, and buildings.

Biomass

Biomass combustion is used by 52% of the global population for cooking and/or heating. When this is conducted indoors on stoves lacking an effective flue, combustion is significantly associated with the development of chronic obstructive pulmonary disease (COPD) and is a risk factor for lung cancer due to DNA damage. Women are at higher risk from biomass combustion because of their exposure to cooking-related fumes and involvement in household chores and their offspring have lower birth. Children under 5 years of age are also at risk of secondary lung function impairment and/or lower respiratory tract infection. The adverse effects of biomass combustion are partly due to PAH that can be metabolized to oxidants such as quinones.[54]

Environmental Tobacco Smoke (ETS) and Electronic Cigarettes (E-cigs)

ETS is the major indoor source of pollutants of respirable size and comprises exhaled mainstream and side-stream smoke from the burning end of cigarettes and related products. The smoke is chemically complex and rich in PAH and oxidants, and both direct exposure and passive exposure exacerbate illnesses affecting the airway lining and increase cancer risk. ETS is a major risk factor for asthma development, and it is likely that multiple mechanisms underlie this effect, including long-term epigenetic changes driven by oxidative stress. Given the importance of ETS in multiple diseases and the scale of tobacco usage, substantial efforts have been directed toward understanding its mechanism of action. Evidence suggests that ETS enhances allergen-induced IgE and IgG_4 by biasing inflammation toward Th_2 (IL-4, -5, and -13-dependent) immune signaling at the expense of Th_1-mediated signaling (interferon (IFN)-γ production).

The usage of E-cigs has grown steadily since their introduction, and this has been actively encouraged in some countries as a means of reducing dependency on conventional cigarettes. It is important to recognize that E-cigs are not a simple, "inert" alternative to conventional tobacco products. The design variations and the range of E-liquid solvents and flavorings available present considerable challenges in understanding their potential health effects. The chemical composition of E-liquid aerosols is complex and variable, and may include aldehydes, volatile organics, and heavy metals.[55,56] Currently, there is a paucity of human data concerning the potential harm of E-cigs, although research in animal models suggests the likelihood of effects that could worsen respiratory allergies, namely, impairment of mucosal barrier defenses, immune receptor activation, and exacerbation of inflammatory signaling.

Lipopolysaccharide (LPS)

LPS is a component of ambient air particulates, including ETS and, as alluded to earlier, its effects are complex. Epidemiological studies have reported data that support the hygiene hypothesis, namely, that LPS exposure in early life is negatively linked to the development of allergy and asthma, possibly through polymorphisms in CD14 (part of the canonical LPS receptor complex). However, LPS also has exacerbating effects; a dichotomy illustrating the complexities of responses to inhaled agents. This possibly arises because the dose–response relationship for LPS may be bell-shaped. It may also reflect the concentration-dependencies of downstream events concerned with (i) LPS inactivation (polymorphism of acyloxyacyl hydrolase is an asthma risk), (ii) TLR4 signal transduction (loss of function polymorphism of toll/interleukin receptor domain-containing activator protein is an asthma risk), or (iii) the operation of noncanonical molecular recognition of LPS. Inhaled LPS causes pathophysiological responses in both allergic and nonallergic airways, through activation of macrophages and neutrophils, but the airways of those with asthma are more sensitive. Although the mechanism is not conclusively established, monocyte and macrophage expression of CD14 is upregulated in asthma and correlates with neutrophil response to LPS. It may also prime the response to inhaled allergens through IgE-dependent mechanisms and the presentation of antigen to mucosal T-cells.[57] In contrast to upregulated CD14, a meta-analysis of epidemiologic studies[58] indicated that the T399I mutation (rs4986791) in TLR4 results in impaired airway expression of TLR4, which is a risk factor for asthma and blunts responses to LPS.

TYPES OF POLLUTANT AND THEIR EFFECTS ON ALLERGENS, ALLERGIC SENSITIZATION, AND ASTHMA

Credible evidence from multiple sources reveals that atmospheric particulates and gases commonly associated with traffic-related air pollution (TRAP) increase the risk of asthma development and lead to asthma exacerbations,[59] particularly in children. The complexity of TRAP makes it difficult to understand what significant components and interactions are responsible for these effects. However, for gaseous pollutants there is little doubt that they can exacerbate asthma by enhancing responses to allergens but, except for ozone, whether any specific gas causes new asthma is unclear. In real life, exposures to pollutants involve both gaseous and particulate components in varying combinations, so the overall response depends upon the combination of materials and the forms in which they are presented to the airways. Although there is an abundance of epidemiologic evidence about pollution, there is little mechanistic understanding of the consequences of exposure to "real-life" mixtures of pollutants and how these contribute to the etiology of asthma. However, that they influence asthma in various ways is not in doubt.

Particulates

Atmospheric particulate matter is heterogeneous, both in composition and in physical behavior, but it is clear that particulates are associated with inflammation, oxidative stress, genotoxicity, and cell death.[60] Compelling evidence gathered across economically developed and less-well developed countries demonstrates that exposure to respirable particulates is associated with a range of major health conditions, including asthma. In urban environments, TRAP is an important source of these particulates, comprising diesel exhaust particulates (DEPs), black carbon (BC), and fine particulate matter, 2.5 μm or less and 10 μm or less in diameter ($PM_{2.5}$ and PM_{10}), and exposure to them is a risk factor for asthma development and exacerbation, particularly in children.

Data show an association between DEP exposure, sensitization, and allergic rhinitis in young children. Other work shows an elevated risk of asthma development in children who were sensitized to aeroallergens and exposed to high levels of TRAP in infancy. This risk was greater than that seen in allergen-sensitized children exposed to only low levels of TRAP.[61,62] This raises the question of whether such an association can be accounted for by the effects of particulates modifying the responses to allergens or by modifying allergens per se. In this regard, particulates and other environmental factors such as climate change–associated temperature rises and increasing CO_2 concentrations, and increasing pollutants such as NO_2 and O_3 have all been shown to influence allergenicity (Table 4.16 and Box 4.4).

The effects of inhaled particulates have been studied in detail, and it is clear that $PM_{2.5}$ particulates impact the whole respiratory tract and, therefore, constitute a potentially high health risk. In contrast, larger particulates (>2.5 < 10 μm aerodynamic diameter) will impact only the larger airways. However, there is no "standard model" for the study of respirable particulates in the lung in vivo, so investigative approaches have ranged from direct respiratory exposure to diluted diesel exhaust to the instillation of DEPs into the bronchial or nasal airways. Collectively, available data suggest that DEPs cause airway inflammation in people regardless of whether they have asthma or not.

In asthma, responses mediated by IgE and IgG may be enhanced, but it is unclear whether this involves elevated IgE levels. Studies in humans and in experimental animal models suggest that DEPs also shift immune responses to a Th_2 phenotype. Challenge studies show that $PM_{2.5}$ particulates elicit a mild inflammatory response in the airways, partly due to the presence of transition metals (e.g., Cu, Ni, Zn) within the particles. Particulate matter, especially DEPs, is also loaded with PAH, which can be converted to quinones and other oxidants. Studies in humans and experimental animal models confirm that the extent of hydrocarbon loading influences responses to particulates. However, particulates may be loaded with many substances, including fungal spores and pollens, which have a direct independent association with asthma. DEPs are also suggested to increase the susceptibility to viral infections and this may be of significance in asthma where interactions between allergens and respiratory viruses are central to the risk of asthma exacerbations. Evidence shows that pollutant exposure increases viral mRNA levels in allergic rhinitis, as well as promoting eosinophilic inflammation. Mechanistically, responses to DEPs may be due to increased expression of TLR3.

TABLE 4.16 **Environmental Modifiers of Allergens and Allergenicity of Outdoor Allergens**

Pollutants[a]	Climate Change[b]
Enhanced allergenicity due to adjuvant properties of particulates	Extended pollen seasons—earlier start, later finish
Differential expression of allergens in pollen grains	Increased pollen production
Increased allergen content in pollen grains, e.g., Bet v 1	Increased allergen expression in pollen grains
Increase in pollen protein expression with possibility of creating new allergens	Increased allergen content in pollen grains
Increased releasability of cytoplasmic allergens and allergen-laden granules from pollen grains	Increase in pollen protein expression with possibility of creating new allergens
Post-translational modification of pollen allergens	Change in distribution of pollen-producing plants
Enhanced antigen presentation	Induction of fungal sporulation
Alteration in pollen germination rate	
Modulation of microbiome	
Modulation of pollen-associated lipid mediators with potential impact on allergen immunogenicity	

[a]Particulates, heavy metals, diesel exhaust particles (DEPs), environmental tobacco smoke (ETS), NO_2, SO_2, O_3.
[b]Temperature, CO_2.
Adapted from Stewart GA, Peden DP, Thompson PJ, Ludwig M. Allergens and air pollutants. In: Holgate ST, Church MK, Broide DH, Martinez FD, editors. Allergy. 4th ed. Edinburgh: Saunders; 2012. For a review, see Ref. 53.

Gaseous Pollutants

Exposure to the gaseous pollutants sulfur dioxide (SO_2), nitrogen dioxide (NO_2), and ozone (O_3) may occur singly, but is more likely to occur in combination with each other and/or particulates. Such pollutants, which influence the integrity of the epithelial lining or which modify innate and/or acquired immune responses, have the potential for interacting with inhaled allergens. This raises the question of whether gaseous pollutants explain the increased incidence of asthma. For reasons, explained earlier, the complexity and variability of TRAP make this a difficult question to answer and, because of this, the increased asthma risk reported in some birth cohort studies is difficult to ascribe to specific components. However, the effects of those components have been characterized in laboratory studies, allowing some inferences to be drawn as illustrated later.

Sulfur Dioxide (SO_2)

SO_2 is a toxic gas with a pungent, rotten odor whose contribution to acid aerosol formation means that it is has been extensively studied.[63] Acute inhalation is associated with shortness of breath and respiratory discomfort, and is linked with ER visits and hospital admissions or premature death. Chronically, it increases the likelihood of developing asthma or COPD and is correlated with the presence of current symptoms. The effects of SO_2 are rapid in onset (<2 min) resulting in a bronchospastic rather than an inflammatory response, which involves wheezing, chest discomfort, and dyspnea, although repeated exposure may result in tachyphylaxis. Because the acute effects of inhaled SO_2 rely on absorption through the bronchial mucosa, they are exacerbated by exercise and are mitigated by nasal breathing, which redirects absorption via the nasal mucosa. However, this mitigation is reduced in asthma patients with nasal co-morbidities (e.g., rhinitis and sinusitis) where nasal airflow is decreased.

BOX 4.4 **Important Effects of Indoor and Outdoor Pollutants on Allergic Disease**

- Air pollutants exacerbate asthma symptoms, and pollution may contribute to the development of asthma.
- Increasing global temperatures and rising carbon dioxide levels affect plant pollination potential and allergen potency. Ambient air pollutants can modify the allergen exposure of allergic persons.
- The WHO declared indoor air pollution one of the most preventable risk factors contributing to the global burden of disease. Indoor pollutants include biomass burning and tobacco smoke.
- Pollutant exposures can induce allergic and nonallergic inflammation in asthmatics.
- Genetic susceptibility to air pollution includes polymorphisms in oxidative stress response genes and in innate immunity genes.
- Public policy approaches to decrease ambient air pollutant levels have improved various parameters of public health outcomes, including asthma morbidity.

Nitrogen Dioxide (NO_2)

Epidemiologic surveys have consistently revealed a strong association between ambient NO_2 concentrations and both acute and chronic changes in lung function and the exacerbation of asthma. While the ability of NO_2 to enhance airway reactivity is equivocal at low exposure levels, at higher concentrations it has more notable effects on lung function in people with asthma in whom it augments the acute response to allergens.[64] The mechanism of NO_2 involves an inflammatory neutrophilic infiltration. Studies in vitro suggest that the airway epithelium has a significant role in orchestrating the inflammatory responses through cytokine production. Although definitive proof is awaited, there is an obvious potential for responses to NO_2 and allergens to interact at this level of inflammatory signaling and injury.

Ozone (O_3)

O_3 is a pungent, pale blue gas; its strongly oxidant action is damaging to mucous and respiratory tissues[65] and, therefore, has the potential to modify responses to inhaled allergens. Some data also suggest that it may be a cause of nascent asthma, in addition to exacerbating established disease, for which stronger evidence exists.[66] In the troposphere, ozone is formed by photochemical reaction between nitrogen oxides and volatile organic compounds from vehicle emissions and industrial discharges. This reaction is promoted by temperature and, consequently, the significance of O_3 as a pollutant increases during warmer months with photochemical smog. In the indoor environment, it may also be formed by electrical discharge in some types of electrical equipment. Ozone is an inherently unstable molecule whose breakdown generates reactive products which per se may possess irritant properties but are currently of unknown relevance to allergic disease.

The gas is a well-recognized trigger for asthma exacerbations, even at low levels of exposure, and there is a significantly increased risk of death from respiratory causes at higher levels.[65] Controlled-exposure studies show that, acutely, O_3 induces a rapid decrease in forced vital capacity (FVC) and forced expiratory volume in 1 s (FEV1), a sensation of chest discomfort on deep breathing, and an increase in nonspecific airway responsiveness mediated by sensory neural reflexes. These changes in lung function are accompanied by, but not correlated with, the onset of a moderately persistent (~24 h) neutrophilic inflammation. The increased susceptibility of people with asthma to O_3 is due to potentiation of allergic inflammation and innate immune responses. Mechanistic studies indicate that some responses are mediated by TLR4,[67] possibly activated by hyaluronic acid release, a known pro-inflammatory DAMP, from the airway epithelium. Levels of hyaluronic acid are increased in airway surface liquid in people with or without asthma when exposed to ozone. Other inflammatory events involve the release of cytokines, prostaglandins, and leukotrienes. As with NO_2, exposure, physical activity (and, thus, raised respiratory rate) increases the effective lung dose of O_3, so it is recommended that persons at risk minimize exertion.

AIR POLLUTION, CLIMATE CHANGE, AND ALLERGENS

Changes in temperature and CO_2 levels have well-documented effects on plant biology and it is reasonable to anticipate that some of these may have relevance to allergy.[68] While laboratory studies indicate that CO_2 levels can increase the numbers and allergenicity of pollen grains, field data are currently limited and conflicting. Similarly, only restricted real-world data exist about pollutants increasing pollen release, although data obtained under controlled conditions for timothy grass suggest this could occur with NO_2 and O_3.[69] Regardless of the effects of pollutants on pollen quantity and potency, interactions between particulates and pollens may have significance in enhancing the tissue delivery of allergens.

CONCLUSIONS

Our knowledge of allergens has grown enormously since the late 1980s, and most, if not all of the major, clinically important allergens have been cloned. We know much about their functions in the original source, and we understand more about how they might interact with components of the innate immune system and modulate IgE responses. Detailed molecular knowledge of allergens is now being translated into the clinical sphere, particularly in diagnostics where microarrayed recombinant indoor, outdoor, and food allergens have become available. Whilst these diagnostics are unlikely to replace skin prick testing in the clinic or single source immunoassays, they are useful in helping differentiate between primary sensitization and cross-reactivity in the diagnosis of food allergy, in rapidly determining whether patients are polysensitized, and in providing guidance in selecting patients for immunotherapy. In parallel, we are now acknowledging that patients do not just inhale benign proteins but rather collections of biologically active containers replete with both eukaryotic and prokaryotic components that contribute either to inflammation or its suppression in exposed individuals via our innate immune systems.

ACKNOWLEDGMENTS

The work of the authors described in this chapter was supported by Australia's National Health and Medical Research Council (NHMRC), The Asthma Foundation WA, Asthma UK, The Medical Research Council (UK), and The Wellcome Trust.

REFERENCES

1. Broeks SA, Brand PL. Atopic dermatitis is associated with a fivefold increased risk of polysensitisation in children. Acta Paediatr. 2017;106(3):485–488.
2. Kim KW, Kim EA, Kwon BC, et al. Comparison of allergic indices in monosensitized and polysensitized patients with childhood asthma. J Korean Med Sci. 2006;21(6):1012–1016.
3. Arbes SJ Jr., Cohn RD, Yin M, Muilenberg ML, Friedman W, Zeldin DC. Dog allergen (Can f 1) and cat allergen (Fel d 1) in US homes: results from the National Survey of Lead and Allergens in Housing. J Allergy Clin Immunol. 2004;114(1):111–117.
4. Filep S, Tsay A, Vailes L, et al. A multi-allergen standard for the calibration of immunoassays: CREATE principles applied to eight purified allergens. Allergy. 2012;67(2):235–241.
5. van Ree R, Chapman MD, Ferreira F, et al. The CREATE project: development of certified reference materials for allergenic products and validation of methods for their quantification. Allergy. 2008;63(3):310–326.
6. Soh WT, Aglas L, Mueller GA, et al. Multiple roles of Bet v 1 ligands in allergen stabilization and modulation of endosomal protease activity. Allergy. 2019;74(12):2382–2393.
7. Marsh DG, Goodfriend L, King TP, Lowenstein H, Platts-Mills TA. Allergen nomenclature. Bull World Health Organ. 1986;64(5):767–774.
8. El-Gebali S, Mistry J, Bateman A, et al. The Pfam protein families database in 2019. Nucleic Acids Res. 2019;47(D1):D427–D432.

9. Radauer C, Bublin M, Wagner S, Mari A, Breiteneder H. Allergens are distributed into few protein families and possess a restricted number of biochemical functions. J Allergy Clin Immunol. 2008;121(4):847–852. e7.

10. Radauer C, Breiteneder H. Pollen allergens are restricted to few protein families and show distinct patterns of species distribution. J Allergy Clin Immunol. 2006;117(1):141–147.

11. Barnes C. Fungi and Atopy. Clin Rev Allergy Immunol. 2019;57(3):439–448.

12. Obersteiner A, Gilles S, Frank U, et al. Pollen-associated microbiome correlates with pollution parameters and the allergenicity of pollen. PLoS One. 2016;11(2):e0149545.

13. Behrendt H, Becker WM. Localization, release and bioavailability of pollen allergens: the influence of environmental factors. Curr Opin Immunol. 2001;13(6):709–715.

14. van Loon LC, Rep M, Pieterse CM. Significance of inducible defense-related proteins in infected plants. Annu Rev Phytopathol. 2006;44:135–162.

15. Simon-Nobbe B, Denk U, Pöll V, Rid R, Breitenbach M. The spectrum of fungal allergy. Int Arch Allergy Immunol. 2008;145(1):58–86.

16. Voorhorst R, Spieksma-Boezeman MI, Spieksma FT. Is a mite (Dermatophagoides sp) the producer of the house dust allergen? Allerg Asthma (Leipz). 1964;10:329–334.

17. Pollart SM, Chapman MD, Fiocco GP, Rose G, Platts-Mills TA. Epidemiology of acute asthma: IgE antibodies to common inhalant allergens as a risk factor for emergency room visits. J Allergy Clin Immunol. 1989;83(5):875–882.

18. Sears MR, Herbison GP, Holdaway MD, Hewitt CJ, Flannery EM, Silva PA. The relative risks of sensitivity to grass pollen, house dust mite and cat dander in the development of childhood asthma. Clin Exp Allergy. 1989;19(4):419–424.

19. Sporik R, Holgate ST, Platts-Mills TA, Cogswell JJ. Exposure to house-dust mite allergen (Der p I) and the development of asthma in childhood. A prospective study. N Engl J Med. 1990;323(8):502–507.

20. Gelber LE, Seltzer LH, Bouzoukis JK, Pollart SM, Chapman MD, Platts-Mills TA. Sensitization and exposure to indoor allergens as risk factors for asthma among patients presenting to hospital. Am Rev Respir Dis. 1993;147(3):573–578.

21. Illi S, von Mutius E, Lau S, Niggemann B, Grüber C, Wahn U. Perennial allergen sensitisation early in life and chronic asthma in children: a birth cohort study. Lancet. 2006;368(9537):763–770.

22. Almqvist C, Larsson PH, Egmar AC, Hedrén M, Malmberg P, Wickman M. School as a risk environment for children allergic to cats and a site for transfer of cat allergen to homes. J Allergy Clin Immunol. 1999;103(6):1012–1017.

23. Reponen T, Vesper S, Levin L, et al. High environmental relative moldiness index during infancy as a predictor of asthma at 7 years of age. Ann Allergy Asthma Immunol. 2011;107(2):120–126.

24. Zhang Z, Reponen T, Hershey GK. Fungal exposure and asthma: IgE and non-IgE-mediated mechanisms. Curr Allergy Asthma Rep. 2016;16(12):86.

25. Tovey ER, Chapman MD, Platts-Mills TA. Mite faeces are a major source of house dust allergens. Nature. 1981;289(5798):592–593.

26. Chan TF, Ji KM, Yim AK, et al. The draft genome, transcriptome, and microbiome of Dermatophagoides farinae reveal a broad spectrum of dust mite allergens. J Allergy Clin Immunol. 2015;135(2):539–548.

27. Kang BC, Johnson J, Veres-Thorner C. Atopic profile of inner-city asthma with a comparative analysis on the cockroach-sensitive and ragweed-sensitive subgroups. J Allergy Clin Immunol. 1993;92(6):802–811.

28. Arruda LK, Barbosa MC, Santos AB, Moreno AS, Chapman MD, Pomés A. Recombinant allergens for diagnosis of cockroach allergy. Curr Allergy Asthma Rep. 2014;14(4):428.

29. Konradsen JR, Fujisawa T, van Hage M, et al. Allergy to furry animals: new insights, diagnostic approaches, and challenges. J Allergy Clin Immunol. 2015;135(3):616–625.

30. Platts-Mills JA, Custis NJ, Woodfolk JA, Platts-Mills TA. Airborne endotoxin in homes with domestic animals: implications for cat-specific tolerance. J Allergy Clin Immunol. 2005;116(2):384–389.

31. Wright GR, Howieson S, McSharry C, et al. Effect of improved home ventilation on asthma control and house dust mite allergen levels. Allergy. 2009;64(11):1671–1680.

32. Munir AK, Einarsson R, Dreborg SK. Indirect contact with pets can confound the effect of cleaning procedures for reduction of animal allergen levels in house dust. Pediatr Allergy Immunol. 1994;5(1):32–39.

33. Gao X, Yin M, Yang P, et al. Effect of exposure to cats and dogs on the risk of asthma and allergic rhinitis: a systematic review and meta-analysis. Am J Rhinol Allergy. 2020;34(5):703–714.

34. Ownby DR, Peterson EL, Wegienka G, et al. Are cats and dogs the major source of endotoxin in homes? Indoor Air. 2013;23(3):219–226.

35. Stewart GA, Richardson JP, Zhang J, Robinson C. The structure and function of allergens. In: Adkinson NF, Bochner BS, Burks AW, Busse WW, Holgate ST, Lemansk eRF, eds. Middleton's allergy—principles and practice. 8th ed. Philadelphia, USA: Elsevier Saunders; 2014:398–429.

36. Wan H, Winton HL, Soeller C, et al. Der p 1 facilitates transepithelial allergen delivery by disruption of tight junctions. J Clin Invest. 1999;104(1):123–133.

37. Zhang J, Chen J, Robinson C. Cellular and molecular events in the airway epithelium defining the interaction between house dust mite group 1 allergens and innate defences. Int J Mol Sci. 2018;19(11):3549.

38. Zhang J, Chen J, Newton GK, Perrior TR, Robinson C. Allergen delivery inhibitors: a rationale for targeting sentinel innate immune signaling of group 1 house dust mite allergens through structure-based protease inhibitor design. Mol Pharmacol. 2018;94(3):1007–1030.

39. Jacquet A, Robinson C. Proteolytic, lipidergic and polysaccharide molecular recognition shape innate responses to house dust mite allergens. Allergy. 2020;75(1):33–53.

40. Millien VO, Lu W, Shaw J, et al. Cleavage of fibrinogen by proteinases elicits allergic responses through Toll-like receptor 4. Science. 2013;341(6147):792–796.

41. Gour N, Lajoie S, Smole U, et al. Dysregulated invertebrate tropomyosin-dectin-1 interaction confers susceptibility to allergic diseases. Sci Immunol. 2018;3(20):eaam9841.

42. Platts-Mills TA, Tovey ER, Mitchell EB, Moszoro H, Nock P, Wilkins SR. Reduction of bronchial hyperreactivity during prolonged allergen avoidance. Lancet. 1982;2(8300):675–678.

43. Platts-Mills TAE. Allergen avoidance in the treatment of asthma: problems with the meta-analyses. J Allergy Clin Immunol. 2008;122(4):694–696.

44. Sanda T, Yasue T, Oohashi M, Yasue A. Effectiveness of house dust-mite allergen avoidance through clean room therapy in patients with atopic dermatitis. J Allergy Clin Immunol. 1992;89(3):653–657.

45. Matsui E, Thomas AE, Platts-Mills TAE. Indoor allergens. In: Burks AW, Holgate S, O'Hehir R, Bacharier L, Broide D, Hershey GK, eds. Middleton's allergy: principles and practice. 1. 9th ed. London: Elsevier; 2019:451–466.

46. Portnoy J, Miller JD, Williams PB, et al. Environmental assessment and exposure control of dust mites: a practice parameter. Ann Allergy Asthma Immunol. 2013;111(6):465–507.

47. Satyaraj E, Wedner HJ, Bousquet J. Keep the cat, change the care pathway: a transformational approach to managing Fel d 1, the major cat allergen. Allergy. 2019;74(Suppl 107):5–17.

48. Phipatanakul W, Matsui E, Portnoy J, et al. Environmental assessment and exposure reduction of rodents: a practice parameter. Ann Allergy Asthma Immunol. 2012;109(6):375–387.

49. Barnes CS, Horner WE, Kennedy K, Grimes C, Miller JD. Home assessment and remediation. J Allergy Clin Immunol Pract. 2016;4(3):423–431. e15.

50. Michel O, Ginanni R, Duchateau J, Vertongen F, Le Bon B, Sergysels R. Domestic endotoxin exposure and clinical severity of asthma. Clin Exp Allergy. 1991;21(4):441–448.

51. Hernandez ML, Peden DB. Air pollution: indoor and outdoor. In: Burks AW, Holgate S, O'Hehir R, Bacharier L, Broide D, Hershey GK, eds. Middleton's allergy: principles and practice. 1. London: Elsevier; 2019:479–499.

52. Peden DB. The epidemiology and genetics of asthma risk associated with air pollution. J Allergy Clin Immunol. 2005;115:213–219.

53. Schiavoni G, D'Amato G, Afferni C. The dangerous liaison between pollens and pollution in respiratory allergy. Ann Allergy Asthma Immunol. 2017;118(3):269–275.

54. Gilmour MI, Jaakkola MS, London SJ, Nel AE, Rogers CA. How exposure to environmental tobacco smoke, outdoor air pollutants, and increased pollen burdens influences the incidence of asthma. Environ Health Perspect. 2006;114(4):627–633.

55. Rawlinson C, Martin S, Frosina J, Wright C. Chemical characterisation of aerosols emitted by electronic cigarettes using thermal desorption-gas chromatography-time of flight mass spectrometry. J Chromatogr A. 2017;1497:144–154.

56. Herrington JS, Myers C. Electronic cigarette solutions and resultant aerosol profiles. J Chromatogr A. 2015;1418:192–199.

57. Peden DB. The role of oxidative stress and innate immunity in O(3) and endotoxin-induced human allergic airway disease. Immunol Rev. 2011;242(1):91–105.

58. Arbour NC, Lorenz E, Schutte BC, et al. TLR4 mutations are associated with endotoxin hyporesponsiveness in humans. Nat Genet. 2000;25(2):187–191.

59. Tiotiu AI, Novakova P, Nedeva D, et al. Impact of air pollution on asthma outcomes. Int J Environ Res Public Health. 2020;17(17):6212.

60. Arias-Pérez RD, Taborda NA, Gómez DM, Narvaez JF, Porras J, Hernandez JC. Inflammatory effects of particulate matter air pollution. Environ Sci Pollut Res Int. 2020;27:42390–42404.

61. Codispoti CD, LeMasters GK, Levin L, et al. Traffic pollution is associated with early childhood aeroallergen sensitization. Ann Allergy Asthma Immunol. 2015;114(2):126–133.

62. Brandt EB, Biagini Myers JM, Acciani TH, et al. Exposure to allergen and diesel exhaust particles potentiates secondary allergen-specific memory responses, promoting asthma susceptibility. J Allergy Clin Immunol. 2015;136(2):295–303. e7.

63. Bernstein JA, Alexis N, Bacchus H, et al. The health effects of non-industrial indoor air pollution. J Allergy Clin Immunol. 2008;121(3):585–591.

64. Trasande L, Thurston GD. The role of air pollution in asthma and other pediatric morbidities. J Allergy Clin Immunol. 2005;115(4):689–699.

65. Jerrett M, Burnett RT, Pope 3rd CA, et al. Long-term ozone exposure and mortality. N Engl J Med. 2009;360(11):1085–1095.

66. Hernandez ML, Lay JC, Harris B, et al. Atopic asthmatic subjects but not atopic subjects without asthma have enhanced inflammatory response to ozone. J Allergy Clin Immunol. 2010;126(3):537–544. e1.

67. Bauer RN, Diaz-Sanchez D, Jaspers I. Effects of air pollutants on innate immunity: the role of Toll-like receptors and nucleotide-binding oligomerization domain-like receptors. J Allergy Clin Immunol. 2012;129(1):14–24. quiz 5–6.

68. Barnes CS. Impact of climate change on pollen and respiratory disease. Curr Allergy Asthma Rep. 2018;18(11):59.

69. Ziska LH, Beggs PJ. Anthropogenic climate change and allergen exposure: the role of plant biology. J Allergy Clin Immunol. 2012;129(1):27–32.

70. Gotzsche PC, Johnasen HK. House dust mite control measures for asthma: systematic review. Allergy 2008; 63:646–659.

5

Principles of Allergy Diagnosis

Anca-Mirela Chiriac and Pascal Demoly

CHAPTER OUTLINE

INTRODUCTION

The cause–effect relationship between allergens and allergic diseases was suspected (and investigated) long before the identification of immunoglobulin E (IgE) antibodies (the "reagins") half a century ago. Thus, chronologically, skin testing took the lead on the detection and quantification of

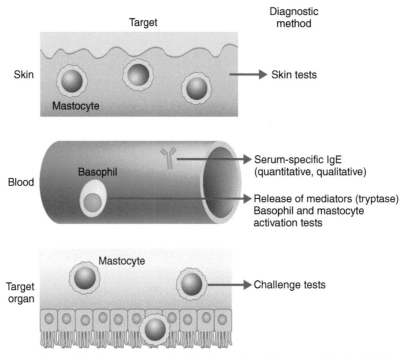

Fig. 5.1 Differences between in vivo and in vitro tests used in the diagnosis of immunoglobulin E (IgE)–mediated diseases.

serum-specific IgE (sIgE) and has been the primary tool for investigation in allergy since its introduction in 1865 by Charles Blackley.

Since the early recognition that allergic diseases (later described as IgE-mediated allergic diseases for their immediate clinical forms) are caused by exposure to allergens, it has been a common practice to establish the presence or absence of sensitization by reexposure of the individual to the allergen. This consists of tests that are performed either in vivo or in vitro (Fig. 5.1).

Skin tests are simple, quick to perform, low cost, and highly sensitive, which explains their key position in allergy diagnosis.[1-3] Nowadays, prick tests are performed with different devices. Needles as well as single or multiheaded devices have been proposed and used in order to decrease the variability of the prick test procedure by different investigators, to increase acceptability (especially in children), and to permit several tests to be performed with one application and thus minimize technician time and increase efficiency. The selection and number of allergen sources should be based on the history provided by the patient and his environment.

With the ongoing technological revolution occurring in biology over the last two decades (Fig. 5.2), in-depth allergic profiles of patients can nowadays be captured.[4] New technologies have facilitated the identification, cloning, and purifying of the most common allergenic molecules, the so-called molecular allergology (component-resolved diagnosis, CRD), whose place in detecting IgE sensitization is ever growing due to the precision it conveys. In contrast to conventional sIgE antibody assays, CRD does not rely upon crude preparations obtained from natural allergen sources (generally poorly defined mixtures containing both allergenic and nonallergenic components) but

on sIgE antibodies directed toward single components purified from natural sources or produced by recombinant techniques.

Today, these allergenic components can be consistently produced. They are not yet widely available in current allergy/clinical practices for in vivo testing, but are available for in vitro testing, either in single or multiplex assays. More than 130 allergenic molecules from more than 50 allergen sources are commercially available for in vitro sIgE testing.[4-6]

As a result of this significant progress in biochemistry and molecular biology during the last two decades, sensitization patterns to hundreds of allergenic components could be studied throughout life and resulting longitudinal trajectories be identified. Data from different cohorts, especially birth cohorts, have proven that patterns of sensitization have different times of occurrence (early life or later on) and different stability (permanent or transient), and that their respective association with clinical expression, including comorbidity and multimorbidity, is different.[7-9] Respiratory and food allergies largely benefit nowadays from allergenic profiling and, to a lesser extent, Hymenoptera venom allergy. Unfortunately, little or no applicable progress has been made in the last decades for drug allergy, whose allergy workup remains mostly in vivo.

Coupled with machine learning, knowledge about in-depth molecular allergenic profile and its timely evolution has entailed a shift of paradigm. The "classical" atopic march referring to a sequential development of symptoms (or diseases) from eczema in infancy to asthma and then allergic rhinitis in later childhood cannot explain the spectrum of allergic phenotypes and endotypes. In the near future, this concept could become completely obsolete, giving way to a mechanism-based framework and incorporating the molecular sensitization march, instead of just the traditional symptom-based criteria.[8,10]

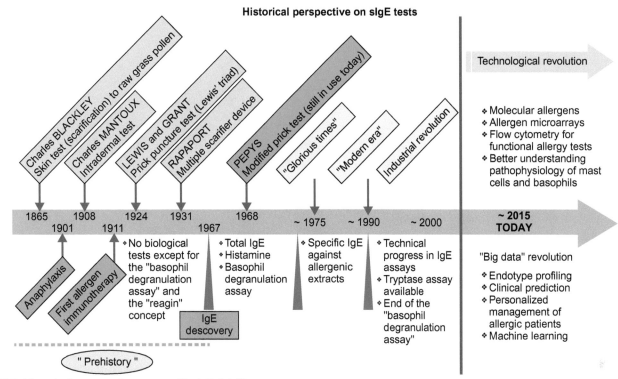

Fig. 5.2 Historical perspective on specific IgE *(sIgE)* tests.

Among nonspecific allergy tests performed in immediate-type reactions, serum tryptase measurement has become a "must" whenever anaphylaxis occurs.[11] The interpretation of acute (i.e., during the presumed allergic reaction) and basal tryptase values guides the clinician through the spectrum of possible diagnoses: IgE-mediated allergy, non-allergic manifestations, and mastocytosis. Tryptase has proven its utility especially in drug and Hymenoptera venom allergy, and to a lesser extent, in food allergy anaphylaxis.

If molecular allergology holds a privileged place, because of its role in phenotyping allergic profiles, the main limitation of IgE sensitization tests is that a positive test does not necessarily mean that patients will experience symptoms, because patients can have allergen-sIgE without clinical symptoms (Fig. 5.3). Therefore, knowledge of and training in interpretation of these tests are mandatory.

The diagnosis and management of allergic diseases is problematic due to their increasing prevalence and complexity. The majority of patients seeking medical advice for allergies are first seen in the primary care setting.[12–14] As a result, primary care physicians are increasingly expected to diagnose and manage allergies. Studies have shown that effective allergy services can not only improve quality of life but can also be cost-saving. An adequate care pathway should clarify and improve referral practices, prompting primary care to manage mild and moderate allergic patients referring only more complex or severe cases to specialist services, thus avoiding delays in patient management.

This chapter is focused on the approach of a patient with a suspected IgE-mediated allergy.

Highly specific allergy tests, namely challenge tests, which are performed in specialized centers, are not within the scope of this chapter.

USE OF IGE SENSITIZATION TESTS IN EPIDEMIOLOGY

Skin tests and sIgE detection (classically in serum but also in other fluids like tears and breast milk for research purposes) have been used to assess the prevalence of sensitizations to common food and respiratory allergens in the general population and how it compares with the prevalence and severity of symptomatic allergic or respiratory diseases, for long-term studies of the development of sensitization and natural desensitization and the factors that influence both. More recently, molecular allergology has been used in epidemiological studies (cross-sectional or longitudinal cohorts) to study the changes in the allergy profile or the prediction of the occurrence allergic disease over time.

PATHOGENESIS AND ETIOLOGY

Skin tests reproduce the IgE-dependent allergic reaction that occurs in the target organs. The IgE-mediated allergic response in the skin results immediately in a wheal and flare reaction that depends on proinflammatory and neurogenic mediators (i.e., immediate reaction). It is irregularly followed by a late-phase reaction (LPR) starting 1 to 2 hours later, peaking at 6 to 12 hours, and resolving in approximately 24 to 48 hours. The LPR is represented by an erythematous inflammatory reaction. It is rarely seen, in common practice.

The immediate reaction is essentially induced by mast cell degranulation after allergen challenge. Histamine and tryptase release begins about 5 minutes after allergen injection and peaks at 30 minutes.

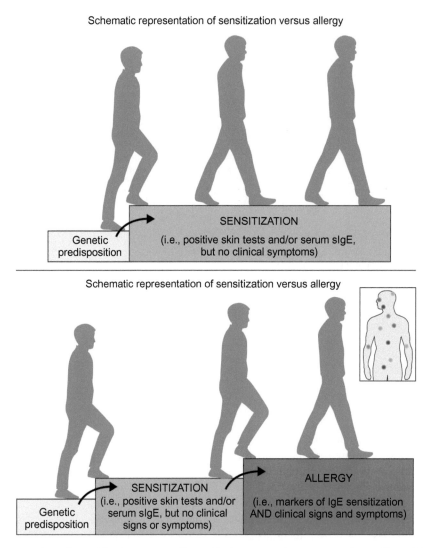

Fig. 5.3 Schematic representation of sensitization versus allergy. Patients who have a genetic predisposition to produce specific IgE toward allergens of the environment become sensitized to different allergens throughout their life. Their sensitization may be proven by skin testing or serum-specific IgE. However, if these patients have no clinical complaint of allergy, they are considered just "sensitized," but not truly allergic. When symptoms and signs evocative of allergy occur for the allergens for which the patient is sensitized, the patient is then considered allergic.

Regarding detection and quantification of serum sIgE, the principle of detection and quantification of sIgE relies on the formation of an antigen-antibody immune complex between the protein extract and the sIgE antibodies in the patients' serum recognizing the antigen. Subsequently, an antihuman-IgE antibody is added. A substrate is then added and its metabolization by the enzyme-conjugated anti-IgE will result in signal, evaluated by image analysis software.[15]

CLINICAL FEATURES

The diagnosis of allergy requires first an appropriate medical history and physical examination.

Suspected IgE-mediated reactions classically occur within 1 hour (immediate reactions) after the last allergen exposure and have characteristic semiology (Fig. 5.4). In peculiar cases and for specific allergens, IgE-mediated reactions

may occur within 6 hours (rarely even later) after allergen exposure (e.g., wheat allergy, red meat allergy, proton pump inhibitor allergy).

PATIENT EVALUATION

Why Test

Why Search for IgE Sensitization?

The term *atopy* describes a heritable propensity to produce IgE antibodies toward innocuous antigens through the process of sensitization. The classical "atopic" diseases, namely asthma, rhinitis, food allergy, and atopic dermatitis, are actually associated with both allergen-sIgE and non-allergic mechanisms that may coexist in the same patient. In addition, they tend to cluster, and patients may present concomitant or consecutive diseases (allergic multimorbidity) as shown in various recent studies.[7–9]

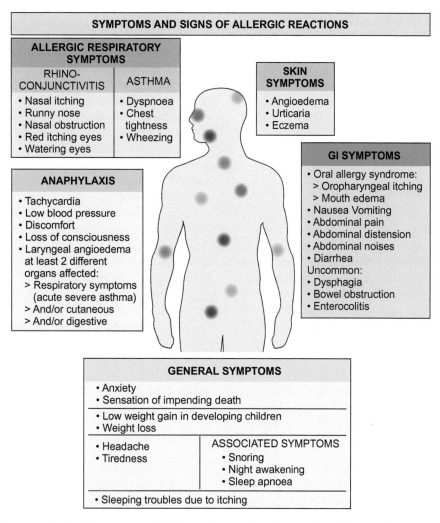

SYMPTOMS AND SIGNS OF ALLERGIC REACTIONS

ALLERGIC RESPIRATORY SYMPTOMS

RHINO-CONJUNCTIVITIS	ASTHMA
• Nasal itching • Runny nose • Nasal obstruction • Red itching eyes • Watering eyes	• Dyspnoea • Chest tightness • Wheezing

SKIN SYMPTOMS
• Angioedema
• Urticaria
• Eczema

ANAPHYLAXIS
• Tachycardia
• Low blood pressure
• Discomfort
• Loss of consciousness
• Laryngeal angioedema at least 2 different organs affected:
> Respiratory symptoms (acute severe asthma)
> And/or cutaneous
> And/or digestive

GI SYMPTOMS
• Oral allergy syndrome:
> Oropharyngeal itching
> Mouth edema
• Nausea Vomiting
• Abdominal pain
• Abdominal distension
• Abdominal noises
• Diarrhea
Uncommon:
• Dysphagia
• Bowel obstruction
• Enterocolitis

GENERAL SYMPTOMS
• Anxiety
• Sensation of impending death
• Low weight gain in developing children
• Weight loss

• Headache • Tiredness	ASSOCIATED SYMPTOMS • Snoring • Night awakening • Sleep apnoea

• Sleeping troubles due to itching

Fig. 5.4 Symptoms and signs of allergic reactions. *GI*, Gastrointestinal. (Adapted from Demoly P, Chabane H, Fontaine JF, et al. Development of algorithms for the diagnosis and management of acute allergy in primary practice. World Allergy Organ J 2019; 12(3):100022, Fig. 4.)

Confirmatory evidence of sIgE sensitization allows the practitioner to reinforce the causal relationship between symptoms and (the suspected) allergens when the patient is exposed to them, prompting counseling on targeted allergen avoidance, symptomatic, and/or specific disease-modifying treatment, when appropriate (e.g., allergen immunotherapy, AIT).

Moreover, testing will address common patient concerns about allergy, predicting exacerbations and response to therapies, and possibly increase compliance with therapy.[14] Positive allergy test results can be considered as one of the referral criteria for specialist care.

The stakes of confirmatory evidence of IgE sensitization are even higher, due to its predictive value of more complex clinical forms:
- Patterns of aeroallergen sensitization help in defining asthma phenotypes;
- monosensitization and polysensitization seem to be different phenotypes;
- asthma-rhinitis multimorbidity is associated with IgE;
- polysensitization in adolescents and adults;
- asthma-rhinitis multimorbidity is associated with IgE;

- polysensitization in adolescents and adults;
- asthma-rhinitis multimorbidity is associated with polysensitization, irrespective of the age (children, adolescents, and adults);
- the multimorbid polysensitized phenotype is associated with (i) food allergy, (ii) atopic dermatitis, (iii) a low probability of remission of IgE sensitization and symptoms, (iv) elevated levels of total and sIgE, (v) high levels of blood eosinophils, and (vi) a high rate of allergy in family history.

On the other hand, the lack of evidence of IgE sensitization prompts a search for other causes of symptoms and the management of a differential diagnosis. In children, negative results do not exclude the possibility of development of upcoming sensitization and allergic diseases in the future and may be repeated (see later).

Whom to Test

Who Would Benefit From Testing?

Classical indications[3] are (i) asthma, (ii) rhinitis/rhinosinusitis/rhinoconjunctivitis/conjunctivitis, suspected (iii) food, (iv) drug, (iv) Hymenoptera venom allergy, (vi) anaphylaxis, and (vii) suspected occupational allergy.

Other indications more likely fall within a case-by-case indication due to the complexity of the diseases: (i) chronic or acute urticaria (when clinical history suggests an allergen as potential trigger/aggravating factor); (ii) eczema/atopic dermatitis (if the underlying presence of IgE hypersensitivity to specific allergens is suspected); (iii) eosinophilic esophagitis, eosinophilic gastroenteritis, or allergic bronchopulmonary aspergillosis, where IgE sensitization is one of the characteristics of the disease's pathogenesis.

When to Test

Is There an Age Limit to Perform Skin Tests?

Skin test wheals increase in size from infancy to adulthood and then often decline after the age of 50. Using prick tests, it has been observed that a significant wheal was detectable after 3 months of age in most infants tested with histamine, codeine phosphate, or allergen extracts. Infants react predominantly with a large erythematous flare and a small wheal. It is therefore possible to perform skin tests to diagnose allergic disorders in infancy, but because the size of the wheal is often reduced, the size of the wheal induced by allergen extracts should always be compared with that elicited by positive control solutions.

Intradermal tests can elicit pain, and this may limit their use in young children. The discomfort may be reduced by the use of a topical anesthetic cream such as the eutectic mixture of local anesthetics (EMLA), which reduces the flare but not the wheal responses.

Does My Patient Need to Be Tested Regularly?

In clinical practice, routine repeated skin testing and serum sIgE dosage are recommended during venom AIT as an indirect measure of acquired tolerance. Otherwise, it is not recommended. However, the search for IgE sensitization may be repeated for a variety of reasons, including (i) the age of the patient (i.e., allergic children have the tendency to acquire new sensitivities over time, beginning with foods and indoor allergens followed by pollens and outdoor molds); (ii) the patient's exposure to new allergens (e.g., acquisition of a new pet, geographic relocation, new job); or (iii) increase and change in symptoms (raising the suspicion of new acquired sensitivities).

Where to Test

The Location: Are Skin Tests Safe to Perform and Can They Be Performed in Office Settings?

Two iatrogenic risks have been evaluated, namely the infectious and the allergic one. Skin tests with necrotizing drugs (e.g., vinorelbine) are not performed.

It could be argued that multiple-use vials of commercialized extracts may raise issues in terms of infectious risk. To date, no report regarding nosocomial infections resulting from skin-prick test procedures has been published. Nevertheless, even if no methicillin-resistant *Staphylococcus aureus* or vancomycin-resistant enterococci were observed in field samples, nosocomial infections may become a concern if skin tests are performed on subjects who are pathogen carriers. Skin bacteria such as *Staphylococcus epidermidis* can survive in allergen extracts for as long as 21 days. Simple prevention measures during pricking and storing of the vials are in place in all practices and explain the absence of reported cases.

The risk of eliciting a generalized reaction during skin test performance is higher with intradermal tests and drugs than with prick tests and commercial inhalant or natural food allergens. Of note, generalized reactions do not necessarily concern allergic ones, since vasovagal reactions are more frequent.

The skin-prick test appears to be safe. Systemic reactions after testing with inhalant allergens, although anecdotal, have been reported. The overall rate of generalized reactions is less than 0.5% in large series (including thousands of pediatric and adult patients undergoing skin-prick tests for inhalant and food allergens).[16] Possible risk factors for adverse reactions during skin testing were suggested: low age and active eczema for generalized allergic reactions; female sex; and multiple skin-prick tests performed on a single patient for vasovagal reactions. No fatalities have been reported.

Intradermal tests, on the other hand, bring a 500 to a 1000 times increase (compared to prick test) in the antigen load that the body is exposed to via the skin and therefore can provoke untoward, large local (immediate and late) and systemic reactions, with an incidence ranging from 0.02% to 1.4% of the tested patients. Some fatalities have been reported, and beta-lactam drugs are most frequently involved in these rare extreme cases.[17] Therefore, several precautionary measures should be taken when using this technique:

- intradermal tests may be performed by a nurse or a technician, but a physician should always be nearby;
- performing skin-prick tests before intradermal tests, and using serial 10-fold dilutions of the usual test concentration, especially in patients with histories of anaphylaxis, are mandatory ways to minimize untoward adverse local and systemic reactions;
- a waiting period of 20 to 30 minutes in the office of the physician is recommended before the patient is released, and this period may be extended for high-risk patients (e.g., patients treated with β-blocking agents, which may interfere with the efficacy of adrenaline, if administered).

In the case of an anaphylactic reaction, a rubber tourniquet should be placed above the test site on the arm and an epinephrine (adrenaline) administered intramuscularly, preferentially in the lateral thigh (i.e., vastus lateralis), according to recommendations.[18]

What to Test

Do All Allergists Test the Same Allergens? Is There a "Standardized" Panel to Be Observed, and If So, How Many Allergens Should Be Tested?

The number of skin tests varies according to the age of the patient (i.e., fewer prick tests are needed in infants for food allergens, house-dust mites, indoor molds, indoor insects, and animal danders versus pollens; acceptability to skin tests in preschool children is essential, and the number of skin tests should indeed be reduced to a minimum based on the available evidence[1-3]); the geographic location of the patient; the availability of commercial extracts; and the history of the allergic disease (e.g., persistent versus intermittent symptoms, clear causative factors).

If the panel of tested allergens generally depends on the allergen exposure of the geographical area, it should be kept in mind that allergic patients are traveling across countries, and this demographic reality influences the patterns of sensitizations found in a certain area. In a large, multicenter European study involving more than 3000 subjects, sensitization rates were comparable for the most frequent inhalant allergens across Europe but depending on the country,[19] 2 to 9 allergens of 18 were sufficient to identify 95% of sensitized subjects, whereas 4 to 13 allergens were required to identify 100% of sensitized subjects (Table 5.1). When testing certain allergens, like grass pollen, it should be kept in mind that the grass pollen mix selected should cover the regionally most dominant grasses, because non–cross-reactive species exist (e.g., tropical grasses).

Detection of serum sIgE by qualitative tests to mixtures of common respiratory or food allergens is commercially available and could be an option when skin testing is not readily possible. However, their sensitivity is generally lower than that of skin testing, and a negative result cannot rule out allergic sensitization.

When using CRD, the number of tests necessary to enable a correct diagnosis increases significantly, thus increasing the complexity of clinical interpretation and the costs, since more than one component needs to be included to allow identification of the exhaustive allergy profile for the sources of allergens

of interest. The microarray technique for CRD enables sIgE antibody testing in a multiplex format and allows the simultaneous quantification of more than a hundred sIgE antibodies. Sensitizations to respiratory and food allergenic components can be studied in parallel, and cross-sensitizations with or without clinical impact can be identified. This is also a way to find hidden allergens and explain some patients' clinical histories. However, correct application and interpretation of multiplexed CRD require training, since some of the information it provides may be clinically irrelevant. For example, it has repeatedly been shown that ubiquitous structures such as cross-reactive carbohydrate determinants present on glycoproteins of plants and Hymenoptera venom, homologues of the major allergen from birch pollen, profilins, and nonspecific lipid transfer proteins can elicit a significant number of positive sIgE results without clinical significance.[1]

Can We Test Anything on the Skin?

When noncommercialized and nonstandardized allergens are tested, hygienic and nonirritant conditions should be observed. It is not acceptable to test with substances that may potentially contain infectious agents. Some substances (e.g., chemotherapeutic drugs like vinorelbine) may elicit skin necrosis and are strictly forbidden. Others should be diluted in order to respect the skin pH.

With respect to commercialized extracts, the quality of the allergen extract is of major importance. Some false-negative reactions are caused by the lack of sufficient allergens in nonstandardized extracts. Although many years ago skin test materials were often made directly in hospital laboratories or in physicians' offices by extracting allergenic raw materials, this practice cannot be recommended anymore. Allergen extracts are marketed with documented potency (standardized using biologic methods and labeled in biologic units), composition, and stability following regulatory agencies' guidelines.[20] They are extracts from a single source material or mixtures of related, cross-reacting allergens, such as grass pollen, deciduous tree pollen, related ragweed pollen, and related mite allergen extracts. Mixtures of unrelated allergens are avoided because their use may result in false-negative responses due to overdiluted allergenic epitopes in some mixes[2] or enzymatic degradation by proteases.

Variations in the quality and potency of commercial extracts, which may or may not be related to the differences between the US and the European standardization systems, are particularly common in extracts for mites, animal danders, molds, and pollens.[1] In addition to problems related to standardization, some extracts (e.g., Hymenoptera venoms) can induce false-positive reactions by nonimmunologic mechanisms. Preservatives used in allergen extracts also may be irritants; thimerosal can elicit a wheal and flare reaction in nonsensitized subjects.

Because of the difficulties in preparing consistently standardized extracts from natural raw material, new technologies have been tried. Starting from allergen-encoding cDNAs, large amounts of highly pure allergens with a high batch-to-batch consistency can be produced that satisfy the quality requirements of medicinal products manufactured by recombinant DNA technology (rAllergens). Recombinant allergens used for

TABLE 5.1 Examples of Panel for Inhalant Allergens (A) and Food Allergens (B)

A	B
Dust mite[a] (*Dermatophagoides pteronyssinus/farinae*)	Cow's milk
	Goat's milk
Cat (*Felis domesticus*)	Sheep's milk
Dog (*Canis familiaris*)	Hen egg white
Cockroach (*Blatella germanica*)	Fish
Alternaria alternata (tenuis)	Crustaceans
Cladosporium herbarum	Mollusk
Aspergillus fumigatus	Wheat
Alder (*Alnus incana*)[b]	Peanut
Birch (*Betula alba/verrucosa*)[b]	Soybean
Cypress (*Cupressus sempervirens/arizonica*)	Lupin
Hazel (*Corylus avellana*)[b]	Hazelnut
Plane (*Platanus vulgaris*)	Walnut
Grass mix[c]	Cashew nut
Olive (*Olea europaea*)	Pine nut
Mugwort (*Artemisia vulgaris*)	Sesame
Ragweed (*Ambrosia artemisiifolia*)	Mustard
Parietaria judaica	Celery
	Avocado
	Kiwi
	Banana
	Apple
	Peach

Panel A adapted from Bousquet PJ, Burbach G, Heinzerling LM, et al. GA2LEN skin test study III: minimum battery of test inhalant allergens needed in epidemiological studies in patients. Allergy 2009;64:1656–1666.
[a]In tropical countries, testing with *Blomia tropicalis* is recommended.
[b]Cross-reactive.
[c]Including *Poa pratensis, Dactilis glomerata, Lolium perenne, Phleum pratense, Festuca pratensis,* and *Helictotrichon pratense.*

in vivo diagnoses should have the same IgE binding activity as their natural counterparts. The rAllergens of various pollens, molds, mites, bee venom, latex, and celery have already been used for skin testing allergic and control individuals, and skin-prick tests and intradermal tests with rAllergens have proved to be highly specific and safe. Although the diagnostic sensitivity of single rAllergens usually is lower than those obtained with allergen extracts, it can be increased by using rAllergen panels covering the most important allergenic structures in a given complex allergen extract. This type of approach with rAllergens may be of great importance for the diagnosis of allergy to unstable allergen extracts such as fruits and cross-reacting allergens. However, to date, although rAllergens are available in some countries where they are approved for allergy diagnostics, they have not made their way into current clinical practice, most likely due to the cost of their production.

My Patient May Be Allergic to Mango Fruit, Is There an Allergen Extract for This Specific Food?

Classically, commercialized allergen extracts should be stored in a refrigeration unit at 2–8 °C to improve stability. The large spectrum of allergies makes it impossible to have commercialized and standardized extracts for all potential allergenic substances. When a suspicion of food allergy arises, it is common practice to perform prick tests with the culprit natural food itself. Thus, patients will be required to bring their own "material" for skin testing, in accordance with the intake that elicited the reaction. However, fresh seasonal fruits, for instance, are not always available throughout the year, so allergists find a solution by using frozen aliquots of these fruits.[21,22] The validity of this method has been confirmed, and skin testing with frozen fruits from different families (e.g., apple, peach) proved to be a reliable alternative, with a performance similar to that of fresh fruits. This reasoning is generally extended to other foods, in daily activity, for practical purposes.

For skin testing with fresh foods, thermal denaturation of allergen structure by cooking has been well established. Therefore, the material used for skin testing should observe the same cooking conditions (raw or cooked food) as the culprit dish. When a skin-prick test to a natural food is positive, allergists often confirm the sensitization by measuring the presence of sIgE to the food source and, when appropriate, the molecular allergen is recognized. Also, when skin testing to fresh foods, it should be kept in mind that, contrary to standardized allergen extracts, the allergen is not equally distributed in the food (e.g., *lipid transfer protein* Pru p 3 is highly condensed in the peach peel). Therefore, precautions should be taken, and all parts of the suspected food should be tested to increase sensitivity.

My Patient Was Referred to the Allergist for a Suspicion of Food Allergy. The Allergist Also Performed Skin Tests to Inhalant Allergens, Although My Patient Does Not Have Any Respiratory Complaints

With the growing knowledge in allergology, especially through the input of rAllergens, allergists now have the possibility to establish an allergic profile that goes all the way to the molecular level. Performing skin tests for inhalant allergens enables the allergist to search for atopic sensitization, as a screening test that may then be completed by in vitro assessments of sIgE. Cross-sensitizations between pollens and fruits/vegetables have been described and are known to lead to major clinical impact.[23] Food allergies do not have the same clinical relevance, according to the geographical area where they are diagnosed (e.g., allergy to apple is generally less severe when sensitization to apple occurs via sensitization to birch pollen, as it is often the case in Northern Europe, as compared to Southern Europe, where primary sensitization responsible for apple allergy is to a different apple protein, known to elicit potentially life-threatening reactions).

Determining the allergen sensitization profiles is a major indication of CRD in food allergy.[1] Whether they are animal-derived (e.g., milk, egg, fish allergy) or plant-derived (by primary or secondary sensitization to the food itself), food allergies have largely benefited from the input of data obtained by CRD. In some allergies (e.g., peanut, hazelnut), CRD may discriminate between true allergy and merely sensitization, allowing an individual risk assessment of severity with impact upon dietary measures. Some secondary plant-derived food allergies are now well characterized: the oral allergy syndrome or "birch-fruit-vegetable" syndrome, due to primary sensitization to the major birch pollen allergen Bet v 1 and its extensive cross-reactivity with its labile homologues in fruits, vegetables and nuts; or the latex-fruit-vegetable syndrome, due to cross-sensitization between the allergenic components present in natural rubber and similar epitopes present in fruits like kiwi or banana.[1]

How to Test

What Skin Tests Are Recommended in Allergy Practice?

Prick and intradermal tests are routinely used for skin testing. In the prick method, the antigen is placed on the skin and introduced into the epidermis with a variety of devices. In the intradermal method, the antigen is injected into the dermis using a hypodermic syringe and needle (Fig. 5.5). Before initiating any skin test procedure, some precautions should be taken (Box 5.1). Common errors in skin tested are listed below (Boxes 5.2 and 5.3).

Are Both Types of Tests Mandatory?

Out of safety concerns and in order to ensure the progressive increase in allergen input, intradermal tests should always be preceded by prick tests. However, the latter are not always followed by intradermal tests. A comparison between prick and intradermal tests is shown in Table 5.2. The starting dose of solutions in patients with a preceding negative prick test result should range between 100-fold and 1000-fold dilutions of the concentrated extract used for prick testing.

What Quantity of Allergen Penetrates the Skin Using These Techniques?

It has been shown that even when performed by a skilled operator and with standardized techniques, the prick test shows great limits of reproducibility, at least as far as the size of the inoculum volume is concerned. The variability of the inoculum depends, in a statistically significant way, not only on the tester skills but also on the subject's individual characteristics and therefore can

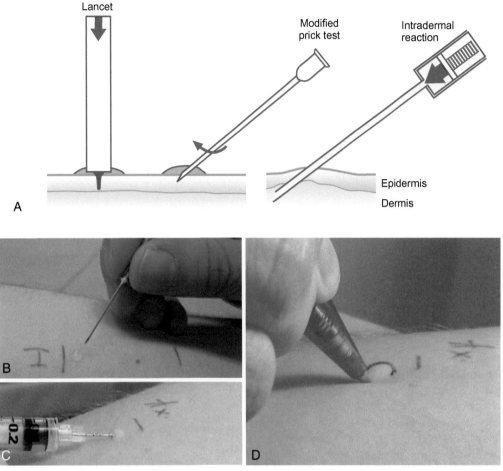

Fig. 5.5 Common methods of skin testing. (A,B) Prick puncture test. (C) For the intradermal test, a volume of appropriately 0.02 to 0.05 mL of allergen extract is injected intracutaneously to produce a small superficial bleb (2 to 4 mm in diameter). (D) The size of skin tests may be outlines with a pen to obtain a permanent record.

BOX 5.1 Skin Testing Precautions

1. Never perform skin tests unless a physician is immediately available to treat systemic reactions.
2. Have emergency equipment, including epinephrine, readily available.
3. Be careful with patients with current allergic symptoms.
4. Determine the potency and stability of the allergen extracts used.
5. Be certain that the test concentrations are appropriate.
6. Include a positive and a negative control solution.
7. Perform tests in normal skin.
8. Evaluate the patient for dermographism.
9. Determine and record medications taken by the patient and time of last dose.
10. Record the reactions at the proper time.

BOX 5.2 Common Errors in Skin-Prick Testing

1. Tests are placed too close together (<2 cm), and overlapping reactions cannot be separated visually.
2. Induction of bleeding can lead to false-positive results.
3. Insufficient penetration of skin by puncture instrument can lead to false-negative results; this occurs more frequently with plastic devices.
4. Allergen solutions can spread during the test or when the solution is wiped away.

BOX 5.3 Common Errors in Intradermal Testing

1. Test sites are too close together, and false-positive results can be observed.
2. Volume injected is too large (>0.1 mL).
3. High concentration of allergen can lead to false-positive results.
4. Splash reaction is caused by air injection.
5. Subcutaneous injection leads to a false-negative test (i.e., no bleb formed).
6. Intracutaneous bleeding site is read as a positive test result.
7. Too many tests performed at the same time may induce systemic reactions.

be reduced only within certain limits by the standardization and perfectibility of the technique. The average volume of the prick test inoculum is equal to 0.016 μL, with a remarkable dispersion of the values around the mean. Regarding intradermal test, a volume of approximately 0.02 to 0.05 mL is injected into the dermis. The concentration of allergen extract required to elicit a positive reaction with intradermal testing is 1000 to 30,000 times smaller than that necessary for a positive prick test.

What Is the Reference to Ensure Reliable Skin Reactivity?

Because of variability in cutaneous reactivity, it is necessary to include negative and positive controls in every skin test evaluation. The negative control solutions are the diluents used to

TABLE 5.2 Relative Advantages of Skin-Prick Tests and Intradermal Tests

Advantages	Skin-prick Test	Intradermal Test
Simplicity	+++	++
Speed	++++	++
Interpretation of positive and negative reactions	++++	++
Discomfort	+	+++
False-positive reactions	Rare	Possible
False-negative reactions	Possible	Rare
Reproducibility	+++	++++
Sensitivity	+++	++++
Specificity	++++	+++
Detection of IgE antibodies	Yes	Yes
Safety	++++	++
Testing of infants	Yes	Difficult

+, Mild; ++, moderate; +++, high; ++++, very high.

TABLE 5.3 Inhibitory Effect of Drugs on IgE-Mediated Skin Tests

Drugs	Degree	Duration (days)	Clinical Significance[a]
H₁ antihistamines			
Azelastine	++++	3–10	Yes
Bilastine	++++	3–10	Yes
Cetirizine	++++	3–10	Yes
Chlorpheniramine	++	1–3	Yes
Clemastine	+++	1–10	Yes
Cyproheptadine	0 to +	1–8	Yes
Desloratadine	++++	3–10	Yes
Diphenhydramine	0 to +	1–3	Yes
Doxepin	++	3–11	Yes
Ebastine	++++	3–10	Yes
Hydroxyzine	+++	1–10	Yes
Ketotifen	++++	>5	Yes
Levocabastine	Possible		Yes
Levocetirizine	++++	3–10	Yes
Loratadine	++++	3–10	Yes
Mequitazine	++++	3–10	Yes
Mizolastine	++++	3–10	Yes
Promethazine	++	1–3	Yes
Rupatadine	++++	3–10	Yes
Tripelennamine	0 to +	1–3	Yes
H₂ antihistamines			
Cimetidine	0 to +		No
Ranitidine	+		No
Imipramines	++++	>10	Yes
Phenothiazines	++		Yes
Corticosteroids			
Systemic, short-term	0		
Systemic, long-term	Possible		Yes
Inhaled	0		
Topical skin	0 to ++		Yes
Theophylline	0 to +		No
Cromolyn	0		
β₂-Agonists			
Inhaled	0 to +		No
Oral, injection	0 to ++		No
Formoterol	Unknown		
Salmeterol	Unknown		
Dopamine	+		
Clonidine	++		
Montelukast	0		
Allergen immunotherapy	0 to ++		No

+, Mild; ++, moderate; +++, high; ++++, very high.
[a]Clinical significance for skin testing.

preserve the allergen extracts. All negative controls should be totally negative. The rare dermographic patient develops wheal and erythema reactions to the negative control. The negative control also detects traumatic reactivity induced by the skin test device (the wheal may approach a diameter of 3 mm with some devices) or the technique of the tester. Although any reaction at a negative control test site makes interpreting allergen sites more difficult, these responses are essential in accurately assessing the presence or absence of true allergic sensitization.

Positive control solutions (histamine or mast cell secretagogues such as codeine phosphate) are used to detect suppression by medications or diseases and to detect exceptional patients who are poorly reactive to histamine. The mean wheal size for positive control solutions is between 5 and 8 mm.

My Patient Is Under Antihistaminic and Antiasthmatic Treatment. How Long Does He Need to Stop the Treatment Before Skin Testing?

Some drugs can interfere with the performance of skin tests and can modulate the wheal or the flare, complicating interpretation of skin tests. Other drugs used in allergic or asthmatic patients do not modify the cutaneous responsiveness, and they can be continued. Tables 5.3 and 5.4 outline the inhibitory effects of therapeutic drugs on skin tests and the delay of suppression of such treatments before performing skin tests. However, it is not reasonable to consider the suppression of antidepressant treatment in psychiatric disorders without consulting the prescribing doctor. In such a scenario, sIgE dosage could be the primary diagnostic tool, since it is not influenced by ongoing treatment.

Antihistamines

The H₁ antihistamines inhibit the wheal and flare response to histamine, allergen, and mast cell secretagogues. The duration

TABLE 5.4   Other Drugs With H1 Antihistamine Effect

Drug Name	Drug Type	Approximative Elimination Half-life[a]
Agomelatine	Atypical antidepressant	1–2 h
Aripiprazole	Atypical antipsychotic	75 h
Clozapine	Atypical antipsychotic	16 h (6 h–30 h)
Dosulepin	Tricyclic antidepressant	30 h
Mianserine	Atypical antidepressant (tetracyclic antidepressant)	40 h (21 h–61 h)
Milnacipran	Serotonin–norepinephrine reuptake inhibitor	8 h
Mirtazapine	Atypical antidepressant (tetracyclic antidepressant)	20 h–40 h
Olanzapine	Atypical antipsychotic	30 h
Paliperidone	Atypical antipsychotic	23 h 25 to 50 days for paliperidone palmitate
Risperidone	Atypical antipsychotic	3–17 h
Quetiapine	Atypical antipsychotic	7 h
Brompheniramine	Antihistamine H1	25 h
Cyproheptadine	Antihistamine H1	10 h to 15 h
Dexchlorpheniramine	Antihistamine H1	14 h to 25 h
Doxylamine	Antihistamine H1	10 h
Fexofenadine	Antihistamine H1	11 h–15 h
Pimethixene	Antihistamine H1	Variable, often prolonged
Triprolidine	Antihistamine H1	3.2 h

The half-life of elimination is given, in absence of clear clinical data on their effect on skin testing.

[a]According to pharmacokinetics, after five to seven half-lives, the amount of the drug in the body is considered negligible.

of the inhibitory effect is linked to the pharmacokinetics of the drug and its active metabolites. First-generation H_1 antihistamines reduce skin reactivity for up to 24 hours or slightly longer (for more than 5 days for ketotifen). Second-generation H_1 antihistamines such as azelastine, bilastine, cetirizine, desloratadine, ebastine, fexofenadine, levocetirizine, loratadine, mizolastine, and rupatadine may suppress skin responses for 3 to 7 days. Some H_1 antihistamines, such as cetirizine, inhibit skin tests more than others do, and this effect correlates with relief of allergic rhinitis symptoms. For other antihistamines, such as loratadine, blunting of skin test reactivity to allergen or histamine is not necessarily predictive of the clinical efficacy of these drugs in seasonal allergic rhinitis treatment.

Topical H_1 antihistamines such as levocabastine or azelastine may suppress skin tests especially if multiple doses are used, and these drugs should be discontinued for at least 48 hours before skin testing.

H_2 antihistamines used alone have a limited, if any, inhibitory effect on skin tests. Discontinuing H_2 antagonists on the day of testing is probably sufficient to prevent significant suppression of skin tests and optional for most allergists.

Imipramines, Phenothiazines, and Tranquilizers

Tricyclic antidepressants exert a potent and sustained reduction in skin responses to histamine. This effect may last for a few weeks. Tranquilizers and antiemetic agents of the phenothiazine class have H_1 antihistaminic activity and can abrogate skin test responses. Topical doxepin hydrochloride abolishes skin reactivity after 1 to 3 days of therapy and for up to 11 days after its discontinuation.

Corticosteroids

Short-term (<1 week) administration of corticosteroids used at therapeutic doses in asthmatic patients does not modify cutaneous reactivity to histamine, or allergens. Long-term corticosteroid therapy does not alter histamine-induced vascular reactivity in skin but affects cutaneous mast cell responses and modifies the skin texture, which makes interpretation of immediate skin tests difficult in some cases. However, it has been shown that allergen-induced skin tests can be accurately performed in asthmatic patients receiving long-term oral corticosteroid treatment. The effects of inhaled corticosteroids have not been directly evaluated, but because therapeutic doses produce fewer systemic effects than oral steroids, their potential for interference is predictably insignificant. In contrast, the application of topical dermal corticosteroids for 1 week reduces the immediate and the late-phase skin reaction induced by allergen.

Other Immunomodulators

Few data are available regarding the effect of other immunomodulating agents, including biologicals, on skin testing. During omalizumab treatment in asthmatic allergic patients, the size of allergen-induced early phase and late-phase skin responses decreases without being abolished. Under ibrutinib therapy, the response in skin test is abolished (except to the positive control).

Other Drugs

Theophylline slightly reduces skin tests, but its administration does not need to be stopped before skin testing.

Short-acting inhaled β_2-agonists in doses approved for the treatment of asthma do not usually inhibit allergen-induced skin tests. Oral terbutaline can decrease the allergen-induced wheal, but this inhibitory effect has little significance in clinical practice. For long-acting inhaled β_2-agonists, such as formoterol and salmeterol, definitive results are lacking. Conversely, β-blocking agents such as propranolol can significantly increase skin histamine reactivity.

Inhaled cromolyn and nedocromil do not alter the skin wheal response to skin tests with allergens or degranulating agents, and neither does cutaneously applied sodium cromoglycate. Dopamine and clonidine can decrease skin test reactivity, whereas this effect has not been observed with nifedipine and montelukast. Angiotensin-converting enzyme inhibitors moderately increase skin reactivity to allergen, histamine, codeine, and bradykinin. Topical pimecrolimus does not seem to modify skin reactivity.

Can Skin Tests Be Performed Despite Ongoing Antihistaminic Treatment?

Upon the allergist's decision, skin tests may be performed under antihistaminic treatment (e.g., in patients with antidepressant treatment having antihistaminic properties, if the risk/benefit analysis is in favor of pursuing the treatment). However, in such circumstances, only positive results must be taken into account, and all negative results must be considered as potentially false negatives. The allergy workup can be supplemented in these cases with in vitro allergen-sIgE tests. Typically, skin tests are more sensitive than the latter, but using standardized extracts, the percentage agreement between in vitro allergen-sIgE tests and skin-prick tests is between 85% and 95%, depending on the allergens being evaluated. Moreover, other in vivo tests (e.g., bronchial, nasal, or oral challenges) can be considered, in an appropriate medical environment. For good clinical practice, H1-antihistamines should be stopped a week before practicing immediate-reading skin tests.

On Which Area of the Body Are Skin Tests Performed?

Skin test can be performed either on the back or on the forearm (or both, at the same time).

The back as a whole is more reactive than the forearm, and this differential effect is more pronounced for allergen extracts than for histamine solutions. Within these two areas, differences of reactivity have been shown: (1) the middle and upper back areas are more reactive than the lower back, and (2) the antecubital fossa is the most reactive portion of the arm, whereas the wrist is the least reactive (therefore, tests should not be placed in areas 5 cm from the wrist and 3 cm from the antecubital fossa). Apart from the practical aspect, performing skin tests on the forearm adds an educational value to the test, because the patients can see the results for themselves. Both forearms can be used. Whichever area is chosen, a safety distance of at least 2 cm between tests should be observed, in order to avoid cross-contamination.

How Much Does It Take to Get the Result of the Skin Tests?

Regardless of which method is used, the immediate skin test induces a wheal and flare response that reaches a peak in 8 to 10 minutes for histamine, 10 to 15 minutes for mast cell secretagogues, and 15 to 20 minutes for allergens. Globally, it takes between 15 and 20 minutes for prick tests and intradermal tests, respectively. Skin tests are read at the peak of their reaction and in a standard manner. When the reactions are mature, the size of each reaction is measured with a millimeter rule. To obtain a permanent record, the size of the reaction is outlined with a pen, blotted onto cellophane tape, and stored on paper or scanned for the patients' electronic health records.

How to Interpret

When Is a Skin Test Considered Positive?

Evaluation of the wheal or erythema is used to assess the positivity of skin tests. The positive control should optimally show a wheal diameter that is 3 mm or larger.[3] Reactions to prick tests are regarded as positive and possibly indicative of clinical allergy if they are greater than 3 mm in wheal diameter and greater than 10 mm in flare diameter. Another criterion is the ratio of the size of the wheal induced by the allergen compared with the positive control. Any degree of positive response (i.e., small wheals of 1 to 2 mm with flare and itching), with appropriate positive and negative controls, indicates the presence of allergic sensitization to a particular allergen. Although significant in immunologic terms, small positive reactions do not necessarily indicate the presence of a clinically relevant allergy. Correlating skin test results with the clinical history is essential in interpreting the clinical significance of the testing procedure.

Can Skin Tests Become Positive Later On? My Patient Developed a Reaction a Few Hours After the Allergy Visit and Skin Tests

The immediate reaction resulting in a wheal and flare is irregularly followed by an LPR starting 1 to 2 hours later, peaking at 6 to 12 hours, and resolving in approximately 24 to 48 hours. The LPR is represented by an erythematous inflammatory reaction. LPRs are not often recorded: not only are their mechanisms insufficiently characterized, but their exact clinical significance is unknown. Histamine accounts for only a limited portion of the LPR. Lymphocytes, predominantly CD4+ T cells, play a key role in the generation and regulation of the LPR by the generation and release of cytokines. These findings are in contrast to delayed hypersensitivity, in which CD8+ T cells are significant participants in the infiltrated erythema that characterizes a positive test. Interestingly, the same cellular pattern may be found after an immediate wheal and flare response that does not lead to a macroscopic LPR.

How Reliable Is Skin Testing?

False-positive and false-negative skin test results may reflect improper technique or material. False-positive results may be provoked by impurities, contaminants, and nonspecific mast cell secretagogues in the extract, as well as by dermatographism and nonspecific enhancement from a nearby strong reaction. False-negative skin test results can be caused by extracts of poor initial potency or subsequent loss of potency; drugs modulating the allergic reaction; diseases attenuating the skin response; decreased reactivity of the skin in infants and elderly patients; improper technique (e.g., no or weak puncture); ultraviolet radiation exposure; a too-short or too-long time interval from the reaction; organ allergy; non–IgE-mediated mechanism; and infections, such as those by helminths. The use of positive and negative control solutions (or even the use of controls subjects) may help to clarify some of the false-negative or false-positive results, because reactions are decreased or abolished in patients with weakly reactive skin but are enhanced in those with dermographism or in cases where irritant extracts are used.

Learned societies across the world agree that when properly performed, prick tests are considered to be the most convenient and least expensive screening method for detecting respiratory and food allergic reactions in most patients. However, until the diagnostic efficacy of prick tests is fully established with standardized allergens and methods, negative prick results may be confirmed by more sensitive intradermal techniques, especially for drugs and stinging insect venoms. Even when false-positive and false-negative results have been eliminated, the proper interpretation of test results requires a thorough knowledge of the history and physical findings, because positive skin test result alone does not confirm definite clinical sensitivity to an allergen.

My Patient Has Positive Skin Tests for Cat Dander but No Allergic Symptoms in the Presence of Cats. Does This Mean He Is Allergic to Cats or Not?

A positive skin test response confirms the presence of allergic sensitization but not the presence of allergic disease. Allergic sensitization with no correlative allergic disease is a common finding, occurring in 8% to 30% of the population when using a local standard panel of aeroallergens. Same holds true for some food and drugs. However, positive skin test results for asymptomatic subjects may foreshadow the subsequent onset of allergic symptoms. Prospective studies have shown that 30% to 60% of sensitized-only individuals subsequently develop allergic symptoms that can be attributed to exposure to allergens that previously elicited positive skin test responses.[24]

With inhalant allergens, the skin-prick test is the cheapest and most effective method to diagnose respiratory allergies. Skin-prick tests give immediate information on sensitivity to individual allergens and should therefore be the primary method clinicians use to assess respiratory allergic diseases. Positive skin test results with a medical history that suggests clinical sensitivity strongly incriminate the allergen as a contributor to the disease process. Conversely, a negative skin test result with a negative history favors a nonallergic disorder.[14] Interpretation of skin tests that do not correlate with the clinical history is more difficult, and in these situations, measurements of allergen-sIgE and provocative challenges are of interest.

My Patient Is Sensitized to Many Respiratory Allergens. Can He Benefit From Allergen Immunotherapy?

Skin testing merely shows sensitization to the tested allergen sources, which are crude allergen extracts containing a mixture of both allergenic and nonallergenic components. In patients polysensitized to pollens, especially to pollens with overlapping pollination seasons, CRD allows the identification of the profile of sensitization,[1] that is, to genuine or cross-reactive allergens, thus allowing to target the patients who are sensitized to major allergens as candidates who would benefit most from AIT.[25] From these studies it emerges that CRD results alter initial prescription of AIT in up to 50% of the patients, in both children and adults.

My Patient Has Undergone Allergen Immunotherapy for 3 Years to House-Dust Mites but Still Has Positive Skin Tests to These Allergens. Does This Mean That the Treatment Was Not Efficacious?

Demonstrating allergen sensitization before starting AIT is mandatory. A decreased wheal and flare reaction has been observed in patients undergoing AIT (to inhalant or food

allergens), as well as in patients who are spontaneously desensitized (e.g., professional beekeepers). However, with the exception of Hymenoptera venom immunotherapy, skin tests are not recommended in immunotherapy follow-up. They cannot be used to assess the efficacy of AIT in practice, nor should they be used to decide on the cessation of immunotherapy.

My Patient Has Suffered From an Anaphylactic Shock a Few Days Ago. The Allergist Prescribed an Emergency Kit, but Did Not Perform Any Skin Tests Yet. Why?

After a systemic allergic reaction, a refractory period of up to 6 weeks has been described. This cutaneous anergy (or hypoergy) is attributed to the mediators' depletion after intense mast cell degranulation. It was first described in systemic allergic reactions induced by Hymenoptera sting, and in the absence of further studies, it has been applied to the exploration of other supposedly IgE-mediated reactions. Therefore, following a systemic reaction, an early evaluation might be performed, but in this case, only positive skin test results should be taken into account. If an early evaluation yields negative results, a retest at 4 to 6 weeks is mandatory. Conversely, for certain allergens (e.g., drugs), skin test reactivity may decrease in time, and waiting too long a time (i.e., months to years) to perform skin tests after an allergic event is considered to be a potential source of false-negative results. Sensitization as assessed by skin tests (and in vitro IgE testing) may disappear after cessation of exposure, but there are few data on whether the loss of skin sensitization serves as a guarantee for systemic tolerance upon allergen challenge.

REFERRAL

Inevitably, competences necessary for the management of allergic patients in primary care are broader and more diverse than a few decades ago.[26,27] Therefore, evidence-based recommendations from clinical guidelines from learned allergy societies or expert groups have to be translated into practical tools, providing step-by-step guidance through the allergy reasoning and assisting the physician in making decision before referral. Figs. 5.6A and B show examples of pathways for suspected IgE-mediated respiratory and drug allergy.[13]

A structured allergy history appears to be insufficient when assessing patients with asthma and rhinitis in general practice. The predictive value of clinical history alone in diagnosis of allergic rhinitis was 82% to 85% for seasonal allergens (at least 77% for perennial allergens) and increased to 97% to 99% when skin tests or IgE specific assays were performed in combination. For other allergies (Hymenoptera venom, food and drug allergies, anaphylaxies), referral to the allergists would probably be the option of choice in most cases. Indeed, strict avoidance without understanding better what is going on could rather be deleterious for the patient. However, prior to referral, a series of actions should be undertaken, to facilitate the work of the allergist.

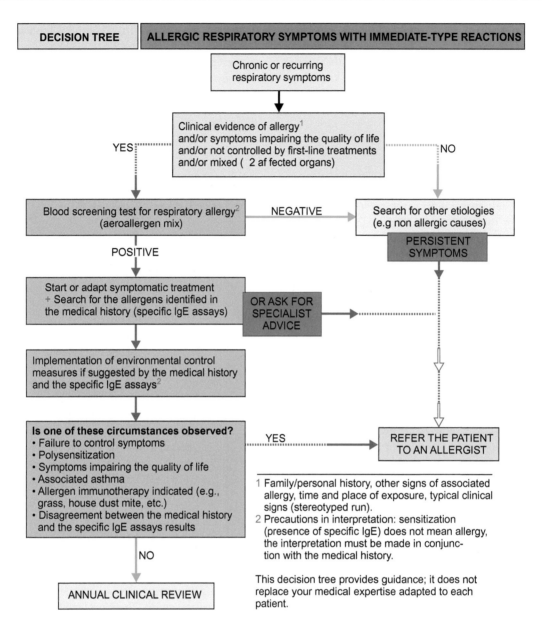

Fig. 5.6 Pathways for suspected IgE-mediated respiratory and drug allergy (A, From Demoly P, Chabane H, Fontaine JF, de Boissieu D, Ryan D, Angier E, Just J. Development of algorithms for the diagnosis and management of acute allergy in primary practice. World Allergy Organ J 2019;12(3):100022, Fig. 2; B, Adapted from Demoly P, Chabane H, Fontaine JF, de Boissieu D, Ryan D, Angier E, Just J. Development of algorithms for the diagnosis and management of acute allergy in primary practice. World Allergy Organ J 2019;12(3):100022, Fig. 3.)

CONCLUSIONS

A major challenge for practitioners working in the allergy field is to create awareness, especially among primary care physicians and other peers, of the value of the tests bringing IgE sensitization to light. Such tests, whether performed in vivo or in vitro,

enable the clinician to confirm or refute sensitization and atopy, which have important prognostic implications. The currently available technologies for detection and quantification of serum sIgE (and in particular molecular allergology) have refined and increased the accuracy of allergy diagnosis, allowing to identify individual sensitization profiles that cannot be achieved by

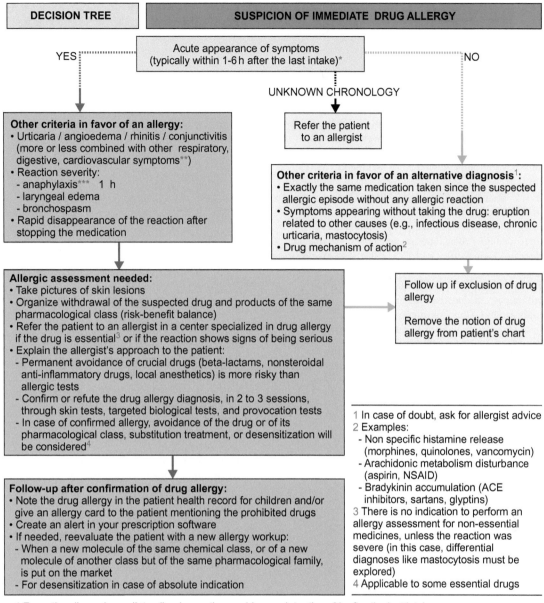

DECISION TREE — SUSPICION OF IMMEDIATE DRUG ALLERGY

Acute appearance of symptoms
(typically within 1-6 h after the last intake)*

YES .... NO

UNKNOWN CHRONOLOGY

Refer the patient
to an allergist

Other criteria in favor of an allergy:
• Urticaria / angioedema / rhinitis / conjunctivitis
  (more or less combined with other respiratory,
  digestive, cardiovascular symptoms**)
• Reaction severity:
  - anaphylaxis*** 1 h
  - laryngeal edema
  - bronchospasm
• Rapid disappearance of the reaction after
  stopping the medication

Other criteria in favor of an alternative diagnosis[1]:
• Exactly the same medication taken since the suspected
  allergic episode without any allergic reaction
• Symptoms appearing without taking the drug: eruption
  related to other causes (e.g., infectious disease, chronic
  urticaria, mastocytosis)
• Drug mechanism of action[2]

Allergic assessment needed:
• Take pictures of skin lesions
• Organize withdrawal of the suspected drug and products of the same
  pharmacological class (risk-benefit balance)
• Refer the patient to an allergist in a center specialized in drug allergy
  if the drug is essential[3] or if the reaction shows signs of being serious
• Explain the allergist's approach to the patient:
  - Permanent avoidance of crucial drugs (beta-lactams, nonsteroidal
    anti-inflammatory drugs, local anesthetics) is more risky than
    allergic tests
  - Confirm or refute the drug allergy diagnosis, in 2 to 3 sessions,
    through skin tests, targeted biological tests, and provocation tests
  - In case of confirmed allergy, avoidance of the drug or of its
    pharmacological class, substitution treatment, or desensitization will
    be considered[4]

Follow up if exclusion of drug
allergy

Remove the notion of drug
allergy from patient's chart

1 In case of doubt, ask for allergist advice
2 Examples:
  - Non specific histamine release
    (morphines, quinolones, vancomycin)
  - Arachidonic metabolism disturbance
    (aspirin, NSAID)
  - Bradykinin accumulation (ACE
    inhibitors, sartans, glyptins)
3 There is no indication to perform an
allergy assessment for non-essential
medicines, unless the reaction was
severe (in this case, differential
diagnoses like mastocytosis must be
explored)
4 Applicable to some essential drugs

Follow-up after confirmation of drug allergy:
• Note the drug allergy in the patient health record for children and/or
  give an allergy card to the patient mentioning the prohibited drugs
• Create an alert in your prescription software
• If needed, reevaluate the patient with a new allergy workup:
  - When a new molecule of the same chemical class, or of a new
    molecule of another class but of the same pharmacological family,
    is put on the market
  - For desensitization in case of absolute indication

* Exceptionally, an immediate allergic reaction could occur later than 6 h after the last intake
** In the case of anaphylaxis / a drop in blood pressure:
    - Ask for urgent advice
    - Dose tryptasemia in the acute phase (30 min to 3 h after symptoms onset)
** In rare cases, anaphylaxis may occur several hours after the last ingestion of the drug, typically for drugs like
proton pump inhibitors

Fig. 5.6–cont'd

skin testing. After allergic sensitization and relevant diseases have been established, proper education regarding allergen avoidance and the prescribing of appropriate medical therapy (including AIT) can be safely and appropriately instituted.

Shared responsibility and communication between the allergist and the general practitioner or the specialist interested in allergology enhance the chances of proper management for the heterogenous spectrum of allergic patients.

REFERENCES

1. Bousquet J, Heinzerling L, Bachert C, et al. Practical guide to skin prick tests in allergy to aeroallergens. Allergy. 2012;67:18–24.

2. Bernstein IL, Li JT, Bernstein DI, et al. American Academy of Allergy, Asthma and Immunology; American College of Allergy, Asthma and Immunology. Allergy diagnostic testing: an updated practice parameter. Ann Allergy Asthma Immunol. 2008;100:S1–S148.

3. Ansotegui IJ, Melioli G, Canonica GW, et al. IgE allergy diagnostics and other relevant tests in allergy: a World Allergy Organization position paper. World Allergy Organ J. 2020;13(2):100080.

4. Steering Committee Authors. Review Panel Members. A WAO-ARIA-GA²LEN consensus document on molecular-based allergy diagnosis (PAMD@): update 2020. World Allergy Organ J. 2020;13(2):100091.

5. Heffler E, Puggioni F, Peveri S, Montagni M, Canonica GW, Melioli G. Extended IgE profile based on an allergen macroarray: a novel tool for precision medicine in allergy diagnosis. World Allergy Organ J. 2018;11(1):7.

6. Potapova E, Bauersachs D, Villella V, et al. Validation study of a new chemiluminescent singleplex IgE assay in a set of Italian allergic rhinitis patients. Clin Exp Allergy. 2020;51:604.

7. Burte E, Bousquet J, Siroux V, Just J, Jacquemin B, Nadif R. The sensitization pattern differs according to rhinitis and asthma multimorbidity in adults: the EGEA study. Clin Exp Allergy. 2017;47(4):520–529.

8. Custovic A, Custovic D, Kljaić Bukvić B, Fontanella S, Haider S. Atopic phenotypes and their implication in the atopic march. Expert Rev Clin Immunol. 2020;16(9):873–881.

9. Siroux V, Ballardini N, Soler M, et al. The asthma-rhinitis multimorbidity is associated with IgE polysensitization in adolescents and adults. Allergy. 2018;73(7): 1447–1458.

10. Lau S, Matricardi PM, Wahn U, Lee YA, Keil T. Allergy and atopy from infancy to adulthood: messages from the German birth cohort MAS. Ann Allergy Asthma Immunol. 2019;122(1):25–32.

11. Valent P, Akin C, Arock M, et al. Definitions, criteria and global classification of mast cell disorders with special reference to mast cell activation syndromes: a consensus proposal. Int Arch Allergy Immunol. 2012;157:215–225.

12. Demoly P, Bossé I, Maigret P. Perception and control of allergic rhinitis in primary care. NPJ Prim Care Respir Med. 2020;30(1):37.

13. Demoly P, Chabane H, Fontaine JF, et al. Development of algorithms for the diagnosis and management of acute allergy in primary practice. World Allergy Organ J. 2019;12(3):100022.

14. Casale TB, Pedersen S, Rodriguez Del Rio P, Liu AH, Demoly P, Price D. The role of aeroallergen sensitization testing in asthma management. J Allergy Clin Immunol Pract. 2020;8(8):2526–2532.

15. Van Gasse AL, Mangodt EA, Faber M, Sabato V, Bridts CH, Ebo DG. Molecular allergy diagnosis: status anno 2015. Clin Chim Acta. 2015;444C:54–61.

16. Liccardi G, D'Amato G, Canonica GW, et al. Systemic reactions from skin testing: literature review. J Investig Allergol Clin Immunol. 2006;16:75–78.

17. Chiriac AM, Vasconcelos MJ, Izquierdo L, Ferrando L, Nahas O, Demoly P. To challenge or not to challenge: literature data on the positive predictive value of skin tests to beta-lactams. J Allergy Clin Immunol Pract. 2019;7(7):2404–2408. e11.

18. Simons FE, Ardusso LR, Dimov V, et al. World Allergy Organization. World Allergy Organization Anaphylaxis Guidelines: 2013 update of the evidence base. Int Arch Allergy Immunol. 2013;162(3):193–204.

19. Bousquet PJ, Burbach G, Heinzerling LM, et al. GA2LEN skin test study III: minimum battery of test inhalent allergens needed in epidemiological studies in patients. Allergy. 2009;64:1656–1662.

20. Klimek L, Hoffmann HJ, Kalpaklioglu AF, et al. In-vivo diagnostic test allergens in Europe: a call to action and proposal for recovery plan-an EAACI position paper. Allergy. 2020;75(9):2161–2169.

21. Bégin P, Des Roches A, Nguyen M, et al. Freezing does not alter antigenic properties of fresh fruits for skin testing in patients with birch tree pollen-induced oral allergy syndrome. J Allergy Clin Immunol. 2011;127:1624–1626.

22. Garriga T, Guilarte M, Luengo O, et al. Frozen fruit skin prick test for the diagnosis of fruit allergy. Asian Pac J Allergy Immunol. 2010;28:275–278.

23. Skypala IJ. Can patients with oral allergy syndrome be at risk of anaphylaxis? Curr Opin Allergy Clin Immunol. 2020;20(5):459–464.

24. Bodtger U, Poulsen LK, Malling HJ. Asymptomatic skin sensitization to birch predicts later development of birch pollen allergy in adults: a 3-year follow-up study. J Allergy Clin Immunol. 2003;111:149–154.

25. Matricardi PM, Dramburg S, Potapova E, Skevaki C, Renz H. Molecular diagnosis for allergen immunotherapy. J Allergy Clin Immunol. 2019;143(3):831–843.

26. Wallengren J. Identification of core competencies for primary care of allergy patients using a modified Delphi technique. BMC Med Educ. 2011;11:12.

27. Jutel M, Papadopoulos NG, Gronlund H, et al. Recommendations for the allergy management in the primary care. Allergy. 2014;69(6):708–718. Erratum in: Allergy 2014;69(8):1118. Braunsthal, G-J [corrected to Braunstahl, G-J]. Erratum in: Allergy 2014;69(10):1428.

6

Allergen-Specific Immunotherapy

Helen E. Smith, Aziz Sheikh, and Robyn E. O'Hehir

SUMMARY OF IMPORTANT CONCEPTS

- Allergen immunotherapy is an effective treatment both for allergic rhinitis and for allergic asthma.
- Sustained clinical effectiveness requires several years of treatment.
- Initially, specific immunotherapy (SIT) induces allergen-specific regulatory T cells that decrease T cell responses to allergens. Over time, there is immune deviation from a predominantly Th2 to a predominantly Th1 pattern of cytokine production.
- Immunotherapy modifies the course of allergic disease, as evidenced by decreases in rates of new allergic sensitizations, and prevention of progression from allergic rhinitis to asthma.
- A minimum of 3 years of SIT will result in persistent benefit for several years after discontinuation.
- Several approaches have been tried to improve the safety and convenience of SIT. These include chemical modifications

of allergen extracts and alternative routes of administration, with sublingual SIT (SLIT) being very popular and effective.

INTRODUCTION

Allergic rhinitis is common and, in many cases, not adequately controlled by standard drug therapy. Specific immunotherapy (SIT) offers a way to desensitize patients, rendering them less sensitive to inhalation of seasonal or perennial allergens. This decreases their symptoms and improves quality of life, as well as decreases the need to use disease-suppressing medication such as nonsedating antihistamines and nasal corticosteroids. SIT also helps in selected patients with allergic asthma, who are especially affected by allergic triggers. SIT provides long-lasting benefits, beyond the period of treatment, but SIT must be administered over several years to achieve maximal efficacy. Traditional SIT involves a course of injections, typically starting with a build-up or initiation phase of 7 to 12 weekly injections followed by monthly maintenance injections for 3 years.

Research has explored modified vaccines to improve efficacy with shorter courses and to minimize the risk of adverse effects. Alternative routes of administration have become popular, with sublingual immunotherapy (SLIT) showing broadly comparable efficacy to subcutaneous injection SIT (SCIT).

HISTORICAL PERSPECTIVE

Interest in the use of vaccination to treat allergy dates back to the late 19th century.[1] It was well recognized that hay fever was a reaction against grass pollen, and that it involved immune recognition of pollen components, so, although the exact mechanisms were unknown, different researchers attempted to immunize patients with pollen extracts. When early attempts invoked anaphylaxis, incremental regimens were tried, starting with a very low dose, and increasing gradually until a large dose could be administered safely. In 1911, Noon and Freeman published the first paper on successful injection immunotherapy. Over the next decade, the practice of injection therapy for hay fever was widely adopted, especially in the US. The scope of immunotherapy was extended to treat perennial rhinitis and asthma, covering additional pollens and perennial allergens such as house-dust mites (HDMs) and animal danders. SIT was one of the first treatments to be subjected to randomized controlled trials, with trials beginning in the 1950s.

For over 100 years, immunotherapy has been given by the same method developed by Noon, with injections at weekly intervals of progressively greater concentrations of extract, followed by a period of several years of maintenance injections. However, in the past 25 years, there has been increasing interest in administering immunotherapy by other routes, especially sublingual/oral, which is intended to decrease the risk of adverse reactions and increase patient convenience. Other areas of research have focused on vaccine modifications so that optimum desensitization can be achieved with fewer injections.

INDICATIONS FOR SPECIFIC ALLERGEN IMMUNOTHERAPY

SIT has three main indications: allergic rhinoconjunctivitis, allergic asthma, and anaphylaxis due to allergy to wasp and bee venom (Box 6.1 and see Chapter 15 Insect Allergy). The efficacy of SIT in seasonal and perennial allergic rhinitis has been established in many well-designed clinical trials.[2]

SIT is also effective as an adjunct therapy in asthma, although its role in treating asthma is less important than in treating allergic rhinitis. In placebo-controlled studies, SIT has been shown to be effective in carefully selected patients with asthma caused by grass pollen, cats, and HDM (Fig. 6.1). The effect is most marked on allergen-specific bronchial hyperresponsiveness,

but effects on lung function have been inconsistent. However, some carefully conducted studies of seasonal and/or perennial asthma have yielded only limited evidence of clinical improvement in patients with asthma. The critical issue is to be sure that the chosen allergen is responsible for causing symptoms in the

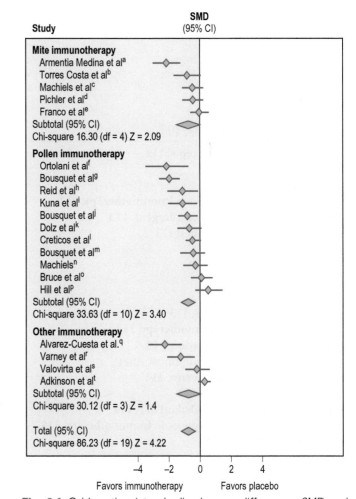

Fig. 6.1 Odds ratios (standardized mean difference, *SMD*) and 95% confidence intervals *(CIs)* for clinical improvement, as evidenced by reduction in asthmatic symptoms after allergen immunotherapy in placebo-controlled studies. *df*, Degrees of freedom. Modified from Abramson M, Puy R, Weiner J. Immunotherapy in asthma: an updated systematic review. Allergy 1999;54:1022–1041. Referenced studies: *a*, Armentia Medina et al. Allergo Immunopathol (Madr) 1995;23:211; *b*, Torres Costa et al. Allergy 1996;51:238; *c*, Machiels et al. J Clin Invest 1990;85:1024; *d*, Pichler et al. Allergy 1997;52:274; *e*, Franco et al. Allergo Immunopathol (Madr) 1995;23:58; *f*, Ortolani et al. J Allergy Clin Immunol 1984;73:283; *g*, Bousquet et al. J Allergy Clin Immunol 1990;85:490; *h*, Reid et al. J Allergy Clin Immunol 1986;78:590; *i*, Kuna et al. J Allergy Clin Immunol 1989;83:816; *j*, Bousquet et al. J Allergy Clin Immunol 1989;84:546; *k*, Dolz et al. Allergy 1996;51:489; *l*, Creticos et al. N Engl J Med 1996;334:501; *m*, Bousquet et al. Clin Allergy 1985;25:179; *n*, Machiels et al. Clin Exp Allergy 1990;20:653; *o*, Bruce et al. J Allergy Clin Immunol 1977;59:449; *p*, Hill et al. BMJ 1982;284:306; *q*, Alvarez-Cuesta et al. J Allergy Clin Immunol 1994;93:556; *r*, Varney et al. Clin Exp Allergy 1997;27:860; *s*, Valovirta et al. Ann Allergy 1986;57:173; *t*, Adkinson et al. N Engl J Med 1997;336:324.

BOX 6.1   Indications for SIT

- Allergic rhinitis
- Allergic asthma (if well controlled)
- Hymenoptera sensitivity

individual patient, and that other contributory treatable traits have already been addressed. Unstable asthma is a risk factor for adverse reactions to SIT, so patients must be carefully selected and optimally managed, and the right allergens must be chosen if immunotherapy is to be of benefit for asthma.[3]

Systemic reactions to hymenoptera venom are relatively rare but can be fatal. If there are no contraindications, SIT is the treatment of choice for this group of patients. The decision to treat is based on exposure risk and likely benefit, so these patients require specialist assessment and careful consideration of the risk-to-benefit ratio (see Chapter 15 Insect Allergy).

CLINICAL EFFICACY WITH SPECIFIC ALLERGENS

Grass, Tree, and Weed Pollens

Patients with seasonal allergic rhinitis are typically sensitized to grass pollen, tree pollens, or ragweed. The specific trigger is usually clear from the history and can be confirmed by detection of serum-specific IgE by skin testing or laboratory testing (sometimes colloquially called "RAST" testing from radio allergosorbent testing, now superceded by immunoassays). Patients with multiple allergies can also benefit from pollen SIT, but the impact is most evident in those with a narrow range of sensitivities.[2] Typically, treatment is given pre-seasonally for 3 years, but sometimes SIT is given all year round, again for a total of 3 years. Improvement can be expected in about 80% of patients if appropriately selected. For these patients, their symptoms may be decreased rather than completely abolished, with a marked decrease in the number of days with severe symptoms and less need for rescue medications (e.g., antihistamines) compared with untreated or placebo-treated controls. Patients who also have pollen-induced seasonal asthma will usually notice an improvement in their chest symptoms, as well as in their nasal symptoms.

House-Dust Mites

HDM sensitization is common and has been implicated as a risk factor for developing asthma. However, unlike pollen allergy, it can be difficult to determine how much of a patient's rhinitis symptoms are attributable to HDM. This is partly because exposure to HDM allergens occurs all year round and partly because many patients with rhinitis also have symptoms due to structural changes and sinusitis that are independent of their HDM allergy and therefore will not respond to mite-specific treatment. Nevertheless, SIT with HDM extracts may be effective in controlling symptoms of perennial allergic rhinitis. Most clinicians would agree that if there is no benefit after 6 months, continuing SIT is unlikely to achieve any benefits. In some cases, an alternative allergen extract may be tried, but more often it is necessary to discontinue SIT and revert to standard pharmacologic treatment.

Domestic Pets

Sensitization to domestic pet allergens is associated with an increased risk of developing asthma. In theory, domestic pet allergen exposure is avoidable and, historically, SIT for pet

allergy was only considered appropriate for people with occupational exposure (e.g., veterinarians and social workers). Clinical trials have shown decreases in asthma symptoms and medication usage, as well as improvements in nonspecific bronchial hyperresponsiveness in cat-allergic patients who do not have cats at home, supporting the use of cat immunotherapy. Currently, there are no corresponding data for dog allergy.

Fungi

Airborne fungal spores are recognized causes of life-threatening asthma attacks and "epidemic outbreaks" of asthma. Unfortunately, there is little accurate information on exposure patterns to most fungal species, and as there are thousands of different species of fungi, it is hard to establish which fungi are relevant to an individual's allergic disease. Diagnosis is made even more difficult because fungal extracts are of variable quality, and there are no allergen extracts available for many genera of fungi because it is impossible to grow them in artificial media. Some benefits on asthma and allergic rhinitis symptoms have been reported in double-blind, controlled studies of SIT with extracts of *Cladosporium herbarum* and *Alternaria alternata*. With fungi, as with any allergen, the decision to use SIT is guided by the patient's sensitization, a pattern of symptoms consistent with the pattern of exposure, and the availability of an extract of sufficient standardization to allow delivery of a therapeutically effective and safe dose. Currently, fungi SIT is seldom prescribed in clinical practice.

Cockroach

Cockroach sensitization is now recognized as a major factor in the pathogenesis of asthma, particularly in those living in inner cities, especially in warmer climates, but there have been no adequately controlled trials of cockroach SIT.

Multiple Allergen Mixtures

Most of the double-blind, placebo-controlled studies that have confirmed the effectiveness of SIT in allergic rhinitis and asthma were performed with single allergen extracts. However, in the US, a typical immunotherapy prescription often contains multiple unrelated allergen extracts. Although current US guidance supports the use of allergen mixtures, it is recommended that patients should only be treated with relevant allergens. The inclusion of too many allergens into a maintenance injection may decrease the overall effectiveness of the treatment.[4] The evidence supporting treatment with multiple allergens comes mainly from trials using mixtures of two allergens; very few studies have examined multi-allergen SIT mixes, and what evidence there is comes from studies performed over 40 years ago, with different mixtures from today. However, clinical experience suggests that SIT with multiple allergen mixes can be effective if the number of allergens used does not dilute out the individual constituents to ineffective concentrations.

SPECIFICITY OF ALLERGEN IMMUNOTHERAPY

SIT is most effective where there is a limited range of allergic sensitivities and where there is clear evidence that those allergens are responsible for triggering symptoms. Clinical improvement is generally only seen in the response to allergens contained within the treatment mixture. However, as some allergens have overlapping proteins, for example, grasses, treatment with pollen from one grass species can decrease responses to pollens from other grasses, but treating with grass pollen has no effect on sensitivity to ragweed, and vice versa.

Clarity about which allergens are triggering symptoms is easier to establish for seasonal pollen allergens and for occupational exposure to domestic animals; it is more difficult to be sure that perennial allergens or people's own pets are truly responsible for ongoing symptoms. Where there is doubt about the role of allergens in causing symptoms or a large number of allergens are implicated, optimizing dose and compliance with nonsedating antihistamines and nasal corticosteroids may be preferable to SIT.

EVIDENCE OF DISEASE MODIFICATION

Part of the argument in favor of SIT is that it may have long-term benefits by modifying the course of the disease, whereas drug therapies only suppress the symptoms for as long as they are taken (Box 6.2). Two outcomes are cited as evidence of disease modification—the prevention of emergent asthma in patients treated for allergic rhinitis and the prevention of new allergic sensitizations. A multicenter European study found that SIT with birch and/or Timothy grass for 3 years decreased the risk of developing asthma by 2.5-fold in children who only had symptoms of rhinitis at the initiation of SIT.[5] This benefit was still apparent 7 years after completing SIT. Several studies have reported decreased rates of development of new sensitizations after SIT, as indicated by newly positive skin-prick test results. In the two larger studies, the rate of new sensitization was decreased by 56%–65% compared with the control group, and this effect persisted for 3 years after completion of 3 to 4 years of treatment with SIT. It seems unlikely that SIT with one allergen directly affects B cells that recognize unrelated allergens. However, SIT might decrease nasal inflammation and thereby alter the local environment, decreasing the likelihood that exposure to other allergens would lead to sensitization. Overall, although there is a promising line of enquiry, there is a need for more evidence from high-quality clinical trials before SIT can be recommended to prevent clinical allergy.[6,7]

Persistence of Clinical Improvement After Cessation of Immunotherapy

Both open and blinded studies have indicated a slow recurrence of grass pollen symptoms after completing 3 or 4 years of SIT. This recurrence reached 31% by the third year after treatment, but with no appreciable increase thereafter. The persistence of benefit is supported by subjective and objective measures,

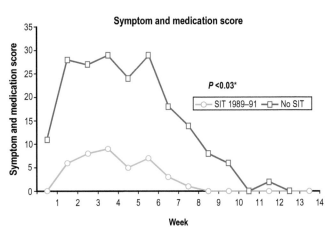

Fig. 6.2 Persistence of the effect of specific immunotherapy *(SIT)* 12 years after completing therapy. The graph shows symptoms' scores during the pollen season in patients treated in childhood 12 years earlier *(blue circles)* compared with matched control group *(red squares)*. From Eng PA, et al. Three-year follow-up after discontinuation of pre-seasonal grass pollen immunotherapy in childhood. Allergy 2006;61:198–201.

including conjunctival and skin sensitivity to grass pollen. The longest follow-up data have been reported in a 12-year open study of grass immunotherapy in children, in which the treated children continued to have decreased symptom and medication scores during the grass season and fewer new sensitizations compared with untreated controls (Fig. 6.2). Similar persistence of the effect was reported after immunotherapy with HDM extract. Over a 3-year period after discontinuation, approximately half experienced a relapse in symptoms, but half remained symptom-free.

PHARMACOECONOMICS OF SIT

The fact that the benefits of SIT extend far beyond the period of treatment is a key element of the economic argument for SIT. The possible cost benefits of SIT in children with newly diagnosed allergic rhinitis have been assessed. Highly significant reductions were achieved in pharmacy claims, outpatient visits, and hospital admissions after SIT, compared with data for similar children not receiving SIT. The total medical costs were reduced by 25%, even when the cost of the immunotherapy was included. Another study compared 2771 children with newly diagnosed allergic rhinitis who received SIT and 11,010 who did not. Healthcare utilization for the 18 months after starting SIT was US$3247 (including the cost of SIT) compared with US$4872 in the control group.

IMMUNOLOGIC RESPONSE TO INHALANT SIT

Much effort has focused on dissecting the mechanisms of successful immunotherapy, partly to try to improve the efficacy and safety of SIT, and partly to try to find markers of treatment failure so that ineffective courses can be stopped early. Box 6.3 summarizes current understanding of the immunologic changes associated with successful injection immunotherapy for inhalant allergies.

BOX 6.2   Evidence of Disease Modification

- Prevention of asthma
- Prevention of new allergic sensitizations

BOX 6.3 The Immunologic Response to Immunotherapy

End-Organ Response

Decreased Early and Late Responses to Specific Allergen

- Conjunctiva
- Skin: early; late
- Nose
- Bronchi: early; late

Decreased Nonspecific Reaction to Bronchial Challenge

- Histamine
- Methacholine

Decreased Tissue Inflammation

- Eosinophils
- Metachromatic cells

Humoral Response

IgE

- Early rise in specific IgE
- Suppression of seasonal rise in specific IgE
- Late decline in specific IgE

IgG

- Increase in specific IgG
- Early predominantly IgG$_1$
- Late predominantly IgG$_4$

Cellular Response

Basophils

- Nonspecific loss of responsiveness

Lymphocytes and Peripheral Blood Mononuclear Cells

- Decreased serum IL-2R
- Decreased lymphocyte proliferation
- Generation of specific suppressor cells
- Regulatory T lymphocytes
  - Increased expression of Foxp3
  - Secreting IL-10
  - Secreting TGF-β

Evidence of Immune Deviation

- Decreased stimulated release of Th2 cytokines
  - IL-4
  - IL-13
- Preferential deletion of Th2 T cells
- Increased stimulated release of Th1 cytokines
  - IFN-γ
- Increased stimulated mRNA for Th1 cytokines
  - IFN-γ
  - IL-12

Other Immunologic Changes

- Decrease in FcεRII/CD23 and B cell activation markers
- Decreased costimulatory molecules
- Decreased release of cytokines
  - IL-2
  - TNF
  - Histamine-releasing factors
  - Platelet-activating factor

IFN, interferon; *IgE, IgG*, immunoglobulins E and G; *IL*, interleukin; *IL-2R*, interleukin type 2 receptor; *mRNA*, messenger RNA; *TGF-β*, transforming growth factor-β; *TNF*, tumor necrosis factor.

OVERVIEW OF THE IMMUNE RESPONSE TO IMMUNOTHERAPY

The effect of SIT on cellular inflammation has been studied extensively with findings on immunologic responses to SIT reported that may appear contradictory. There are some studies reporting induction of regulatory T cells (Treg) that suppress both Th1 and Th2 cytokine responses to specific allergen stimulation, whereas other studies report an immune deviation from a Th2 to a Th1 response such that allergen stimulation of T cells results in increased synthesis of IL-12 and interferon-γ (IFN-γ) and decreased synthesis of IL-4. Current perspectives are that the Treg response occurs very early in the course of subcutaneous immunotherapy (SCIT), but with time there is a more general suppression of T cell reactivity to the injected allergen. While a detailed discussion of the immunologic mechanisms of SIT is beyond the scope of this chapter, the mechanisms involved can be summarized briefly as follows:

- Eosinophils, basophils, and mast cells are the main effector cells of the allergic response.
- The increased levels of eosinophils seen during natural allergen exposure are decreased by SIT.
- Seasonal increases in nasal basophils and mast cells are also blunted.
- Allergen-specific IgE levels increase early and then decrease slowly after SIT, but the rate of change is much less than would be expected if this were an important mechanism.
- In contrast, allergen-specific IgG4 levels rise steeply after SIT. This is generally considered to be a direct consequence of the injection of foreign material rather than the mechanism by which SIT works. The immediate cause of IgG4 production is likely to be induction of Treg producing IL-10.

Both during and after SIT, there is a general suppression of allergen-specific T cell responses, which is now thought to be due to induction of allergen-specific Treg, which produce two key cytokines: IL-10 and transforming growth factor-β (TGF-β). In parallel, there is suppression of allergen-specific lymphocyte proliferation and decreased production of IFN-γ, IL-5, and IL-13. IL-10 is an inhibitor of proliferative and cytokine responses in T cells, which inhibits IgE production and enhances IgG4 production. TGF-β induces an isotype switch toward IgA. At present, increased allergen-specific IL-10 production is considered a marker of successful SIT and may also be a marker of adherence.

Two types of CD4$^+$ helper T lymphocytes have been described: Th2 cells, which preferentially secrete IL-4; and Th1 cells, which preferentially secrete IFN-γ in response to allergen stimulation. Allergic individuals have increased numbers of allergen-specific Th2 cells in their peripheral circulation but normal levels of antigen-specific Th1 and Treg. SIT leads to a decrease in allergen-specific Th2 cells, suggesting that SIT may work by deviating the immune response away from the Th2 pattern. This may be mediated through induction of cells producing IL-12. Increased numbers of cells expressing IL-12 mRNA have been noted in skin sites challenged with allergen after SIT. IL-12 promotes Th1 lymphocyte proliferation and suppresses Th2 cells, so the finding of increased IL-12-secreting cells is consistent with a shift from Th2 to Th1 allergen-specific responses after SIT.

INDICATIONS FOR SIT

While anaphylaxis to *Hymenoptera* venom is an absolute indications for SIT, there are no such absolute indications for inhalant allergens. Broadly speaking, SIT should be considered for patients who have troublesome symptoms of allergic rhinitis, rhinoconjunctivitis, or allergic asthma after natural exposure to allergens and who demonstrate specific IgE antibodies to relevant allergens. Other factors to consider are the severity and duration of symptoms, medication requirements, and patient preference. Because of the increased risk of adverse effects in patients with poorly controlled asthma, SCIT should only be offered to patients with asthma if their asthma is well controlled and their forced expiratory volume in 1 second (FEV_1) is greater than 80% predicted.

Outside the US, most SIT injections involve single allergens, which are obtained commercially and used individually. In contrast, in the US, it is common to use combinations of extracts and to mix the allergens in a single maintenance vial tailored to that patient. However, some caution is needed, because extracts from fungi and cockroaches contain proteases that can degrade the proteins in other extracts they are mixed with. Current best advice is not to mix cockroach or any fungal extract with extracts of pollens, HDM, or danders, but other combinations may be acceptable.

Effective SIT requires administration of sufficient allergenic protein. A variety of methods have been used to define the potency of allergen extracts. Experience gained over many years and many trials has shown that a maintenance dose of approximately 6–20 μg of major allergen is needed to achieve clinical efficacy. The actual amount varies between manufacturers and between allergens, and the lack of clarity on this point remains a matter of concern to practitioners and regulators alike.

Injection Schedules

A SIT schedule consists of two phases: the build-up or initiation phase going from very low dose to the full maintenance dose, and then a maintenance phase, in which the same dose is given at intervals over a number of years. Typically, the build-up phase is achieved by injections twice-weekly, weekly, or alternate weeks (Box 6.4, Table 6.1). Various alternative regimens have been devised, with clusters of injections given at intervals or rush protocols, in which the full build-up phase is achieved in 1 to 2 days. Once patients reach the maintenance dose of their immunotherapy extract, injection frequencies are decreased

to typically every 4 weeks. The basic treatment regimen may require modification because of either missed visits or reactions to the previous injection. Dosage reductions are usually not needed during a pollen season.

BOX 6.4   Example of a Conventional US-Style Allergen Extract Treatment Schedule

The following schedule should be used, with modification if necessary, as outlined in the accompanying instructions.

Instructions for the Injection of Allergenic Extracts
Begin with vial **#4** and progress to vial **#1**, which is the most concentrated or "maintenance" solution. The injections should be given every **week**. Once maintenance is reached, the injection should be given every **3–4** weeks, with the following exceptions: **give weekly for first month and every 2 weeks for the second month**.

Schedule

Vial #5	Vial #4	Vial #3	Vial #2	Vial #1
0.05 mL	0.05 mL	0.05 mL	0.05 mL	0.05 mL
0.10 mL	0.10 mL	0.10 mL	0.07 mL	0.07 mL
0.20 mL	0.20 mL	0.20 mL	0.10 mL	0.10 mL
0.40 mL	0.40 mL	0.40 mL	0.15 mL	0.15 mL
			0.25 mL	0.20 mL
			0.35 mL	0.30 mL
			0.50 mL	0.40 mL
				0.50 mL

The **bold-underlined** entries are representative instructions that would be placed in the blank spaces in the schedule.

TABLE 6.1   A European-style Injection Immunotherapy Schedule for Hay Fever, Giving Two Injections Each Week for 6 Weeks

Week no.	Injection no.	Allergen concentration	Volume (mL)	Amount of allergen (SQ-U)
1	1	1000	0.1	100
1	2	10,000	0.1	1000
2	3	10,000	0.2	2000
2	4	10,000	0.4	4000
3	5	10,000	0.6	6000
3	6	100,000	0.1	10,000
4	7	100,000	0.1	10,000
4	8	100,000	0.2	20,000
5	9	100,000	0.3	30,000
5	10	100,000	0.3	30,000
6	11	100,000	0.5	50,000
6	12	100,000	0.5	50,000

Adapted from Frew et al. Clinical efficacy and safety of specific allergy vaccination with Alutard grass in seasonal allergic rhinoconjunctivitis: a large-scale randomised double-blind placebo-controlled multi-centre study [UKIS—The UK Immunotherapy Study]. J Allergy Clin Immunol 2006;117:319–25. 2006.[2]

Adverse Reactions to SIT

Localized and systemic reactions may occur after SIT. Local reactions are more frequent during the build-up phase than during maintenance and, if large, may warrant adjustment to the schedule (e.g., repeating the previous dose before progressing to the next and higher dose) or premedication with nonsedating antihistamines. The occurrence of local reactions after SIT does not predict subsequent systemic reactions, so if the concern is solely about the possible occurrence of a systemic reaction, no dose adjustment is needed after a local reaction.

Systemic reactions are more serious and can occasionally prove fatal. The fatality rate in the US between 1985 and 2001 has been estimated to be about 1 per 2.5 million injections. In a national survey, three-quarters of systemic reactions were cutaneous or upper respiratory, while one-quarter exacerbated asthma, and 3% involved life-threatening respiratory compromise or hypotension. Although it used to be thought that patients were at increased risk for systemic reactions during the relevant pollen season, this has not been substantiated in large observational studies. Patients with asthma are at greater risk of adverse reactions, especially if their asthma is labile or symptomatic at the time of the injection, requires oral corticosteroid treatment, or has resulted in recent hospitalization or emergency room visits. With proper care and attention, it is reasonable to treat people whose asthma is mild and stable, but symptoms and peak flow readings should be checked prior to each dose. Almost all severe reactions start within 20 min of the injection, and a minimum observation period of 30–45 min after injections is widely accepted as appropriate. Late-onset systemic reactions are relatively rare, but when they do occur, they are usually mild and subside spontaneously, without requiring epinephrine (adrenaline) or emergency department attendance.

SIT in Pregnancy

There are two specific concerns during pregnancy: the risk to the fetus should there be an anaphylactic reaction to SIT, and the potential effects of SIT on the development of the fetus's immune system. Current advice is that SIT should not be initiated during pregnancy, but maintenance treatment may be continued in the absence of a history of systemic reactions. There is no evidence of any increase in the rates of prematurity, toxemia, abortion, neonatal death, or congenital malformations when SIT is continued in pregnancy. Whether maternal SIT has any beneficial effects on the unborn child in terms of preventing the development of allergic disease is not known, and it is unlikely ever to be studied formally.

Adherence to SIT

The long duration of SIT and dosing fatigue are important contributors to patients stopping their therapy prematurely. The number of patients not completing their course of SIT ranges from 10% to 46%. These poor completion rates have stimulated research into developing vaccines that can achieve the same benefits as conventional SIT but within a shorter time frame and using alternative routes of administration that are easier for the patient.

SUBLINGUAL IMMUNOTHERAPY

It has been known for many years that immunologic tolerance can be achieved by mucosal application of proteins. SLIT exploits this by applying relatively large doses of allergen to the buccal mucosa before swallowing. As this is safe and can be done at home, it is much more convenient for patients than standard injection immunotherapy (SCIT). The immunologic mechanisms of successful SLIT are like those of SCIT, but dendritic cells in the buccal mucosa are thought to play a key role in inducing tolerance, most likely through Treg (Fig. 6.3). SLIT achieves decreased symptoms and medication requirements, as well as disease modification, similar to the outcomes associated with successful SCIT. Economic considerations may influence the type of immunotherapy used, as the vaccine costs are relatively expensive compared with SCIT.

Recent interest in SLIT has been driven in part by a perception that injection SCIT is hazardous. When treating a relatively benign disease such as allergic rhinitis, the risk of serious adverse reactions weighs more heavily than when treating cancer or life-threatening autoimmune disease.

Over the past 30 years, several different preparations of aqueous allergen extracts have been tried for sublingual use, including sprays and drops. Standardized extracts for SLIT are available for HDM (*Dermatophagoides farinae* and *Dermatophagoides pteronyssinus*), cat dander, weeds (ragweed, *Parietaria*, mugwort), grasses, and tree pollens. To improve reliability of dosing and compliance, tablet formulations were developed; grass pollen SLIT tablets have been commercially available and approved for treating allergic rhinitis since 2009. The tablet formulation increases the stability of the product and improves standardization of doses; tablets also simplify SLIT administration and minimize the potential risks of errors in dose administration.

Several large clinical trials have shown SLIT to be clinically effective, improving allergic rhinitis and asthma symptoms and reducing requirements for rescue medication.[8] SLIT is now widely used in Europe, especially in France, Germany, and Italy, but also in the US and Oceania. Different regimens are employed: some include a rapid build-up phase, while others start directly at the maintenance dose. Depending on the manufacturer and preparation, SLIT doses are 50–110 times those used in SCIT. SLIT has a safer profile than SCIT; serious side effects are very rare, and the more common local side effects are usually confined to the early weeks of treatment and are responsive to intercurrent nonsedating antihistamines. In addition to its safer profile, SLIT is administered at home after the first dose under observation—an additional advantage over SCIT, which requires clinic visits.

Long-term data are lacking, but based on SCIT practice and available clinical trials with seasonal allergens, 3 years or more of treatment is recommended.[9]

Mechanisms of SLIT

When allergens are placed in contact with the oral mucosa for several minutes before swallowing, a small amount of the allergenic material is absorbed into the mucosa (the rest is swallowed and digested, never reaching immunocompetent cells).

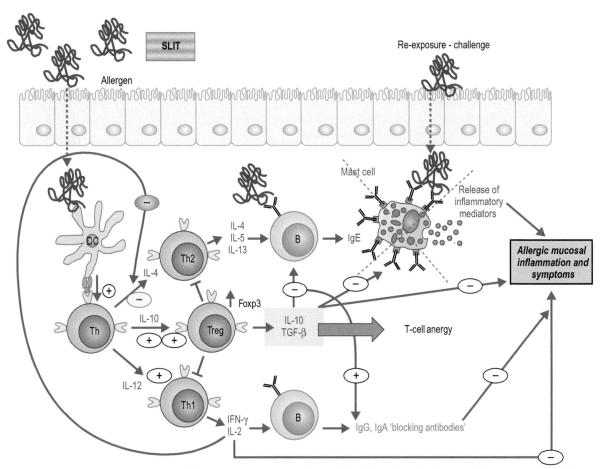

Fig. 6.3 Immunologic mechanisms of specific sublingual immunotherapy *(SLIT)*. Locally administered allergen using SLIT is taken up by mucosal dendritic cells *(DCs)* and then presented to T cells together with interleukin (IL)-12, biasing the response toward a Th1-like profile and away from the pro-IgE Th2 profile arbitrated by protolerogenic mechanisms mediated by the increased release of IL-10. There is enhanced secretion of interferon-γ (IFN-γ) and IL-2, which drive specific B cell production of nonpathogenic and protective IgG1 and IgG4 antibodies and decreased release of the Th2 pro-IgE cytokine IL-4. Oral mucosal DCs actively upregulate regulatory T cell (Treg) subtypes, including Forkhead box P3 protein *(Foxp3)*-expressing T cells, contributing to T cell anergy mediated by IL-10 and transforming growth factor-β *(TGF-β)*. These interconnected pathways lead to reduction in allergic inflammation and symptoms.

The fraction that is retained in the oral mucosa is taken up by dendritic cells that migrate to the regional lymph nodes. Both standard allergens and chemically modified allergoids persist in the mouth for several hours, and small amounts can still be identified in the oral cavity up to 20 hours later. In theory, absorption from sites other than the oral mucosa might also contribute to the immunologic stimulus from SLIT, but there is minimal clinical benefit from allergens given orally and simply swallowed without a period of retention under the tongue.

The immunologic changes associated with successful SLIT are similar to those observed with SCIT (Fig. 6.3). These include enhanced suppressor activity of IL-10-secreting Treg; suppression of eosinophils, mast cells, and basophils; and antibody isotype switching from IgE to IgG4 and possibly IgG2. Current data suggest that IL-10-producing Treg are pivotal to the various changes induced by SIT. Once induced, chronic allergen exposure may favor expansion of Tr1 cells through IL-12 and IL-27 synthesis. Recruitment of these cells into areas of inflammation will lead to amplification of local cytokine responses, including IL-12, IL-10, and TGF-β1. The IL-12 will skew any Th2 and Th17

cells toward the Th1 phenotype, whereas IL-10 suppresses allergen-specific Th2 and Th17 responses, induces IgG4, and inhibits recruitment of mast cells, basophils, and eosinophils. Lastly, TGF-β1 blocks the Th2 response and decreases the activation of mast cells and eosinophils. Research in this area is now focused on identifying more efficient ways of inducing allergen-specific Treg, including the use of appropriate immunologic adjuvants.

Most of these phenomena are also found after SLIT (Box 6.5), albeit with smaller changes in specific IgE, specific IgG, and cytokines compared with those identified in patients treated by injection SIT.[10] Induction of allergen-specific IgG4 is a consistent finding in most SLIT studies using large doses of allergen, but some studies reporting good clinical responses to SLIT have not detected any change in allergen-specific IgE, IgG, or IgG4. This may partly reflect the timing of the immunologic analysis relative to administration of SLIT, but some doubts remain about the relationship between changes in these immunologic measures and the delivery of clinical benefit.[11] Current and ongoing research suggests late induction of allergen-specific IgG2, which may provide a biomarker of effective SLIT.[12]

BOX 6.5 Possible Mechanisms of SLIT

- Induction of IgG antibodies (early sustained IgG4 and late IgG2)
- Reduction in specific IgE (long-term)
- Reduced recruitment of effector cells
- Altered helper T cell cytokine balance (shift to Th1 from Th2)
- T cell anergy
- B cell suppression
- Increased regulatory T cell (Treg) function

Although there is considerable overlap in the immune responses found in individual studies of SCIT and SLIT, some differences have been identified between SCIT and SLIT. Because not all the phenomena reported after SCIT occur after SLIT, it is possible that different or additional mechanisms may occur in SLIT.

Side Effects of SLIT

SLIT has a much safer profile than SCIT, but local side effects are common, most frequently local irritation of the oral mucosa and sometimes local swelling. Systemic reactions are extremely rare, but caution is advised in patients who have experienced systemic side effects to other forms of SIT. Local side effects ease with accompanying nonsedating antihistamines during early weeks and repeated use, and rarely lead patients to discontinue therapy. To avoid unnecessary discontinuation, patients should be supervised when they take their first doses. This allows any potential side effects to be discussed and the therapeutic regimen to be explained.

Efficacy of SLIT

Several well-conducted clinical trials have shown 30%–40% decreases in symptom score and rescue medication use in patients with seasonal allergic rhinitis after SLIT. In general, the trials show that clinically significant benefits are achieved in the first year of SLIT, and the magnitude of benefit does not increase much in the second and third years. However, it is likely that the second and third years of SLIT contribute to the overall durability of the response, which we know from double-blind, placebo-controlled trials extends for at least 2 years after 3 years of therapy (Fig. 6.4), supporting reports from open-label clinical

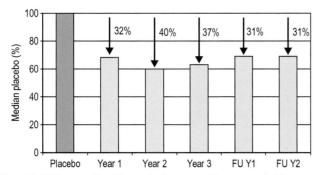

Fig. 6.4 Efficacy of sublingual allergen tablets on rhinitis symptoms over 3 years of treatment and 2 further years on placebo. Adapted from Durham SR et al. SQ-standardised sublingual grass immunotherapy: confirmation of disease modification 2 years after 3 years of treatment in a randomised trial. J Allergy Clin Immunol 2012;129:717–725.

practice that benefits are maintained for at least 7 years after ceasing SLIT. Lasting benefit seems to be more likely in those with more severe disease at enrolment.

SLIT with grass pollen tablets has also been studied in children and adolescents, in both Europe and North America. Grass pollen tablets were well tolerated, and the levels of benefit achieved were comparable with those found in adults.

SLIT has been most extensively tested in grass pollen allergy, but tablet-based therapies are now available for HDM, and ones for tree pollen allergy and animal dander are under development. Further large-scale trials are needed in well-defined patient groups.

SLIT for Asthma

Most clinical trials of SLIT have focused on evaluating its efficacy in allergic rhinitis.[13] Some trials included patients with asthma, and SLIT appears to decrease asthma symptoms and medication scores after 2 years of treatment. A study of HDM SLIT tablets in patients with asthma who were not well controlled in Global Initiative for Asthma (GINA) treatment steps 2–4 demonstrated efficacy and has resulted in inclusion of consideration of HDM SIT in the GINA guidelines for asthma management.[14] SLIT is currently recommended for patients with allergic rhinitis, with or without asthma, but is not currently recommended specifically for treatment of asthma. Importantly, current guidelines recommend that SLIT should only be initiated in patients with asthma who are stable with an FEV1 >70% predicted.

SIT for grass pollen allergy may offer protection against epidemic thunderstorm asthma in regions that are geographically susceptible and where ryegrass is the prevalent pasture grass associated with seasonal rhinitis.[15]

Durability of Treatment

A key question in deciding whether to use SLIT is how long the benefits of therapy extend beyond the period of treatment. Maintaining double-blind trials for years is extremely difficult,[16] both for the investigators and for the control group participants who have to go without treatment for years to answer the question properly. Evidence from long-term follow-up of open-label therapy has shown that the longer the course of treatment, the longer the benefit persists. Five years of SLIT gave benefits for at least 7 years, whereas the benefit of 3 to 4 years of SLIT seemed to wane more quickly. The more recent double-blind, placebo-controlled studies continued for 2 years after completing therapy have demonstrated a durable response. Unfortunately, accurate cost–benefit analysis requires an estimate of the durability of therapeutic effect, so the lack of long-term data remains a problem for policymakers and manufacturers alike.

Effects of SLIT on the Natural History of Allergic Disease

As discussed earlier, there is considerable interest in the possibility that SIT may modify the course of allergic disease. If unequivocally substantiated, this effect would dramatically swing the economic argument in favor of SIT because one could discount the costs of treatment against the costs of the future

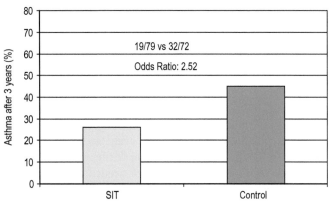

Fig. 6.5 Pollen SIT reduces asthma in children with seasonal allergic rhinitis. Adapted from Möller C et al. Pollen immunotherapy reduces the development of asthma in children with seasonal rhinoconjunctivitis (the PAT-study). J Allergy Clin Immunol 2002; 109:251–256.

condition that has been avoided. Data have been presented in two areas: prevention of new sensitizations and prevention of asthma. As with SCIT, atopic children treated with SLIT acquire fewer new sensitizations over 3 years, compared with untreated children.[17] SLIT also may prevent children with rhinitis from developing asthma later. In a 3-year study, 18 of 44 control children developed asthma versus only 8 of 45 SLIT-treated children (Fig. 6.5).

Thus, both SCIT and SLIT appear to modify the course of allergic disease by decreasing the incidence of new sensitizations, preventing the development of clinical asthma, and/or accelerating its resolution. The mechanism remains unclear but probably involves a combination of immunologic effects and downstream changes to the structure and function of the small airways. Better data are needed, but if confirmed, these disease-modifying and preventive effects of SIT would have a major impact on any cost–benefit analysis.

Safety and Cost-Effectiveness of SLIT

One of the main drivers behind the development of SLIT was awareness of risks associated with SCIT. Although SCIT is usually quite safe in patients without asthma, occasional serious adverse events do occur, but these are rarely fatal. In most reports, the rate of serious systemic reactions in patients with rhinitis is about 1 in 500 injections. Most clinical trials of SLIT report local side effects, particularly itching of the mouth and palate, but there were few serious systemic side effects. Since SLIT preparations became available commercially, a small number of serious adverse events have been reported, mainly in patients who had already experienced problems with conventional SCIT. These isolated episodes were typically not witnessed by medical personnel, so some doubt remains regarding their precise nature, but clearly some caution is required if SLIT is given to such patients. The first dose of SLIT should normally be taken in the physician's office, particularly in patients who previously experienced problems with SCIT. In some series, up to 11.6% of patients had experienced wheezing or worsening of nasal symptoms on one or more occasions after a SLIT dose, although the overall frequency of systemic adverse reactions was only 1 in 3000 doses.

No discussion of new therapeutic options is complete without consideration of the economic aspects. Rhinoconjunctivitis is a common condition, and standard therapies such as non-sedating antihistamines and even nasal corticosteroids are relatively inexpensive compared with forms of SIT. SLIT offers improvements that cannot be achieved by standard pharmacotherapy, but it is relatively expensive compared with antihistamine therapy, which is adjusted according to symptoms. Cost-effectiveness analysis requires assumptions on the likely durability of benefits and the period of impact on relevant financial outcomes. Some evidence of cost-effectiveness has been presented, indicating a cost of 13,000–18,000 Euros (US$17,000–25,000) per quality-adjusted life year (QALY) gained. The benefit consisted of decreases in rescue medication and fewer hours lost from work (production loss). The analysis used a horizon of 9 years and assumed that the clinical benefit achieved in the first years of therapy would be sustained throughout. On this basis, tablet-based SLIT could be considered as cost-effective at current prices compared with standard thresholds applied by national regulatory bodies.[18,19]

In summary, there is evidence of favorable cost–benefit analysis, but this has not yet resulted in major changes in the development and reconfiguration of allergy health services. SLIT is relatively expensive, especially compared with standard drug treatment for allergic rhinitis. Currently, SLIT needs to be targeted to patients with significant disease.[17]

MODIFIED ALLERGEN EXTRACTS AND ADJUVANTS (BOX 6.6)

A major disadvantage of conventional SIT is the considerable investment in time and money required on the part of the patient to achieve and maintain effective doses of allergen extract. To address this, allergists began experimenting over 60 years ago with ways of slowing the absorption of allergen from the injection site to both decrease the number of injections

---

BOX 6.6 Modifications to Allergen Extracts and Routes of Administration

- Depot preparations
  - Aluminum adsorption
  - Tyrosine adsorption
  - Liposome-encapsulated
- Allergoids
- Recombinant technology
  - Unmodified major allergens
  - Mutated or deleted major allergens
- TLR stimulation
  - 3-Deacylated MPL
  - CpG (type A and type B): combined with allergen or administered without allergen
- Transcutaneous
- Transmucosal
  - Oral
  - Intranasal
  - Sublingual

required and to improve safety. Various depot preparations have been tried; alum precipitation reduces the risk of systemic side effects, but trials indicate that even with modified vaccines 3 years of treatment is still needed for maximum efficacy.

Various adjuvants have been tried to increase the immunologic effect of a given amount of allergen. Two of these involved stimulation of Toll-like receptors (TLRs), which are cell surface receptors that recognize molecular patterns commonly found in bacteria and viruses. When allergens are given together with TLR stimulation, the immunologic effect is altered, biasing the response toward a Th1 pattern. Unmethylated CpG DNA motifs stimulate TLR9, and lipopolysaccharides and a derivative, monophosphoryl lipid A (MPL), stimulate TLR4. SIT studies using MPL as an adjuvant have shown clinical efficacy after only four injections, but further data on durability are needed before this can be adopted into routine use. Immunostimulation with CpG-containing DNA sequences has been tested for ragweed and HDM allergy. Initial trials were promising, although later ragweed studies proved less effective.

Allergenic proteins can be cross-linked with formaldehyde or glutaraldehyde to produce larger molecules, which are less able to react with IgE antibodies. Such allergen extracts are called "allergoids" and have proved effective in clinical trials, although their clinical use has been limited to the US. In contrast, allergoids have proved more popular in Europe, allowing rapid build-up regimens and delivery of large amounts of allergen in fewer injections. Encapsulation of unmodified HDM allergen extracts in liposomes has also been investigated. Liposomes are lipid vesicles formed by one or more phospholipid bilayers that entrap the water-soluble extract in their internal aqueous compartment. They are biodegradable and stable and prolong the half-life of the encapsulated drug while acting as an adjuvant, inducing a Th1 response.

Recombinant Allergen Vaccines

In theory, recombinant technology offers the possibility of improving the standardization and safety of allergen SIT. Most of the key components of inhaled allergens have been identified, cloned, sequenced, and expressed in various systems. This allows production of virtually unlimited quantities of allergenic proteins, mutated proteins, or fragments of allergenic proteins.

Unmodified Allergens

There have been several trials of SIT with unmodified purified major allergens. To date, the trials have shown efficacy but no real superiority to standard SIT. In theory, SIT vaccines could be personalized to the individual's serologic pattern of reaction, but this approach raises awkward regulatory questions yet to be addressed.

Modified Allergens

Genetic modification can produce hypoallergenic variants of allergenic proteins, which may decrease the risk of IgE-mediated side effects while retaining desired T cell effects. This approach has mainly been studied for birch pollen. Other reported genetically modified allergens include hybrid molecules derived from HDM, Timothy grass, and cat dander.

THE FUTURE OF SLIT

Future developments in SLIT may take several forms, including mucoadhesives, allergoids, adjuvants, and new allergens (latex, foods). The delivery of allergen to the mucosa may be improved by creating formulations that adhere better to the mucosa and deliver the necessary amount of allergen more efficiently. Such mucoadhesives could allow smaller amounts of allergen, thereby decreasing the risk of local side effects and adverse reactions. The efficiency of SLIT might also be improved by more persistent presence of the allergen.

As with SCIT, it may be possible to use modified allergens, for example, allergoids, which retain the ability to stimulate T cells while having decreased binding to IgE. This should decrease side effects, and has been tested in patients with grass pollen allergy, in whom it appears effective, both when given all year round and when used pre-seasonally. Adjuvants that selectively induce IL-10 could also enhance the efficacy of SLIT vaccines. Another adjuvant, *Lactobacillus plantarum*, deviates T cells toward a mixed Th1/Treg pattern. Both these adjuvants have enhanced the efficacy of SLIT in a mouse model of asthma.

CONCLUSIONS

Allergen immunotherapy has been practiced with only relatively modest changes for more than 100 years. The clinical effectiveness of adequate doses in appropriate patients for both allergic rhinitis and bronchial asthma has been repeatedly confirmed. Treatment by the sublingual route is becoming increasingly popular. SLIT appears to be as effective as SCIT for allergic rhinitis and is certainly more convenient for patients. The precise mechanisms of SIT action remain uncertain. Both SCIT and SLIT are associated with induction of Treg, expression of IL-10 and TGF-β1, and secretion of allergen-specific IgG4 and possibly IgG2. The major threat to future use of SCIT and SLIT is the lack of comprehensive cost-effectiveness data, which are increasingly required by healthcare commissioners when deciding which treatments to fund. Future developments will include a wider range of allergens, adaptations with mucoadhesives and adjuvants to refine the immunologic response, and research into the durability of responses to determine cost-effectiveness.

As well as confirming primary efficacy, clinical trials of SCIT and SLIT have confirmed a persisting beneficial effect after immunotherapy is discontinued. These findings suggest that immunotherapy has the potential to be used more widely. Increased utilization would be facilitated by alternative extracts and better methods of administration making SIT safer and more convenient for the patient.

REFERENCES

1. Frew AJ. Hundred years of immunotherapy. Clin Exp Allergy. 2011;41:1221–1225.
2. Frew AJ, Powell RJ, Corrigan CJ, et al. Clinical efficacy and safety of specific allergy vaccination with Alutard grass in seasonal allergic

rhinoconjunctivitis: a large-scale randomised double-blind placebo-controlled multi-centre study (UKIS—The UK Immunotherapy Study). J Allergy Clin Immunol. 2006;117:319–325.

3. Abramson MJ, Puy RM, Weiner JM. Injection allergen immunotherapy for asthma. Cochrane Database Syst Rev. 2010;8:CD001186.

4. Cox L, Nelson H, Lockey R. Allergen immunotherapy: a practice parameter third update. J Allergy Clin Immunol. 2011;127:S1–S55.

5. Jacobsen L, Niggemann B, Dreborg S, et al. Specific immunotherapy has long-term preventive effect on seasonal and perennial asthma: 10-year follow-up on the PAT study. Allergy. 2007;62:943–948.

6. Kristiansen M, Dhami S, Netuveli G, et al. Allergen immunotherapy for the prevention of allergy: a systematic review and meta-analysis. Pediatr Allergy Immunol. 2017;28(1):18–29.

7. Halken S, Larenas-Linnemann D, Roberts G, et al. EAACI guidelines on allergen immunotherapy: prevention of allergy. Pediatr Allergy Immunol. 2017;28(8):728–745.

8. Dhami S, Nurmatov U, Arasi S, et al. Allergen immunotherapy for allergic rhinoconjunctivitis: a systematic review and meta-analysis. Allergy. 2017;72(11):1597–1631.

9. Roberts G, Pfaar O, Akdis CA, et al. EAACI guidelines on allergen immunotherapy: allergic rhinoconjunctivitis. Allergy. 2018;73(4):765–798.

10. Bohle B, Kinaciyan T, Gerstmayr M, et al. Sublingual immunotherapy induces IL-10-producing T regulatory cells, allergen-specific T-cell tolerance, and immune deviation. J Allergy Clin Immunol. 2007;120:707–713.

11. Novak N, Bieber T, Allam JP. Immunologic mechanisms of sublingual allergen-specific immunotherapy. Allergy. 2011;66:733–739.

12. Heeringa JJ, McKenzie CI, Varese N, et al. Induction of IgG2 and IgG4 B-cell memory following sublingual immunotherapy for ryegrass pollen allergy. Allergy. 2020;75:1121–1132.

13. Dhami S, Kakourou A, Asamoah F, et al. Allergen immunotherapy for allergic asthma: A systematic review and meta-analysis. Allergy. 2017;72(12):1825–1848.

14. Virchow JC, Bacher V, Kuna P, et al. Efficacy of a house dust mite sublingual allergen immunotherapy tablet in adults with allergic asthma: a randomized clinical trial. JAMA. 2016;315:1715–1725.

15. O'Hehir RE, Varese N, Deckert K, et al. Epidemic thunderstorm asthma protection with five grass pollen tablet sublingual immunotherapy. Am J Resp Crit Care Med. 2018;198:126–128.

16. Durham SR, Emminger W, Kapp A, et al. SQ-standardized sublingual grass immuno-therapy: confirmation of disease modification 2 years after 3 years of treatment in a randomized trial. J Allergy Clin Immunol. 2012;129:717–725.

17. Asaria M, Dhami S, van Ree R, et al. Health economic analysis of allergen immunotherapy for the management of allergic rhinitis, asthma, food allergy and venom allergy: a systematic overview. Allergy. 2018;73(2):269–283.

18. Hankin CS, Cox L, Lang D, et al. Allergen immunotherapy and health care cost benefits for children with allergic rhinitis: a large-scale, retrospective, matched cohort study. Ann Allergy Asthma Immunol. 2010;104:79–85.

19. Bachert C, Vestenbaek U, Christensen J, et al. Cost-effectiveness of grass allergen tablet (Grazax) for the prevention of seasonal grass pollen induced rhinoconjunctivitis: a Northern European perspective. Clin Exp Allergy. 2007;37:772–779.

SUGGESTED READING

Alvaro-Lozano M, Akdis CA, Akdis M, et al. EAACI allergen immunotherapy user's guide. Pediatr Allergy Immunol. 2020;31(Suppl. 25):1–101.

Agache I, Lau S, Akdis CA, et al. EAACI Guidelines on allergen immunotherapy: house dust mite driven allergic asthma. Allergy. 2019;74:855–873.

Bousquet J, Pfaar O, Togias A, et al. 2019 ARIA care pathways for allergen immunotherapy. Allergy. 2019;74:2087–2102.

Breiteneder H, Peng Y, Agache I, et al. Biomarkers for diagnosis and prediction of therapy responses in allergic diseases and asthma. Allergy. 2020;75(12):3039–3068.

Calderon MA, Cox L, Casale TB, et al. Multiple-allergen and single-allergen immunotherapy strategies in polysensitized patients: looking at the published evidence. J Allergy Clin Immunol. 2012;129:929–934.

Calderon MA, Waserman S, Bernstein DI, et al. Clinical practice of allergen immunotherapy for allergic rhinoconjunctivitis and asthma: an expert panel report. J Allergy Clin Immunol Pract. 2020;S2213-2198(20) 30479-7.

Incorvaia C, Al-Ahmad M, Ansotegui I, et al. Personalized medicine for allergy treatment: allergen immunotherapy still a unique and unmatched model. Allergy. 2020 https://doi.org/10.1111/all.14575.

Jensen-Jarolim E, Bachmann M, Bonini S, et al. State-of-the-art in marketed adjuvants and formulations in allergen immunotherapy: a position paper of the European Academy of Allergy and Clinical Immunology (EAACI). Allergy. 2020;75:746–760.

Mahler V, Esch RE, Kleine-Tebbe J, et al. Understanding differences in allergen immunotherapy products and practices in North America and Europe. J Allergy Clin Immunol. 2019;143:813–828.

Mosbech H, Deckelmann R, de Blay F, et al. Standardized quality (SQ) house dust mite sublingual immunotherapy tablet (ALK) reduces inhaled corticosteroid use while maintaining asthma control: a randomized, double-blind, placebo-controlled trial. J Allergy Clin Immunol. 2014;134:568–575.

Pfaar O, Agache I, de Blay F, et al. Perspectives in allergen immunotherapy: 2019 and beyond. Allergy. 2019;74(Suppl. 108):3–25.

Pfaar O, Angier E, Muraro A, et al. Algorithms in allergen immunotherapy in allergic rhinoconjunctivitis. Allergy. 2020;75(9):2411–2414.

Reitsma S, Subramaniam S, Fokkens WW, Wang DY. Recent developments and highlights in rhinitis and allergen immunotherapy. Allergy. 2018;73:2306–2313.

Van Zelm MC, McKenzie CI, Varese N, et al. Recent developments and highlights in immune monitoring of allergen immunotherapy. Allergy. 2019;74:2342–2354.

Wheatley LM, Wood R, Nadeau K, et al. Mind the gaps: clinical trial concepts to address unanswered questions in aeroallergen immunotherapy. An NIAID/AHRQ workshop. J Allergy Clin Immunol. 2019;14:1711–1726.

Zielen S, Devillier P, Heinrich J, et al. Sublingual immunotherapy provides long-term relief in allergic rhinitis and reduces the risk of asthma: a retrospective, real-world database analysis. Allergy. 2018;73:165–177.

7

Asthma

Stephen T. Holgate

CHAPTER OUTLINE

SUMMARY OF IMPORTANT CONCEPTS

- Asthma is a common but complex clinical syndrome affecting people of all ages, characterized by variable airflow obstruction, bronchial hyperresponsiveness, and airway inflammation, and manifesting as differing phenotypes.
- Almost all asthma results from inflammation of the conducting airways most frequently Type 2 inflammation (mast cells, eosinophils, and Type 2 lymphocytes [Th2 and ILC2 cells]) and most often involving allergic mechanisms, especially in child-onset disease.
- The symptoms of asthma are nonspecific, and diagnosis may not be straightforward in community settings. Spirometry is used to demonstrate the airflow obstruction, and patient-held peak expiratory flow (PEF) meters to show variable airflow obstruction.
- Symptoms and airflow limitation vary between individuals and over time, either spontaneously, in response to triggers (such as allergens, air pollution, and viral infection), or as a result of treatment.
- Stepwise treatment is advocated, with step-up if control is inadequate and step-down when stable. Inhaled corticosteroids (ICS) are the primary treatment of all patients with asthma irrespective of severity, with short-acting inhaled bronchodilators only used as rescue medication.
- Many patients have inadequate asthma control for a variety of reasons. These include severe disease, continued exposure to environmental drivers, inadequate or ineffective treatment, nonadherence to treatment, and the influence of comorbidities. On excluding treatment nonadherence, new biologics are now available for targeting the Type 2 causal pathways of asthma and moving disease management closer to personalized care.

INTRODUCTION AND OVERVIEW

Background

Asthma is a complex clinical syndrome characterized by variable airflow obstruction, bronchial hyperresponsiveness (BHR), and cellular inflammation. Asthma is defined by the Global Initiative in Asthma (GINA)[1] as "a heterogeneous disease, usually characterized by airway inflammation. It is defined by the presence of respiratory symptoms such as wheeze, shortness of breath, chest tightness and cough that vary over time and in intensity, together with variable expiratory airflow limitation."

Asthma is a common and potentially serious condition affecting an estimated 300 million individuals of all ages worldwide, comprising 1% to 18% of the population in different countries; highest in economically developed countries but rising over time in low- and middle-income countries.[2,3] It poses a major burden on patients, their families and communities, and on health economies.[4]

Asthma results in variable respiratory symptoms and variable airflow limitation, leading to activity and quality of life (QoL) impairment and sometimes in episodic flare-ups ("asthma attacks" or exacerbations) that may result in emergency healthcare utilization, hospitalization, and, in rare cases, even death. Classic asthma symptoms include breathlessness, wheezing, chest tightness, phlegm production, and cough, particularly at night or early morning. Asthma may manifest only as a chronic cough (cough-variant asthma) or as exercise-induced shortness of breath and wheezing.

Symptoms and airflow limitation vary between individuals and over time, either spontaneously, in response to triggers, or as a result of treatment. Although treatable with effective inhaled, oral, and parental therapies, and with the exception of occupational asthma (OA) where a single sensitizing agent is responsible and can be avoided, there is as yet no cure. Asthma therefore imposes a major burden on health systems, on societies through costs of treatment and lost productivity, and on personal and family life. As it is such a common condition, the bulk of diagnosis and management occurs in primary care in most economically developed countries, with specialist care generally reserved for those with more severe disease, poor control, or diagnostic uncertainty.

The airways in people with asthma usually show persistent but therapeutically modifiable inflammation, the most frequent being Type 2 inflammation involving activated T lymphocytes, and eosinophils and in those who are allergic, mast cells and immunoglobulin (Ig) E directed to specific allergens to which the individual is sensitive. People with asthma also demonstrate bronchial (airway) hyperresponsiveness (BHR, i.e., increased sensitivity to physical and/or chemical bronchoconstrictor stimuli). BHR is found in almost all symptomatic asthmatic patients,[5] can increase after sensitizing exposures, and can decrease after antiinflammatory treatment. Provocation of asthma can occur through interaction with a variety of trigger factors, including allergens, airborne irritants, stress, viral respiratory infections, air pollution, and occupational exposure, each of which likely acts through different pathways to produce the same end result: multicellular inflammation limited to the conducting airways, BHR, and airflow obstruction. Exposure to triggers can result in contraction of airways' smooth muscle (bronchospasm), respiratory symptoms, and asthma attacks, particularly in those with uncontrolled or under-treated asthma.

Diagnosis

The symptoms of asthma are nonspecific and shared with other respiratory and nonrespiratory conditions, and diagnosis may not be straightforward. Airway inflammation and BHR are fundamental to the underlying mechanisms of asthma leading to the characteristic variable airflow obstruction that defines the disease but currently are rarely measured in primary care settings. Spirometry is used to demonstrate the presence and reversibility of airflow obstruction, and patient-held peak expiratory flow (PEF) meters can be used to show variable airflow obstruction over a period of time (e.g., 2–4 weeks). Variable and reversible airflow obstruction is specific but insensitive in the diagnosis of asthma, as airway physiology may be normal in the absence of asthma triggers.[6] Although there is evidence of "under-diagnosis," based on the presence of suggestive symptoms and findings in population-based surveys in people without a diagnosis of asthma,[7] there is also growing evidence that a considerable minority of patients diagnosed and treated for asthma in the community lack objective evidence of the disease.[8,9] Lung function testing with spirometry and PEF monitoring is possible in primary care settings, but needs to be of a high standard. Lung function can be difficult to measure in younger children. The criteria for the diagnosis of asthma should be (but are often not) recorded in the medical record.

Airway Inflammation and Remodeling

Airway inflammation is the principal mechanism of asthma, and the principal treatment target. Typical features of airway inflammation are increased eosinophils, mast cells, and lymphocytes and a predominance of Type 2 helper T lymphocytes (Th2 cells), which produce mediators such as interleukin-3 (IL-3), IL-4, IL-5, IL-13, and granulocyte-macrophage colony-stimulating factor (GM-CSF). In more severe allergic and in non-allergic asthma, as encountered in adult onset, the tissue eosinophilia has been linked to recruitment and activation of innate lymphoid cells (ILCs) capable of secreting large amounts of IL-5 and IL-13[10] (Fig. 7.1). However, some patients exhibit different patterns of inflammation, including neutrophilic inflammation either alone or with eosinophils,[11] or, less frequently, few inflammatory cells (pauci-granulocytic phenotype).[12]

Asthma is characterized by structural changes in the airway that may precede the development of asthma. These include epithelial damage, subepithelial fibrosis, increased airway vasculature, nerve proliferation, and increased smooth muscle mass.[13] Mucous hypersecretion is associated with an increase in the number of submucosal secretory glands and epithelial goblet cells.

Treatment

For many years, a stepwise approach to treatment is generally applied and advocated in guidelines[14,15] based on the effectiveness, safety, cost, and availability of medication. Treatment step is increased in those not achieving control and reduced after a period (e.g., 3–6 months) of full control. Regular "controller" therapy with inhaled corticosteroids (ICS) is advocated for most, for symptom control and risk reduction. Inhaled short-acting inhaled bronchodilators (SABAs) are provided as "rescue" medication to temporarily reverse bronchospasm, usually in the form of short-acting inhaled β_2-agonists.

However, there has been a recent important change in the advice offered by the 2020 update of the Global Initiative for Asthma (GINA)[16] for managing "mild asthma." Inhaled SABA taken as required has been first-line treatment for asthma for 50 years dating back to an era when asthma was considered primarily to be a disease of bronchoconstriction (bronchospasm). As pointed out by GINA, regular or frequent use of short-acting inhaled b-agonists as bronchodilators (SABA) is accompanied by b-receptor downregulation,

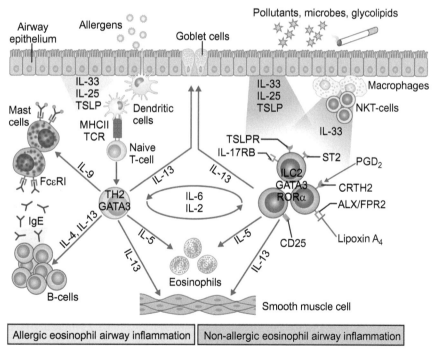

Fig. 7.1 Two different pathways lead to eosinophilic airway inflammation in asthma. In allergic asthma, dendritic cells present allergens to CD4+ T-cells, inducing T-helper *(Th)2* cells, which produce interleukin *(IL)-*4, IL-5, and IL-13, and leading to IgE switching in B-cells, airway eosinophilia, and mucous hypersecretion. In non-allergic eosinophilic asthma, air pollutants, microbes, and glycolipids induce the release of epithelium-derived cytokines, including IL-33, IL-25, and thymic stromal lymphopoietin *(TSLP)*, which activate innate lymphoid cells *(ILCs)* in an antigen-independent manner via their respective receptors (IL-17 receptor B *[IL-17RB]*, Il1rl1 (also known as ST2), a member of the IL-1 superfamily, and TSLP receptor *[TSLPR]*). Activated ILC2s produce high amounts of IL-5 and IL-13, leading to eosinophilia, mucus hypersecretion, and airway hyperreactivity. *CRTH2,* Chemoattractant receptor homologous molecule expressed on Th2 cells; *ALX/FPR2,* receptor for lipoxin A$_4$; *FcεRI,* high-affinity receptor for IgE; *GATA3,* GATA-binding protein 3; *PG,* prostaglandin; *ROR,* retinoic acid receptor–related orphan receptor; *NK,* natural killer; *MHC,* major histocompatibility complex; *TCR,* T-cell receptor. (Reproduced with permission from Brusselle GG, Maes T, Bracke KR. Eosinophils in the spotlight: eosinophilic airway inflammation in nonallergic asthma. Nat Med 2013;19:977–979.)

decreased broncho-protection, rebound hyperresponsiveness, decreased bronchodilator response,[16,17] and an increased allergic and eosinophilic airway inflammation.[18] Higher use of SABA is also linked to serious adverse clinical outcomes such as a higher risk of emergency department (ED) presentations and a greater risk of death.[19,20] Patient satisfaction with, and reliance on, regular SABA use is reinforced by its rapid relief of symptoms, its prominence in emergency and hospital management of exacerbations, and its low cost. GINA now recommends that all adults and adolescents with asthma should receive ICS as an antiinflammatory controller treatment, to modulate the baseline level of airways inflammation and reduce the risk of serious exacerbations. In those uncontrolled on standard doses of ICS, long-acting bronchodilators (usually as long-acting β_2-agonists, LABA) may be added to ICS, often in the form of a fixed dose ICS-LABA combination inhaler. Other add-on treatments may be used in those not achieving control, including leukotriene receptor antagonists (LTRA), theophylline, and inhaled long-acting antimuscarinic cholinergic antagonists (LAMA), but with each of these their need must be traded off against their side effects. Newer treatments for specific groups of patients with difficult-to-control asthma include parenteral monoclonal antibodies targeted at different parts of the complex inflammatory pathway.

Prevalence and Impact of Asthma

Asthma prevalence has ranged from 3% to 5% in developing countries to >20% in developed countries, affecting people of all ages. The disability-adjusted life years lost due to asthma are estimated to be 15 million per year, which equates to 1% of total global health impairment and compares with those of diabetes, cirrhosis of the liver, and schizophrenia. Although some countries have reported a reduction in hospitalization and deaths in recent years, for many economically developed countries, the improvements seen over the last decades of the last century have plateaued or even increased in the new millennium. The prevalence of asthma is increasing in many developing countries. In clinical trials, most (but not all) patients are able to achieve high levels of control,[21] yet surveys repeatedly show that in "real life," most patients continue to suffer significant levels of symptoms and many have asthma attacks.[22] This is sometimes related to biologically severe, therapy-resistant disease, but more often to exacerbations triggered by environmental exposures, infection avoidable and behavioral factors such as poor adherence to treatment, poor inhaler technique, or to unaddressed comorbidities. A recent UK national review of asthma deaths[23] reported preventable factors in the majority.

HISTORICAL PERSPECTIVE

While originally considered a disease of bronchospasm treated purely with bronchodilators, overuse of inhaled β-agonist bronchodilators in the 1970s and 1980s and an associated increase in mortality led to a reevaluation of the disease as one of airway inflammation in genetically susceptible individuals driven by environmental exposures mostly to inhaled allergens, viral infections, and air pollution. Allergic-type asthma is frequently accompanied by other manifestations of allergy such as allergic rhinitis, conjunctivitis, food allergy, and atopic dermatitis (AD).

EPIDEMIOLOGY

Most asthma (Fig. 7.2) begins in early childhood, although it may later remit sometimes for years before returning in later life. Of asthma sufferers, 95% have their first episode of wheezing before the age of 6 years.[24] Adult-onset asthma is less common and should raise consideration of OA (see below). Adult-onset asthma occurs more in women and is associated with more persistent airflow obstruction, a lack of association with atopy, a range of comorbidities, and a worse prognosis.[25]

Early-life wheezing often remits, but asthma lasting into adult life is likely to be persistent. Asthma is more common in boys than girls, but more common in women than men, the sex switch occurring in adolescence.[26] Asthma has become more common in all ages in recent decades, paralleled by similar increases in sensitization and allergic diseases as a whole. This increase in allergy and asthma is associated with Western lifestyles and prevalence increases as populations adopt such lifestyles and become urbanized. While there is much still to discover for this association, early life programming involving the gut and respiratory microbiome seems important.[27]

Incidence

Currently, there are no international measures of asthma incidence, or the risk of developing asthma within a specified time. A US study found the incidence of asthma in the first year of life was 3%, dropping to 0.9% and then to 0.1% in the age group 1 to 4 years and after the age of 15 years, respectively. A New Zealand cohort study reported that at age 9 years, 27% of all children had a history of at least one episode of wheezing, and 4.2% were receiving asthma therapy. These figures are similar in the US and Australian cohort studies[28,29]; in all, the age of first reported wheeze was greatest in the first year and levelled off in the teenage years linked to the hormonal changes of puberty.[30] Adult-onset asthma has an estimated incidence of 4.6 cases per 1000 person-years in females and 3.6 in males.

Prevalence

Due to the intermittent nature of asthma, wheezing at any time in the previous 12 months is often used to define asthma. The recognition of differing wheezing phenotypes, particularly in younger children, hampers the definitive labeling of asthma. The International Study of Asthma and Allergies in Childhood (ISAAC) reported the 12-month prevalence of symptoms ranged from 3% to 5% in countries that included Indonesia, China, and Greece, to >20% in Canada, Australia, New Zealand, and the UK.[31] The prevalence of childhood asthma in Western countries either remained steady or decreased in the 7 years between the ISAAC surveys, but increased in many low-prevalence non-Western countries. The plateau in Western countries may represent the population having achieved its

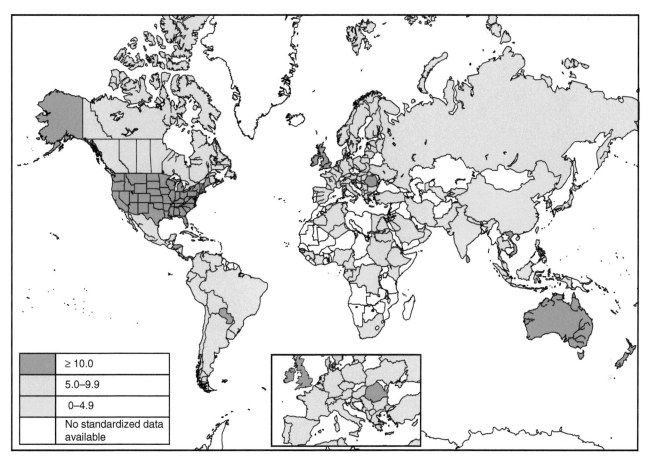

Fig. 7.2 World map of the prevalence of current asthma in children aged 13 to 14 years. Map provided by Richard Beasley. Data are based on International Study of Asthma and Allergies in Childhood (ISAAC III).[3] The prevalence of current asthma in the 13 to 14 year age group is estimated as 50% of the prevalence of self-reported wheezing in the previous 12 months. (From Global Initiative For Asthma, Online Appendix, Global Strategy For Asthma Management and Prevention, Revised 2014.)

genetic potential: all children predisposed to develop asthma now do so. The increase in low-prevalence countries appears as the economy develops and the countries become more "Westernized." Some insight has been uncovered through studying discreet populations with widely differing lifestyles such as those of the Amish and Hutterite farming people of common European decadency. Exposure to high concentrations of microbial products from livestock farming at crucial stages during development seems to be a powerful driver for protecting against allergy and asthma.[27,32] Other lifestyle factors in such communities also operate in the Amish including diet (e.g., unpasteurized milk, high vegetable, fruit, and fiber) and reduced exposure to transport-related air pollution and other environmental chemicals.[33]

Changing Trends

Asthma in many countries is increasing in prevalence. The proportion of US children up to 17 years with asthma over a 12-month period increased from 3.6% in 1980 to 7.5% in 1995. According to the Centers for Disease Control and Prevention (CDC), in 2018, 24,753,379 (7.7% ± 0.20%), SE, US citizens, had a diagnosis and were receiving treatment for asthma. This comprises 5,530,131 (7.5% ± 0.37%) children and young adults (age <18 years) and 19,223,248 (7.7% ± 0.22 %) adults (age 18+ years).

Boys experience an elevated prevalence rate until 17 years, from when prevalence in girls is higher. There is much debate about why this sex-linked change in prevalence occurs, but hormonal changes and growth patterns seem most likely.[26,34] Children of Indigenous American or Alaska Native descent have asthma prevalence rates 25% higher than Black and 60% higher than White children. Puerto Rican children have the highest prevalence of all groups, 140% higher than non-Hispanic White children, whereas Mexican and Asian children have low reported rates. The increases in asthma prevalence in Africa, Latin America, and Asia result in a growing global burden of asthma.[35]

PATHOGENESIS AND ETIOLOGY

Asthma is a complex syndrome manifesting through an interaction of genetic and environmental factors. While persistent airway inflammation is a key feature, structural changes occur in the airways referred to as airway wall remodeling. Remodeling occurs primarily in the major bronchi but as asthma becomes severe, it spreads distally to involve smaller bronchi and bronchioles and even down the alveoli.[36,37] At least two-thirds of asthmatics have features of allergy, constituting *allergic* or *extrinsic asthma*, accompanied by elevated levels of circulating allergen-specific and total serum immunoglobulin

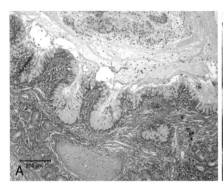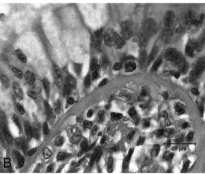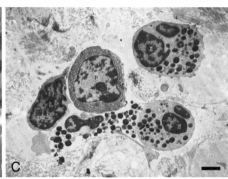

Fig. 7.3 (A) A low-magnification light micrograph of the bronchial wall in a person with moderate asthma shows mucosal inflammation, increased airway smooth muscle and bronchial gland mass, mucous cell hyperplasia in the surface epithelium, and a prominent mucus plug in the lumen. (B) Higher magnification of a region of epithelium shown in (A) demonstrates eosinophils in the epithelial layer and lamina propria, with thickening of the reticular basement membrane. (C) Transmission electron micrograph of cells in the mucosa from a patient with mild asthma shows a lymphocyte *(L)*, plasma cell *(P)*, and adjacent eosinophils *(E)* (bar = 2 μm).

E (IgE), and most often beginning in childhood. In contrast, *non-allergic* asthma is not associated with atopy with onset later in life.

Inflammatory Changes

Airway inflammation is the dominant abnormality even in the earliest stages of the disease. Airway mucosa inflammatory cells include lymphocytes, plasma cells, mast cells, and macrophages, and most typically eosinophils (Fig. 7.3).[38] The neutrophilic non-eosinophilic asthma phenotype is less-well defined although may be present in up to 50% of patients with symptomatic asthma.[11,39] This phenotype is described as high neutrophil counts in sputum ranging from 40% to 76% of sputum cells and associated with severe asthma, corticosteroid insensitivity, chronic airflow obstruction, and during acute exacerbations. There is increasing evidence that a proportion of neutrophilic asthma is driven by bacteria in an altered airway microbiome.[40] In allergic asthma, most cells exhibit a helper T cell Type 2 (Th2) profile of cytokine secretion, characterized by production of interleukin-4 (IL-4), IL-5, IL-9, IL-13, and GM-CSF.[41] These cytokines are secreted by a variety of cells including Th2 and innate lymphocytes, mast cells, and eosinophils. In allergic asthma, allergen is recognized by dendritic cells that span the epithelium and through co-stimulation activate naïve T lymphocytes converting them to Th2 lymphocytes which are virtual "factories" for producing Th2 cytokines along with a range of chemoattractant molecules (chemokines). Chemokines such as RANTES, eotaxin, TARC, CCL17, and CCL22 along with molecules called alarmins (IL-25, TSLP, and IL-33) are produced by a perturbed epithelium and enhance allergen induced Th2 responses.[42]

However, some patients do not show eosinophilic inflammation and or Th2 cytokine responses. These respond less well to ICS[43] and other interventions targeting Th2 cytokines. They have a predominantly mononuclear inflammatory cell airway response, with T lymphocytes and activated macrophages. Neutrophils may be prominent in some. Such inflammation is less associated with allergic responses and more a response to bacterial, viral, or chemical pollutant interactions with the epithelium.

Structural Changes and Airway Remodeling

Structural alterations of the lung are termed *airway remodeling* (see Chapter 1).[44] Airway wall thickening in large and small airways is characteristic, involving all airway wall components. The epithelium is hyperplastic and injured (Fig. 7.4), and autopsies in fatal asthma show epithelial sloughing. Epithelial cells lie on a basement membrane thickened by subepithelial fibrosis, with hyperplasia and hypertrophy of mucus-secreting cells. The airway walls have increased vascularity and smooth muscle hypertrophy or hyperplasia. Stiffness and loss of elasticity of the parenchyma occur, contributing to air trapping and hyperinflation. The normal parenchyma is linked to the airway by alveolar septa, which apply traction to the airway (Fig. 7.5), but their effectiveness is affected by subepithelial fibrosis and inflammation. There is evidence that a leaky and dysfunctional airway epithelium underlies the sensitivity of the asthmatic lung to the inhaled environment including allergens, microbes, and chemical pollutants. The asthmatic epithelium also behaves like a chronic wound in repairing when damaged by "secondary intention" with the laying down of new matrix and secretion of growth factors that drive remodeling changes.[45]

Immunologic Factors

With asthma onset being in early childhood, immunologic and early life immune development factors play a crucial role in its development along with other allergic (atopic) diseases. Early events and exposures shape and inform the developing immune system, with early life microbial programming being fundamental. Microbial diversity and the relative abundances of *Veillonella* and *Prevotella* in the airways at age 1 month predict asthma by age 6 years.[46] The gut microbiome may also be involved in this immune programming towards allergy and asthma. One-year-old children with an immature gastrointestinal microbial composition have an increased risk of asthma at age 5 years.[47] This association is only found among children born to asthmatic mothers, suggesting that lacking microbial stimulation during the first year of life triggers the expression of their inherited asthma risk. In addition to microbial contact, a range of factors

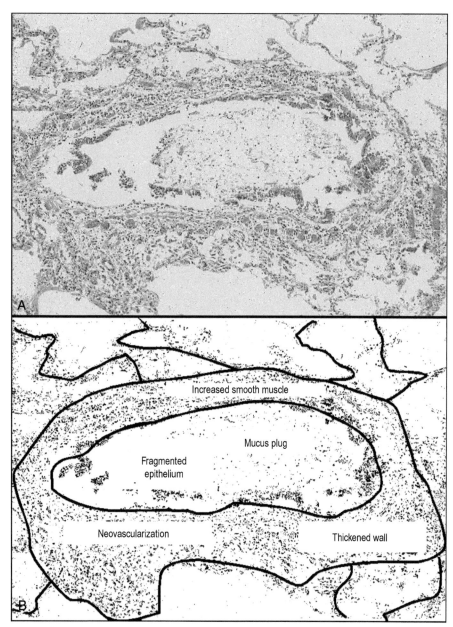

Fig. 7.4 (A) Airway specimen from the lung of a patient who died of asthma (i.e., status asthmaticus) shows profound structural changes (i.e., remodeling). (B) The airway wall is thickened by cellular infiltration, extracellular matrix deposition, and expansion of smooth muscle, and there is pronounced neovascularization. The epithelium is friable and disintegrating, and a mucus plug occupies the airway lumen (hematoxylin-eosin stain, ×100).

such as diet, cigarette smoke, and other airborne pollutant exposure increase the risk of allergic disease (Figs. 7.6 and 7.7).[48]

Genetics and Epigenetics

It has long been known that asthma and allergies run in families. Asthma has high heritability involving multiple genes, each with a modest effect, combine with environmental factors to produce the phenotypes of asthma. Genome-wide association studies (GWAS) have provided insights into pathogenesis, but so far these have not translated into novel therapeutic or preventative interventions. Of the many susceptibility genes uncovered through this hypothesis-free approach (Table 7.1), there are shared and distinct genetic risk factors for childhood-onset and adult-onset asthma.[49] A number of genes identify known immunological molecules involved in asthma pathogenesis, for example, IL1RL1 which encodes ST2, the receptor for IL-33, TSLP, and IL-33 itself.[50,51] Gene–environment interaction studies have demonstrated the importance of environmental triggers for initiation, exacerbation, and persistence of asthma, with the epithelium playing a sentinel orchestrating role.[52] Candidate gene association studies evaluate genetic variation in genes involved in disease pathogenesis (e.g., genes encoding cytokines, chemokines, and receptors). There are also genes linked to remodeling such as *ADAM33*, with polymorphism associated with early-life measures of lung function, BHR, and decline in lung function over time.[53]

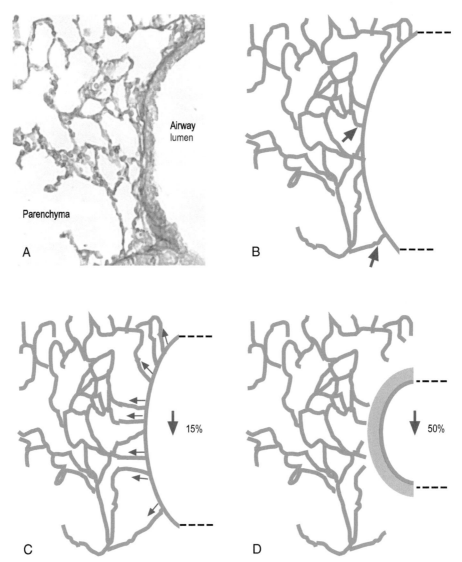

Fig. 7.5 Parenchyma-airway interdependence. (A) The airway and parenchyma are apparent in the stained histologic section of a lung. (B) The alveolar septa attach to the outer portion of the airway wall *(arrows)*. (C) The attachments function as tethers that apply outward tension *(small arrows)* when a normal (unremodeled) airway constricts. (D) When an airway is remodeled *(shaded area)*, the tethers are effectively broken, allowing the airway to constrict more than occurs in an unremodeled airway.

Pharmacogenetics refers to the relationship between genetic variation and drug response, with research focused on the β_2-adrenoceptor encoded by the gene ADRB2. Specific alleles for this gene predict response to short-acting β-agonists.[54] Responses to ICS and leukotriene antagonists also vary between individuals, and polymorphisms in steroid-signaling and other pathways being important.[55] In the future, systems incorporating genetic predictors of response may enable targeted treatment.

Epigenetic processes result from modifications of DNA structure without a change in the sequence in response to environmental exposures and as such, may be passed between generations. Epigenetic factors are a particular focus of interest in current research involving gene/environmental interactions such as methylation of specific sites within the promoter regions of genes, modification of the chromatin histone structure increasing or decreasing access of genes to specific promoter molecules, cutting and splicing of RNA prior to protein transcription and micro RNAs which are small non-coding

RNA molecules that function in RNA silencing and post-transcriptional regulation of gene expression.[56]

CLINICAL FEATURES AND PHENOTYPES OF ASTHMA

Phenotypes of Adult Asthma

Asthma is not a single disease but a group of clinical entities that share common features. The term *phenotype* refers to the observable characteristics of an individual or group resulting from interaction of its genotype with its environment and reflect the heterogeneity of asthma.[57] Phenotypes are defined by clinical features, pattern of inflammation, pulmonary function, triggers, or comorbidity (Box 7.1). Variability is noted in age of onset, allergy versus no allergy, inflammatory patterns, and response to treatment. Cluster analyses have identified clinically distinct phenotypes in adults,[58] but phenotype overlap is

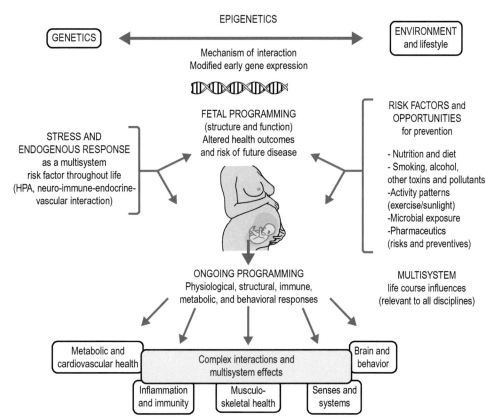

Fig. 7.6 Importance of early life events in the programming of structural and functional development. Physiologic, immune, metabolic, and behavioral patterns of response are determined early in development and may be modified by events and exposures early in life. Epigenetic effects provide a mechanism for gene–environment interactions, which may alter future disease risk with potentially greater effects in early life, when systems are developing. The same developmental plasticity provides opportunities early in life for disease prevention. *HPA,* Hypothalamic–pituitary axis. (Adapted from the University of Western Australia Developmental Origins of Health and Disease [DOHaD] Consortium, Perth, Australia, 2012.)

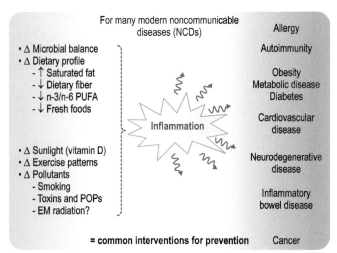

Fig. 7.7 Common risk factors for many noncommunicable diseases (NCDs); inflammation is a common element. Lifestyle changes are associated with an increase in inflammatory diseases, suggesting common risk factors and a central role for the immune system. Many risk factors for allergic disease are also implicated in many other NCDs, highlighting the need for a multidisciplinary approach to disease prevention. *EM,* Electromagnetic; *POPs,* persistent organic pollutants; *PUFA,* polyunsaturated fatty acid.

extremely common in asthmatic patients.[59] An *endotype* is a subtype defined by distinct functional or pathophysiologic mechanisms, and addresses etiology and pathophysiology.[60] Assessment of phenotypes potentially allows effective targeting of therapy. Beyond atopy, asthma is often associated with comorbidities such as rhinitis, sinusitis, nasal polyposis, gastroesophageal reflux disease (GERD), obstructive sleep apnea (OSA), hormonal disorders, and psychological disturbances (Table 7.2).[61]

Phenotypes in Children

Symptoms and clinical features are broadly similar in children, but childhood phenotypes of wheezing illnesses are complex, particularly in younger children. The Tucson Children's Respiratory Study (TCRS)[62] identified four wheezing phenotypes: (1) never (51%); (2) transient early (20%), with onset of wheezing before age 3 years and wheezing resolved by age 6; (3) persistent (14%), with onset of wheezing before age 3 years with continued wheezing at age 6; and (4) late onset (15%), with onset of wheezing between 3 and 6 years of age, and differences in risk factors and persistence between atopic and non-atopic wheezers. Early transient wheezing is the most prevalent phenotype, characterized by recurrent episodes in the first year. Of children who wheeze in the first 3 years, 60% have resolution

TABLE 7.1 Genome-Wide Association Studies for Asthma and Allergic Disease

Study	Discovery Population	Study Size	Phenotype Analyzed	Genes or Loci[a]	Gene Product and Functional Role
Moffatt et al. (2007)[30]	UK (White) German	994 asthmatics and 1243 controls; replicated in 2320 (German) and 3301 (UK) individuals	Childhood-onset asthma	ORMDL3, GSDMA, or GSDMB	Orosomucoid 1–like 3: transmembrane protein anchored in the endoplasmic reticulum but function unknown gasdermin A and B: expressed in epithelium and gut but function unknown; locus also associated with Crohn disease and ulcerative colitis
Weidinger et al. (2008)[31]	European	1530 Individuals, replication in four independent samples ($n = 9769$)	IgE levels, allergic sensitization	FCER1A	Fc fragment of IgE high-affinity receptor 1, alpha polypeptide: IgE receptor α unit initiates inflammation and hypersensitivity responses to allergens
				RAD50	RAD50 homolog (Saccharomyces cerevisiae): important for DNA double-strand break repair, cell cycle checkpoint activation, telomere maintenance, and meiotic recombination; adjacent to the IL-4, IL-13 cytokine locus
Gudbjartsson et al. (2009)[32]	Icelandic, European, East Asians, 10 different populations	9392 (Icelandic); 12,118 (European); 5212 (East Asian); 7996 cases and 44,890 controls (10 populations)	Blood eosinophil counts	IL1RL1	IL-1 receptor–like 1: murine studies suggest receptor is induced by proinflammatory stimuli and may be involved in helper T cell function
				WDR36, TSLP	WD repeat domain 36: may facilitate formation of heterotrimeric or multiprotein complexes; family members involved in many cellular processes, including cell cycle progression, signal transduction, apoptosis, and gene regulation; gene adjacent to TSLP Thymic stromal lymphopoietin: epithelial cell–derived cytokine with a key role in induction of allergic inflammation
				RAD50	See earlier
				MYB	Myeloblastosis viral oncogene homolog: nuclear transcription factor implicated in proliferation, survival, and differentiation of hematopoietic stem and progenitor cells
				IL33	IL-33: epithelial cell–derived IL-1–like cytokine ligand for the IL-1 receptor–related protein ST2; activates mast cells and Th2 lymphocytes
Kim et al. (2009)[33]	Korean	84 TDI asthma cases and 263 unexposed, healthy controls	TDI asthma	CTNNA3	Catenin (cadherin-associated protein), alpha 3: key molecule in the E-cadherin–mediated cell–cell adhesion complex; α-catenin suppresses invasion and tumor growth and inhibits RAS-MAPK activation; genetic polymorphisms may disturb defense systems of the airway epithelium, increasing airway hyperresponsiveness to environmental toxins such as TD
Moffatt et al. (2010)[34]	European	10,365 persons with physician-diagnosed asthma and 16,110 unaffected persons	Asthma	IL18R1	IL-18 receptor 1: member of the IL-1 receptor family; DC-derived IL-18 drives Treg differentiation and plays a role in airway inflammation in murine asthma models; IL-18 expression increased in asthma; adjacent to IL1RL1 (see earlier)

(Continued)

TABLE 7.1   Genome-Wide Association Studies for Asthma and Allergic Disease—cont'd

Study	Discovery Population	Study Size	Phenotype Analyzed	Genes or Loci[a]	Gene Product and Functional Role
				HLA-DQ	MHC class II, DQ members: due to extensive linkage disequilibrium across the HLA region, difficult to identify specific genes that underlie association signals in this locus; extended haplotypes across the HLA region have been studied in relation to specific allergen sensitization and production of TNF-α, which is encoded in the HLA class III region
				IL33	See earlier
				SMAD3	SMAD family member 3: transcription modulator activated by TGF-β, a cytokine that controls proliferation, differentiation, and other functions in many cell types, including Tregs; Smad3-deficient mice have increased levels of proinflammatory cytokines in lungs; potential role in airway remodeling
				IL2RB	IL-2 receptor, beta: IL-2 controls survival and proliferation of Tregs; implicated in differentiation and homeostasis of effector T cell subgroups, including Th1, Th2, Th17, and memory CD8+ T cells
				IL13	IL-13: Th2 cytokine that drives IgE production by B cells and goblet cell differentiation and mucus production by airway epithelial cells
				RORA	RAR-related orphan receptor A: encodes member of NR1 subfamily of nuclear hormone receptors; expressed at high levels in keratinocytes with cluster of proteins that form the structural and innate immune defenses of the epithelial barrier
				SLC22A5	Solute carrier family 22 (organic cation transporter), member 5: encodes a carnitine transporter
			IgE levels	IL13	See earlier
				HLA locus	See earlier
				STAT6	Signal transducer and activator of transcription 6: transcription factor critical to IL-4 and IL-13 intracellular signaling regulating IgE and Th2 cytokine production
				IL4R, IL21R	IL-4 receptor: a subunit of the IL-4/IL-13 receptorIL-21 receptor: IL-21 and its receptor (IL-21R) are upregulated in skin lesions of patients with active AD and in murine models; they play a critical role in sensitization and allergic inflammation in skin
Sleiman et al. (2010)[35]	US	793 asthmatic children and 1988 matched controls of European ancestry (discovery set); 917 asthmatics and 1546 matched controls of European ancestry (replication 1); 1667 North American children of African ancestry who had asthma and 2045 ancestrally matched controls (replication 2)	Asthma	DENND1B	DENN/MADD domain–containing 1B: gene is expressed by NK cells and DCs; DENND1B protein predicted to interact with the TNF-α receptor

(Continued)

TABLE 7.1 Genome-Wide Association Studies for Asthma and Allergic Disease—cont'd

Study	Discovery Population	Study Size	Phenotype Analyzed	Genes or Loci[a]	Gene Product and Functional Role
Li X et al. (2010)[36]	US (White)	473 severe asthmatics and 1892 general population controls	Severe or difficult-to-treat asthma	RAD50-IL13 and HLA-DR and -DQ regions	See earlier
Ferreira et al. (2011)[37]	Australian (White)	2669 physician-diagnosed asthmatics and 4528 controls from Australia, combined with data from Moffatt et al. (2010) ($n = 26,475$; further replication in additional 25,358 independent samples	Asthma	IL6R	IL-6 receptor: increased sIL-6R level in serum and airways of asthma patients; correlates with Th2 cytokine production in the lung; selective blockade of sIL-6R in mice suppresses IL-4, IL-5, and IL-13 production and decreases eosinophil numbers in the lung
				11q13.5 near C11orf30, LRRC32	Leucine-rich repeat containing 32: this locus is also associated with AD (see later) and Crohn disease
Hirota T et al. (2011)[38]	Japanese	7171 cases, 27,912 controls	Adult asthma	USP38 and GAB1	Ubiquitin-specific peptidase 38: function is unclear GRB2-associated binding protein 1: scaffolding adapter protein that plays an important role in the signaling pathway activated by cytokine receptors for IL-3, IL-6, IFN-αl, IFN-γ, and B cell and T cell receptors
				A locus on chromosome 10p14	Region contains no reported genes but is located 1 Mb downstream of GATA3, a master regulator of Th2 cell differentiation
				A gene-rich region on chromosome 12q13	Associated with type 1 diabetes and alopecia areata; strongest associated SNP is located 2 kb upstream from IKZF4 (i.e., EOS), which is involved in differentiation of regulatory T cells
Torgerson et al. (2011)[39]	European-American, African-American or African-Caribbean, and Latino ancestry	3246 cases with asthma, 3385 nonasthmatic controls, 1702 asthma case-parent trios, and 355 family-based cases and 468 family-based controls	Asthma	PYHIN1	Pyrin and HIN domain family member 1: asthma susceptibility specific to persons of African descent
Tantisira et al. (2011)[40]	US (White)	Four independent populations totaling 935 persons	Improvement in lung function in response to glucocorticoid therapy for asthma	GLCCI1	Glucocorticoid-induced transcript 1: expressed in lung and immune cells; expression is significantly enhanced by glucocorticoids in asthma-like conditions
Du et al. (2012)[41]	US (White)	403 subjects and trios; replication in 584 children from a Costa Rican cohort	Gene–vitamin D interaction in asthma exacerbations	CRTAM	Cytotoxic and regulatory T cell molecule: this class I MHC-restricted T cell–associated molecule is highly expressed in activated human CD8+ and NK T cells, both implicated in asthma pathogenesis
Esparza-Gordillo et al. (2009)[42]	European	939 cases, 975 controls. 270 complete nuclear families with two affected siblings	AD	C11orf30 locus	See earlier
Paternoster et al. (2011)[43]	European	5606 cases and 20,565 controls from 16 population-based cohorts; replication in 5419 cases and 19,833 controls from 14 studies	AD	OVOL1	Ovo-like 1: belongs to highly conserved family of genes that regulate development and differentiation of epithelial tissues and germ cells; regulates epidermal proliferation and differentiation

(Continued)

TABLE 7.1 Genome-Wide Association Studies for Asthma and Allergic Disease—cont'd

Study	Discovery Population	Study Size	Phenotype Analyzed	Genes or Loci[a]	Gene Product and Functional Role
				Locus near *ADAMTS10* and *ACTL9*	ADAM metallopeptidase with thrombospondin type 1 motif and actin-like 9: most strongly associated SNP is upstream of ADAMTS10 and downstream of ACTL9 (encoding a hypothetical protein); ADAMTS proteins are complex, secreted, zinc-dependent metalloproteinases that bind to and cleave extracellular matrix components and are involved in connective tissue remodeling and extracellular matrix turnover
				KIF3A	Kinesin family member 3A: located within the Th2 cytokine cluster at 5q31.1
Sun et al. (2011)[44]	Chinese Han	1012 cases and 1362 controls; replication in 3624 cases and 12,197 controls	AD	*TMEM232* and *SLC25A46*	Transmembrane protein 232: encodes a protein belonging to the functional class of tetraspan transmembrane proteins. Solute carrier family 25, member 46: this family encodes mitochondrial carrier proteins, which may shuttle metabolites across the inner mitochondrial membrane
				TNFRSF6B and *ZGPAT*	Tumor necrosis factor receptor superfamily, member 6B decoy: important role in adaptive immune responses. Zinc finger, CCCH type with G patch domain: located at 20q13.3; limited analysis of variants found no significant association
Ramasamy et al. (2012)[45]	European	3933 self-reported cases and 8965 controls	Allergic rhinitis	*HLA-DRB4* C11orf30 locus *TMEM232* and *SLC25A46*	HLA locus (see earlier) See earlier See earlier

[a]Genes or loci identified in addition to those previously identified in GWAS.

DC, Dendritic cell; *HLA*, human leukocyte antigen; *IFN-γ*, interferon-γ; *IgE*, immunoglobulin E; *IL*, interleukin; *MAPK*, mitogen-activated protein kinase; *MHC*, major histocompatibility complex; *NK*, natural killer; *sIL-6R*, soluble IL-6 receptor; *SMAD*, derived from *Drosophila* mothers against decapentaplegic (Mad) and *Caenorhabditis elegans* Sma genes; *SNP*, single-nucleotide polymorphism; *TDI*, toluene diisocyanate induced; *TGF-β*, transforming growth factor-β; *Th1*, helper T cell type 1; *Th2*, helper T cell type 2; *Th17*, helper T cell type 17; *TNF-α*, tumor necrosis factor-α; *Treg*, regulatory T cell; *US*, United States.

BOX 7.1 Phenotypes of Asthma

Based on Airway Inflammation
- Eosinophilic
- Neutrophilic
- Paucigranulocytic

Based on Clinical Features
- Mild, moderate, or severe asthma
- Exacerbation-prone
- Treatment-resistant
- Early-onset or late-onset asthma
- Asthma in the elderly

Based on Pulmonary Function
- With a component of fixed airway obstruction
- With marked/rapid fluctuations of airway caliber
- With marked hyperinflation

Based on Triggers
- Allergic or non-allergic asthma
- Aspirin or nonsteroidal antiinflammatory drugs
- Occupational allergens or irritants
- Hormones: premenstrual and menopausal asthma
- Exercise- or cold air–induced asthma
- Asthma in the high-level athlete
- Asthma in the smoker

Based on Associated Comorbid Conditions
- Rhinitis/rhinosinusitis, nasal polyps, and aspirin intolerance
- Psychological disturbances (e.g., depression, anxiety disorders)
- With dysfunctional breathing (hyperventilation syndrome, vocal cord dysfunction)
- With associated chronic obstructive pulmonary disease
- Asthma in the obese

TABLE 7.2 Tests for Asthma-Related Comorbidities

Comorbidity	Potentially Useful Tests
Rhinitis	
Allergic	Allergy skin-prick test
	Serum-specific IgE
Non-allergic	ENT examination
Associated with nasal polyps	Sinus radiography/CT scan
CRS and sinusitis	
GERD	Proton-pump inhibitor treatment trial
	24-h esophageal pH measurement
	Imaging techniques
Obesity	BMI and other obesity measures
	Detection of metabolic syndrome
OSA	Sleep studies: polysomnography
Psychopathologies	Psychological evaluation
Dysfunctional breathing	Nijmegen questionnaire[30]
VCD	Flow-volume loop
	Visualization of the pharynx: laryngoscopy
Hormonal and metabolic disorders	Hormone measurements
COPD and smoking	Pulmonary function tests
	Chest radiography/CT scan
	Biomarkers
Infections	
Viral	Specific serologies
Bacterial	Various identification measures
Fungal	Precipitins for *Aspergillus*/fungal cultures/*Aspergillus* serology

BMI, Body mass index; *COPD*, chronic obstructive pulmonary disease; *CRS*, chronic rhinosinusitis; *CT*, computed tomography; *ENT*, ear, nose, and throat; *GERD*, gastroesophageal reflux disease; *IgE*, immunoglobulin E; *OSA*, obstructive sleep apnea; *VCD*, vocal cord dysfunction.
Adapted from Boulet LP, Boulay MÈ. Asthma-related comorbidities. Expert Rev Respir Med 2011;5:377–393.

of their symptoms by 6 years of age. Transient wheezing has no significant relationship to atopy but is associated with maternal smoking during pregnancy (odds ratio [OR], 2.2; 95% confidence interval [CI], 1.3–3.7). Transient wheezing is associated with lower levels of lung function. Less than one-quarter of transient wheezers continue to wheeze during adolescence. Children with transient wheezing do not have increased methacholine reactivity or PEF variability at age 11 years.

Non-atopic persistent wheezing is associated with the first episode of wheezing occurring before the age of 1 year, representing 20% of wheezy children under 3 years of age. Episodes become less frequent by teenage years. Children have a lower level of prebronchodilator lung function and enhanced airway reactivity. IgE-associated atopic persistent wheezing is found in 20% of children who wheeze during the first 3 years, with symptoms first presenting after age 1 year and an association with early sensitization to food or aeroallergens. Risk factors include

male sex, parental asthma, AD, eosinophilia at 9 months, and history of wheezing with infections. Early onset sensitization to a range of aeroallergens in the first 3 years of life is a major predictor of more severe asthma.[63]

Persistent wheezers continue to have symptoms and lower airflow as they reach teenage years, but no progressive deficits in lung function. Other longitudinal birth cohort studies have reported similar results, although these have suggested additional phenotypes. The European Respiratory Society has defined symptom-based phenotypes: "episodic" (or "viral") and "multi-trigger" wheeze.[64] Children with episodic (viral) wheeze have discrete symptomatic periods. Children with multi-trigger wheeze have wheezing both during exacerbations and between episodes in response to various triggers, including viruses, allergens, exercise, and cigarette smoke, and also exhibit lower airway function.[65]

EVALUATION AND DIAGNOSIS

The lack of a simple gold standard diagnostic test and limited availability of diagnostic tests may lead to difficulties in primary care, and there is evidence of both over- and under-diagnosis.[66]

Diagnosis in Adults
Risk Factors

Potential risk factors for the development of asthma should be ascertained and documented. These include (1) family history, sex, and age; (2) allergies—especially to aeroallergens house dust mite, pet dander, mold, grass and tree pollen, and certain foods; (3) smoking—smokers have a high risk of asthma and those whose mothers smoked during pregnancy or who were exposed to secondhand smoke are also more likely to develop asthma; (4) air pollution—constant exposure to air pollution raises the risk for asthma and those who grew up or live in urban areas have a higher risk for asthma; (5) obesity—although the reasons are unclear, some experts point to low-grade inflammation in the body that occurs with extra weight; and (6) viral respiratory infections (Box 7.2).[67]

History and Examination

Asthma is a symptomatic condition characterized by episodic wheeze, shortness of breath, cough sputum production, and chest tightness exacerbated by triggers. Symptom pattern and triggers should be documented. However, symptoms do not accurately predict pulmonary function and are not reliable to establish a diagnosis in isolation.[8,68] Physical examination is often normal unless the disease is severe or the examination is performed during an exacerbation or exposure to triggers, when wheezes can be heard on auscultation, with prolonged expiratory time.

Lung Function

Pulmonary function tests should always be performed in the diagnosis of asthma (Box 7.3). Spirometry is the preferred method to measure airway obstruction.[15] A ratio of forced expiratory volume in 1 s (FEV_1) to forced vital capacity (FVC) of <0.7 defines airflow obstruction. FEV_1 is an absolute measure

BOX 7.2 Suggested Items for Medical History[a]

A detailed medical history of the new patient who is known, or thought, to have asthma should address the following items:

1. Symptoms
   - Cough
   - Wheezing
   - Shortness of breath
   - Chest tightness
   - Sputum production
2. Pattern of symptoms
   - Perennial, seasonal, or both
   - Continual, episodic, or both
   - Onset, duration, frequency (number of days or nights, per week or month)
   - Diurnal variations, especially nocturnal and on awakening in early morning
3. Precipitating and/or aggravating factors
   - Viral respiratory infections
   - Environmental allergens, indoor (e.g., mold, house-dust mite, cockroach, animal dander, or secretory products) and outdoor (e.g., pollen)
   - Characteristics of home, including: age, location, cooling and heating system, wood-burning stove, humidifier, carpeting over concrete, presence of molds or mildew, characteristics of rooms where patient spends time (e.g., bedroom and living room with attention to bedding, floor covering, stuffed furniture)
   - Smoking (patient and others in home or day-care)
   - Exercise
   - Occupational chemicals or allergens
   - Environmental change (e.g., moving to new home; going on vacation; alterations in workplace, work processes, or materials used)
   - Irritants (e.g., tobacco smoke, strong odors, air pollutants, occupational chemicals, dusts and particulates, vapors, gases, aerosols)
   - Emotions (e.g., fear, anger, frustration, hard crying, or laughing)
   - Stress (e.g., fear, anger, frustration)
   - Drugs (e.g., aspirin and other nonsteroidal antiinflammatory drugs, β-blockers including eye drops, others)
   - Food, food additives, and preservatives (e.g., sulfites)
   - Changes in weather, exposure to cold air
   - Endocrine factors (e.g., menses, pregnancy, thyroid disease)
   - Comorbid conditions (e.g., sinusitis, rhinitis, GERD)
4. Development of disease and treatment
   - Age of onset and diagnosis
   - History of early-life injury to airways (e.g., bronchopulmonary dysplasia, pneumonia, parental smoking)
   - Progression of disease (better or worse)

- Present management and response, including plans for managing exacerbations
- Frequency of using SABA
- Need for oral corticosteroids and frequency of use
5. Family history
   - History of asthma, allergy, sinusitis, rhinitis, eczema, or nasal polyps in close relatives
6. Social history
   - Day-care, workplace, and school characteristics that may interfere with adherence
   - Social factors that interfere with adherence, such as substance abuse
   - Social support/social networks
   - Level of education completed
   - Employment
7. History of exacerbations
   - Usual prodromal signs and symptoms
   - Rapidity of onset
   - Duration
   - Frequency
   - Severity (need for urgent care, hospitalization, ICU admission)
   - Life-threatening exacerbations (e.g., intubation, ICU admission)
   - Number and severity of exacerbations in the past year
   - Usual patterns and management (what works?)
8. Impact of asthma on patient and family
   - Episodes of unscheduled care (ED, urgent care, hospitalization)
   - Number of days missed from school/work
   - Limitation of activity, especially sports and strenuous work
   - History of nocturnal awakening
   - Effect on growth, development behavior, school or work performance, and lifestyle
   - Impact on family routines, activities, or dynamics
   - Economic impact
9. Assessment of patient's and family's perceptions of disease
   - Patient's, parents', and spouse's or partner's knowledge of asthma and in the chronicity of asthma and in the efficacy of treatment
   - Patient's perception and beliefs regarding use and long-term effects of medications
   - Ability of patient and parents, spouse, or partner to cope with disease
   - Level of family support and patient's and parents', spouse's, or partner's capacity to recognize severity of an exacerbation
   - Economic resources
   - Sociocultural beliefs

[a]This list does not represent a standardized assessment or diagnostic instrument. The validity and reliability of this list has not been assessed.
ED, Emergency department; *GERD*, gastroesophageal reflux disease; *ICU*, intensive care unit; *SABA*, short-acting β-agonists.
From National Heart, Lung, and Blood Institute. Expert Panel Report 3 (EPR-3): Guidelines for the Diagnosis and Management of Asthma: Full Report 2007. Available at: <https://www.ncbi.nlm.nih.gov/books/NBK7232/>; accessed August 30, 2020.

BOX 7.3 Diagnosis of Asthma in Adults

Symptoms of episodic breathlessness, wheezing, cough, chest tightness, phlegm production (one or more)
PLUS[a]
Increase in FEV_1 after a bronchodilator or after a course of controller therapy ≥12% (and a minimum ≥200 mL)
OR

Increase in PEF after a bronchodilator or after a course of controller therapy of 60 L/min (minimum ≥20%) or an increase ≥20%, based on multiple daily readings
OR
Methacholine PC_{20} <4 mg/mL (4–16 mg/mL is borderline)
OR
Decrease in FEV_1 after exercise challenge ≥10%–15%[b]

[a]Ideally with an FEV_1/FVC less than the lower limit of normal value (<0.075–0.8).
[b]If exercise-induced asthma is suspected, eucapnic voluntary hyperpnea or mannitol/hyperosmolar challenges may be used if available.
FEV_1, Forced expiratory volume in 1 s; *FVC*, forced vital capacity; *PC_{20}*, provocative concentration that induces a 20% fall in FEV_1; *PEF*, peak expiratory flow.
Adapted from Global Initiative for Asthma (GINA) 2020. Available at: <2020 GINA Report, Global Strategy for Asthma Management and Prevention. P.O. Box 558 Fontana, WI 53125, USA. Online. Available: https://ginasthma.org/wp-content/uploads/2020/06/GINA-2020-report_20_06_04-1-wms.pdf> and from Lougheed MD, Lemiere C, Ducharme FM, et al.; Canadian Thoracic Society Asthma Clinical Assembly. Canadian Thoracic Society 2012 guideline update: diagnosis and management of asthma in preschoolers, children and adults. Can Respir J 2012;19:127–164.

of the volume of air exhaled in the first second of forced expiration, and normative tables are available for groups, stratified by ages and sex, allowing the determination of the percent predicted FEV_1. A reduced percent predicted FEV_1 with a low FEV_1/FVC ratio indicates the presence of airway obstruction. Significant reversibility (usually defined as an increase in FEV_1 of 12% or more with at least a 200-mL change) after inhalation of a b_2-agonist bronchodilator and/or following 4 weeks of antiinflammatory treatment with ICS is strongly indicative of asthma. Spirometry is reliable and reproducible when performed correctly[69] and is entirely possible to perform in primary care settings especially with the availability of hand-held portable instruments some equipped for remote monitoring.[70] However, staff require training, quality assurance is needed, and equipment requires maintenance and calibration. Ideally, spirometers should produce a visible or hard-copy "flow-volume" or "volume-time" trace to allow inspection of the adequacy of the test. It has been recommended to use the 5th percentile as the "lower limit of normal" because these values are not always proportional to the percent of predicted value. However, fixed-ratio lower limit of normal for FEV_1/FVC (70%) and percent of predicted FEV_1 are still commonly used.

PEF measurements with a portable peak flow meter is useful, although are more dependent on patient effort. Domiciliary morning and night monitoring of PEF (usually as the best of three tests) can be used to demonstrate PEF variability over a period of time (e.g., 2 weeks) to support the diagnosis of asthma. PEF should be compared with the patient's best value, as normative values can be less reliable. Characteristically in asthma, monitoring in untreated patients produces a "saw-tooth" pattern, with significant diurnal variability (lower values on morning readings). Diurnal PEF variability is calculated as the highest PEF of the day minus the lowest PEF reading divided by the mean of the day's highest and lowest readings and averaged over a 1- to 2-week period. Average diurnal variability is >10%, and the greater the variation, the greater is the support for the diagnosis.[70]

Bronchial Hyperreactivity (BHR or Bronchial Hyperresponsiveness)

Bronchial provocation testing provides an objective measure of the constriction thresholds or "twitchiness" of the airways.[71] In these tests, patients inhale (usually via a nebulizer) increasing concentrations or cumulative doses of a bronchoconstrictor substance, and spirometry is repeated until a 20% reduction in baseline FEV_1 is observed. In patients with normal pulmonary function or nonsignificant reversibility of airway obstruction, a bronchoprovocation test is useful to confirm BHR to support an asthma diagnosis. Direct challenges involve the inhalation of a bronchoconstrictor; the lower the concentration or dose required, the more hyperreactive are the airways. Direct bronchial challenge tests are highly sensitive judged against a gold standard of a subsequent diagnostic review made by an experienced clinician with the aid of all diagnostic tests and response to treatment over some months, and negative tests help exclude asthma. The commonest test used is the methacholine inhalation test, measuring the provocative concentration of methacholine

inducing a 20% fall in FEV_1 (PC_{20}). The test is sensitive but not specific and may be positive in conditions such as rhinitis or chronic obstructive pulmonary disease (COPD). Regular use of ICS may normalize the test by suppressing underlying inflammation.

Indirect bronchial stimuli such as exercise, hypertonic aerosols such as saline or mannitol, adenosine monophosphate (AMP), and eucapnic voluntary hyperpnea (EVH) have also been used, and correlate better with airway inflammation.[71]

Determination of the Allergic Status

Asthma is often allergic in nature and allergy skin-prick tests help identify specific sensitizing allergens in a particular patient. The temporal relationship of symptoms with allergen exposure should be documented, but subclinical inflammation after allergen exposure may be insufficient to induce acute symptoms. Measurement of specific IgE in the serum (e.g., by a radioallergosorbent test [RAST] or ImmunoCAP®) can also identify sensitization to a particular allergen. Component-resolved diagnostics (CRD) has facilitated the development of products in which sIgE to more than 100 allergen components can be measured simultaneously by using small volumes of serum.[72] Although elevated serum total IgE levels suggest an atopic status, increased total IgE can occur in the absence of atopy and, therefore, does not really help in establishing a diagnosis of asthma.

Assessment of Airway Inflammation

Noninvasive assessments of airway inflammation are helpful in cases of diagnostic difficulty, including induced sputum analysis and measurement of fractional nitric oxide concentration in exhaled breath (FeNO). In general, they are underused.[73] Nebulized hypertonic saline is used to induce sputum, from which inflammatory cell numbers and types are recorded, generally reserved for patients with severe asthma in research and hospital settings. Levels of FeNO are increased in asthma and correlate with the presence of eosinophilic airway inflammation.[74] Production of nitric oxide (NO) by airway epithelial cells is driven by inducible NO synthase (iNOS) and is upregulated in Type 2 asthmatic inflammation, and inhibited by corticosteroid therapy. Clinical guideline stated that FeNO may help to detect eosinophilic inflammation, assess the likelihood of corticosteroid responsiveness, contribute to the monitoring of corticosteroid needs, and detect nonadherence.[75] This test is simple to perform and relatively inexpensive and can be effectively performed in primary care settings.[76]

Imaging

Imaging studies are not particularly useful in the diagnosis or follow-up of asthma but can be used to investigate diagnostic difficulties when they arise such as allergic bronchopulmonary aspergillosis, COPD (and emphysema), bronchiectasis, and interstitial diseases. Imaging is a useful research tool.[77] Lung hyperinflation, a mosaic perfusion pattern at full inspiration (reflecting ventilation-perfusion inequalities), and increased airway wall thickness are more prevalent on high-resolution chest computed tomography in severe asthma.

Asthma Diagnosis in Specific Settings
Occupational Asthma

There is growing recognition that work-related asthma is a major public health concern and frequently goes unrecognized.[78] *Work-related asthma* is a broad term indicating asthma worsened by the workplace, encompassing OA, which is caused by a specific workplace agent, and *work-exacerbated asthma* (WEA), which is asthma worsened by stimuli at the workplace (Fig. 7.8). A widely cited definition emphasizes the causal relationship between asthma and the workplace: "Occupational asthma is characterized by airway inflammation, variable airflow limitation, and airway hyperresponsiveness due to causes and conditions attributable to a particular occupational environment and not to stimuli encountered outside the workplace."

A pooled analysis indicates that 17.6% of all cases of adult-onset asthma are attributable to workplace exposures.[63] Cohort studies reported incidence rates of 2.7 to 3.5 cases of OA per 100 person-years amongst workers exposed to laboratory animals; 4.1 per 100 person-years amongst those exposed to wheat flour; and 1.8 per 100 person-years amongst dental health apprentices exposed to latex gloves. The pathophysiology in most cases is an allergic IgE-dependent mechanism. Some forms of OA are not linked to IgE responses such as that driven by diisocyanate exposure.[79] The agents and occupations most commonly implicated in this type of asthma are listed in Table 7.3.

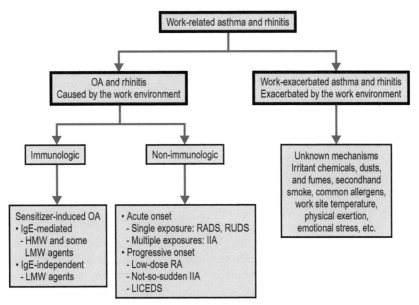

Fig. 7.8 Classification of work-related asthma and rhinitis. *HMW,* High-molecular-weight; *IgE,* immunoglobulin E; *IIA,* irritant-induced asthma; *LICEDS,* low-intensity chronic exposure dysfunction syndrome; *LMW,* low-molecular-weight; *OA,* occupational asthma; *RADS,* reactive airways dysfunction syndrome; *RUDS,* reactive upper airways dysfunction syndrome.

TABLE 7.3 Principal Agents Causing Immunologic OA

Agent		Workers/Occupations at Risk
High-molecular-weight agents		
Cereals (flour)	Wheat, rye, barley, buckwheat	Millers, bakers, pastry makers
Latex	Gloves	Healthcare workers, laboratory technicians
Animals	Mice, rats, cows, seafood	Laboratory workers, farmers, seafood processors
Enzymes	α-Amylase, maxatase, alcalase, papain, bromelain, pancreatin, amylases, lipases and proteases.	Baking products manufacture, bakers, detergent production, pharmaceutical industry, food industry, laundry products
Low-molecular-weight agents		
Isocyanates	Toluene diisocyanate (TDI), methylene diphenyl-diisocyanate (MDI), hexamethylene diisocyanate (HDI)	Polyurethane production, plastic industry, molding, spray painters, insulation installers
Metals	Chromium, nickel, cobalt, platinum	Metal refinery, metal alloy production, electroplaters, welders
Biocides	Aldehydes, quaternary ammonium compounds	Healthcare workers, cleaners
Persulfate salts	Hair bleach	Hairdressers
Acid anhydrides	Phthalic, trimellitic, maleic, tetrachlorophthalic acids	Epoxy resin workers
Reactive dyes	Reactive black 5, pyrazolone derivatives, vinyl sulfones, carmine	Textile workers, food industry workers
Acrylates	Cyanoacrylates, methacrylates, di- and triacrylates	Manufacture of adhesives, dental and orthopedic materials, sculptured fingernails, printing inks, paints and coatings
Wood dusts	Red cedar, iroko, obeche, oak	Sawmill workers, carpenters, cabinet and furniture makers

The diagnosis is difficult and requires specialist referral. It is important, as early removal of the sensitizing factor may allow full resolution. OA may be suspected from the temporal relationship between asthma symptoms and exposure to workplace sensitizers. To confirm the diagnosis, serial measures of airway responsiveness and PEF can be used, or specific bronchoprovocation tests performed.[80]

Asthma in the Elderly

Elderly patients may have difficulty in performing pulmonary function tests and may show a different pattern of asthma, mostly a combined neutrophilic and eosinophilic inflammatory pattern with more severe airway obstruction and physiologic features related to the aging of the lung. COPD is often misdiagnosed in this population.[81]

Asthma in the Athlete

Athletes may present with asymptomatic BHR or asthma that is less responsive to therapy.[82] Because symptoms are unreliable and expiratory flows are often normal, bronchoprovocation tests are often needed.

Conditions That May Mimic Asthma

Many conditions may be confused or associated with asthma and can influence its manifestations (Box 7.4). These conditions include dysfunctional breathing syndromes such as vocal cord dysfunction and hyperventilation syndrome, upper airways diseases, deconditioning, obesity-related symptoms, pulmonary embolism, OSA, and airway neoplasms. Smoking-induced COPD and cardiac insufficiency may manifest with asthma-like symptoms in elderly patients. Less common masqueraders include bronchiectasis, vasculitis (e.g., Churg–Strauss syndrome), cystic fibrosis, and mastocytosis.

Diagnosis in Children

The natural history of pediatric wheezing is complex. The evaluation is made more complicated by difficulty in obtaining

---

BOX 7.4   Differential Diagnosis of Asthma

- Bronchiolitis
- Cardiac condition (e.g., heart failure)
- Chronic obstructive pulmonary disease
- Cystic fibrosis
- Deconditioning
- Dysfunctional breathing (e.g., hyperventilation syndrome)
- Foreign body aspiration
- Laryngotracheomalacia, tracheal stenosis
- Obstructive sleep apnea
- Other causes of cough (e.g., chronic eosinophilic bronchitis, GERD, ACE-inhibitor)
- Pulmonary embolism
- Pulmonary infiltrate with eosinophilia (PIE syndrome)
- Tracheobronchial tumor
- Upper airways diseases (e.g., upper airway cough syndrome)
- Vocal cord dysfunction

ACE, Angiotensin-converting enzyme; *GERD*, gastroesophageal reflux disease.

BOX 7.5   Key Symptom Indicators for Considering a Diagnosis of Asthma

1. Wheezing—high-pitched wheezing sounds when breathing out (normal chest exam without wheezing does not exclude asthma)
2. History of any of the following:
   - Cough (worse particularly at night)
   - Recurrent wheeze
   - Recurrent difficulty breathing
   - Recurrent chest tightness
3. Symptoms occur or worsen in the presence of:
   - Exercise
   - Viral infection
   - Inhalant allergens (e.g., animals with fur or hair, house-dust mites, mold, pollen)
   - Irritants (tobacco or wood smoke, airborne chemicals)
   - Changes in weather
   - Strong emotional expression (laughing or crying hard)
   - Stress
   - Menses
4. Symptoms occur or worsen at night, waking the patient

Modified from National Heart, Lung, and Blood Institute. Expert Panel Report 3 (EPR-3): Guidelines for the Diagnosis and Management of Asthma: Full Report 2007. Available at: <https://www.ncbi.nlm.nih.gov/books/NBK7232/>; accessed August 30, 2020.

---

objective lung function measurements and the complexity of wheezing phenotypes.

History and Examination

The presence of multiple key indicators increases the probability that a child has asthma (Box 7.5). Documenting risk factors, symptoms, triggers, and reversible airflow obstruction where possible are needed, as with adults. Risk factors include a personal or family history of atopic disease. Age of onset, timing and pattern of wheezing, relationship of episodes to viral illness and feeding, comorbidities, response to previous treatments, and socioenvironmental factors contributing to morbidity should be documented (see Box 7.2).

Atypical features suggesting an alternative diagnosis include symptoms starting at birth, continuous wheezing, failure to thrive, failure to respond to medications, and no association with typical triggers such as viral upper respiratory infections or exposure to allergens after sensitization. Box 7.6 lists the differential diagnosis of asthma and comorbid diseases, and Table 7.4 shows their relative frequency by age. Physical examination may be normal; however, findings that increase the probability of asthma are chest hyperinflation, use of accessory muscles, hunched shoulders, barrel chest, wheezing during normal breathing or forced expiration, rhinitis, and dermatitis. Unilateral wheezing may indicate foreign body aspiration.

Radiographic Studies

Radiographic studies are not required in routine diagnosis, although may be useful in cases of diagnostic uncertainty.

Pulmonary Function Tests

Pulmonary function testing (PFT) with spirometry should be possible in primary care in the majority of children over the age

BOX 7.6 Differential Diagnosis for Asthma in Infants and Children

Upper Airway Diseases
- Allergic rhinitis and sinusitis

Obstructions Involving Large Airways
- Foreign body in the trachea or bronchus
- Vocal cord dysfunction
- Vascular rings or laryngeal webs
- Laryngotracheomalacia, tracheal stenosis, or bronchostenosis
- Enlarged lymph nodes or tumor

Obstructions Involving Small Airways
- Viral bronchiolitis or obliterative bronchiolitis
- Cystic fibrosis
- Bronchopulmonary dysplasia (chronic lung disease of prematurity)
- Heart disease

Other
- Recurrent cough not caused by asthma (infection, habit cough, postnasal drip)
- Aspiration from swallowing mechanism dysfunction or gastroesophageal reflux disease

Modified from National Heart, Lung, and Blood Institute. Expert Panel Report 3 (EPR-3): Guidelines for the Diagnosis and Management of Asthma: Full Report 2007. Available at: <https://www.ncbi.nlm.nih.gov/books/NBK7232/>; accessed August 30, 2020.

TABLE 7.4 Age-Related Differential Diagnosis for Wheezing

Condition	Infancy	Childhood	Adolescence
Asthma	+	+++	+++
Airway malacia	++	+	−
Cystic fibrosis	+++	+	±
Foreign body	++	+++	±
Airway infection	+++	++	+
Bronchopulmonary dysplasia	+++	+	−
Primary ciliary dyskinesia	+	++	+
Bronchiectasis	+	+	+
Congenital anomalies (vascular ring)	+++	+	−
Vocal cord dysfunction	−	±	++
Tumors	±	±	±
Aspiration syndromes	+	±	±
Pulmonary edema	+	+	+

−, Unlikely to present in this age group; +, likely to present in this age group; ± may present in this age group.
Modified from Bierman CW, Pearlman DS, editors. Allergic diseases from infancy to adulthood. 2nd ed. Philadelphia: Saunders; 1988.

of 6 years. PEF is well suited for monitoring trends in asthma control over time in children aged 4 years and older, but less useful in diagnosing asthma or classifying severity. FEV_1 is generally normal in children with asthma, but FEV_1/FVC decreases as asthma severity increases. Pre- and postbronchodilator determinations can be obtained with improvements of 12% or greater for FEV_1 clinically significant, although many will not reach this degree of reversibility.[83] Specialized PFTs include body plethysmography, impulse oscillometry, and infant lung function testing and are available in most pediatric medical centers, but not in primary care. Plethysmography allows the measurement of lung volumes and airway mechanics (resistance, conductance, specific conductance). Impulse oscillometry (IOS) measurements are based on respiratory system resistance and reactance produced by a loudspeaker on the child's respiratory system during quiet tidal breathing.[84] A lung function test using rapid thoracoabdominal compression has similar results in infants as produced by voluntary maneuvers performed by adults. These tests require sedation but are well tolerated. If the diagnosis is not clear bronchial provocation testing may be useful.

Laboratory Evaluation

These are not generally needed in the diagnosis of childhood asthma. The presence of eosinophilia in the presence of atopy is supportive, but not necessarily diagnostic, of asthma. Evaluation of immune competence might disclose an immune deficiency. Sweat chloride testing, a biopsy to evaluate ciliary structure, and bronchoscopy are important in diagnosing other diseases. Allergen-specific IgE to mites, tree pollen, grass pollen, or animal dander is uncommon during the first year of life but increases during the preschool years. However, early onset multiple allergen sensitization predicts more severe asthma later in childhood. A total of 60% of children at high risk for development of asthma were sensitized to aeroallergen and/or food allergen by ages 2 and 3 years. The presence of allergen-specific IgE is determined using the radioallergosorbent test (RAST or ImmunoCAP) or skin-prick testing. An elevated FeNO is very helpful in confirming asthma in childhood in the absence of corticosteroid treatment.[85]

Monitoring Asthma

Asthma is a variable condition, and monitoring is required to ensure both current control and reduction in future risk. According to GINA, asthma is controlled if there are no daytime symptoms, no limitations of activities, no nocturnal symptoms or awakenings, no need for reliever medication, normal or near-normal pulmonary function, and no exacerbations (Table 7.5). The goal of therapy is to maintain control with the least amount of medication. Assessment of control is based on the patient's response to treatment (Table 7.6); categories are *well controlled*, *not well controlled*, and *very poorly controlled*. Although high levels of control are possible for most patients with mild to moderate asthma in clinical trials, in "real-world" asthma care, poor control is not uncommon and often not volunteered by patients or fully appreciated by clinicians. Structured proactive care by primary care clinicians, with at least an annual assessment of control and including instruction in self-management, improves asthma outcomes.[86,87]

Since asthma is primarily an inflammatory disorder of the airways, disease activity can be monitored by using

TABLE 7.5   Levels of Asthma Control

A. Assessment of Current Clinical Control (Preferably Over 4 weeks)

Characteristic	Controlled (All of the Following)	Partially Controlled (Any Measure Present)	Uncontrolled
Daytime symptoms	None (twice or less/week)	More than twice/week	Three or more features of partially controlled asthma[a,b]
Limitation of activities	None	Any	
Nocturnal symptoms/awakening	None	Any	
Need for reliever/rescue treatment	None (twice or less/week)	More than twice/week	
Lung function (PEF or FEV$_1$)[c]	Normal	<80% Predicted or personal best (if known)	

B. Assessment of Future Risk (Risk of Exacerbations, Instability, Rapid Decline in Lung Function, Side Effects)

Features that are associated with increased risk of adverse events in the future include poor clinical control, frequent exacerbations in past year,[a] ever admission to critical care for asthma, low FEV$_1$, exposure to cigarette smoke, high-dose medications.

[a]Any exacerbations should prompt review of maintenance treatment to ensure that it is adequate.
[b]By definition, an exacerbation in any week makes that "an uncontrolled asthma" week.
[c]Without administration of bronchodilator. Lung function is not a reliable test for children 5 years and younger.
From Global Initiative for Asthma (GINA), 2012. Available at: <http://www.ginasthma.org/guidelines-gina-report-global-strategy-for-asthma.html>.

TABLE 7.6   Assessment of Asthma Control in Patients 12 Years of Age and Older

Control Category/Component	Asthma Control Classification: Frequency/Nature of Component		
	Well Controlled	Not Well Controlled	Very Poorly Controlled
Impairment			
Symptoms	≤2 day/week	>2 day/week but not daily	Throughout the day
Nighttime awakenings	≤2×/month	3–4×/month	7×/week
Interference with normal activity	None	Minor limitation	Extremely limited
SABA use for symptom control	≤2 day/week	>2 day/week	Several times a day
FEV$_1$ or peak flow	>80% predicted or personal best	60%–80% predicted or personal best	<60% predicted or personal best
Validated Questionnaire Scores			
ATAQ	0	1–2	1–2
ACQ	≤0.75	≥1.5	N/A
ACT	≥20	16–19	≤15
RISK			
Exacerbations requiring oral systemic corticosteroids	0–1/year	≥2/years	
	Consider severity and interval since last exacerbation.		
Progressive loss of function	Evaluation requires long-term follow-up care.		
Treatment-related adverse effects	Medication side effects can range in intensity from none to very troublesome and worrisome. The level of intensity does not correlate with specific levels of control but should be considered in the overall assessment of risk.		
Recommended action for treatment	Maintain current level of step care. Regular follow-up every 1–6 months to maintain control. Consider step-down if asthma is well controlled for at least 3 months.	Step-up 1 step and re-evaluate in 2–6 weeks. For side effects, consider alternative treatment options.	Consider short course of oral systemic corticosteroids. Step-up 1–2 steps and reevaluate in 2 weeks. For side effects, consider alternative treatment options.

ACQ, Asthma Control Questionnaire; ACT, Asthma Control Test; ATAQ, Asthma Treatment Assessment Questionnaire; FEV$_1$, forced expiratory volume in 1 s; FVC, forced vital capacity; N/A, not applicable; SABA, short-acting β_2-agonist.
From National Heart, Lung, and Blood Institute. Expert Panel Report 3 (EPR-3): Guidelines for the Diagnosis and Management of Asthma: Full Report 2007. Available at: <http://www.nhlbi.nih.gov/files/docs/guidelines/asthgdln.pdf>; accessed July 7, 2015.

inflammatory biomarkers such as sputum eosinophils and FeNO. While the former is more difficult to perform in primary care, FeNO is now feasible using the modern smaller measurement devices.

Severity

Asthma severity reflects underlying disease activity, and definition is based on intensity and frequency of symptoms and degree of impairment of pulmonary function.[88] Severity is assessed

BOX 7.7 Domains of Outcomes Used in the Assessment of Asthma Severity and Disease Control

Impairment
- Symptoms
- Night-time awakenings
- Use of short-acting β_2-agonists for symptom control
- Interference with normal activity
- Lung function

Risk
- Exacerbations
- Progressive loss of lung function
- Side effects from medications

From National Heart, Lung, and Blood Institute. Expert Panel Report 3 (EPR-3): Guidelines for the Diagnosis and Management of Asthma: Full Report 2007. Available at: <https://www.ncbi.nlm.nih.gov/books/NBK7232/>; accessed August 30, 2020.

prior to commencing therapy or by the level of medication needed to achieve asthma control. Severity can vary over time, reflecting changes in response to treatment or in the intrinsic nature of the disease.

As referred to earlier, GINA has recently stated that all forms of asthma once diagnosed should be treated with an ICS irrespective of severity.[16] Thus, it is no longer acceptable for milder disease to be treated with intermittent or regular inhaled SABA.[89] Mild persistent asthma is defined as requiring a low dose of ICS to achieve control, moderate asthma as requiring a higher dose of ICS or additional medication, and severe asthma as requiring high ICS doses plus add-on medication with or without oral corticosteroids. Based on two large clinical trials, GINA guidelines now recommend that at step 1, which includes people with asthma who only require their reliever medication twice a month or less, patients use a combined ICS/LABA therapy on an as-needed basis.[90]

Within the scope of asthma severity and control are two major domains: impairment and risk (Box 7.7). *Impairment* refers to the frequency and intensity of current symptoms, based on five factors: daytime symptoms, nighttime awakenings, SABA use for symptom control, interference with activity, and lung function. *Risk* focuses on three elements: exacerbations; progressive loss of lung function; and side effects from medications.

Symptom Control

Validated questionnaires (such as the Asthma Control Questionnaire, ACQ; the Asthma Control Scoring System, ACSS; the Asthma Control Test, ACT; and pediatric equivalents, such as the Pediatric ACT) have been standardized to quantify asthma control.[91] These are preferable to single questions, because they assess overall control of the disease. Cutoff thresholds for "controlled," "partially controlled," and "not controlled" asthma are available for most questionnaires. Uncontrolled patients require an assessment of adherence, inhaler technique, and self-management behavior, but escalation of treatment may be needed. By contrast, for well-controlled patients, it may be possible to reduce the level of treatment.

Exacerbations

Exacerbations are defined by the need for short courses of oral corticosteroids and/or for emergency care. Frequency of oral corticosteroid use, ED visits, hospital admissions, and unscheduled healthcare use should all be recorded.[92] Whenever possible, the frequency, severity, and causes of asthma exacerbations should be documented. Exacerbation occurring in the recent past is a strong predictor of future exacerbations.[93] All patients who have experienced an exacerbation need to have their disease self-management behavior investigated and an updated written self-management plan provided. Poor adherence with ICS medication, overuse of SABA medication (hence the recent GINA recommendation that SABAs should never be used alone), at-risk behaviors such as smoking, and poor inhaler technique may be important and potentially reversible factors increasing exacerbation risk.

Asthma-Related Quality of Life

QoL is a patient-centered dimension of asthma that may not correlate well with current control, pulmonary function or biomarkers, but reflects how the patient experiences asthma in their life. QoL and symptoms are overlapping but discrete domains of asthma control; for instance, it is possible to have low symptoms but impaired QoL, for example, in the case of a patient who avoids physical exercise or sport to prevent exercise-induced asthma symptoms. Validated QoL questionnaires, either "generic," measuring overall health status (e.g., SF36, EQ5D), or "disease-specific," measuring the specific impact of asthma (e.g., Asthma QoL Questionnaire[91]), help to predict healthcare use and future exacerbations and to characterize the impact of disease on the individual. The online versions of the ACQ and AQLQ show high levels of agreement with the paper versions and can therefore be safely used in eHealth applications to respectively monitor asthma control and QoL.[94]

Lung Function

Measures of PEF should be used for monitoring control. PEF should ideally be compared with the patient's best value and can be used for domiciliary monitoring. It is most useful in labile, severe asthma or when patients have difficulties in interpreting their respiratory symptoms (so-called "under-perceivers," who may only become aware of bronchoconstriction when it is advanced). It is also helpful in documenting the effects of therapy or environmental triggers, particularly in the workplace. Such patients can benefit from an asthma action plan based on PEF in addition to or instead of symptoms. Repeated spirometry (e.g., on an annual basis) can demonstrate the development of fixed or deteriorating lung function, which may indicate an asthma-COPD overlap syndrome (ACOS) in smokers[95] or the development of airway remodeling and the possible need for more intensive treatment.

Rescue Medication Use

When asthma is well-controlled, use of short-acting rescue bronchodilators should be occasional or absent. The requirement for rescue medication use on more than 2 days a week is indicative of suboptimal control and the need for a review of maintenance therapy. The frequency of ordering of refill prescriptions for SAB medication is a useful guide to SAB use, which is frequently under-reported by patients. Overuse of SABA medication is associated with increased risk of exacerbation, hospitalization, and mortality; reasons why GINA has made its recent recommendation for using ICS even in those with mild disease.

Adherence With Regular Medication and Inhaler Technique

An important and often neglected aspect of monitoring asthma is an assessment of whether the prescribed medication is being used correctly. Underuse of regular medication, particular with ICS preparations, is very common and is associated with poor control.[96] One-quarter of asthma exacerbations are attributable to ICS medication nonadherence and 60% of asthma-related hospitalisations.[97] The reasons for nonadherence are complex and may be broadly categorized as "non-intentional" and "intentional" nonadherence.[98] In non-intentional nonadherence, the patient forgets to take the medication, is unable to obtain medication, or has poor inhalational technique, resulting in inadequate lung deposition of medication. "Intentional non-adherence" occurs when a patient makes a conscious decision not to use the medication as prescribed, usually affecting ICS medication. This is often due to an under-appreciation of the effectiveness of ICS and over-perception of side-effect risks ("steroid phobia"), and points to the need for improved self-management education.[97] Detection of ICS nonadherence through refill prescription monitoring or other methods, and a following discussion with the patient, has been shown to improve both adherence and asthma outcomes.[99] The need for objective real-time methods of measuring adherence to ICS medication is clear, and going forward, electronic monitoring devices (EMDs) now offer a solution with the potential of becoming the gold standard for asthma care.[100] EMDs together with electronic text messaging (SMS) have been implemented in other chronic disease states such as diabetes and congestive heart failure, with marked success. Benefits of EMDs include the ability to track exact numbers of doses taken without a patient needing to add extra steps to their care plan, to provide new data for clinical decision making, and to increase motivation and engagement by patients.[101]

Personal Asthma Action Plan

According to the 2020 GINA guidance, a partnership between the patient and their health care providers is important for effective asthma management. Training health care providers in communication skills may lead to increased patient satisfaction, better health outcomes, and reduced use of health care resources. A key factor in successful asthma care is effective self-management, and all patients should have asthma education and the provision of a written personal asthma action plan.[102] This should be reviewed and reinforced annually and after any episode of loss of control. Asthma management involves a continuous cycle to assess, adjust treatment, and review response. Any action plan should include instructions on daily management, as well as specific strategies to deal with worsening of asthma symptoms and loss of disease control. A written action plan should be provided (Fig. 7.9). Traditionally, the action plan includes three levels: "I feel good" (green zone); "I do not feel good" (yellow zone); and "I feel awful" (red zone). An action plan includes symptoms and may include lung function, usually with a peak flow meter. It is critical to provide understandable and acceptable instructions on actions to take in the face of a loss of control.

ASTHMA MANAGEMENT

Long-Term Management in Adults

As a long-term variable condition, a key factor is a successful partnership between patient and clinician, involving education in self-management. GINA advocates that patients should be trained in essential skills and guided asthma self-management, including asthma information, inhaler skills, adherence, written asthma action plan, self-monitoring of symptoms and/or PEF, regular medical review. The patient's response should be evaluated whenever treatment is changed. Assess symptom control, exacerbations, side-effects, lung function, and patient (and parent, in the case of children with asthma) satisfaction.

Control of Environmental Factors

It is important to identify environmental factors that may affect asthma control. Allergens can be identified by means of skin or serologic testing, and by correlation of exposure to symptoms. Efforts should be made to reduce exposure to allergens whenever possible, although this can prove difficult. Avoidance of active and passive cigarette smoke exposure should be minimized, as smoking increases asthma severity and reduces response to ICS.[103] Surprisingly, little attention has been given to outdoor and indoor air pollution as a driver of asthma and exacerbations.[104] Avoidance of places where air pollution is known to be high, for example, close to traffic, urban canyons, and poorly ventilated spaces, is advised. Asthmatic patients and their parents can also play a key role in advocating for local clean air strategies and associated interventions.[105]

Comorbidity

Treatment of coexisting conditions, such as chronic rhinosinusitis and nasal polyposis, gastroesophageal reflux, obesity and psychosocial issues, as well as other organ manifestations of atopy, should be addressed. Obesity with increases in body mass index (BMI) have become a significant public health problem and may compromise pulmonary physiology. Obese patients have increased asthma risk while obese asthmatic patients have more symptoms, more frequent and severe exacerbations, reduced response to asthma medications, and decreased QoL.[106] Psychological problems are up to six-times more common in people with asthma than in the general population, and outcomes of all varieties are associated with poor asthma control. The mechanisms underlying this relationship and the effectiveness of psychological interventions are poorly understood. There is a complex and negative effect of psychological factors on QoL in asthma.[107] Psychological factors may affect immunologic pathways, perception of symptoms, and behavior.[108]

My Asthma Action Plan

Patient name: _____

Medical record #: _____

Physician's name: _____   DOB: _____

Physician's phone #: _____   Completed by: _____   Date: _____

Long-Term-Control Medicines	How Much To Take	How Often	Other Instructions
		_____ times per day EVERY DAY!	
		_____ times per day EVERY DAY!	
		_____ times per day EVERY DAY!	
		_____ times per day EVERY DAY!	

Quick-Relief Medicines	How Much To Take	How Often	Other Instructions
		Take ONLY as needed	NOTE: If this medicine is needed frequently, call physician to consider increasing controller medications.

Special instructions when I feel ⬤ *good,* ◯ *not good*, and ⬤ *awful*.

GREEN ZONE

I feel *good.*
(My **peak flow** is in the **GREEN** zone.)

Peak Flow
My Personal Best

Prevent asthma symptoms every day:
☐ Take my long-term-control medicines (above) every day.
☐ Before exercise, take _____ puffs of
_____
☐ Avoid things that make my asthma worse like: _____
_____

YELLOW ZONE

I do *not* feel *good.*
(My **peak flow** is in the **YELLOW** zone.)
My symptoms may include one or more
of the following:
• Wheeze
• Tight chest
• Cough
• Shortness of breath
• Waking up at night with asthma symptoms
• Decreased ability to do usual activities
• _____
• _____

80% Personal Best

CAUTION: I should continue taking my long-term-control asthma medicines every day AND:

☐ Take _____
_____

If I still do not feel good, or my peak flow is not in the *Green Zone* within 1 hour, then I should:

☐ Increase _____
☐ Add _____
☐ Call _____

RED ZONE

I feel *awful* :
(My **peak flow** is in the **RED** zone.)
Warning signs may include one or more
of the following:

• It's getting harder and harder to breathe.

• Unable to sleep or do usual activities because of trouble breathing.

50% Personal Best

Liters/Min.
Peak Flow Meter

MEDICAL ALERT! Get help!

☐ Take _____
  until I get help immediately!
☐ Take _____
☐ Call _____

DANGER!
Get help immediately!

Call 9-1-1 if you have trouble walking or talking due to shortness of breath or lips or fingernails are gray or blue.

Source: Adapted and reprinted with permission from the Regional Asthma Management and Prevention (RAMP) initiative, a program of the Public Health Institute. http://www.calasthma.org/uploads/resources/actionplanpdf.pdf. San Francisco Bay Area Regional Asthma Management Plan.

Fig. 7.9 Sample asthma action plan—adult, as presented in the Expert Panel Report 3 (EPR-3). (From National Heart, Lung, and Blood Institute. Expert Panel Report 3 (EPR-3): Guidelines for the Diagnosis and Management of Asthma: Full Report 2007. Available at: <https://www.ncbi.nlm.nih.gov/books/NBK7232/>; accessed August 30, 2020.)

Breathing control exercises, encouraging slow steady nasal diaphragmatic breathing, and discouraging hyperventilation, may be helpful as adjuvant treatment in patients with symptoms and QoL impairment, to complement standard pharmacotherapy.[109]

Pharmacologic Treatment in Adults

Medications used in asthma treatment are categorized as *quick-relief* and *long-term control* (Box 7.8). Quick-relief drugs (e.g., SABAs) act to rapidly reduce airflow obstruction, and

BOX 7.8 Classification of Asthma Treatment Medications

Quick-Relief Medications
- Short-acting β₂-agonists
- Anticholinergics
- Systemic corticosteroids

Long-Term Controllers
- Corticosteroids—inhaled and systemic
- Long-acting β₂-agonists
- Leukotriene receptor antagonists
- Cromolyn/nedocromil
- Anticholinergics
- Biologics: Omalizumab, mepolizumab, reslizumab, benralizumab, and dupilumab

TABLE 7.7 Estimated Comparative Daily Dosages for Inhaled Corticosteroids for Older Children[a] and Adults With Asthma

Drug	Low Daily Dose, Adult	Medium Daily Dose, Adult	High Daily Dose, Adult
Beclomethasone HFA 40 or 80 μg/puff	80–240 μg	241–480 μg	>480 μg
Ciclesonide MDI 80 μg/ puff, 160 μg/puff	80–240 μg	241–320 μg	>320 μg
Budesonide DPI 90, 180, or 200 μg/inhalation	180–600 μg	601–1200 μg	>1200 μg
Flunisolide 250 μg/puff	500–1000 μg	1001–2000 μg	>2000 μg
Flunisolide HFA 80 μg/ puff	320 μg	321–640 μg	>640 μg
Fluticasone			
HFA/MDI: 44, 110, or 220 μg/puff	88–264 μg	265–440 μg	>440 μg
DPI: 50, 100, or 250 μg/inhalation	100–300 μg	301–500 μg	>500 μg
Mometasone DPI 200 μg/inhalation	200 μg	400 μg	>400 μg
Triamcinolone acetonide 75 μg/puff	300–750 μg	751–1000 μg	>1500 μg

[a]12 Years of age and older.
DPI, Dry powder inhaler; *HFA,* hydrofluoroalkane; *MDI,* metered-dose inhaler.
From National Heart, Lung, and Blood Institute. Expert Panel Report 3 (EPR-3): Guidelines for the Diagnosis and Management of Asthma: Full Report 2007. Available at: <http://www.nhlbi.nih.gov/files/docs/guidelines/asthgdln.pdf>; accessed July 7, 2015.

long-term control medications (e.g., corticosteroids) reduce airway inflammation and its consequences.

Quick-Relief Medications

Short-Acting β₂-Agonists. The SABAs, albuterol (salbutamol), levalbuterol, terbutaline, and pirbuterol, are effective inhaled bronchodilators and the agents of choice for the acute relief of symptoms. However, contrary to the way these drugs have been used in the past, they should now never be used in isolation but in the presence of ICS irrespective of asthma severity to reduce their risk of serious exacerbations and to control symptoms.

Anticholinergics. Ipratropium bromide is a muscarinic cholinergic antagonist and is used in asthma, primarily in patients who either are intolerant of β₂-agonists or are experiencing limited benefit from SABA use.[110] Tiotropium is a long-acting anticholinergic agent used in COPD, but data are emerging for its use in asthma. Evidence from Phase III trials in the adult and pediatric population has shown that tiotropium is well tolerated and improves a range of endpoints as an add-on treatment to ICS therapy, regardless of asthma characteristics and clinical phenotypes.[111]

Long-Term Control Medications

Medications for long-term control are used on a daily basis to control airway inflammation.

Corticosteroids. Corticosteroids are the primary antiinflammatory medication used in long-term control of asthma. They improve both impairment and risk but do not have disease-modifying activities, and effects recede once discontinued.[112] Their antiinflammatory actions are broad-based and affect lymphocyte function, principally helper T cell Type 2 (Th2) generation, and inflammatory cell migration and activation.

ICSs have minimal long-term side effects in low to moderate doses. Multiple formulations are available; these may be used in low, medium, or high doses, depending on underlying severity (Table 7.7). Oral corticosteroids are used in short-term bursts for acute exacerbations, but their regular use causes potentially serious systemic side-effects.

Leukotriene Modifiers. Leukotriene modifiers interfere with the leukotriene pathway, and included LTRAs montelukast and zafirlukast. Leukotriene modifiers, such as montelukast, are used in combination with ICS in more severe asthma. However, it has been reported that montelukast rarely causes serious psychiatric side effects and as a consequence, the United States Food and Drug Administration (FDA) has strengthened its warning about mental health side effects linked to montelukast.[113]

Long-Acting β₂-Agonists. LABAs—salmeterol and formoterol (Table 7.8)—are inhaled bronchodilators that improve airflow for at least 12 hours. They must not be used alone in asthma for safety reasons, but given in combination with an ICS (e.g., fluticasone-salmeterol [Advair]; budesonide-formoterol [Symbicort]; and mometasone-formoterol [Dulera]) (Table 7.9). Combination ICS-LABA medications are available in low, medium, and high doses, based on ICS dose and lead to greater control of impairment and exacerbations.[114] Indacaterol is an ultra-LABA with 24-hour duration of bronchodilation. Indacaterol inhalation is for use only in people with COPD and should not be used to treat asthma.

Biologics. The first biologic used to treat allergic-type asthma is directed towards blocking the effects of IgE (omalizumab, Xolair) by interfering with IgE binding to its high-affinity receptor on mast cells and other inflammatory cells and leading to loss of this receptor. It is given by subcutaneous injection in accordance with body weight. Omalizumab is recommended

TABLE 7.8 Usual Dosages of Long-Acting β₂-Agonists (LABAs) for Older Children[a] and Adults With Asthma

Medication	Formulation	Dose	Comments
			Inhaled LABAs should not be used alone for symptom relief or exacerbations. Use with ICS.
Salmeterol	DPI 50 µg/blister	1 Blister q12h	Decreased duration of protection against EIB may occur with regular use.
Formoterol	DPI 12 µg/single-use capsule	1 Capsule q12h	Each capsule is for single use only; additional doses should not be administered for at least 12 h. Capsules should be used only with the Aerolizer inhaler and should not be taken orally.

DPI, Dry powder inhaler; *EIB*, exercise-induced bronchospasm; *ICS*, inhaled corticosteroid; *LABA*, long-acting β₂-agonists.
[a]12 Years of age and older.
Modified from National Heart, Lung, and Blood Institute. Expert Panel Report 3 (EPR-3): Guidelines for the Diagnosis and Management of Asthma: Full Report 2007. Available at: <http://www.nhlbi.nih.gov/files/docs/guidelines/asthgdln.pdf>; accessed July 7, 2015.

TABLE 7.9 Usual Dosages for ICS-LABA Treatment for Older Children[a] and Adults With Asthma

Combination Agent	Formulation	Dose	Comments
Fluticasone–salmeterol (Advair)	DPI 100 µg/50 µg, 250 µg/50 µg, or 500 µg/50 µg	1 inhalation BID; dose depends on severity of asthma	*100/50 DPI or 45/21 HFA*: for patient whose asthma is not controlled on low- to medium-dose ICS
	HFA 45 µg/21 µg, 115 µg/21 µg, or 230 µg/21 µg		*250/50 DPI or 115/21 HFA*: for patients whose asthma is not controlled on medium- to high-dose ICS
Budesonide–formoterol (Symbicort)	HFA, MDI 80 µg/4.5 µg, 160 µg/4.5 µg	2 inhalations BID; dose depends on severity of asthma	*80/4.5*: for patients whose asthma is not controlled on low- to medium-dose ICS *160/4.5*: for patients whose asthma is not controlled on medium- to high-dose ICS
Mometasone–formoterol (Dulera)	HFA, MDI 50 µg/5 µg, 100 µg/5 µg, or 200 µg/5 µg,	2 inhalations BID; dose depends on the severity of asthma	*50/5*: for patients whose asthma is not controlled on low-dose ICS *100/5*: for patients whose asthma is not controlled on medium-dose ICS *200/5*: for patients whose asthma is not controlled on high-dose ICS

DPI, Dry powder inhaler; *HFA*, hydrofluoroalkane; *ICS-LABA*, combination inhaled corticosteroid and long-acting β₂-agonist; *MDI*, metered-dose inhaler.
[a]12 Years of age and older.
From National Heart, Lung, and Blood Institute. Expert Panel Report 3 (EPR-3): Guidelines for the Diagnosis and Management of Asthma–Full Report 2007. Available at: <http://www.nhlbi.nih.gov/files/docs/guidelines/asthgdln.pdf>; accessed July 7, 2015.

for patients with severe asthma by GINA at Step 5, in those with poor control, raised IgE, and evidence of allergen-specific IgE.

The recent understanding of the Type 2 inflammatory pathways involved in asthma has opened up a search for novel agents that block components of this using monoclonal antibodies. Beyond IgE, two pathways have emerged as prime targets—IL-5 and its receptor (IL5r) involved in eosinophil recruitment and activation in the airways and IL-4 and IL-13 that are variably involved in the allergic cascade (involving T helper Type 2 lymphocytes) and the non-allergic (involving Type 2 innate lymphocytes) that also involve eosinophil recruitment (reviewed in Ref. 115).

As described by the AAAAI, in addition to omalizumab there are four new biologics for the treatment of severe Type 2 asthma—mepolizumab, reslizumab, benralizumab, and dupilumab—with several others currently in development. Mepolizumab, reslizumab, and benralizumab all target the IL-5

pathway to reduce the number and/or inflammatory effects of eosinophils. Dupilumab targets a receptor for two molecules IL-4 and IL-13 that drive allergic inflammation.[116] Although some differences exist between countries, in the US, omalizumab is approved for patients as young as 6 years old, while all the other biologics with the exception of reslizumab (approved for adults 18 and over) are approved for patients as young as 12 years old. Overall, studies have shown biologics to be very safe mainly because they are human(ized) proteins and are highly targeted, so that any adverse reactions are likely to be linked to their primary molecular mechanistic target. There are currently no set recommendations on how long a patient should be treated with a biologic. Guidelines recommend trialing the medication for at least four months and assess progress at intervals. In the case of omalizumab and mepolizumab, there is now a need to see if any of these antibody treatments induce long-term remission if treatment discontinued, as occurs with biologics used in early rheumatoid arthritis.[117] When compared to other controller medications for asthma biologics are expensive and therefore each country has developed specific clinical criteria for their indication and reimbursement.[118]

Methylxanthines. Sustained-release theophylline has modest bronchodilator activity, and its use in asthma is limited by its toxicity and modest efficacy and the need for monitoring of serum theophylline levels (reviewed in Ref. 119).

Cromolyn Sodium and Nedocromil Sodium. Cromolyn sodium and nedocromil sodium interfere with mast cell activation mechanisms to reduce inflammatory mediator release. Although these compounds are extremely safe, their use in patients older than 12 years of age is limited, and in some countries their availability is now limited (reviewed in Ref. 119). In the US, neither cromolyn nor nedocromil is available in HFA-containing MDIs, and no formulation of nedocromil is marketed for asthma. As a result, the only remaining formulations for asthma are solutions of cromolyn (10 mg/mL) for nebulization. However, dry-powder inhaler formulations for cromolyn and nedocromil are still available in other countries.

Step Care Approach to Asthma Management

Guidelines recommend that therapy be tailored to needs, circumstances, and responsiveness of the individual patient. The step care approach to asthma (Fig. 7.10) is based on the premise that increasing severity is most effectively controlled by greater amounts of medication, particularly of antiinflammatory agents.

Intermittent Asthma

Step 1 Care. Intermittent asthma characterized by symptoms on less than 3 days per week; night-time awakenings less than twice per month; use of SABA no more than 2 days per week; normal activity; normal lung function; exacerbation frequency of 0 to 1 per year (Table 7.10).

Until recently, SABAs have been recommended as effective in relieving symptoms and normalizing pulmonary function in mild asthma. Previous versions of GINA suggested that mild asthma in adults can be well managed with either reliever medications, for example, SABA alone or with the additional use of regular low-dose ICS. Given the low frequency or perceived non-bothersome nature of symptoms in mild asthma, patients' adherence towards their controller medications, especially to ICS is usually not satisfactory. Such patients often rely on SABA alone to relieve symptoms, which contributes to SABA overreliance with poor asthma outcomes especially exacerbations and even deaths. The new GINA 2020 asthma treatment recommendations[16] describe a significant change in asthma management at Steps 1 and 2 of the five treatment steps. The report acknowledges the mounting evidence showing safety problems with SABAs overuse in the absence of concomitant controller

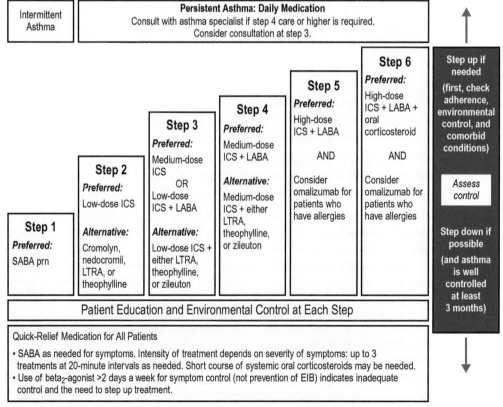

Fig. 7.10 Step-care approach to asthma treatment according to disease severity, as presented in the Expert Panel Report 3 (EPR-3). *EIB,* Exercise-induced bronchospasm; *ICS,* inhaled corticosteroid; *LABA,* long-acting β-agonist; *LTRA,* leukotriene receptor antagonist; *SABA,* short-acting β₂-agonist. (From National Heart, Lung, and Blood Institute. Expert Panel Report 3 (EPR-3): Guidelines for the Diagnosis and Management of Asthma: Full Report 2007. Available at: <https://www.ncbi.nlm.nih.gov/books/NBK7232/>; accessed August 30, 2020.)

TABLE 7.10 Assessment of Asthma Severity in Patients 12 Years of Age and Older

Severity Category/Component	Asthma Severity Classification: Frequency/Nature of Component			
	Intermittent	Persistent		
		Mild	Moderate	Severe
Impairment				
Symptoms	≤2 day/week	>2 day/week but not daily	Daily	Throughout the day
Night-time awakenings	≤2×/month	3–4×/month	>1×/week but not nightly	7×/week
SABA use for symptom control	≤2 day/week	>2 day/week but not >1×/day	Daily	Several times a day
Interference with normal activity	None	Minor limitation	Some limitation	Extremely limited
Lung function *Normal FEV$_1$/FVC:* 8–19 years: 85% 20–39 years: 80% 40–59 years: 75% 60–80 years: 70%	Normal FEV$_1$ between exacerbations FEV$_1$ >80% predicted FEV$_1$/FVC normal	FEV$_1$ ≥80% predicted FEV$_1$/FVC normal	FEV$_1$ >60% but <80% predicted FEV$_1$/FVC reduced 5%	FEV$_1$ <60% predicted FEV$_1$/FVC reduced >5%
Risk				
Exacerbations requiring oral systemic corticosteroids	0–1/year	≥2/years		
	Consider severity and interval since last exacerbation. Frequency and severity may fluctuate over time for patients in any severity category. Relative annual risk of exacerbations may be related to FEV$_1$			
Recommended step for initiating treatment	Step 1	Step 2	Step 3	Step 5
				Consider short course of oral corticosteroids.
	In 2–6 weeks, evaluate level of control that is achieved and adjust therapy accordingly.			

FEV$_1$, Forced expiratory volume in 1 s; FVC, forced vital capacity; SABA, short-acting β$_2$-agonist.
From National Heart, Lung, and Blood Institute. Expert Panel Report 3 (EPR-3): Guidelines for the Diagnosis and Management of Asthma–Full Report 2007. Available at: <http://www.nhlbi.nih.gov/files/docs/guidelines/asthgdln.pdf>; accessed July 7, 2015.

medication and does not support SABA-only therapy in mild asthma and has included new off-label recommendations such as symptom-driven (as-needed) low-dose ICS-formoterol combination or low-dose ICS taken whenever SABA is taken. The SYGMA 1 and 2 trials compared as-needed versus maintenance regimens for the budesonide-formoterol combination indicated that as-needed budesonide–formoterol combinations provided a similar effect on annual rate of exacerbation reduction and overall, in a lower exposure to ICSs compared to a maintenance ICS regimen although budesonide–formoterol used as needed was inferior in terms of conferring ongoing asthma control (i.e., proportion of weeks with good asthma control).[120]

Persistent Asthma (see Fig. 7.10)

Step 2 Care: Mild Persistent Asthma. Mild persistent asthma characterized by symptoms less than 3 days per week, nighttime awakenings three to four times per month, use of SABA on less than 3 days per week, no activity limitation, normal lung function between exacerbations (FEV$_1$ of 80%; 0 to 1 exacerbation in the preceding year (see Table 7.10).

Low-dose daily ICS (see Table 7.7) is by far the preferred treatment, resulting in fewer symptoms, a decreased exacerbation risk, and improved lung function.[121] For patients requiring Step 2 treatment, GINA 2020 recommends controller treatment

as daily low-dose ICS with as needed SABA. This is based on evidence that regular low-dose ICS use substantially reduces asthma symptoms, increases lung function, improves QoL, and reduces risks of severe exacerbations,

LTRAs relieve symptoms and improve lung function but are less effective than ICSs[122] as first-line treatment but may be an option in nonadherent patients.[123] Theophylline has limited antiinflammatory effects and a narrow therapeutic profile and is no longer recommended.

Step 3 Care: Moderate Persistent Asthma. As described previously, for most adults or adolescents with asthma, treatment can be started with either regular daily low-dose ICS or as-needed low-dose ICS-formoterol (or, if not available, low-dose ICS whenever SABA is taken). If, at initial presentation, the patient has troublesome asthma symptoms on most days or is waking from asthma once or more a week, according to GINA 2020, starting at Step 3 involves daily low-dose ICS with the addition of a LABA separately or as combination therapy.

Moderate persistent asthma is characterized by daily symptoms, night time awakening more than once per week, need for daily SABA use, limitation in daily activity, and compromises in lung function (FEV1 >60% but <80%) and an average of two exacerbations in the previous year (see Table 7.10). Guidelines combination therapy with low-dose ICS and an LABA (see

Table 7.9). The observation that the addition of LABA to low-dose ICS had greater efficacy than doubling the dose of ICS has been substantiated by many subsequent studies.[124] Effects include improvement in lung function, symptoms, exacerbations, and a lessened need for SABA. Evidence also supports increasing the dose of ICS to achieve improved lung function, symptoms and exacerbations. However, GINA Step 3 recommends low-dose ICS plus LABA as the preferred treatment. Both options improve control, but the addition of LABA has been consistently found to be superior and is the preferable treatment. In observational data,[125] LABA addition proved superior in symptom control, but an increase in ICS dose more effective in reducing exacerbations, plausibly explained by improved inflammation control translating into fewer exacerbations.

There have been concerns over life-threatening events, including death, associated with LABA use following the Salmeterol Multicenter Asthma Research Trial (SMART) study, a randomized controlled trial involving 26,355 asthma subjects randomized to receive salmeterol alone or albuterol, along with ICS; among patients in the salmeterol treatment group, an increased incidence in life-threatening events and respiratory-related or asthma-related deaths was noted.[126] A metaanalysis performed by the US FDA also found an added risk with LABA use.[127] As a result, the FDA issued an advisory statement and a "black box" warning label to all LABA inhalers, advising that LABAs should never be used as monotherapy. The FDA further recommended that once control is achieved, step-down should be considered, with discontinuation of LABA therapy if possible.[128] However, the increased risks were mostly noted when LABAs were used as monotherapy.

GINA also recommends that the combination therapy of budesonide and formoterol can be used for both maintenance and rescue treatment in a "single maintenance and reliever therapy" (SMART) regimen. This involves regular once or twice daily combination inhaler use, with additional inhalations for relief of symptoms. Although not approved by the US FDA, the SMART regimen has been shown to reduce exacerbations, and is used in other parts of the world.

Acceptable, nonpreferred alternatives for add-on therapy include a LTRA, but theophylline is no longer recommended. In one study, the addition of LTRA to ICS was found to be equivalent to doubling ICS.[129] However, a systematic review of studies comparing the add-on of a LABA with ICS and of LTRA with ICS found superiority with the LABA-ICS combination.[130]

Steps 4 and 5 Care: Severe Persistent Asthma.

Patients at Steps 4 and 5 care have severe persistent asthma (see Fig. 7.10). Their impairment includes symptoms throughout the day, sleep disturbance, need for frequent daily SABA, activity limitations, and compromised lung function (FEV_1 <60% predicted). These patients also have frequent exacerbations.

Guidelines now recommend medium-dose ICS in combination with LABA, especially in those with exacerbations, ED visits, or hospitalizations. Nonpreferred options include add-on therapy with LTRA or inhaled ipratropium. Control achieved in patients at Steps 4 and 5 care is often worse than in milder disease. At high ICS doses, adrenal function is suppressed and cataracts or osteoporosis develops in some patients, although risks are far less than continuous use of oral or injected corticosteroids.

Step 5 Care in Severe Persistent Asthma.

For patients at Step 5, it is recommended to advance the ICS dose to higher doses (see Table 7.9), although evidence for added effectiveness is limited.[131] In the past, it is this group of patients who are at the greatest risk of corticosteroid side effects especially if receiving continuous or frequent oral/systemic corticosteroids to manage their disease at the lowest possible dose, with monitoring for adverse effects, while attempting to reduce dose once control is achieved.

This group of patients also contain a proportion who are refractory to corticosteroids.[132] In this subgroup, associations have been revealed between specific respiratory infections and steroid-resistance in adults. A stratified medicine approach has enabled the identification of new therapies using macrolides, as well as several novel disease mechanisms creating the potential of new therapeutic targets.[133]

However, it is in the severe persistent asthma subpopulation that the new generation of biologics targeting IgE, IL-5, and the IL-4/ IL-13 signaling pathways is revolutionizing (Figs. 7.1 and 7.11). While such treatments are initiated by asthma/allergy specialists, the choice of a particular monoclonal antibody for any particular patient is still evolving. Respiratory experts recognize the role of phenotypes, biomarkers, and treatable traits in guiding treatment decisions and patient identification. The majority of experts stated that they use two to three biomarkers routinely in their clinical practice; blood eosinophils and FeNO were identified as the most practical for the diagnosis and management of severe asthma and that a combination of these two biomarkers provides the best overall assessment of Type 2 airway inflammation.[134] A precision medicine approach driven by treatable traits may be the new standard approach for treating asthma in the near future.[133] In the case of severe Type 2 asthma, the use of anti-IgE, -Il-5/IL5Receptor, and IL-4Receptor/Il-13Receptor has the distinct advantage of enabling oral corticosteroid reduction and, in some cases, treating other organ manifestations of Type 2 inflammatory disease (e.g., dupilumab in severe AD, omalizumab in urticaria, and mepolizumab in eosinophilic gastroesophagitis).[135] Of the currently available monoclonal antibodies omalizumab (anti-IgE); mepolizumab, reslizumab and benralizumab (anti-IL-5 pathways), and dupilumab (anti-IL-4/IL-13), choosing one over the other is proving difficult since head-to head comparisons have not been undertaken.

As William Busse recently stated[136] "the primary, and important benefit, of biologics in severe asthma has been an achievement of disease control, reflected by a significant reduction in exacerbations. The implementation of biologics in asthma treatment marks a new era in asthma treatment and provides effective options where nothing was previously available. The next steps with biologics will be to determine their efficacy in moderate disease, and eventually when safety issues are established, to determine disease modification or possibly asthma prevention."

Bronchial Thermoplasty.

In 2010, bronchial thermoplasty was approved. The aim of bronchial thermoplasty for severe asthma is to reduce the smooth muscle mass and nerves lining

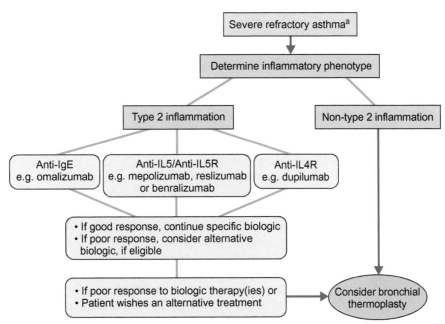

Fig. 7.11 Algorithm to guide the selection of patients with severe refractory asthma for treatment with biologics and bronchial thermoplasty. Note: Biologics and bronchial thermoplasty are treatment options for patients with severe asthma (Step 5) who have uncontrolled asthma despite high-dose ICS plus long-acting β2-agonist and the long-acting muscarinic antagonist tiotropium and after assessment and management of causes of difficult-to-control asthma, such as nonadherence, poor inhaler technique, comorbidities, under treatment, and other behavioral factors. *ICS*, Inhaled corticosteroid; *LABA*, long-acting β₂-agonist; *LTRA*, leukotriene receptor antagonist; *SABA*, short-acting β-agonist. (Reproduced with permission from Thomson NC. Recent developments in bronchial thermoplasty for severe asthma. J Asthma Allergy 2019;12:375–387.)

the airways, thereby reducing bronchospasm. The procedure requires sedation or general anesthesia. A catheter is introduced into the bronchial tree and short pulses of radiofrequency energy are applied circumferentially to sequential portions of the airway wall (transiently heating them to 65 °C) and moving from the distal to the proximal bronchi. The procedure is usually undertaken in specialist centers on three separate occasions one month apart with an interval of at least 3 weeks between each treatment. Bronchial thermoplasty modestly improves clinical outcomes in severe asthma such as asthma QoL and risk of exacerbations. Its clinical indication is in **non-Th2** asthma especially paucigranulocytic subtype[137] (Fig. 7.11). Follow-up studies provide reassurance on the long-term safety of the procedure. However, uncertainties remain about predictors of response, mechanism(s) of action, and place in management of severe asthma.[137]

Step-up and Step-down Considerations. After initiation or adjustment, follow-up evaluation should occur in 2 to 6 weeks. If asthma remains uncontrolled, advancement to the next step is indicated—or a course of oral corticosteroids initiated to achieve control. According to GINA (2020), sustained step-up for at least 2 to 3 months is indicated when symptoms and/or exacerbations persist despite 2 to 3 months of controller treatment. Before deciding to increase medication, the following should be assessed: incorrect inhaler technique, poor adherence, modifiable risk factors, for example, smoking, symptoms due to comorbid conditions, for example, allergic rhinitis.

If controlled for 3 months, stepping down treatment should be considered to find the lowest therapeutic regimen controlling both symptoms and exacerbations and minimizing side-effects.

After selecting an appropriate time for step-down, risk factors, including history of previous exacerbations or ED visit, and low lung function, should be assessed and baseline symptom control and lung function recorded followed by a written asthma action plan, close monitoring, and a follow-up visit arranged.[16] Step-down aims to reduce ICS dosing by 25% to 50% at 2- to 3-month intervals. If asthma is well-controlled on low-dose ICS or LTRA, as-needed low-dose ICS-formoterol is a step-down option. Low-dose ICS taken whenever a SABA is taken (with combination or separate inhalers) is more effective as a stepdown strategy than SABA alone and in adults or adolescents with asthma, ICS should not be stopped unless this is needed temporarily to confirm the diagnosis of asthma. A follow-up appointment to review progress is important.

Immunotherapy

Allergen immunotherapy (AIT) is the only treatment modality that is able to change the natural history of allergic disease by inducing allergen-specific immunological tolerance and is therefore a therapeutic option for selected patients whose asthma has a strong allergic basis.[138] There is increasing evidence of the clinical efficacy of AIT in the treatment of allergic asthma.[139] The GINA guidelines on the management of asthma have recently been updated to include AIT as an additional option for the treatment of asthma.[140] Unfortunately, most published reports of AIT in asthma comprised secondary outcomes in patients with allergic rhinitis. A recent "real-world" asthma trial in South Korea[141] in which subcutaneous AIT was used has shown that, irrespective of the type of allergen, AIT had a significant ICS-sparing effect and reduced acute exacerbation in patients with allergic asthma.

There continues to be uncertainty over the role of sublingual AIT. Guidelines suggest it could be used as add on therapy when the asthma is known to be driven strongly by a single allergen such as house dust mite or grass pollen. A recent systematic review, involving 54 randomized controlled trials (RCTs) on efficacy: 31 SCIT, 18 SLIT, and 5 on SCIT versus SLIT, concluded that "overall, SLIT and SCIT were beneficial for the majority of asthma-related outcomes assessed. Local and systemic allergic reactions were common but infrequently required changes in treatment. Life-threatening events (such as anaphylaxis) were reported rarely."[142] However, most studies were conducted in mild asthma in which allergic rhinitis was the major target. What is needed are more studies in patients with severe persistent allergic asthma rather than mild disease. However, in children SLIT does seem to produce clear benefits especially in preventing the onset of the "allergic march" across childhood towards asthma.[143]

Vaccination. It is advised that people with moderate or severe asthma should receive an annual influenza vaccine.[144] Inactivated influenza vaccines are associated with fewer side effects and are safer to administer to adults and to children over the age of 3 years, including those with "difficult to control" asthma. People with asthma should receive other vaccinations according to the local schedules and recommendations unless there are specific contraindications.

Food Allergy and Anaphylaxis. Food allergy is uncommon as an exacerbating factor in asthma, occurring primarily in children and young people.[145] Food avoidance should not be recommended until allergy has been clearly demonstrated that may include an oral challenge. Acute bronchoconstriction is a frequent clinical manifestation of food-induced anaphylaxis in those in whom asthma has not been diagnosed as well as those with known asthma. Anaphylaxis is a life-threatening condition that can both mimic and complicate severe asthma and can occur in any situation in which medication or biological substances are given, particularly by injection. The symptoms include flushing, pruritus, urticaria, angioedema, dyspnea, stridor, wheezing, gastrointestinal symptoms, and hypotension. Prompt treatment is vital and includes injected epinephrine and antihistamines followed by systemic corticosteroids, with bronchodilators oxygen and circulatory support if required.[146] Everyone experiencing anaphylaxis should undergo a full specialist assessment to identify triggers and instigate avoidance measures and training in self-administration of emergency treatment with preloaded epinephrine syringes.

Separate from IgE-triggered food allergy, food additives and preservatives (such as sulfites, tartrazine and monosodium glutamate) may occasionally cause worsening of asthma, but confirmation requires referral and blinded oral challenges.

Asthma Management in Infants and Children

Uncontrolled pediatric asthma is accompanied by increased exacerbation rate, impaired QoL, and persisting airflow obstruction. Current clinical practice guidelines do not always adequately address pediatric asthma as a result of the limited availability of clinical efficacy and safety data in younger patients and the practice of extrapolating adult recommendations to children. The direct application of the GINA or other definitions of asthma to pediatric patients is problematic, especially in patients <6 years of age. Wheeze, a characteristic of pediatric asthma, is a symptom of other lung conditions not infrequently misdiagnosed as asthma and leading to the inappropriate prescription of ICS. Furthermore, the relationship between preschool wheeze and asthma remains debatable. Outside of an acute exacerbation setting, a 12% improvement in FEV_1 can be difficult to demonstrate in children with asthma, because FEV_1 levels are mostly in the normal range. Under this constraint, the diagnosis of asthma is most often based on clinical criteria.

As with adults, the goals of asthma in children are adequate symptom control and reduced risks of exacerbations. Natural history modification and possible disease prevention are also of high importance in children, but there remains much debate about what interventions are required to achieve this.[147] Once attention has been made to environmental triggers,[148] achieving asthma control requires pharmacological intervention, including the use of controller medication, rescue medication, and add-on therapy, in the case of severe asthma.

As with adults, there are four categories of asthma severity: intermittent, mild persistent, moderate persistent, and severe persistent. Control level is used to adjust therapy by category: well-controlled, not well-controlled, and poorly controlled. Severity and control are evaluated as *impairment* (current asthma symptoms and pulmonary function) and *risk* (exacerbations and side to effects). A stepwise approach is recommended in three age ranges: 0 to 4 years (infants and young children), 5 to 11 years, and 12 years of age and older (Figs. 7.12–7.14, respectively).

As with adults, *long-term control medications* are taken daily to achieve and maintain control, and *quick-relief, rescue* or *reliever medications* produce rapid reversal of acute airflow obstruction. Therapy should be maintained for 3 to 6 months if stable, after which "step-down" is considered. Unfortunately, robust data to help guide step-down are lacking. Giving daily long-term controller therapy only during specific exposures or seasons can also be considered. For example, in children who experience episodes related to viral infections, stepping up therapy at high-risk times of the year (school attendance) or social situations (day-care settings) may be appropriate. Patient education and environmental control should be discussed at every step.

Nonpharmacologic Management in Children
Environmental Control

Aeroallergen sensitization is associated with risk of developing asthma. Dust mite exposure in older children correlates with wheezing and BHR.[149] Pet dander exposure can occur without the presence of an animal in the home and may trigger worsening asthma in sensitized children.[150] Reduction of house-dust mite exposure may decrease symptoms and BHR in sensitized children, although can be hard to achieve in practice.[149] Children with persistent asthma should be evaluated by history for seasonal fluctuations with substantiation by allergy skin testing or

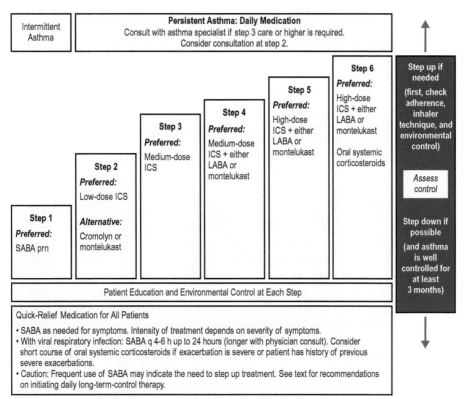

Fig. 7.12 Stepwise approach to therapy in children 0 to 4 years of age, as presented in the Expert Panel Report 3 (EPR-3). *ICS,* Inhaled corticosteroid; *LABA,* long-acting β₂-agonist; *SABA,* short-acting β-agonist. (From National Heart, Lung, and Blood Institute. Expert Panel Report 3 (EPR-3): Guidelines for the Diagnosis and Management of Asthma: Full Report 2007. Available at: <https://www.ncbi.nlm.nih.gov/books/NBK7232/>; accessed August 30, 2020.)

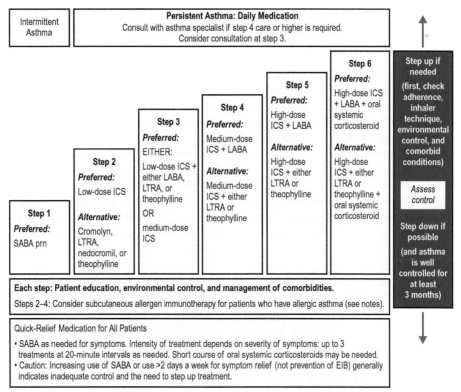

Fig. 7.13 Stepwise approach to therapy in children 5 to 11 years of age, as presented in the Expert Panel Report 3 (EPR-3). *EIB,* Exercise-induced bronchospasm; *ICS,* inhaled corticosteroid; *LABA,* long-acting β₂-agonist; *LTRA,* leukotriene receptor antagonist; *SABA,* short-acting β-agonist. (From National Heart, Lung, and Blood Institute. Expert Panel Report 3 (EPR-3): Guidelines for the Diagnosis and Management of Asthma: Full Report 2007. Available at: <https://www.ncbi.nlm.nih.gov/books/NBK7232/>; accessed August 30, 2020.)

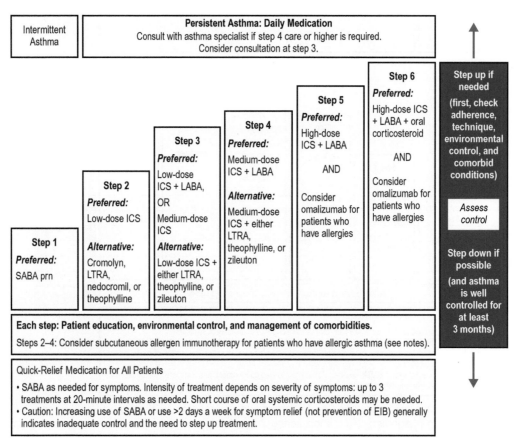

Fig. 7.14 Step-wise approach to therapy in patients 12 years of age and older, as presented in the Expert Panel Report 3 (EPR-3). *EIB*, Exercise-induced bronchospasm; *ICS*, inhaled corticosteroid; *LABA*, long-acting β₂-agonist; *LTRA*, leukotriene receptor antagonist; *SABA*, short-acting β-agonist. (From National Heart, Lung, and Blood Institute. Expert Panel Report 3 (EPR-3): Guidelines for the Diagnosis and Management of Asthma: Full Report 2007. Available at: <https://www.ncbi.nlm.nih.gov/books/NBK7232/>; accessed August 30, 2020.)

specific IgE antibodies. Passive smoke exposure adversely influences asthma in many ways, yet many parents and caregivers continue to smoke. The indoor environment, where allergen and chemical pollutant levels can be high and where moisture (damp) and temperature play adjunctive roles, is an import place to encourage environmental interventions.[151,152]

Psychosocial Factors

Observational studies have identified an association between stress and depression and poorly controlled asthma. Stress is also associated with an increased prevalence[153] and risk of exacerbations in children with negative life events.[154] Emotions can influence airway function, interpretation of symptoms, and the ability to react appropriately to them. Conversely, asthma may influence psychosocial adaptations in the home and at school. Even maternal stress can increase the chance of offspring developing asthma.[155] Asthmatic children have significantly more anxiety disorders, lower self-esteem, greater functional impairment, greater school problems, psychiatric illnesses, and intrafamily stress. Psychosocial factors such as conflict between family and the medical staff, inappropriate self-care, depressive symptoms, behavioral problems, and disregard of symptoms may occur.[156] Parental mental status is a predictor of asthma morbidity, hospitalization, and poor adherence to therapy.

Asthma Education

Education of children with asthma and their caregivers on skills of self-assessment, use of medications, and actions to prevent or control exacerbations is associated with reduction in urgent care visits and hospitalizations, reduction in school absences, and improvement in health status (Fig. 7.15).[157]

Pharmacologic Therapy in Children

Inhaled Corticosteroids. As for adults, the mainstay controller medication in pediatric asthma is an ICS to limit airway inflammation and improve lung function[158] and reduce exacerbations.[159] Indeed, ICSs are the first-line prophylactic therapy in all pediatric age groups.[16] However, ICS dose regimens for the pediatric population vary with different guidelines, as do the thresholds used to define low-, medium-, and high-dose ICS and high variability of dose delivered according to device choice. For persistent disease, options for step-up and step-down are more variable. Features relevant include age, dosing, delivery system, the risk–benefit ratio, and cost-effectiveness of each medication by itself and in combination.

Effectiveness must be weighed against toxicity, particularly regarding growth. Although numerous studies have established the safety of ICS in children, potential to decrease growth rate remains[160] influenced by dose and potency of specific ICS;

Asthma Action Plan

Name: _____

Date of birth: _____

My best peak-flow is: _____

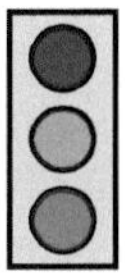

Quick Relief Medication: _____

Controlled Asthma Is:
1. No cough or wheeze during day or night.
2. Sleep through the night.
3. No missed school/work/play.
4. No emergency visits for asthma.

Rescue or quick-relief medication is used as needed for relief of asthma symptoms (cough, wheezing, chest tightness or shortness of breath). It may also be used 5–15 minutes before exercise if needed.

Green Zone: Doing Well	Use these controller medications everyday		
Medicine	How much to take	When to take it	Special Instructions

→ Take quick-relief medication for asthma symptoms

Peak Flow: from _____ to _____

Yellow Zone: Asthma Getting Worse	Begin yellow zone medications at first signs of a cold or asthma symptoms
Asthma Symptoms • Cough, wheezing • Starting to cough during sleep • Can do some, but not all, usual activities • Decreased response to albuterol Peak Flow: from _____ to _____	→ Take quick-relief medication up to every 4 hours as needed for asthma symptoms → Continue Green Zone medication ☐ → Add/Change to the following medication(s): _____ _____ _____ (use for 5–7 days or until 2 days of being symptom free or back in green zone)

Red Zone: Severe Asthma Signs	Take quick-relief medication and CALL YOUR DOCTOR NOW
• Yellow Zone medications are not helping • Constant cough and/or wheezing • Coughs during sleep most nights • Fast breathing and shortness of breath • Poor response to albuterol Peak Flow: less than _____	→ Take quick-relief medication for asthma symptoms (repeat in 15 minutes if needed) Continue quick-relief medication every 2–4 hours as needed → Continue Green Zone medication ☐ → Add the following medication: _____ _____ _____

If you see any of the following call 911 or go to the EMERGENCY ROOM now:
• Pulling in neck or chest muscles to breathe   • Not able to speak or talk because of asthma • No response to albuterol (rescue medication)   • Lips or fingernails look blue or gray

Provider/Doctor's Name _____   Clinic's Phone Number _____

Return to Clinic _____   Hospital/Emergency Room _____

Signature: _____   Date: _____   Time: _____

Fig. 7.15 Sample asthma action plan for home management of asthma, as presented in the Expert Panel Report 3 (EPR-3). (From National Heart, Lung, and Blood Institute. Expert Panel Report 3 (EPR-3): Guidelines for the Diagnosis and Management of Asthma: Full Report 2007. Available at: <https://www.ncbi.nlm.nih.gov/books/NBK7232/>; accessed August 30, 2020.)

delivery device; age, sex weight; individual susceptibility. The small risk of side effects must be balanced against the ability of ICSs to improve impairment and risk with long-term use. Systemic bioavailability results from the oral (swallowed fraction) and lung components. A balanced approach between the extremes of refusing to prescribe ICS because of steroid phobia and insistence that all need to be on these is advised, and approaches must reflect the observation in adults that the regular use of low-dose ICS decreases mortality. As the incidence of adverse events is dose-dependent, the minimum effective dose in order to achieve uncompromised asthma control should always be considered.[161]

Long-Acting Bronchodilators (LABAs). Salmeterol and formoterol that have been evaluated in children. In the US, salmeterol delivered by metered-dose inhaler (MDI) has been approved for children aged 12 and older; and by dry powder inhaler (DPI) for those 4 years and older; and formoterol has been approved for 5 years and older. Salmeterol has a delayed

(10–15 min) onset of action but the duration of 12 to 18 hours versus 3 to 6 hours for albuterol. Formoterol has a similar onset of action to short-acting bronchodilators. Meta-analyses of trials in patients 12 years and older report greater benefit in improving symptoms, exacerbations and lung function with addition of LABA than with ICS dose.[162,163] The bronchodilator effect of LABAs, however, may diminish with time.[164] Use of LABAs as monotherapy is definitely contraindicated.

In patients 12 years of age and older, the ICS-LABA combination therapy permit reduction in ICS without worsening of control. LABAs should therefore be used as adjunctive therapy in patients older than 5 years not controlled on low-dose ICS. Equal consideration can be given to increasing ICS dose to the addition of a LABA or LTRA to ICS.

Leukotriene Modifiers. Only one leukotriene modifier is now available for use in children younger than 12 years of age, that is, montelukast, in those at least 1 year of age. The overall efficacy of montelukast in comparison with low-dose ICS is, however, lower and strongly favoring ICS.

Montelukast can be used as an alternative, not a preferred, treatment option for mild persistent asthma, and as alternative, not preferred, adjunctive treatment with ICS in moderate or severe asthma.

Cromolyn Sodium and Nedocromil Sodium. Cromolyn sodium is available only in nebulized form and is approved for use in children older than 2 years of age. Nedocromil sodium is no longer available in the US but may be available in other countries. Clinical studies evaluating the efficacy of cromolyn sodium and nedocromil sodium in children and adolescents have demonstrated some efficacy, but again less than ICS.[119]

Theophylline. Theophylline is effective as monotherapy for persistent asthma and has a steroid-sparing effect in children with moderate to severe persistent asthma, although the efficacy of theophylline is less than that of ICS in controlling persistent asthma. As an adjunctive therapy to ICS, theophylline produces a small improvement in lung function similar to that obtained with doubling the dose of ICS. Sustained-release theophylline be used as an alternative, not a preferred, adjunctive agent with ICS.[119] When prescribed, monitoring of serum theophylline levels is needed (target level of 5–15 µg/mL).

Immunomodifiers. Studies of omalizumab in children have demonstrated efficacy in those 5 to 18 years of age.[165] As an add-on to ICS or an ICS-LABA combination, omalizumab leads to improvement in symptoms but has greatest benefit in the prevention of exacerbations. Despite studies demonstrating efficacy, omalizumab is not FDA-approved for use in children younger than 12 years of age. Currently, omalizumab should be considered as adjunctive therapy in persons 12 years of age and older who have severe asthma (Step 5 or 6; Fig. 7.14). However, clinical trials in 6 to 11-year old children with moderate-severe asthma have had some positive outcomes on asthma control and exacerbations and appeared safe suggesting that children younger than 12 years could benefit from this biologic.[166] In the era of new biologicals designed to target specific inflammatory phenotypes of severe asthma there is an urgent need for more trials in children. Recently, mepolizumab has been approved by European Medicines Agency for 6 to 11- year-old children as well as those 12 years and older.

Immunotherapy. Subcutaneous allergen immunotherapy (SCIT) is the only childhood treatment shown to potentially modify allergic sensitization and reduce allergic asthma in regard to specific exposures. A meta-analysis has confirmed the effectiveness of immunotherapy in asthma, with reductions in symptoms, medication use, and bronchial hyperreactivity.[167] Sublingual allergen immunotherapy is now included in pediatric asthma guidelines as an add-on therapy for single allergens such as asthma associated with house dust mite allergy if clear association between symptoms and allergen exposure can be established.[168,169] There is accumulating evidence to suggest that SLIT can attenuate the "allergic march" and, therefore, influence the natural history of asthma in young people.[143]

ACUTE ASTHMA AND REFERRAL FOR HOSPITAL CARE

Introduction

Severe episodes are described as *asthma attacks* or *exacerbations*, with a distinction between an acute flare-up and the day-to-day fluctuations. In the US in 2018, 11.9 million, or 48.2% of those ever diagnosed with asthma by a health professional and still had asthma had at least one asthma attack.[170] The highest attack prevalence is among children 5 to 17 years of age.

Although most exacerbations are mild and can be managed at home, severe exacerbations prompt ED visits and occasionally hospitalization. ED visits and hospitalizations together account for approximately 15% to 50% of the billions of US dollars spent on asthma each year.[171] Indirect costs (e.g., lost productivity) add additional billions. In the US, acute asthma accounts for approximately 1.7 million ED visits and 444,000 hospitalizations annually. Acute presentations are precipitated by many factors, commonly upper respiratory tract infections, air pollution episodes, and exposure to specific allergens.

Exacerbations are important events for patients and their families, associated with morbidity, disruption and, occasionally, mortality. Exacerbations persist for many days, and patients remain at risk for subsequent relapses for weeks after.[172] Frequently, ED visits are followed by inadequate subsequent care; in an observational study, 50% of patients seen in Canadian EDs had not had a follow-up examination within 3 weeks.[173]

The US National Asthma Education and Prevention Program (NAEPP) Coordinating Committee (CC) Expert Panel Report 3 (EPR-3) provides general strategies to manage an exacerbation (Box 7.9). This is also described in GINA 2020.[16]

Evaluation

Key elements in the history include details of the current exacerbation (e.g., time of onset, potential causes), severity of symptoms (especially compared with previous exacerbations), response to treatment, current medications, asthma history (i.e., number of previous unscheduled office visits, ED visits, and hospitalizations), and other comorbid conditions (e.g., other pulmonary or cardiac diseases).

Key elements of the initial physical examination are assessment of overall status (e.g., alertness, fluid status, respiratory

BOX 7.9 Risk Factors for Death From Asthma

Asthma History
- Previous severe exacerbation (e.g., intubation or ICU admission for asthma)
- Two or more hospitalizations for asthma in the past year
- Three or more ED visits for asthma in the past year
- Hospitalization or ED visit for asthma in the past month
- Using more than two canisters of SABA a month
- Difficulty perceiving asthma symptoms or severity of exacerbations
- Other risk factors: lack of a written asthma action plan, sensitivity to *Alternaria*

Social History
- Low socioeconomic status or inner-city residence
- Illicit drug use
- Major psychosocial problems

Comorbid Conditions
- Cardiovascular disease
- Other chronic lung diseases
- Chronic psychiatric diseases

ED, Emergency department; *ICU*, intensive care unit; *SABA*, short-acting β_2-agonist.
(From National Heart, Lung, and Blood Institute. Expert Panel Report 3 (EPR-3): Guidelines for the Diagnosis and Management of Asthma: Full Report 2007. Available at: <https://www.ncbi.nlm.nih.gov/books/NBK7232/>; accessed August 30, 2020.)

distress); vital signs (including pulse oximetry); and chest findings (e.g., use of accessory muscles, wheezing). Examination should also focus on identification of complications (e.g., pneumonia, pneumothorax). In children, the examination should also rule out upper airway obstruction (e.g., foreign bodies). Pulse oximetry can be useful in determining hypoxia.

Pulmonary function should be measured. Although FEV_1 is preferred, serial PEF measurements can provide an estimate of severity and can be used to guide emergency management. PFT is not necessary for patients in extreme respiratory distress. The percentage of predicted FEV_1 or PEF cutoffs for asthma exacerbation severity are 40% for severe and 70% for mild episodes.

Treatment

Table 7.11 summarizes essential information for the major therapeutic options: inhaled, short-acting β_2-agonists (SABAs); systemic (injected) β_2-agonists; anticholinergics; and systemic corticosteroids.

Adults: Home Management of Asthma Exacerbation

Home management (Fig. 7.16) includes an assessment of severity (Fig. 7.17). Initial treatment begins with an increase in frequency of SABA use, usually two to six puffs, 20 minutes apart. Initiation of an oral corticosteroid course can reduce duration of the exacerbation, prevent hospitalizations, and reduce relapse rates. Some patients may be provided with self-held oral corticosteroid courses as part of an action plan. Response to initial treatment is graded as good, incomplete, or poor, based on a reassessment of symptoms and airflow obstruction. With a good response, SABA can be used frequently over the

next 24 to 48 hours, along with a short course of prednisone if appropriate. The most effective dosing schedule and duration for systemic corticosteroids are unclear, but a commonly suggested regimen is 0.5 to 1.0 mg of prednisone/kg of body weight for 3 to 7 days. Depending on the individual patient, prednisone can be stopped or rapidly tapered once control has been reestablished.

For patients experiencing an incomplete response, the approach is continued SABA use and initiation of a course of prednisone, and the clinician should be involved in supervision of treatment. In patients with a poor response to inhaled SABAs, oral corticosteroids should be started, and transfer to a medical facility is indicated.

Although commonly recommended, doubling the dose of ICS is not beneficial, although some data suggest a four-fold increase in ICS may be beneficial.[174]

Adults: Hospital and Emergency Department Care

For patients with severe potentially life-threatening asthma exacerbations, assessment and treatment in hospital settings are needed. The goal of emergency care is to ensure adequate oxygenation, to reverse the obstruction, and to initiate antiinflammatory therapy. Laboratory studies (e.g., arterial blood gas testing) are used for detection of actual or impending respiratory failure and to detect conditions complicating emergency management (e.g., electrocardiogram to rule out cardiac ischemia, chest radiograph to rule out pneumonia).

Oxygen. Supplemental oxygen is recommended for initial ED or inpatient treatment, administered by nasal cannula or mask, to maintain an arterial oxygen saturation (SaO_2) of $\geq 90\%$ or $\geq 95\%$ in pregnant women and those with cardiac disease.

Inhaled, Short-Acting β_2-Agonists. Early treatment is with inhaled selective SABAs (i.e., albuterol [salbutamol], levalbuterol, pirbuterol) because of the rapid effect on bronchospasm. Whether the drug is most effective delivered through a nebulizer or through a metered-dose inhaler (MDI) with a holding chamber or spacer remains an area of research. A Cochrane systematic review[175] found that either delivery method produced similar outcomes. In children, but not adults, MDI with holding chamber or spacer appeared to offer advantages in terms of ED length of stay and adverse effects (e.g., tachycardia). Nebulizer therapy may still be preferred, however, for patients who are unable to cooperative effectively in using an MDI because of their age, agitation, or severity of acute asthma. For patients with life-threatening exacerbations, continuous nebulization[176] may be considered. EPR3 recommendations are summarized in Figs. 7.16 and 7.18 and in Table 7.11.

Inhaled Anticholinergic Agents. There is support, particularly in children, for adding the anticholinergic agent ipratropium bromide to β_2-agonist therapy in severe asthma exacerbations.[177] Multiple doses of ipratropium bromide result in a clinically significant improvement in FEV_1 and reduced the risk of hospitalization by 25%.

Systemic Corticosteroids. Early use of systemic corticosteroids (i.e., within 1 hour of the presentation) delivered by oral or intravenous routes continues to be the principal treatment choice. Early use of corticosteroids in the ED reduces admission

TABLE 7.11   Dosages of Drugs for Asthma Exacerbations

Medications	Dosages		Comments
	Children[a]	Adults	
Inhaled short-acting β₂-agonists			
Albuterol			
Nebulizer solution (0.63 mg/3 mL, 1.25 mg/3 mL, 2.5 mg/3 mL, 5.0 mg/mL)	0.15 mg/kg (minimum dose, 2.5 mg) every 20 min for 3 doses, then 0.15–0.3 mg/kg up to 10 mg every 1–4 h as needed, or 0.5 mg/kg per h by continuous nebulization	2.5–5 mg every 20 min for 3 doses, then 2.5–10 mg every 1–4 h as needed, or 10–15 mg/h continuously	Only selective β₂-agonists are recommended. For optimal delivery, dilute aerosols to minimum of 3 mL at gas flow of 6–8 L/min. Use large-volume nebulizers for continuous administration; may mix with ipratropium nebulizer solution
MDI (90 μg/puff)	4–8 puffs every 20 min for 3 doses, then every 1–4 h inhalation maneuver as needed; use VHC; add mask for children <4 years	4–8 puffs every 20 min up to 4 h, then every 1–4 h as needed	In mild-to-moderate exacerbations, MDI plus VHC is as effective as nebulized therapy with appropriate administration technique and coaching by trained personnel
Bitolterol			
Nebulizer solution (2 mg/mL)	See albuterol dose; thought to be half as potent as albuterol on mg basis	See albuterol dose	Has not been studied in severe asthma exacerbations; do not mix with other drugs
MDI (370 μg/puff)	See albuterol MDI dose	See albuterol MDI dose	Has not been studied in severe asthma exacerbations
Levalbuterol (R-albuterol)			
Nebulizer solution (0.63 mg/3 mL, 1.25 mg/0.5 mL, 1.25 mg/3 mL)	0.075 mg/kg (minimum dose, 1.25 mg) every 20 min for 3 doses, then 0.075–0.15 mg/kg up to 5 mg every 1–4 h as needed	1.25–2.5 mg every 20 min for 3 doses, then 1.25–5 mg every 1–4 h as needed	Levalbuterol administered in one-half (mg) of the albuterol dose provides comparable efficacy and safety; has not been evaluated by continuous nebulization
MDI (45 μg/puff)	See albuterol MDI dose	See albuterol MDI dose	
Pirbuterol			
MDI (200 μg/puff)	See albuterol MDI dose; thought to be one-half as potent as albuterol on a milligram basis	See albuterol MDI dose	Has not been studied in severe asthma exacerbations
Systemic (Injected) β₂-agonsts			
Epinephrine 1:1000 (1 mg/mL)	0.01 mg/kg up to 0.3–0.5 mg every 20 min for 3 doses SQ	0.3–0.5 mg every 20 min for 3 doses SQ	No proven advantage of systemic therapy over aerosol
Terbutaline (1 mg/mL)	0.01 mg/kg every 20 min for 3 doses SQ, then every 2–6 h as needed	0.25 mg every 20 min for 3 doses SQ	No proven advantage of systemic therapy over aerosol
Anticholinergics			
Ipratropium bromide			
Nebulizer solution (0.25 mg/mL)	0.25–0.5 mg every 20 min for 3 doses, then as needed	0.5 mg every 20 min for 3 doses, then as needed	May mix in same nebulizer with albuterol; should not be used as first-line therapy; should be added to SABA therapy for severe exacerbations; addition of ipratropium not shown to provide further benefit after patient is hospitalized
MDI (18 μg/puff)	4–8 puffs every 20 min as needed up to 3 h	8 puffs every 20 min as needed up to 3 h	Should use with VHC and face mask for children <4 years; studies have examined ipratropium bromide MDI for up to 3 h
Ipratropium with Albuterol			
Nebulizer solution (each 3 mL vial contains 0.5 mg ipratropium bromide and 2.5 mg albuterol)	1.5 mL every 20 min for 3 doses, then as needed	3 mL every 20 min for 3 doses, then as needed	May be used for up to 3 h in initial management of severe exacerbations; addition of ipratropium to albuterol not shown to provide further benefit after patient is hospitalized
MDI (each puff contains 18 μg ipratropium bromide and 90 μg of albuterol)	4–8 puffs every 20 min as needed up to 3 h	8 puffs every 20 min as needed up to 3 h	Should use with VHC and face mask for children <4 years

(Continued)

TABLE 7.11   Dosages of Drugs for Asthma Exacerbations—cont'd

Medications	Dosages Children[a]	Adults	Comments
Systemic Corticosteroids[b]			
Prednisone Methylprednisolone Prednisolone	1 mg/kg in 2 divided doses (maximum, 60 mg/day) until PEF is 70% of predicted or personal best	40–80 mg/day in 1 or 2 divided doses until PEF reaches 70% of predicted or personal best	For outpatient burst, use 40–60 mg in single dose or 2 divided doses for total of 5–10 days in adults (children: 1–2 mg/kg per day maximum, 60 mg/day for 3–10 days)

ED, Emergency department; *ICs*, inhaled corticosteroids; *MDI*, metered-dose inhaler; *PEF*, peak expiratory flow; *SABA*, short-acting β₂-agonists; *VHC*, valved holding chamber.

[a]Children ≤12 years of age.

[b]Dosages and comments apply to all three corticosteroids. There is no known advantage for higher doses of corticosteroids in severe asthma exacerbations, nor is there any advantage for intravenous administration over oral therapy if gastrointestinal transit time or absorption is not impaired. The total course of systemic corticosteroids for an asthma exacerbation requiring an ED visit or hospitalization may be 3–10 days. For corticosteroid courses of less than 1 week, there is no need to taper the dose. For slightly longer courses (e.g., up to 10 days), there probably is no need to taper, especially if patients are concurrently taking ICs. The ICs can be started at any point in the treatment of an asthma exacerbation. From National Heart, Lung, and Blood Institute. Expert Panel Report 3 (EPR-3): Guidelines for the Diagnosis and Management of Asthma: Full Report 2007. Available at: <http://www.nhlbi.nih.gov/files/docs/guidelines/asthgdln.pdf>; accessed July 7, 2015.

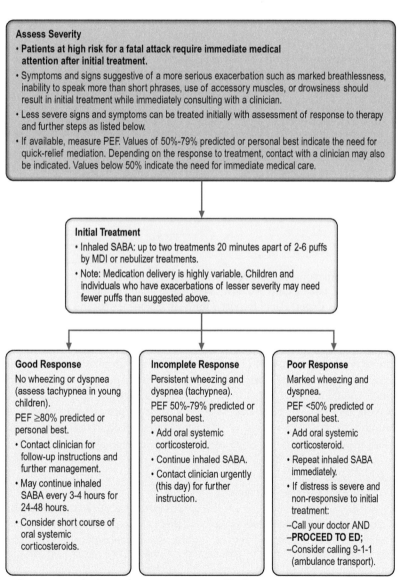

Fig. 7.16 Management of asthma exacerbations: home treatment. *ED*, Emergency department; *MDI*, metered-dose inhaler; *PEF*, peak expiratory flow; *SABA*, short-acting β₂-agonist (quick-relief inhaler). (From National Asthma Education and Prevention Program. Expert Panel Report 3: Guidelines for the Diagnosis and Management of Asthma. Full Report 2007. Washington, DC: US Government Printing Office; 2007.)

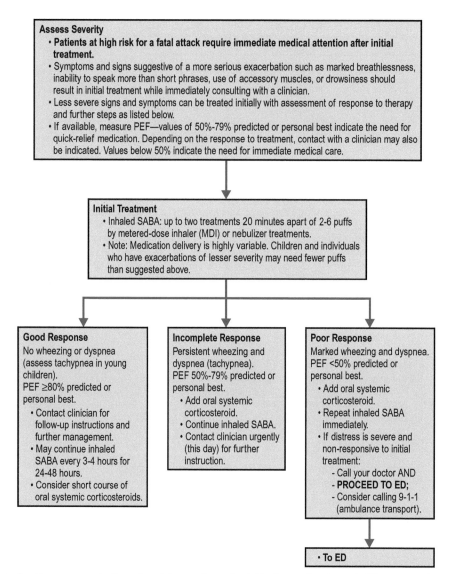

Fig. 7.17 Management of asthma exacerbations in adolescents and adults: home treatment. (Figure numbers refer to those in cited source.) *ED*, Emergency department; *PEF*, peak expiratory flow; *SABA*, short-acting β-agonist (quick-relief medication). (Modified from National Heart, Lung, and Blood Institute. Expert Panel Report 3 (EPR-3): Guidelines for the Diagnosis and Management of Asthma: Full Report 2007. Available at: <https://www.ncbi.nlm.nih.gov/books/NBK7232/>; accessed August 30, 2020.)

rates (OR = 0.40), with a number needed to treat (NNT) of 8, particularly for those not already receiving systemic corticosteroids. Intravenous corticosteroids should be reserved for those who are too breathless to swallow, obtunded or intubated, or unable to tolerate oral medications.

Magnesium Sulfate. Magnesium sulfate ($MgSO_4$) is used in unresponsive acute asthma, with immediate bronchodilator and mild antiinflammatory effects.[178,179] EPR3 recommend consideration of intravenous $MgSO_4$ in patients with life-threatening exacerbations.

Heliox. Heliox, a helium–oxygen mixture, which has been used sporadically since the 1930s. A 2006 Cochrane review yielded a borderline-significant group difference. EPR3 guidelines recommend consideration of heliox only in patients who have life-threatening exacerbations.

Other Therapies. The benefits of agents such as aminophylline are limited.[180] There is presently little evidence to support the use of parenteral aminophylline in addition to standard therapy for acute asthma in adults.[181] Antibiotics should not be used routinely for acute asthma.[182] Despite this, many clinicians continue to prescribe antibiotics for the viral upper respiratory tract infections triggering asthma, a focus for future quality improvements to decrease inappropriate antibiotic use and encouraging antimicrobial resistance.

Care After Hospitalization and ED Visits

Approximately 10% to 20% of ED patients treated for acute asthma and sent home will relapse within 2 weeks of discharge. The use of oral corticosteroids for a short period (e.g., 5–7 days) is appropriate for patients discharged after an acute asthma episode, with a medical review arranged prior to discontinuation. All should also receive ICS if they were not already receiving them. However, in the US, only 11% of discharged patients were prescribed ICS.[183]

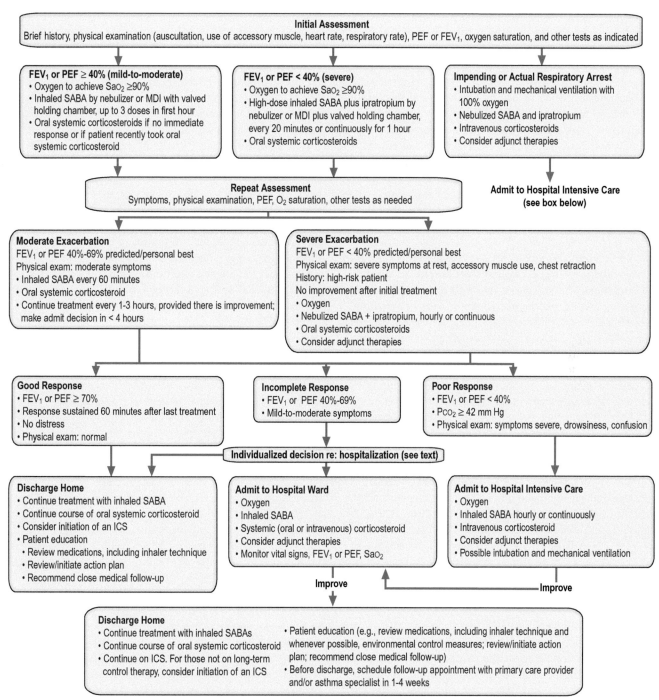

Fig. 7.18 Management of asthma exacerbations: ED and hospital-based care. *FEV₁*, Forced expiratory volume in 1 s; *ICs*, inhaled corticosteroids; *MDI*, metered-dose inhaler; *PCO₂*, partial pressure of carbon dioxide; *PEF*, peak expiratory flow; *SABA*, short-acting β₂-agonist (quick-relief inhaler); *SaO₂*, arterial oxygen saturation. (From National Heart, Lung, and Blood Institute. Expert Panel Report 3 (EPR-3): Guidelines for the Diagnosis and Management of Asthma–Full Report 2007. Available at: <https://www.ncbi.nlm.nih.gov/books/NBK7232/f>; accessed August 30, 2020.)

Managing Exacerbations in Children

In the Childhood Asthma Management Program study of school-aged children with asthma,[184] 40% of the children in the ICS treatment group experienced exacerbation, compared with 75% in those receiving placebo. Many can be managed at home, but as with adults, more severe exacerbations require ED and hospital care.

Home Management

Inhaled SABAs can be delivered by MDI with or without a spacer device, as dry powder formulations, or by handheld nebulizer. Children younger than 5 years of age require the use of a mask with nebulizer treatments or with an MDI and valved spacer system for effective delivery of medication into the airways. Some patients and families prefer nebulizer treatments, which require only slow tidal breathing. Both high-dose MDI and nebulized delivery, however, have been shown to be equally efficacious. If the attack is severe and unresponsive to therapy, the family caregiver and/or the patient should be instructed to contact a healthcare provider. Home therapy may involve the introduction of short-course oral corticosteroids, which reduce the duration and severity of the exacerbation and prevent hospitalization.[185] Quadrupling but not doubling the dose of ICS at the first sign of worsening symptoms in patients already receiving ICS may prevent exacerbations requiring oral corticosteroids.[186] The increased SABA use during an exacerbation should continue until the level of asthma symptom control and PEF values return to the patient's baseline.

Office or Emergency Department Management in Children

If early intervention at home fails, the family should be instructed to take the child to an urgent care center, or hospital ED for further management. The initial assessment should include a brief history, physical examination focused on the work of breathing, PEF determination or spirometry, and measurement of oxygen saturation. Blood gas analysis is not routinely indicated. Routine chest radiographs are not necessary.

In a mild to moderate exacerbation (FEV_1 or PEF of $\geq$40%), initial therapy includes oxygen to keep oxygen saturations higher than 90% and up to three doses in the first hour of inhaled SABA delivered by either nebulizer or MDI with spacer, and oral corticosteroids if no immediate response to bronchodilators is obtained. In severe exacerbations (FEV_1 or PEF <40%), therapy should include prompt administration of oxygen, high-dose inhaled SABA plus ipratropium bromide every 20 minutes or continuously for the first hour and oral corticosteroids. Severe exacerbations are life-threatening, so transfer to an ED is required in most cases to permit close observation for deterioration, repeated assessments, and frequent administration of indicated treatments. Most studies evaluating the use of intravenous aminophylline in the treatment of acute exacerbations have been unable to demonstrate any additional benefit.[181]

Hospital Management in Children

An incomplete response in symptoms or lung function (FEV_1 or PEF of 40%–69%), despite aggressive treatment, warrants hospitalization for continued inhaled SABA, systemic corticosteroids, oxygen (if needed), and close monitoring. Hospitalization should be considered for infants with oxygen saturation <92% on room air.

Posthospital Care

In addition to acute management, a most important aspect should be preventing exacerbation recurrence. Asthma education is warranted in the clinic, ED, and hospital settings, and communication with primary care health providers is crucial.

CONCLUSIONS

Asthma care has seen remarkable developments over the last few decades, with greater understanding of the diverse factors comprising the asthma syndrome leading to therapeutic advances and to improved outcomes. However, asthma remains common, incurable, the global prevalence continues to increase, and the improvements in outcomes seen over the last decades of the last century have stalled in most economically developed countries. Although we have superior insights into the biologic basis of asthma, the complex genetic and environmental factors interacting to manifest as asthma in susceptible individuals, and greater understanding of the immunologic pathways underpinning asthma, translating this knowledge into patient benefit, has lagged. The complexity of asthma is now appreciated, with the various phenotypes and endotypes comprising the asthma syndrome progressively becoming clearer. Asthma guidelines are based on group mean data from clinical trials, and use a stepped approach for all, based on severity and control, yet the heterogeneity of individual responses to different interventions is increasingly apparent. Future developments in asthma care, as with other long-term conditions, are likely to involve "stratified" or "personalized" approaches to asthma care. Since the final manifestation of the various pathologic processes involved in asthma can be very similar, yet the drivers diverse, it is likely that further improvements in asthma outcomes will rely on targeting interventions onto appropriately identified individuals with specific characteristics and endotypes. This will involve better characterization at an individual patient level and an approach that encompasses this diversity by detecting poor control, assessing the reasons for it and directing the most appropriate treatments to improve it. Such a "stratified" approach is already occurring in severe asthma, where the development of expensive new biological treatments that are proving highly effective for appropriately characterized patients including application of biomarkers or treatable traits (e.g., FeNO, blood and sputum eosinophils, and neutrophils) to help identify causal pathways amenable to targeted intervention.[187] While much of this is currently occurring at specialist centers as new ways of intervening in asthma are discovered, such approaches will become part of standard practice in the community management of this disease.

ASTHMA DIAGNOSIS AND MONITORING

There is concern that the diagnosis of asthma is sometimes inappropriately applied, and that asthma is inadequately monitored. The symptoms of asthma are not specific and supporting objective criteria, such as reversible variable airflow obstruction, BHR, or airway inflammation, are often not measured or recorded. General practitioners and community-based nonspecialists frequently lack access to the more sophisticated diagnostic tests needed to confirm or refute the diagnosis in the (frequent) cases of diagnostic uncertainty. This may result in patients with nonspecific respiratory symptoms being labeled as having asthma and commenced on anti-asthma medication (commonly antiinflammatory treatment with ICS) without evidence of a corticosteroid-responsive disease. Lack of response often leads to escalation of treatment rather than a review of the diagnosis. Asthma is defined as an inflammatory disease of the airways characterized by BHR, yet inflammation and hyperreactivity are commonly not assessed outside of research or specialist settings. Recent advances in technology potentially allow

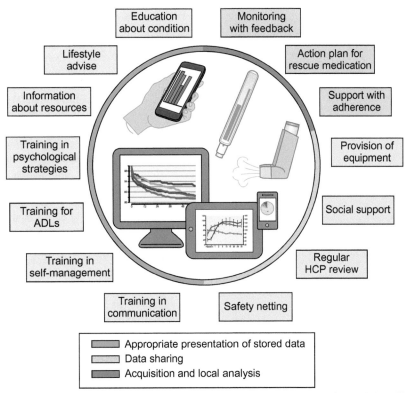

Fig. 7.19 Connected asthma: the potential for technology to transform care. *ADLs,* Activities of daily living. (Reproduced with permission from Clift J. Connected asthma report. Asthma UK; 2016. Available at: <https://www.asthma.org.uk/connectedasthma/>; accessed August 30, 2020.)

greater use of objective testing in routine community settings (including blood biomarkers, exhaled biomarkers such as FeNO, and even bronchial challenge tests such as with inhaled manni-tol), which may have significant implications for the diagnosis, monitoring, and therapeutic decision making in asthma care.[188]

Poor control is frequently not detected by clinicians and not volunteered by patients, who have come to accept the status quo as a fact of life. Novel technologies, such as wearables and intelligent inhalers, are enabling real-time remote monitoring of asthma thereby creating a unique opportunity for personal-ized healthcare[187] (Fig. 7.19). EMDs offer have the potential to become the gold standard in asthma care for the 21st century. Benefits of EMDs include the ability to track exact numbers of inhaled ICS and b2-agonist doses taken, provide new data to assist in clinical decision making, and increase motivation and engagement in patients.[189]

Asthma Treatment

Improvements in asthma therapeutics are likely to involve both more effective use of currently available therapies, and the devel-opment of new treatments for the small but important subgroup with genuine therapy resistant disease.

Better Use of Current Treatments

The most common reasons for suboptimal outcomes in asthma relate to poor adherence and poor inhaler technique. Greater awareness of these important factors and greater partner-ship with patients (including wider use of self-management

education) is a challenge for primary care asthma providers. Improved patient characterization is likely to assist in the bet-ter targeting of current therapies. For instance, in the case of a patient receiving low-dose ICS who remains uncontrolled, cur-rent guidelines suggest that addition of a LABA is the preferred option. However, the ability to measure airway inflammation could guide the decision-making process; evidence of ongoing inflammation could point to inadequate delivery of ICS (e.g., nonadherence or poor inhaler technique) or to the need for increased doses or potency of antiinflammatory medication, whereas normal inflammatory indices would support the use of a bronchodilator or other approaches to achieve control.

Considerable interest exists in the use of combination ICS-fast acting bronchodilator inhalers as rescue medication, in theory allowing increased delivery of antiinflammatory medi-cation as symptoms (and inflammation) worsen; the "single maintenance and reliever" inhaler approach is now possible with more than one product, and as required use at "Step 1" as recommended by GINA 2020. The effectiveness and positioning of these strategies will become clearer in coming years

Current trends in chronic disease management of involv-ing patients (where possible) in decision making and sharing uncertainty are likely if applied effectively to improve adher-ence, patient outcomes, expectations, and satisfaction.

New Treatments

There continues to be new products (Fig. 7.20) for treating asthma reaching the market, although most consist of new

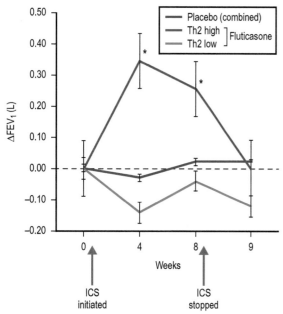

Fig. 7.20 Responsiveness of "Th2 high" asthma to inhaled corticosteroids *(ICS)* and placebo in a randomized controlled trial. FEV_1 measured at baseline (week 0), after 4 and 8 weeks on daily fluticasone (500 µg twice a day), and 1 week after the cessation of fluticasone (week 9). No significant change in FEV_1 in response to placebo is seen at any time point in either group, Th2 low, and placebo. (From Woodruff PG, Modrek B, Choy DF, et al. T-helper type 2-driven inflammation defines major subphenotypes of asthma. Am J Respir Crit Care Med 2009;180:388–395.)

versions of existing therapy classes. The availability of more potent and longer-acting molecules within currently available drug classes (e.g., once daily ICS and LABAs) potentially have limited incremental benefits that may be helpful to some patients. New inhaler devices and delivery systems that are easier for patients to use and for professionals to teach, may again benefit some patients and allow existing classes of medications to be used more effectively.

Prevention

The causes of the increasing global prevalence of asthma remain incompletely understood, with a number of large birth cohort studies ongoing in different parts of the world. These have provided important new information on factors associated with asthma (e.g., early-life microbial exposure; family size and birth rank; early contact with animals) but have not yet provided public health strategies for prevention. The complexity and interdependence of factors promoting or protecting against asthma are slowly being unraveled. Interventions studied have included environmental (e.g., intensive aeroallergen avoidance measures in the home), vaccination, and diet, with generally disappointing results. Advances in computing techniques in large databases are allowing databases to be combined, and it is likely that important new information will become available in the coming years. So, looking to the future, the big challenge is to find new ways of intervening to prevent asthma in the first place and to reverse it once diagnosed, without the need for continued therapy.

REFERENCES

1. GINA. Global Strategy for Asthma Management and Prevention. 2014; Vancouver USA: Global Initiative for Asthma, 1–134.
2. The International Study of Asthma and Allergies in Childhood (ISAAC) Steering Committee. Worldwide variation in prevalence of symptoms of asthma, allergic rhinoconjunctivitis, and atopic eczema: ISAAC. Lancet. 1998;351:1225–1232.
3. Asher MI, Montefort S, Björkstén B, et al. Worldwide time trends in the prevalence of symptoms of asthma, allergic rhinoconjunctivitis, and eczema in childhood: ISAAC Phases one and three repeat multicountry cross-sectional surveys. Lancet. 2006;368:733–743.
4. Masoli M, Fabian D, Holt S, et al. The global burden of asthma: executive summary of the GINA Dissemination Committee report. Allergy. 2004;59:469–478.
5. Cockcroft DW. Bronchoprovocation methods: direct challenges. Clin Rev Allergy Immunol. 2003;24:19–26.
6. Shaw D, Green R, Berry M, et al. A cross-sectional study of patterns of airway dysfunction, symptoms and morbidity in primary care asthma. Prim Care Respir J. 2012;21(3): 283–287.
7. To T, Stanojevic S, Moores G, et al. Global asthma prevalence in adults: findings from the cross-sectional world health survey. BMC Public Health. 2012;12:204.
8. Thomas M, Wilkinson T. Asthma diagnosis in the community: time for a change? Clin Exp Allergy. 2014;44:1206–1209.
9. Aaron SD, Vandemheen KL, Boulet LP, et al. Overdiagnosis of asthma in obese and non-obese adults. CMAJ. 2008;179: 1121–1131.
10. Huang C, Li F, Wang J, Tian Z. Innate-like lymphocytes and innate lymphoid cells in asthma. Clinic Rev Allerg Immunol. 2019;59(3):359–370.
11. Gibson PG, Foster PS. Neutrophilic asthma: welcome back! Eur Respir J. 2019;54:1901846.
12. Tliba O, Panettieri Jr. RA. Paucigranulocytic asthma: uncoupling of airway obstruction from inflammation. J Allergy Clin Immunol. 2019;143:1287–1294.
13. Bergeron C, Boulet LP. Structural changes in airway diseases: characteristics, mechanisms, consequences, and pharmacologic modulation. Chest. 2006;129:1068–1087.
14. Updated BTS/SIGN national Guideline on the management of asthma. 24 July 2019. Online. Available: <https://www.brit-thoracic.org.uk/about-us/pressmedia/2019/btssign-british-guideline-on-the-management-of-asthma-2019/>.
15. National Asthma Education and Prevention Program (NAEPP) Expert panel report 3 (EPR-3): guidelines for the diagnosis and management of asthma. NIH Publication no. 07-4051. Bethesda, MD: US Department of Health and Human Services, National Institutes of Health; 2007.
16. 2020 GINA report, global strategy for asthma management and prevention. P.O. Box 558 Fontana, WI 53125, USA. Online. Available: <https://ginasthma.org/wp-content/uploads/2020/06/GINA-2020-report_20_06_04-1-wms.pdf>.
17. Hancox RJ, Cowan JO, Flannery EM, et al. Bronchodilator tolerance and rebound bronchoconstriction during regular inhaled beta-agonist treatment. Respir Med. 2000;94:767–771.
18. Aldridge RE, Hancox RJ, Robin Taylor D, et al. Effects of terbutaline and budesonide on sputum cells and bronchial hyperresponsiveness in asthma. Am J Respir Crit Care Med. 2000;161:1459–1464.

19. Stanford RH, Shah MB, D'Souza AO, et al. Short-acting β-agonist use and its ability to predict future asthma-related outcomes. Annals of Allergy, Asthma & Immunology. 2012;109:403–407.

20. Suissa S, Ernst P, Boivin JF, et al. A cohort analysis of excess mortality in asthma and the use of inhaled beta-agonists. Am J Respir Crit Care Med. 1994;149:604–610.

21. Bateman ED, Boushey HA, Bousquet J, et al. Can guideline-defined asthma control be achieved? The Gaining Optimal Asthma Control study. Am J Respir Crit Care Med. 2004;170:836–844.

22. Demoly P, Gueron B, Annunziata K, et al. Update on asthma control in five European countries: results of a 2008 survey. Eur Respir Rev. 2010;19:150–157.

23. Levy M, Andrews R, Buckingham R, et al. Why asthma still kills: the National Review of Asthma Deaths (NRAD) Confidential Enquiry report. London: RCP; 2014. Online. Available: <https://www.rcplondon.ac.uk/sites/default/files/why-asthma-still-kills-full-report.pdf>.

24. Guilbert TW, Mauger DT, Lemanske RFJr. Childhood asthma-predictive phenotype. J Allergy Clin Immunol Pract. 2014;2:664–670.

25. de Nijs SB1, Venekamp LN, Bel EH. Adult-onset asthma: is it really different? Eur Respir Rev. 2013;22:44–52.

26. Arathimos R, Granell R, Henderson J, Relton CL, Tilling K. Sex discordance in asthma and wheeze prevalence in two longitudinal cohorts. PLoS One. 2017;12:e0176293.

27. Frati F, Salvatori C, Incorvaia C, et al. The role of the microbiome in asthma: the gut-lung axis. Int J Mol Sci. 2018;20(1):123.

28. Martinez FD, Wright AL, Taussig LM, et al. Asthma and wheezing in the first six years of life. The Group Health Medical Associates. N Engl J Med. 1995;332:133–138.

29. Guilbert T, Moss MH, Lemanske RF Jr, et al. Approach to infants and children with asthma. In: Adkinson NF, Busse WW, Bochner BS, eds. Middleton's allergy: principles and practice. 7th ed. St Louis: Mosby; 2009:1319–1343.

30. Arathimos R, Granell R, Henderson J, et al. Sex discordance in asthma and wheeze prevalence in two longitudinal cohorts. PLoS One. 2017;12:e0176293.

31. Pearce N, Ait-Khaled N, Beasley R, et al. Worldwide trends in the prevalence of asthma symptoms: Phase III of the International Study of Asthma and Allergies in Childhood (ISAAC). Thorax. 2007;62:758–766.

32. Hufnagl K, Pali-Schöll I, Roth-Walter F, et al. Dysbiosis of the gut and lung microbiome has a role in asthma. Semin Immunopathol. 2020;42:75–93.

33. Ober C, Sperling AI, von Mutius E, Vercelli D. Immune development and environment: lessons from Amish and Hutterite children. Curr Opin Immunol. 2017;48:51–60.

34. Holguin F. Sex hormones and asthma. Am J Respir Crit Care Med. 2020;201:127–128.

35. The global asthma report 2018. Online. Available: <http://www.globalasthmareport.org/index.html>.

36. Fehrenbach H, Wagner C, Wegmann M. Airway remodeling in asthma: what really matters. Cell Tissue Res. 2017;367:551–569.

37. Kraft M, Djukanovic R, Wilson S, et al. Alveolar tissue inflammation in asthma. Am J Respir Crit Care Med. 1996;154:1505–1510.

38. Shaver JR, Zangrilli JG, Cho SK, et al. Kinetics of the development and recovery of the lung from IgE-mediated inflammation: dissociation of pulmonary eosinophilia, lung injury, and eosinophil-active cytokines. Am J Respir Crit Care Med. 1997;155:442–448.

39. Chung KF. Neutrophilic asthma: a distinct target for treatment? Lancet Respir Med. 2016;4:765–767.

40. Loverdos K, Bellos G, Kokolatou L, et al. Lung microbiome in asthma: current perspectives. J Clin Med. 2019;8:1967.

41. Akdis CA, Arkwright PD, Brüggen MC, et al. Type 2 immunity in the skin and lungs. Allergy. 2020;75:1582–1605.

42. Nagata M, Nakagome K, Soma T. Mechanisms of eosinophilic inflammation. Asia Pac Allergy. 2020;10:e14.

43. Woodruff PG, Modrek B, Choy DF, et al. T-helper type 2-driven inflammation defines major subphenotypes of asthma. Am J Respir Crit Care Med. 2009;180:388–395.

44. Bosse Y, Reisenfeld EP, Pare PD, et al. It's not all smooth muscle: non-smooth-muscle elements in control of resistance airflow. Annu Rev Physiol. 2010;72:937–962.

45. Holgate ST. The sentinel role of the airway epithelium in asthma pathogenesis. Immunol Rev. 2011;242:205–219.

46. Thorsen J, Rasmussen MA, Waage J, et al. Infant airway microbiota and topical immune perturbations in the origins of childhood asthma. Nat Commun. 2019;10:5001.

47. Stokholm J, Blasé Jr M, Thorsen J, et al. Maturation of the gut microbiome and risk of asthma in childhood. Nat Commun. 2018;9:141.

48. Burbank AJ, Sood AK, Kesic MJ, et al. Environmental determinants of allergy and asthma in early life. J Allergy Clin Immunol. 2017;140:1–12.

49. Pividori M, Schoettler N, Nicolae DL, et al. Shared and distinct genetic risk factors for childhood-onset and adult-onset asthma: genome-wide and transcriptome-wide studies. Lancet Respir Med. 2019;7:509–522.

50. Demenais F, Margaritte-Jeannin P, Barnes KC, et al. Multiancestry association study identifies new asthma risk loci that colocalize with immune-cell enhancer marks. Nat Genet. 2018;50:42–53.

51. Divekar R, Kita H. Recent advances in epithelium-derived cytokines (IL-33, IL-25, and thymic stromal lymphopoietin) and allergic inflammation. Curr Opin Allergy Clin Immunol. 2015;15:98–103.

52. Heijink IH, Kuchibhotla VNS, Roffel MP, et al. Epithelial cell dysfunction, a major driver of asthma development. Allergy. 2020;75:1898–1913.

53. Holgate ST. ADAM metallopeptidase domain 33 (ADAM33): identification and role in airways disease. Drug News Perspect. 2010;23:381–387.

54. Turner S, Francis B, Vijverberg S, et al. Childhood asthma exacerbations and the Arg16 β2-receptor polymorphism: a meta-analysis stratified by treatment. J Allergy Clin Immunol. 2016;138:107–113, e5.

55. Hernandez-Pacheco N, Farzan N, Francis B, Karimi L, et al. Genome-wide association study of inhaled corticosteroid response in admixed children with asthma. Clin Exp Allergy. 2019;49:789–798.

56. DeVries A, Vercelli D. Epigenetic mechanisms in asthma. Ann Am Thorac Soc. 2016;13 (Suppl 1):S48–S50.

57. von Mutius E. Gene-environment interactions in asthma. J Allergy Clin Immunol. 2009;123:3–11.

58. Moore WC, Meyers DA, Wenzel SE, et al. Identification of asthma phenotypes using cluster analysis in the Severe Asthma Research Program. Am J Respir Crit Care Med. 2010;181:315–323.

59. Han YY, Zhang X, Wang J, et al. Multidimensional assessment of asthma identifies clinically relevant phenotype overlap: a

cross-sectional study. J Allergy Clin Immunol Pract. 2020;S2213–2198:30806-0.

60. Holgate ST, Wenzel S, Postma DS, et al. Asthma. Nat Rev Dis Primers. 2015;1:15025.

61. Boulet LP. Influence of comorbid conditions on asthma. Eur Respir J. 2009;33:897–906.

62. Taussig LM, Wright AL, Holberg CJ, et al. Tucson children's respiratory study: 1980 to present. J Allergy Clin Immunol. 2003;111:661–675.

63. Deliu M, Fontanella S, Haider S, et al. Longitudinal trajectories of severe wheeze exacerbations from infancy to school age and their association with early-life risk factors and late asthma outcomes. Clin Exp Allergy. 2020;50:315–324.

64. Brand PL, Baraldi E, Bisgaard H, et al. Definition, assessment and treatment of wheezing disorders in preschool children: an evidence-based approach. Eur Respir J. 2008;32:1096–1110.

65. Sonnappa S, Bastardo CM, Wade A, et al. Symptom-pattern phenotype and pulmonary function in preschool wheezers. J Allergy Clin Immunol. 2010;126:519–526.

66. Saglani S, Menzie-Gow AN. Approaches to asthma diagnosis in children and adults. Front Pediatr. 2019;7:148.

67. Morgan WJ, Martinez FD. Risk factors for developing wheezing and asthma in childhood. Pediatr Clin North Am. 1992;39:1185–1203.

68. Thomas M. Asthma diagnosis: not always simple or straightforward. J Thorac Dis. 2014;6:409–410.

69. Miller MR, Hankinson J, Brusasco V, et al. Standardisation of spirometry. Eur Respir J. 2005;26:319–338.

70. Jindal SK, Aggarwal AN, Gupta D. Diurnal variability of peak expiratory flow. J Asthma. 2002;39:363–373.

71. Anderson SD, Brannan JD. Bronchial provocation testing: the future. Curr Opin Allergy Clin Immunol. 2011;11:46–52.

72. San Miguel-Rodríguez A, Armentia A, Martín-Armentia S, et al. Component-resolved diagnosis in allergic disease: utility and limitations. Clin Chim Acta. 2019;489:219–224.

73. Pavord ID, Bush A, Holgate S. Asthma diagnosis: addressing the challenges. Lancet Respir Med. 2015;3(5):339–341.

74. Schmid J, Hviid-Vyff B, Skjold T, et al. The usefulness of blood eosinophil count and FeNO to predict sputum eosinophilia in the diagnosis of severe eosinophilic asthma. Eur Respir J. 2019;54(suppl 63):OA2150.

75. Dweik RA, Boggs PB, Erzurum SC, et al. An official ATS clinical practice guideline: interpretation of exhaled nitric oxide levels (FeNO) for clinical applications. Am J Respir Crit Care Med. 2011;184:602–615.

76. Stonham C, Baxter N. FeNO testing for asthma diagnosis: a PCRS consensus. Primary care research society; primary care respiratory update. 2019. Online. Available: <https://www.pcrs-uk.org/sites/pcrs-uk.org/files/pcru/articles/2019-Autumn-Issue-18-FeNo-testing-asthma-diagnosis.pdf>.

77. Eddy RL, Svenningsen S, Licskai C, et al. Hyperpolarized gelium 3 MRI in mild-to-moderate asthma: prediction of postbronchodilator reversibility. Radiology. 2019;293:212–220.

78. Cullinan P, Cannon J. Occupational asthma often goes unrecognised. Practitioner. 2012;256:15–18, 2.

79. Wisnewski AV, Jones M. Pro/con debate: is occupational asthma induced by isocyanates an immunoglobulin E-mediated disease? Clinical and Experimental Allergy. 2010;40:1155–1162.

80. Vandenplas O, Suojalehto H, Aasen TB, et al. Specific inhalation challenge in the diagnosis of occupational asthma: consensus statement. Eur Resp J. 2014;43 1573–158.

81. Tzortzaki EG, Proklou A, Siafakas NM. Asthma in the elderly: can we distinguish it from COPD? J Allergy. 2011;2011:843543.

82. Fitch KD, Sue-Chu M, Anderson SD, et al. Asthma and the elite athlete: summary of the International Olympic Committee's consensus conference, Lausanne, Switzerland, January 22–24, 2008. J Allergy Clin Immunol. 2008;122:254–260.

83. Galant SP, Morphew T, Amaro S, et al. Value of the bronchodilator response in assessing controller naive asthmatic children. J Pediatr. 2007;151:457–462.

84. Galan SP, Komarow HD, Hye-Won S, et al. The case for impulse oscillometry in the management of asthma in children and adults. Ann Allergy Asthma Immunol. 2017;118:664–671.

85. Petsky HL, Kew KM, Chang AB, Cochrane Airways Group Exhaled nitric oxide levels to guide treatment for children with asthma. Cochrane Database Syst Rev. 2016;2016:CD011439.

86. Baishnab E, Karner C. Primary care based clinics for asthma. Cochrane Database Syst Rev. 2012;2012(4):CD003533.

87. Pinnock H, Thomas M. Does self-management prevent severe exacerbations? Curr Opin Pulm Med. 2015;21(1):95–102.

88. Cockcroft DW, Swystun VA. Asthma control versus asthma severity. J Allergy Clin Immunol. 1996;98:1016–1018.

89. Reddel HK, Ampon RD, Sawyer SM, Peters MJ. Risks associated with managing asthma without a preventer: urgent healthcare, poor asthma control and over-the-counter reliever use in a cross-sectional population survey. BMJ Open. 2017; 7:e016688.

90. Muneswarao J, Hassal MA, Ibrahim B, et al. It is time to change the way we manage mild asthma: an update in GINA 2019. Respir Res. 2019;20:183.

91. Barnes PJ, Casale TB, Dahl R, et al. The Asthma Control Questionnaire as a clinical trial endpoint: past experience and recommendations for future use. Allergy. 2014;69:1119–1140.

92. Loymans RJ, Ter Riet G, Sterk PJ. Definitions of asthma exacerbations. Curr Opin Allergy Clin Immunol. 2011;11(3):181–186.

93. Adams RJ, Smith BJ, Ruffin RE. Factors associated with hospital admissions and repeat emergency department visits for adults with asthma. Thorax. 2000;55:566–573.

94. Khusial RJ, Honkoop PJ, van der Meer V, Snoeck-Stroband JB, Sont JK. Validation of online Asthma Control Questionnaire and Asthma Quality of Life Questionnaire. ERJ Open Research. 2020;6(1):00289–02019.

95. Nielsen M, Bårnes CB, Ulrik CS. Clinical characteristics of the asthma–COPD overlap syndrome: a systematic review. Int J Chron Obstruct Pulmon Dis. 2015;10:1443–1454.

96. Suissa S, Ernst P, Benayoun S, et al. Low-dose inhaled corticosteroids and the prevention of death from asthma. N Engl J Med. 2000;343:332–336.

97. Engelkes M, Janssens HM, de Jongste JC, et al. Medication adherence and the risk of severe asthma exacerbations: a systematic review. Eur Respir J. 2015;45:396–407.

98. Horne R. Compliance, adherence, and concordance: implications for asthma treatment. Chest. 2006;130(1 Suppl.):65S–72S.

99. Gamble J, Stevenson M, Heaney LG. A study of a multi-level intervention to improve non-adherence in difficult to control asthma. Respir Med. 2011;105:1308–1315.

100. Melvin E, Cushing A, Tam A, et al. Assessing the use of BreatheSmart® mobile technology in adult patients with asthma: a remote observational study. BMJ Open Resp Res. 2017;4:e000204.

101. Howard S, Lang A, Sharples S, et al. What are the pros and cons of electronically monitoring inhaler use in asthma? A multistakeholder perspective. BMJ Open Respir Res. 2016;3:e000159.

102. Gibson PG, Coughlan J, Wilson AJ, et al. Self-management education and regular practitioner review for adults with asthma. The Cochrane Library. 2003;2003(1):CD001117.
103. Bel EH. Smoking: a neglected cause of glucocorticoid resistance in asthma. Am J Respir Crit Care Med. 2003;168:1265–1266.
104. Orellano P, Quaranta N, Reynoso J, Balbi B, Vasquez J. Effect of outdoor air pollution on asthma exacerbations in children and adults: systematic review and multilevel meta-analysis. PLoS One. 2017;12(3):e0174050.
105. Bradley N, Dobney A, Exley K, et al. Review of interventions to improve outdoor air quality and public health. London: Public Health England, Wellington House; 2019. Online. Available: <https://assets.publishing.service.gov.uk/government/uploads/system/uploads/attachment_data/file/795185/Review_of_interventions_to_improve_air_quality.pdf>.
106. Peters U, Dixon AE, Forno E. Obesity and asthma. J Allergy Clin Immunol. 2018;141:1169–1179.
107. Stanescu S, Kirby SE, Thomas M, et al. A systematic review of psychological, physical health factors, and quality of life in adult asthma. NPJ Prim Care Respir Med. 2019;29:37.
108. Thomas M, Bruton A, Moffat M, et al. Asthma and psychological dysfunction. Prim Care Respir J. 2011;20:250–256.
109. Thomas M, McKinley RK, Mellor S, et al. Breathing exercises for asthma: a randomised controlled trial. Thorax. 2009;64:55–61.
110. Westby M, Benson M, Gibson P. Anticholinergic agents for chronic asthma in adults. Cochrane Database Syst Rev. 2004;2004(3):CD003269.
111. Chari VM, McIvor MA. Tiotropium for the treatment of asthma: patient selection and perspectives. Can Respir J. 2018;2018:3464960.
112. Adams N, Bestall J, Jones PW. Budesonide for chronic asthma in children and adults. Cochrane Database Syst Rev. 2001;2001(1):CD003274.
113. FDA requires Boxed Warning about serious mental health side effects for asthma and allergy drug montelukast (Singulair); advises restricting use for allergic rhinitis. March 2020. Online. Available: <https://www.fda.gov/drugs/drug-safety-and-availability/fda-requires-boxed-warning-about-serious-mental-health-side-effects-asthma-and-allergy-drug>.
114. Nelson HS, Busse WW, Kerwin E, et al. Fluticasone propionate/salmeterol combination provides more effective asthma control than low-dose inhaled corticosteroid plus montelukast. J Allergy Clin Immunol. 2000;106:1088–1095.
115. Gandhi N, Bennett B, Graham N, et al. Targeting key proximal drivers of type 2 inflammation in disease. Nat Rev Drug Discov. 2016;15:35–50.
116. McGregor MC, Krings JG, Nair P, Castro M. Role of biologics in asthma. Am J Respir Crit Care Med. 2019;199:433–445.
117. Ajeganova S, Huizinga T. Sustained remission in rheumatoid arthritis: latest evidence and clinical considerations. Ther Adv Musculoskelet Dis. 2017;9:249–262.
118. Anderson WC 3rd. Szefler SJ. Cost-effectiveness and comparative effectiveness of biologic therapy for asthma: to biologic or not to biologic? Ann Allergy Asthma Immunol. 2019;122:367–372.
119. Page CP, Edwards AM, Holgate ST. Xanthines, phosphodiesterase inhibitors and chromones. In: Burks AW, Holgate ST, O'Hehir RE, Broide DH, Bacharier LB, Hershey GKK, Peeples Jr. RS, eds. Middleton's allergy: principles and practice. 9th ed. New York: Elsevier; 2019:1525–1546.
120. O'Byrne PM, FitzGerald JM, Bateman ED, et al. Inhaled combined budesonide-formoterol as needed in mild asthma. N Engl J Med. 2018;378:1865–1876.
121. Pauwels RA, Pedersen S, Busse WW, et al. Early intervention with budesonide in mild persistent asthma: a randomised, double-blind trial. Lancet. 2003;361:1071–1076.
122. Emerman CL, Woodruff PG, Cydulka RK, et al. Prospective multicenter study of relapse following treatment for acute asthma among adults presenting to the emergency department. Chest. 1999;115:919–927.
123. Price D, Musgrave SD, Shepstone L, et al. Leukotriene antagonists as first-line or add-on asthma-controller therapy. N Engl J Med. 2011;364:1695–1707.
124. Greening AP, Ind PW, Northfield M, et al. Added salmeterol versus higher-dose corticosteroid in asthma patients with symptoms on existing inhaled corticosteroid. Allen & Hanburys Limited UK Study Group. Lancet. 1994;344:219–224.
125. Thomas M, von Ziegenweidt J, Lee AJ, et al. High-dose inhaled corticosteroids versus add-on long-acting beta-agonists in asthma: an observational study. J Allergy Clin Immunol. 2009;123:116–121.
126. Nelson HS, Weiss ST, Bleecker ER, SMART Study Group The Salmeterol Multicenter Asthma Research Trial: a comparison of usual pharmacotherapy for asthma or usual pharmacotherapy plus salmeterol. Chest. 2006;129:15–26.
127. McMahon AW, Levenson MS, McEvoy BW, et al. Age and risks of FDA-approved long-acting beta(2)-adrenergic receptor agonists. Pediatrics. 2011;128:e1147–e1154.
128. Chowdhury BA, Dal Pan G. The FDA and safe use of long-acting beta-agonists in the treatment of asthma. N Engl J Med. 2010;362:1169–1171.
129. Price DB, Hernandez D, Magyar P, et al. Randomised controlled trial of montelukast plus inhaled budesonide versus double dose inhaled budesonide in adult patients with asthma. Thorax. 2003;58:211–216.
130. Ram FS, Cates CJ, Ducharme FM. Long-acting beta2-agonists versus anti-leukotrienes as add-on therapy to inhaled corticosteroids for chronic asthma. Cochrane Database Syst Rev. 2005;2005(1):CD003137.
131. Faurschou P, Steffensen I, Jacques L. Effect of addition of inhaled salmeterol to the treatment of moderate-to-severe asthmatics uncontrolled on high-dose inhaled steroids. European Respiratory Study Group. Eur Respir J. 1996;9:1885–1890.
132. Wadhwa R, Dua K, Adcock IM, et al. Cellular mechanisms underlying steroid-resistant asthma. Eur Respir Rev. 2019;28:190021.
133. Galeone C, Scelfo C, Bertolini F, et al. Precision medicine in targeted therapies for severe asthma: Is there any place for "Omics" technology? Biomed Res Int. 2018;2018:4617565.
134. Pavord I, Bahmer T, Braido F, et al. Severe T2-high asthma in the biologics era: European experts' opinion. Eur Respir Rev. 2019;28:190054.
135. Casale TB. Biologics and biomarkers for asthma, atopic dermatitis, urticaria, and nasal polyposis. World Allergy Organization (WAO); April 2018. Online. Available: <https://www.worldallergy.org/education-and-programs/education/allergic-disease-resource-center/professionals/biologics-and-biomarkers>.
136. Busse WW. Biological treatments for severe asthma: A major advance in asthma care. Allergol Int. 2019;68:158–166.
137. Thomson NC. Recent developments in bronchial thermoplasty for severe asthma. J Asthma Allergy. 2019;12:375–387.
138. Passalacqua G, Rogkakou A, Mincarini M, Canonica GW. Allergen immunotherapy in asthma; what is new? Asthma Res Pract. 2015;1:6.

139. Reddel HK, FitzGerald JM, Bateman ED, et al. GINA 2019: a fundamental change in asthma management: treatment of asthma with short-acting bronchodilators alone is no longer recommended for adults and adolescents. Eur Respir J. 2019;53:1901046.

140. Asamoah F, Kakourou A, Dhami S, et al. Allergen immunotherapy for allergic asthma: a systematic overview of systematic reviews. Clin Transl Allergy. 2017;7:25.

141. Rhyou HI, Nam YH. Efficacy of Allergen immunotherapy for allergic asthma in real world practice. Allergy Asthma Immunol Res. 2020;12:99–109.

142. Lin SY, Azar A, Suarez-Cuervo C, et al. The role of immunotherapy in the treatment of asthma. Report No. 17(18)-EHC029-EF. Rockville, MD: Agency for Healthcare Research and Quality (USA); 2018.

143. Porcaro F, Corsello G, Pajno GB. SLIT's prevention of the allergic march. Curr Allergy Asthma Rep. 2018;18:31.

144. Schwarze J, Openshaw P, Jha A, et al. Influenza burden, prevention, and treatment in asthma-a scoping review by the EAACI Influenza in asthma task force. Allergy. 2018;73:1151–1181.

145. Sherenian MG, Singh AM, Arguelles L, et al. Food allergy is an independent risk factor for decreased lung function in children with asthma. Ann Allergy Asthma Immunol. 2018;121:588–593, e1.

146. Campbell RL, Kelso JM. Anaphylaxis: emergency treatment. UpToDate. 2020. Online. Available: <https://www.uptodate.com/contents/anaphylaxis-emergency-treatment>.

147. Szefler SJ, Chmiel JF, Fitzpatrick AM, et al. Asthma across the ages: knowledge gaps in childhood asthma. J Allergy Clin Immunol. 2014;133:3–13.

148. Gautier C, Charpin D. Environmental triggers and avoidance in the management of asthma. J Asthma Allergy. 2017;10:47–56.

149. Zuiani C, Custovic A. Update on house dust mite allergen avoidance measures for asthma. Curr Allergy Asthma Rep. 2020;20:50.

150. Tsou P-Y, McCormack MC, Matsui EC, et al. The effect of dog allergen exposure on asthma morbidity among inner-city children with asthma. Pediatr Allergy Immunol. 2020;31:210–213.

151. Research and Evidence Team RCPCH and RCP. Holgate ST and J Grigg, Working Party Co-chairs. The inside story: health effects of indoor air quality on children and young people. Online. Available: <https://www.rcpch.ac.uk/resources/inside-story-health-effects-indoor-air-quality-children-young-people>.

152. Morgan WJ, Crain EF, Gruchalla RS, et al. Inner-City Asthma Study Group. Results of a home-based environmental intervention among urban children with asthma. N Engl J Med. 2004;351:1068–1080.

153. Wright RJ, Cohen S, Carey V, et al. Parental stress as a predictor of wheezing in infancy: a prospective birth-cohort study. Am J Respir Crit Care Med. 2002;165:358–365.

154. Sandberg S, Paton JY, Ahola S, et al. The role of acute and chronic stress in asthma attacks in children. Lancet. 2000;356:982–987.

155. Douros K, Moustaki M, Tsabouri S, et al. Prenatal maternal stress and the risk of asthma in children. Front Pediatr. 2017;5:202.

156. Strunk RC. Death due to asthma. New insights into sudden unexpected deaths, but the focus remains on prevention. Am Rev Respir Dis. 1993;148:550–552.

157. Everard ML, Wahn U, Dorsano S, et al. Asthma education material for children and their families; a global survey of current resources. World Allergy Organ J. 2015;8:35.

158. Verberne AA, Frost C, Roorda RJ, et al. One year treatment with salmeterol compared with beclomethasone in children with asthma. Am J Respir Crit Care Med. 1997;156:688–695.

159. Castro-Rodriguez JA, Rodrigo GJ. Efficacy of inhaled corticosteroids in infants and preschoolers with recurrent wheezing and asthma: a systematic review with meta-analysis. Pediatrics. 2009;123:e519–e525.

160. Murray CS, Woodcock A, Langley SJ, et al. Secondary prevention of asthma by the use of Inhaled Fluticasone propionate in Wheezy INfants (IFWIN): double-blind, randomised, controlled study. Lancet. 2006;368:754–762.

161. Hossny E, Rosario N, Lee BW, et al. The use of inhaled corticosteroids in pediatric asthma: update. World Allergy Organ J. 2016;9:26.

162. Ni CM, Greenstone IR, Ducharme FM. Addition of inhaled long-acting beta2-agonists to inhaled steroids as first line therapy for persistent asthma in steroid-naive adults. Cochrane Database Syst Rev. 2005;2005(2):CD005307.

163. Masoli M, Weatherall M, Holt S, et al. Moderate dose inhaled corticosteroids plus salmeterol versus higher doses of inhaled corticosteroids in symptomatic asthma. Thorax. 2005;60:730–734.

164. Simons FE. A comparison of beclomethasone, salmeterol, and placebo in children with asthma. N Engl J Med. 1997;337:1659–1665.

165. Busse WW, Morgan WJ, Gergen PJ, et al. Randomized trial of omalizumab (anti-IgE) for asthma in inner-city children. N Engl J Med. 2011;364:1005–1015.

166. Henriksen DP, Bodtger U, Sidenius K, et al. Efficacy of omalizumab in children, adolescents, and adults with severe allergic asthma: a systematic review, meta-analysis, and call for new trials using current guidelines for assessment of severe asthma. Allergy Asthma Clin Immunol. 2020;16:49.

167. Abramson MJ, Puy RM, Weiner JM. Allergen immunotherapy for asthma. Cochrane Database Syst Rev. 2003;2003(4):CD001186.

168. Dorofeeva Y, Shilovskiy I, Tulaeva I, et al. Past, presence, and future of allergen immunotherapy vaccines. Allergy. 2020;76(1):131–149.

169. Del Giudice M, Licari A, Brambilla I, et al. Allergen immunotherapy in pediatric asthma: a pragmatic point of view. Children (Basel). 2020;7:58.

170. American Lung Association. Asthma trends and burden. 2020. Online. Available: <https://www.lung.org/research/trends-in-lung-disease/asthma-trends-brief/trends-and-burden#:~:text=a%20section...-,Asthma%20Mortality,higher%20among%20women%20than%20men>.

171. Barnett SB, Nurmagambetov TA. Costs of asthma in the United States: 2002–2007. J Allergy Clin Immunol. 2011;127:145–152.

172. Emerman CE, Cydulka RK, Crain EF, et al. Prospective multicenter study of relapse following treatment for acute asthma among children presenting to the emergency department. J Pediatr. 2001;138:318–324.

173. Rowe BH, Voaklander DC, Wang D, et al. Asthma presentations by adults to emergency departments in Alberta, Canada: a large population-based study. Chest. 2009;135:57–65.

174. Brenner BE, Chavda KK, Camargo CA Jr. Randomized trial of inhaled flunisolide versus placebo among asthmatics discharged from the emergency department. Ann Emerg Med. 2000;36:417–426.

175. Cates CJ, Crilly JA, Rowe BH. Holding chambers (spacers) versus nebulisers for beta-agonist treatment of acute asthma. Cochrane Database Syst Rev. 2006;2006(2):CD000052.

176. Camargo CA Jr, Spooner CH, Rowe BH. Continuous versus intermittent beta-agonists for acute asthma. Cochrane Database Syst Rev. 2003;4:CD001115.

177. Plotnick LH, Ducharme FM. Combined inhaled anticholinergic agents and beta-2-agonists for initial treatment of acute asthma in children. Cochrane Database Syst Rev. 2000;2000(2):CD000060.

178. Zaidan MF, Ameredes BT, Calhoun WJ. Management of acute asthma in adults in 2020. JAMA. 2020;323:563–564.

179. Rowe BH, Bretzlaff JA, Bourdon C, et al. Magnesium sulfate for treating exacerbations of acute asthma in the emergency department. Cochrane Database Syst Rev. 2000;2000(1):CD001490.

180. Parameswaran K, Belda J, Rowe BH. Addition of intravenous aminophylline to beta2-agonists in adults with acute asthma. Cochrane Database Syst Rev. 2000;2000(4):CD002742.

181. Hart SP. Should aminophylline be abandoned in the treatment of acute asthma in adults? QJM. 2000;93:761–765.

182. Graham V, Lasserson T, Rowe BH. Antibiotics for acute asthma. Cochrane Database Syst Rev. 2001;2001(3):CD002741.

183. Rowe BH, Bota GW, Clark S, et al. Comparison of Canadian versus American emergency department visits for acute asthma. Can Respir J. 2007;14:331–337.

184. Covar RA, Fuhlbrigge AL, Williams P, Kelly HW, Childhood Asthma Management Program Research Group The Childhood Asthma Management Program (CAMP): contributions to the understanding of therapy and the natural history of childhood asthma. Curr Respir Care Rep. 2012;1:243–250.

185. Rachelefsky G. Treating exacerbations of asthma in children: the role of systemic corticosteroids. Pediatrics. 2003;112:382–397.

186. Foresi A, Morelli MC, Catena E. Low-dose budesonide with the addition of an increased dose during exacerbations is effective in long-term asthma control. On behalf of the Italian Study Group. Chest. 2000;117:440–446.

187. Holgate ST, Walker S, West B, Boycott K. The future of asthma care: personalized asthma treatment. Clin Chest Med. 2019;40:227–241.

188. NICE asthma guideline: diagnosis and monitoring. National Institute for Health and Care Excellence (NICE). 20 February 2020. Online. Available: <https://www.guidelines.co.uk/respiratory/nice-asthma-guideline-diagnosis-and-monitoring/453872.article>.

189. Howard S, Lang A, Sharples S, et al. What are the pros and cons of electronically monitoring inhaler use in asthma? A multi-stakeholder perspective. BMJ Open Respir Res. 2016;3:e000159.

8

Allergic Rhinitis and Conjunctivitis

Jonathan Corren and Fuad M. Baroody

SUMMARY OF IMPORTANT CONCEPTS

- The incidence of chronic rhinitis has increased significantly since 2000, particularly in developed countries.
- Moderate to severe rhinitis has been shown to adversely affect performance at work and school, thereby contributing significantly to the indirect economic costs of this disease.
- Approximately 50% to 60% of patients with allergic rhinitis have associated symptoms of allergic conjunctivitis.
- The presence of rhinitis has significant effects on the development and severity of other disorders, including bronchial asthma, sinusitis, middle ear disease, and dental malocclusion.
- The two most common rhinitis syndromes are allergic rhinitis and idiopathic rhinitis, and differentiation of these two disorders requires an assessment of specific immunoglobulin E (IgE).
- A small subset of patients with rhinitis may have symptoms caused by strictly localized allergic mechanisms with no systemic evidence of specific IgE.
- Although rhinitis can be treated effectively with a number of medications, both over-the-counter and prescription products, allergen immunotherapy remains the only disease-modifying treatment capable of causing long-term improvement with respect to nasal symptoms and reduction in incident cases of asthma.

INTRODUCTION

Chronic rhinitis is an increasingly common condition that is now recognized to have a major impact on human health. Persistent nasal dysfunction may have significant effects on physical and emotional functioning, which result in absences from school and work, reduced worker productivity, and impaired school performance. In addition, chronic nasal inflammation may aggravate or lead to the development of other significant disorders, including asthma, rhinosinusitis, and middle ear disease. Recent improvements in current understanding of the pathologic mechanisms of rhinitis are providing key insights into the development of new treatments, including novel immunologic therapies. This chapter presents an overview of the epidemiology, diagnosis, pathophysiology, and treatment of allergic and non-allergic rhinitis and conjunctivitis.

HISTORIC PERSPECTIVE

John Bostock was an English physician who personally suffered from symptoms of "summer catarrh" every June, since childhood. He first described the symptoms of this new malady in 1819, which included nasal congestion, sneezing, and tiredness, which he believed were brought on by the exhausting heat of summer. In 1859, Charles Blackley, who also suffered from this recurrent ailment, became convinced that pollen was linked to these summer nasal symptoms, and that a toxin was the most likely culprit. In his 1873 volume *Experimental Researches on the Cause and Nature of Catarrhus Aestivus*, he reported the results of the first intranasal challenge with rye grass pollen and noted the immediate occurrence of profuse coryza followed by nasal blockage.[1] He then attempted the first effort at pollen immunotherapy by repeatedly applying pollen grains to his abraded skin, which was not effective. In 1911, Noon published the first seminal trial of immunotherapy with a grass pollen extract.[2] Following this study, injections of grass pollen extracts became accepted as an important treatment for seasonal rhinitis, and in 1954, Augustin presented the first double-blind, placebo-controlled trial of pollen extract injection to demonstrate efficacy.[3]

EPIDEMIOLOGY

Incidence and Prevalence

The increase in the prevalence of allergic diseases began to garner attention from epidemiologists in the late 1980s. The International Study of Asthma and Allergies in Childhood (ISAAC) was initiated to establish the prevalence of allergic diseases in 257,800 schoolchildren aged 6 to 7 years and in 463,801 children aged 13 to 14 years, using standardized, validated questionnaires.[4] The prevalence rates for rhinitis collected across all centers ranged from 0.8% to 14.9% (median, 6.9%) in the 6- to 7-year-olds and from 1.4% to 39.7% (median, 13.6%) in the 13- to 14-year-olds.[4] The highest prevalence rates for rhinitis were observed in parts of Western Europe, North America, and Australia, whereas the lowest rates were found in parts of Eastern Europe and south and central Asia. Select analyses revealed that the prevalence rates had increased, with 12-month

> ## BOX 8.1 Factors That Influence the Development of Allergic Rhinitis
>
> **Increased Risk**
> - Female sex
> - Particulate air pollution
> - Maternal smoking
>
> **Decreased Risk**
> - Increased number of siblings
> - Grass pollen exposure
> - Farm environment
> - Mediterranean diet

prevalence rates of 1.8% to 24.2% in children aged 6 to 7 years (median, 8.5%) and 1.0% to 45% (median, 14.6%) in 13- to 14-year-olds[5]; these findings strongly indicated that the prevalence of rhinitis had increased over a relatively short period of time, mostly in Westernized countries with a higher standard of living. In a subgroup analysis of 2810 German children followed from age 9 to 11 years until age 15 to 18 years,[6] the incidence of allergic rhinitis increased from an initial rate of 7% to 14%. These longitudinal data offer compelling evidence that the incidence of allergic rhinitis increases significantly as children grow from childhood into adolescence. A number of exposures in early childhood may act to increase the risk of developing rhinitis (Box 8.1).

Historically, the available data regarding the epidemiology of chronic rhinitis in adults are much more limited. Based on data for 15,394 adults of 20 to 44 years of age, in the European Community Respiratory Health Survey I (ECRHS I), the prevalence of allergic rhinitis ranged from 4.6% in Oviedo, Spain, to 31.8% in Melbourne, Australia.[7] In the most recent (US) National Health and Nutrition Examination Survey (NHANES), conducted from 2005 to 2006, the 12-month prevalence of rhinitis for the entire cohort was 23.5%, with a peak of 31.3% in patients 40 to 49 years of age.[8] For the group as a whole, 24% had seasonal rhinitis and 10% had perennial rhinitis.

Quality of Life and Economic Impact

Large, population-based studies have revealed that chronic rhinitis significantly impairs health-related quality of life. Questionnaires that focus on general quality of life (as used in the SF 36 Health Survey) have demonstrated significant decreases in physical functioning, energy, general health perception, social functioning, emotions, mental health, and pain in patients with moderate to severe perennial allergic rhinitis compared with control subjects.[9] Sleep loss may play a key role in determining quality of life, in that it may lead to daytime fatigue and poor concentration in school, resulting in learning impairment.[10]

Quality-of-life questionnaires have shown that chronic rhinitis may also influence mood and cognitive function. Studies conducted during and after the allergy season reveal that subjects with seasonal allergic rhinitis had significant decreases in verbal learning, decision-making speed, psychomotor speed, reaction time tests, and positive affect scores, as well as workplace productivity compared with those reported for non-allergic control subjects.[11]

Associated Diseases

Approximately 40% of patients with chronic rhinitis have asthma, and 80% of patients with asthma suffer with persistent nasal symptoms.[12] Allergic rhinitis, particularly perennial disease, is a significant independent risk factor for the development of asthma.[13] Nasal disease is also an important risk factor for worsening asthma in patients who have both rhinitis and asthma; the frequency of both emergency department visits and hospitalizations is greater in patients with moderate to severe rhinitis than in patients who have mild or no rhinitis.[14]

Rhinosinusitis is commonly identified in patients with allergic rhinitis. As many as 30% of patients with acute sinusitis, 67% with unilateral chronic sinusitis, and 80% with bilateral chronic sinusitis, have allergic rhinitis.[15] Nasal allergy most likely precipitates acute sinusitis by inducing sinus ostial edema, resulting in impairment of sinus drainage, a shift to anaerobic conditions inside of the sinus cavity, and finally bacterial proliferation. The relationship between allergy and chronic sinus disease is more complex and involves anti-staphylococcal IgE antibodies in some patients and persistent type-2 inflammation of the sinus mucosa.[16]

A considerable proportion of patients with allergic rhinitis have concomitant otitis media with effusion (OME).[17] Pollen exposure has been shown to cause eustachian tube dysfunction, which induces negative pressure in the middle ear space, followed by transudation of fluid.[18]

Adults and children with allergic rhinitis frequently have poor-quality sleep, including difficulty getting to sleep, waking up during the night, and lack of a "good night's sleep."[19] Nasal obstruction associated with allergic rhinitis has been shown to be a risk factor for a variety of problems during sleep, including microarousals, hypopneas, and apnea. Persistent, severe rhinitis in children may also cause chronic mouth breathing, particularly at night, which has been linked to alterations in the palatal anatomy and dental malocclusion.[20]

PATHOGENESIS AND ETIOLOGY

Sensitization of the nasal mucosa to certain airborne allergens entails multiple interactions between antigen presenting cells (i.e., dendritic cells), CD4 Th2 lymphocytes, and B cells that lead to the production of antigen-specific IgE antibodies, which then bind to mast cells and basophils.[21] Subsequent allergen exposure leads to cross-linking of specific IgE molecules on mast cells and their resultant degranulation, with the release of preformed mediators (e.g., histamine) and synthesis of newly generated mediators (e.g., leukotriene C4, prostaglandin D2). Other proinflammatory substances are also generated after allergen exposure, including toxic eosinophil products (e.g., eosinophil cationic protein) and cytokines (e.g., IL-4, -5, and -13). Cytokines are thought to be generated by both Th2 lymphocytes and by mast cells. Cytokines upregulate adhesion molecules on the vascular endothelium, and possibly on marginating leukocytes, and lead to the migration of these inflammatory cells,

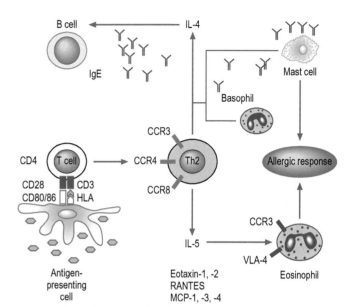

Fig. 8.1 Overview of pathophysiology of allergic rhinitis. *CCR,* Chemokine (C–C motif) receptor; *HLA,* human leukocyte antigen; *IgE,* immunoglobulin E; *IL,* interleukin; *MCP,* monocyte chemoattractant protein; *RANTES,* regulated on activation, normal T expressed and secreted; *Th2,* helper T cell type 2; *VLA-4,* very late antigen 4.

including lymphocytes, eosinophils, and basophils, into the site of tissue inflammation. Various cytokines will also promote the chemotaxis and survival of these recruited inflammatory cells and lead to a secondary immune response by virtue of their capability to promote IgE synthesis by B cells. The nervous system also plays an important role by amplifying and perpetuating allergic reactions. These inflammatory changes lower the threshold of mucosal responsiveness to various specific and nonspecific stimuli, making allergic patients more responsive to stimuli to which they are exposed every day (Fig. 8.1).

Clinical Features

Typical signs and symptoms of allergic rhinitis with or without conjunctivitis include some combination of congestion, sneezing, rhinorrhea (anterior and/or posterior), and pruritus of the nose, eyes, oral mucosa, or face and watering and redness of the eyes. Nasal congestion frequently alternates between both sides of the nose as a function of the physiologic nasal cycle.[22] In addition, during sleep, the dependent side of the nose may become preferentially obstructed. Persistent unilateral obstruction strongly suggests the possibility of an anatomic defect (e.g., nasal septal deviation, concha bullosa of the middle turbinate), inflammatory mass (e.g., nasal polyp), or tumor. Sneezing may be extremely variable but in allergic disease often marked by explosive paroxysms of 5 to 10 sneezes or more. In allergic rhinitis, rhinorrhea most often is clear to white in color, and the presence of purulent secretions strongly indicates the possibility of chronic sinusitis or atrophic rhinitis. Ocular signs and symptoms, including redness, itching, and watering, constitute a major cause of suffering in at least half of the patients with allergic rhinitis,[23] the presence of which will dramatically alter which therapy is selected. Other signs and symptoms, such as headache, a feeling of facial fullness, reduction in or loss of sense of smell, cough, and halitosis, should be noted because the presence of any of these will affect both the diagnosis and choice of treatment. When anosmia is the most prominent symptom and nasal or ocular symptoms are minimal or absent, primary central nervous system lesions should be considered.[24]

Once the spectrum of symptoms has been established, the presence of temporal patterns and specific triggers should be sought. Symptoms of allergic rhinitis often are most intense during the early morning hours as a consequence of circadian variations in inflammation.[25] Aggravation of symptoms while indoors and after exposure to house dust, furry pets, mildew, or cockroaches suggests the presence of IgE-mediated allergy to those specific allergens. Conversely, clear-cut worsening of symptoms in outside environments indicates the probability of allergy to an outdoor allergen such as pollen or mold. Occurrence of symptoms during well-demarcated seasons, as documented in the medical history, usually is diagnostic of allergic rhinitis that is due to an outdoor allergen. Symptoms that occur during the spring usually are ascribed to tree pollen exposure, in summer to grass and outdoor molds, and in fall to weeds and outdoor molds; precise start and stop dates of specific pollination seasons vary geographically.

A large number of triggers may act as irritants rather than as allergens, including volatile organic compounds (e.g., perfumes, paints, cleaning fluids)[26] and particulates (e.g., certain types of outdoor air pollution, construction dust). These substances may be important in provoking nasal symptoms in both allergic and non-allergic rhinitis patients (see below). Changes in climatic factors, such as temperature, humidity, and barometric pressure, are most important in patients with non-allergic rhinitis.[27]

Patient Evaluation, Diagnosis, and Differential Diagnosis

Physical Examination

The routine physical examination provides important information regarding both the cause and severity of rhinitis, as well as potential comorbid conditions, such as conjunctivitis, otitis media, and asthma. Additionally, in young children, the examination may suggest the presence of dental malocclusion and/or facial deformities (e.g., retracted mandible, high-arched palate) that may result from chronic, severe nasal obstruction.[28]

The nose should first be examined for outward signs of prior bony fractures (seen as deformities of the nasal bridge), asymmetry of the nostrils, and in children, a transverse crease over the lower portion of the nose caused by repetitive pushing of the nose upward in response to nasal itching or discharge. The interior of each nostril should be carefully examined using either a handheld otoscope or nasal speculum and headlamp. In patients with moderate to severe mucosal swelling of the inferior or middle turbinates, the examination also should be conducted after the instillation of a topical decongestant such as oxymetazoline. The nasal airway should be examined systematically, to look for and establish the degree of swelling and color of the mucosa; the presence, color, and consistency

of secretions; alterations in internal structures (e.g., septal deviation or perforation); and the presence of any abnormal mass lesions (e.g., nasal polyp) or foreign body. The mucosa in patients with symptomatic allergic rhinitis most often is swollen and pale in color, whereas patients with idiopathic rhinitis more typically have pink or erythematous mucous membranes. Great variability in appearance of the nasal airway is the rule, however, and these characteristics are not reliable for establishing a diagnosis. In patients with allergic rhinitis, the discharge is clear to white in color; the presence of discolored secretions suggests chronic rhinosinusitis (CRS). Crusting, particularly with dried blood, should alert the physician to the possibility of atrophic rhinitis. An anterior nasal septal deviation may be easily visible, whereas more posterior abnormalities may be detected only with flexible rhinoscopy or computed tomography (CT) imaging. Nasal polyps most commonly are seen coming from the superior portion of the airway and are not difficult to distinguish from turbinates by virtue of their gray, glistening, "grape-like" appearance.

Examination of the eyes reveals conjunctival injection in approximately half of patients with allergic rhinitis, which may be associated with erythema and bogginess of the upper and lower eyelids brought on by frequent rubbing. Cyanosis of the infraorbital tissues ("allergic shiners") is thought to be caused by venous stasis and may be seen with any chronic nasal or sinus disorder and is not pathognomonic of allergy.[29]

Fiberoptic Rhinoscopy

Visualization of the nasal airway with a rhinoscope may serve as a very useful adjunct to the routine examination.[30] Flexible rhinoscopes are employed regularly by otorhinolaryngologists, as well as some allergists and primary care physicians, and provide an enhanced view of structures in the superior and posterior regions of the nose. These normally unseen regions include the posterior nasal septum, superior nasal turbinates, middle meatus, adenoid gland, and eustachian tube orifices. Flexible rhinoscopy should therefore be considered in cases of rhinitis in which nasal obstruction is unilateral or refractory to therapy in the absence of any discernible anatomic cause on routine examination. Rigid rhinoscopes are used nearly exclusively by otorhinolaryngologists for visualizing the ostiomeatal complexes of the paranasal sinuses as well as performing nasal or sinus surgery.

Laboratory Testing

Testing for Specific Immunoglobulin E

Assessments of allergen-specific IgE are necessary to distinguish allergic rhinitis from non-allergic rhinitis. Allergy skin testing using the prick-puncture method is considered to provide the best combination of sensitivity and specificity, although in vitro testing has demonstrated comparable performance characteristics for some but not all allergens[31] (see Chapter 5 for a complete discussion of skin and in vitro testing). Although IgE most commonly is distributed systemically and can be identified by allergy skin testing or blood assays, in a subset of patients with allergic rhinitis, specific IgE can be identified only in the nose. This finding, referred to as *local allergic rhinitis*, or entopy, has been suspected for several decades but has only recently undergone rigorous investigation.[32] Nasal allergen challenge is required to clinically confirm this diagnosis, which is performed primarily in research settings. In the near future, this procedure may become part of the clinically accepted evaluation for patients with suspected local allergic rhinitis.

Blood Eosinophils and Total Serum Immunoglobulin E

Large, population-based studies reveal that mean concentrations of total serum IgE and circulating blood eosinophils are increased in allergic rhinitis. Although recent analyses have demonstrated utility using a combination of threshold values for total IgE and blood eosinophils,[33] a great deal of overlap with values in asymptomatic persons is typical, thereby limiting the diagnostic value of these markers.

Radiographic Imaging

The most accurate test for evaluating possible inflammation of the paranasal sinuses is CT.[34] Frequently, mild mucoperiosteal thickening can be seen in patients with uncomplicated allergic rhinitis and non-allergic rhinitis.[35] Radiographic studies should be considered in patients with symptoms that are not typical of rhinitis and are unresponsive to medical therapy, such as chronic purulent rhinorrhea, alterations in sense of smell, or headaches.

While both plain sinus films and ultrasonography of the maxillary sinuses have been shown to accurately predict acute maxillary sinusitis, neither method is useful for chronic disease.[36]

Other Tests

Histologic analyses of blown nasal secretions or scrapings taken from the inferior turbinates have been used historically but are no longer employed routinely in clinical practice. Similarly, tests of nasal patency, such as rhinomanometry or nasal peak flow, are not utilized frequently in clinical practice and are relegated primarily to research studies.

Differential Diagnosis of Allergic Rhinitis

For the classification of chronic rhinitis, see Box 8.2.

Work-Related Rhinitis

Rhinitis related to the workplace is characterized by intermittent or persistent nasal symptoms attributable to exposures incurred in a particular work environment.[37] Work-related rhinitis may be due to immunologic hypersensitivity, including the presence of IgE, or may be non-allergic in etiology. Occupations that carry a high risk for development of work-related rhinitis include laboratory workers, furriers, and bakers (Table 8.1). Diagnosis of work-related rhinitis relies heavily on a history of symptomatic worsening during the work week, with improvement over the weekend and during vacations, when the putative trigger is absent. Eventually, symptoms may persist during periods away from work as mucosal inflammation becomes more established. In situations in which the workplace exposure is a protein, skin or blood testing for specific IgE may be very helpful (see Chapter 14 for detailed commentary).

BOX 8.2 Differential Diagnosis of Chronic Rhinitis

Allergic
- Systemic
- Local (entopy)

Work-related
- Irritant
- Corrosive
- Immunologic

Infectious (Rhinosinusitis)
- Allergic
- Non-allergic

Non-allergic
- Idiopathic (vasomotor)
- Non-allergic with eosinophilia
- Atrophic
  - Primary
  - Secondary
- Medication-related
  - Topical vasoconstrictors (rhinitis medicamentosa)
  - Oral medications
- Exercise-induced
- Cold air–induced
- Gustatory
- Hormonal
- Aging
- Systemic diseases

TABLE 8.1 Occupations with Increased Prevalence of Work-Related Rhinitis

Category	Occupation	Likely Trigger
Irritant	Drywall installer	Gypsum dust
	Makeup artist	Cosmetic powder, perfume
Corrosive	Janitor	Ammonia
	Chemistry technician	Hydrochloric acid
Immunologic		
Immunoglobulin E	Baker	Grain flour
	Furrier	Animal dander
	Livestock breeder	Animal dander
	Veterinarian	Animal dander
	Food processing worker	Foodstuffs
	Pharmacist	Medication powders
Low-molecular-weight substances	Boat builder	Anhydrides

Chronic Rhinosinusitis With and Without Nasal Polyps

CRS is an inflammatory disease of the paranasal sinuses that has been present for 12 weeks or longer.[38] The four cardinal symptoms of CRS are mucopurulent drainage, nasal obstruction, facial discomfort, and decreased sense of smell; two of these must be present, along with CT or endoscopic evidence of sinus mucosal inflammation, in order to establish this diagnosis. Up to one-third of patients with CRS present with nasal polyps, and this subgroup of patients is more likely to experience alterations in the senses of smell and taste than patients without nasal polyps.[39] Usually, patients with CRS are less likely to have symptoms of sneezing and itching of the nasal, ocular, or oral cavity than patients with allergic rhinitis.

Non-Allergic Rhinitis

Idiopathic Non-Allergic Rhinitis (Vasomotor Rhinitis). Idiopathic non-allergic rhinitis, also referred to as vasomotor rhinitis, manifests with chronic or intermittent symptoms of nasal congestion and/or watery rhinorrhea that worsen acutely in response to non-specific provocateurs, including cold air, exercise, pungent odors, smoke, alcohol, and specific physiologic states, such as sexual arousal and emotional upset.[40] One trigger, which deserves special mention, is eating, which most often causes isolated watery discharge and has been referred to as gustatory rhinitis. Patients with idiopathic rhinitis have negative responses on skin or blood tests for specific IgE, including to potential food allergens, although occasionally patients may exhibit a small number of positive reactions that do not correlate with the clinical pattern of symptoms and are considered clinically irrelevant.

Non-Allergic Rhinitis with Eosinophilia. Studies of nasal histopathology reveal that one-third of patients with non-allergic rhinitis have an increased percentage of eosinophils, a condition that has previously been referred to as "non-allergic rhinitis with eosinophilia" or "eosinophilic non-allergic rhinitis."[41] Nasal congestion and discharge are the most frequently reported symptoms, and these patients develop nasal polyps more frequently than other groups of rhinitis patients. It has been speculated, that at least in some cases, non-allergic rhinitis with eosinophilia may represent local allergic rhinitis with local IgE to an unknown allergen. As cytologic analyses of nasal mucus or epithelium are not performed routinely in clinical practice, this subtype of non-allergic rhinitis is not usually identified by physicians.

Atrophic Rhinitis. Atrophic rhinitis is a chronic condition characterized by symptoms of nasal crusting, purulent discharge, nasal obstruction, and halitosis.[42] Primary atrophic rhinitis is most prevalent in areas with prolonged warm seasons, including south Asia and the Middle East and is more common in women. Although primary atrophic rhinitis has no known specific cause, many patients are found to have chronic bacterial infection of the nose and sinuses due to any of a large number of organisms, the most common of which is *Klebsiella ozaenae*. Secondary atrophic rhinitis presents with symptoms similar to those noted above and is the more common form of this disease in the developed world. It is most likely to occur in older patients who have undergone multiple or aggressive nasal surgeries,[42] nasal trauma, or nasal irradiation; in the case of nasal surgery, it has been referred to as the "empty nose syndrome."

Rhinitis Associated With Drugs. Repetitive use of topical α-adrenergic decongestant nasal sprays (e.g., oxymetazoline, phenylephrine) for more than a few days may result in rebound nasal congestion,[43] most likely secondary to downregulation of the α-agonist receptor. With long-term use of these agents, patients may develop a chronic form of rhinitis referred to as

TABLE 8.2 Medications Associated With Chronic Nasal Symptoms

Category	Example(s)
Antihypertensives	Angiotensin-converting enzyme inhibitors
	β-Adrenergic blockers
	Amiloride
	Prazosin
	Hydralazine
Psychotropics	Risperidone
	Chlorpromazine
	Amitriptyline
Phosphodiesterase-5 inhibitors	Sildenafil
	Tadalafil
	Vardenafil
Nonsteroidal antiinflammatory drugs	Ibuprofen
Others	Gabapentin

rhinitis medicamentosa. This disorder most often manifests with severe nasal congestion and occasionally nasal discomfort without other significant symptoms. Cocaine use also has been implicated in causing rhinitis medicamentosa but usually results in significantly more crusting, bleeding, and ultimately septal perforation than topical decongestant drugs. Physical examination in patients with rhinitis medicamentosa often reveals swollen, red nasal mucous membranes with minimal discharge.[43]

A number of systemic medications have been shown to be associated with increased nasal symptoms, particularly congestion and rhinorrhea.[44] General classes of medications that have been implicated in causing rhinitis symptoms include antihypertensives, drugs for erectile dysfunction, psychiatric drugs, and nonsteroidal antiinflammatory drugs (Table 8.2).

Hormonal Rhinitis. Approximately 20% to 30% of pregnant women will develop rhinitis of pregnancy, defined as new-onset nasal symptoms (usually congestion and/or rhinorrhea) in the absence of another known cause that lasts ≥6 weeks and resolves within 2 weeks after delivery.[45] Uncontrolled rhinitis during pregnancy may be a cause of severe snoring, which has been associated with an increased risk of gestational hypertension, preeclampsia, and intrauterine growth retardation.[46] Although abundant data are available to link pregnancy to nasal symptoms, much less is known regarding the relationship between the menstrual cycle or use of exogenous ovarian hormones (i.e., oral contraceptives, hormone replacement therapy) and rhinitis.

The relationship between rhinitis and hypothyroidism and other abnormal hormonal states has not been substantiated by research.

Rhinitis Related to Systemic Disease. A number of systemic diseases may be occasionally associated with symptoms of rhinitis. These include granulomatous diseases (e.g., granulomatosis with polyangiitis, sarcoidosis, midline granuloma), cystic fibrosis, ciliary dyskinesia syndromes, and immunodeficiencies. In most of these conditions, both the nose and sinus cavities are affected. In these disorders, patients often present with

BOX 8.3   Anatomic Abnormalities Causing Nasal Obstruction

- Concha bullosa
- Nasal septal deviation
- Adenoidal enlargement
- Nasal polyps
- Nasal cancer
- Nasal foreign body

multisystem involvement, particularly the lungs and associated constitutional complaints, such as fatigue and poor appetite.

Nasal and Pharyngeal Structural Abnormalities

A number of anatomic abnormalities in the nose and pharynx can cause chronic partial or complete nasal blockage without other significant symptoms (Box 8.3). Concha bullosa (aeration of the middle turbinate bones with expansion of the turbinates) has been shown to be present in varying degrees in approximately two-thirds of the general population; in a small number of affected persons, however, the condition is extensive enough to result in unilateral or bilateral nasal obstruction.[47] Nasal septal deviation can be identified in nearly 20% of people, but only a small fraction of that group will have significant symptoms.[47] Adenoidal enlargement may cause some degree of nasal obstruction in approximately 50% of children; the majority of these will resolve spontaneously without the need for surgical intervention.[48] Children presenting with chronic unilateral nasal obstruction should be evaluated for a possible foreign body in the nose, with the most common examples including peanuts, beads, and buttons. Nasal cancers are very rare with a prevalence of 0.001%.[49] Nasal cancer should be suspected in older persons with unilateral nasal obstruction and bleeding of gradual onset.

Differential Diagnosis of Allergic Conjunctivitis
Other Allergy-Associated Forms of Conjunctivitis

Three allergy-associated forms of conjunctivitis may occasionally be difficult to differentiate from typical allergic conjunctivitis. Vernal keratoconjunctivitis is usually a more severe conjunctival disorder that most often affects young males living in warm climates.[50] Symptoms include ocular itching, mucus discharge, and cobblestoning of the eye, which may vary in severity according to the seasons. Giant papillary conjunctivitis represents a hypersensitivity reaction to medical appliances placed on or into the eyes, including contact lenses and ocular implants. The most common symptoms include itching and a gritty sensation.[51] Atopic keratoconjunctivitis can affect the conjunctiva, cornea, and eyelid, and is most commonly diagnosed in middle-aged adults (30–50 years of age) with atopic dermatitis.[52] Patients usually complain of severe itching of the eyes with associated thickening and lichenification of the eyelids.

Infectious Conjunctivitis

Viral infections may be either unilateral or bilateral, while bacterial conjunctivitis usually affects one eye.[53] Most types of bacterial and viral conjunctivitis are self-limited and do not have significant pruritus. In most cases, bacterial infections are associated with purulent discharge, while viral conjunctivitis is characterized by a clear, watery discharge and may be occasionally difficult to distinguish from acute allergic conjunctivitis.

Dry Eye Syndrome

Dry eye syndrome, or xerophthalmia, may present as an isolated finding or may present as part of a systemic disease, such as Sjögren syndrome or sarcoidosis.[54] Dry eyes are capable of minimal tear production, creating a sensation of grittiness and discomfort. Medications, particularly those with anticholinergic side effects, are a frequent cause of dry eye syndrome and patients should undergo a trial of discontinuation before embarking on an in-depth evaluation. A Schirmer test is a convenient and inexpensive method for documenting dry eyes.

Blepharitis

Anterior blepharitis occurs at the front edge of the eyelid where the eyelashes are attached, while posterior blepharitis affects the inner edge of the eyelid that comes in contact with the eyeball.[55] Individuals with blepharitis experience a gritty or burning sensation in their eyes, excessive tearing, itching and swelling of the eyelids, or crusting of the eyelids. The prominent inflammation of the lids and lesser degree of eye involvement help distinguish blepharitis from allergic conjunctivitis.

Toxic Conjunctivitis

Toxic conjunctivitis is an irritant reaction to ocular medications, which usually occurs after long periods of use.[56] The most commonly implicated agents are preservatives in eye medications, contact lens solutions, and artificial tears. The findings are non-specific and consist of conjunctival erythema, mucus discharge, and itching. The eyelids can eventually become swollen, thickened, and excoriated, findings that are uncommon in allergic conjunctivitis.

Ocular Rosacea

Ocular rosacea commonly presents with burning, itching, sensation of a foreign body, dryness, tearing, or photophobia and may occasionally occur in the absence of rosacea elsewhere on the face.[57] Physical findings include conjunctival erythema, blepharitis, and lid margin telangiectasias.

Keratitis

Keratitis, defined as inflammation of the cornea, most often occurs in response to contact lens use but may also be associated with Herpes simplex infections.[58] This condition typically presents with unilateral findings, often consisting of intense erythema and pain, and may be associated with vision loss. The presence of corneal infiltrates distinguishes this condition from allergic conjunctivitis.

Angle Closure Glaucoma

Angle closure glaucoma may present with injection of the affected eye, but is most always associated with severe unilateral eye pain and vision loss due to corneal edema.[59]

TREATMENT

Allergen Avoidance

Multiple measures for allergen avoidance have been advocated and are most commonly directed at house-dust mites, animal danders, and molds. All environmental control recommendations should be predicated upon a positive finding to an allergy skin test or in vitro test.

House-dust mites (*Dermatophagoides farinae* and *Dermatophagoides pteronyssinus*) are found in most places with relative indoor humidity levels higher than 45%. These microscopic arachnids are found in highest concentrations in carpeting, pillows, mattresses (including foam mattresses), and upholstered furniture. As mite allergen proteins are quite large and heavy, they are unlikely to become airborne for any significant lengths of time. Recent studies have demonstrated that single measures, such as pillow encasings, are not effective in reducing symptoms in patients with allergic rhinitis.[60] However, the simultaneous combination of multiple interventions, including pillow and mattress encasings, acaricidal sprays and powders for carpeting, and frequent washing of bed linens in hot water are beneficial in reducing rhinitis symptoms due to dust mites.[61] High-efficiency particulate air (HEPA) filters have never been shown to be helpful in dust mite-induced rhinitis.

Nearly 50% of American households own at least one cat, and 25% of allergic rhinitis sufferers are allergic to cats. One study of cat allergen avoidance measures demonstrated that a combination of carpet removal, frequent washing of bedding, and washing the cat resulted in large reductions of levels of major cat allergen with an attendant reduction of rhinitis symptoms.[62] HEPA filters used as a solitary measure, however, have not been found to be effective.[63] Overall, the most practical and effective approach to reduction of indoor cat allergen is removal of the cat from the indoor environment. Even this measure, however, may not be immediately effective because residual allergen may remain at relatively high levels in the carpeting and upholstered furniture for several months or longer.[63] After removal of the cat, therefore, all carpeting should be removed and upholstered furniture cleaned.

Indoor mold growth usually results from water intrusion into the living space. Air sampling can accurately identify relevant species and numbers of spores in water-damaged buildings. When mold growth affects large areas of the indoor environment, abatement of damaged areas and corrective measures to prevent future water leakage are often beneficial in reducing rhinitis symptoms in mold-allergic individuals.

Exposure to outdoor allergens, such as grass, tree and weed pollens, and outdoor mold spores, is very difficult to control. Avoidance of outdoor activity during peak pollen hours (usually between 11:00 h and 15:00 h) may be helpful in some patients. In general, however, allergy to these ubiquitous triggers is therefore best addressed with pharmacotherapy and/or immunotherapy.

Pharmacotherapy

Antihistamines

H_1-antihistamines act as inverse agonists that combine with and stabilize the inactive conformation of the H1-receptor, shifting the equilibrium toward the inactive state.[64] They are commonly used in the treatment of allergic rhinitis and conjunctivitis.

Oral H_1-antihistamines have been shown to reduce histamine-mediated symptoms and signs such as sneezing, itching, rhinorrhea, and eye symptoms but are not as effective in alleviating nasal congestion.[65] They are rapidly absorbed after oral administration and usually begin to provide relief within 1 to 2 h. Oral H_1-antihistamines also have been shown to be safe and effective in children, and many are available in liquid form.[66] The side effects of first-generation antihistamines (e.g., diphenhydramine) can be bothersome and include sedation and anticholinergic effects, such as constipation, dry mouth and eyes, and urinary outlet obstruction. Newer antihistamines have a low reported incidence of sedation as well as minimal or no anticholinergic effects. First-generation antihistamines produce significant performance impairment in school and while driving, and their use has been associated with increased car and occupational accidents.[67] Furthermore, the anticholinergic effects of these agents (and those of other medications with anticholinergic effects) have recently been associated with a higher risk of dementia.[68] Based on the unfavorable side effect profile, newer practice parameters support the use of second-generation over first-generation antihistamines for the treatment of allergic rhinitis.

H_1-antihistamines are also available for intranasal administration. Azelastine hydrochloride and olopatadine hydrochloride both have a more rapid onset of action than oral antihistamines, usually within 15 to 30 min, and result in significant reduction of nasal congestion as well as itching, sneezing, and runny nose. These medications may cause alteration of taste sensation and occasionally somnolence.[69,70]

Decongestants

Decongestants reduce nasal congestion but have no other significant effects on the symptoms of rhinitis. Both topical and systemic decongestants act by α-adrenergic stimulation, which results in vascular constriction and a reduction of nasal blood supply to the sinusoids. Topical decongestants can be either catecholamines (such as phenylephrine) or imidazoline derivatives (such as xylometazoline or oxymetazoline) and have a more rapid onset of action and stronger effect than systemic decongestants. Topical decongestants do not have systemic side effects; however, in children there have been rare case reports of seizures. When these agents are used for longer than 5 days, rebound nasal congestion may develop in some patients. Therefore, topical decongestants should be used primarily to reduce nasal congestion in patients with acutely severe rhinitis in order to facilitate the penetration of intranasal corticosteroids or antihistamines.

Oral decongestants do not cause rebound congestion but are not as effective as topical formulations. Agents that combine an oral decongestant, usually pseudoephedrine, with an antihistamine are frequently used for the treatment of acute and chronic rhinitis due to a variety of causes. Phenylephrine, another oral decongestant, is available over-the-counter, but a meta-analysis has shown lack of efficacy on objective and subjective measures of nasal congestion compared to placebo.[71] The most common side effects of oral decongestants are insomnia and irritability, which can occur in as many as 25% of patients taking these medications. At normal doses, aggravation of hypertension and cardiac arrhythmias may occur. Taken in overdose, these agents may result in renal failure, psychosis, strokes, and seizures. They should therefore be largely avoided in patients with hypertension, heart disease, seizure disorders, hyperthyroidism, and prostatic hypertrophy and in those taking monoamine oxidase inhibitors. Because of the potential of converting pseudoephedrine into methamphetamines, products containing this decongestant are sold behind the counter in the US.

Intranasal Corticosteroids

Intranasal corticosteroids are the most potent drugs available for the management of allergic rhinitis, and have been shown to significantly reduce all nasal symptoms of allergic rhinitis. In comparative studies in allergic rhinitis, intranasal steroids (INSs) have been shown to be superior in efficacy to both H_1-antihistamines[72] and leukotriene receptor antagonists.[73] An unexpected benefit of use of INSs in patients with allergic rhinitis is a significant reduction in concomitant allergic ocular symptoms[74] (see Medications for Ocular Symptoms, later). INSs begin to have effects within 7 to 8 hours of dosing, although some reports demonstrate an effect within 2 hours.[75] Although continuous use is usually recommended, some studies have demonstrated that as-needed use of intranasal fluticasone propionate is superior to placebo.[76] The main side effects of INSs include local nasal irritation (in 5%–10% of patients) and epistaxis (4%–8%). In patients with perennial rhinitis treated with fluticasone propionate or mometasone furoate continuously for 1 year, nasal mucosal biopsy specimens showed no evidence of atrophy and normalization of the epithelium.[77] Rarely, septal perforations and *Candida* overgrowth have been reported. With regard to potential systemic effects, INSs that have been subjected to rigorous study have not been shown to affect parameters such as growth in children.[78] Despite these reassuring findings, it is recommended that pediatric patients receiving INSs be evaluated every 6 months using a stadiometer to monitor growth.

INSs also have been shown to be effective in the treatment of non-allergic rhinitis. Among the available preparations, fluticasone propionate and fluticasone furoate are approved by the Food and Drug Administration (FDA) for the treatment of non-allergic rhinitis in addition to allergic rhinitis.

Systemic Corticosteroids

The role of systemic steroids in the treatment of rhinitis is limited because of their adverse effects and the limited morbidity of the disease. They are best reserved for patients with any type of rhinitis who present initially with severe nasal obstruction. A short course of oral prednisone, 30 mg daily for 3 to 5 days, usually will significantly decrease nasal edema and allow for enhanced penetration of INS.

Intramuscular injections of corticosteroids have been a popular therapy, dating back many years. Data demonstrating efficacy are limited, however. Use of intramuscular injections of depot steroids generally should be avoided for the treatment of seasonal allergic rhinitis because of the risk of rare but potentially catastrophic side effects, particularly aseptic necrosis of the femoral head. In addition, as seasonal rhinitis is usually a life-long disease, patients who request and receive this treatment

multiple times per year for many years may be at increased risk for long-term effects of systemic corticosteroids, such as cataracts and osteoporosis.

Leukotriene Inhibitors

Montelukast has comparable efficacy with oral antihistamines for the relief of all ocular and nasal symptoms of allergic rhinitis, including congestion, rhinorrhea, and sneezing.[79] It is less effective than INSs. As montelukast is also approved for the treatment of asthma, it may be an effective first-line treatment in patients with both allergic rhinitis and asthma. Newer guidelines do not recommend montelukast as monotherapy for the initial treatment of allergic rhinitis and reserve its use for patients who are not treated effectively, or cannot tolerate alternative therapies.[67] When using montelukast, one should be aware of postmarketing reports of rare drug-induced neuropsychiatric events.[80]

Cromolyn Sodium

Intranasal cromolyn sodium 4% solution is available over-the-counter and has been shown to be clinically effective in the treatment of allergic rhinitis. As with antihistamines, it is more helpful for sneezing, itching, and rhinorrhea and less effective in relieving nasal congestion. Treatment is most effective when dosing is started before the onset of symptoms. The recommended dosage frequency is four times daily, leading to compliance problems, but the drug is very safe, especially in children and pregnant women.

Anticholinergics

Anticholinergic drugs are useful in the treatment of those patients in whom rhinorrhea is the predominant complaint. Ipratropium bromide has little or no systemic effect when administered intranasally and has been shown to be effective in controlling watery nasal discharge in perennial allergic rhinitis.[81] It has no effect, however, on sneezing, itching, or nasal congestion. Ipratropium can be used in conjunction with drugs of other classes, such as antihistamines or INSs, for the treatment of rhinorrhea in patients with allergic rhinitis.

Ipratropium bromide also is useful for the treatment of watery discharge that occurs in patients with perennial non-allergic rhinitis.[82] In addition, ipratropium has been found to effectively reduce rhinorrhea associated with gustatory rhinitis and rhinorrhea induced by exposure to cold, dry air.[83]

Medications for Ocular Symptoms

Oral H_1-antihistamines and leukotriene receptor antagonists have demonstrated efficacy in reducing ocular redness, tearing, and itch. Topical ocular antihistamines frequently are prescribed as adjunctive agents for patients with rhinoconjunctivitis and as the primary medication for patients with isolated allergic conjunctivitis.[84] As would be expected with topical therapy, these drugs begin to work within a few minutes and have a 12- to 24-hour duration of action. The various agents are available as both over-the-counter and prescription products.

INSs also have been shown to have significant effects in reducing allergic eye symptoms. In a meta-analysis comparing oral H_1-antihistamines and INSs for the control of ocular symptoms, no difference was found in the efficacy of these two classes.[72] The mechanism of this favorable effect of INSs is speculated to be reduced intranasal inflammation, which in turn inhibits the nasal ocular reflex initiated by allergen contact to the nasal mucosa.

Combinations of Medications

Often, a single pharmacologic agent does not effectively reduce symptoms of rhinitis. As noted above, oral antihistamines are frequently combined with oral decongestants to treat allergic rhinitis. The combination of an INS plus an intranasal antihistamine, including both azelastine and olopatadine, has been shown to be more effective than either agent given alone.[85] A combination spray composed of fluticasone propionate and azelastine hydrochloride is commercially available. In clinical practice, oral antihistamines frequently are combined with INSs in patients who do not respond to antihistamines alone. Nevertheless, studies of INS given together with oral H_1-antihistamines, including loratadine and cetirizine, have not shown that the combination is significantly better than INS given alone.[86] Recent guidelines do not recommend the combination of oral antihistamines and INSs. When an oral antihistamine (with or without decongestant) does not provide relief for allergic rhinitis symptoms, one should switch to an INS and discontinue the oral antihistamine. Similarly, when an INS alone is not sufficient to control symptoms, one should add an intranasal antihistamine, and not an oral one.[67]

With respect to combination treatment of eye symptoms, intranasal fluticasone propionate plus intraocular olopatadine was significantly more effective than the combination of fluticasone and fexofenadine, tested using an ocular challenge model.[87]

Allergen Immunotherapy

Specific allergen immunotherapy has been shown to be effective in seasonal and perennial allergic rhinitis.[67] The principal advantages of immunotherapy over pharmacotherapy are that it generally is more efficacious and that two consecutive years of treatment results in persistent tolerance.[88] Immunotherapy should be considered in a number of clinical scenarios, including severe allergic rhinitis unresponsive to usual pharmacotherapy and allergen avoidance measures; allergic rhinitis complicated by other disorders, particularly new-onset or worsening asthma; and occurrence of significant adverse effects from medications for rhinitis. In addition, in patients who desire a more lasting improvement in their allergic rhinitis, a strong case can be made that immunotherapy is a cost-effective alternative to pharmacotherapy.[89] Subcutaneous immunotherapy is the predominant route of administration employed in the US, although sublingual immunotherapy is now commercially available with ragweed, northern pasture grasses, and house-dust mites. Experimental comparisons between these two modes of delivery, as well as studies of which allergens provide optimal efficacy, are ongoing and conceivably will resolve many of the controversies that currently exist (see Chapter 6 for detailed commentary).

Surgery

Individuals with a significant anatomic nasal defect (e.g., nasal septal deviation) may require surgery if nasal obstruction is of a degree that adversely affects quality of life. In patients with chronic rhinitis, in the absence of a structural abnormality, surgery is rarely indicated. Turbinate reduction surgery should be used in patients with refractory mucosal edema only if pharmacotherapy and immunotherapy have been tried and failed.

Overall Approach to Treatment
Allergic Rhinitis

The following approach to treatment is based on recent national and global recommendations (Fig. 8.2).[67] In patients with *mild, intermittent* symptoms of allergic rhinitis who complain primarily of rhinorrhea or sneezing, an oral or topical intranasal antihistamine, taken as needed, often is very effective. In patients with intermittent symptoms of nasal congestion, an intranasal antihistamine or an antihistamine-decongestant combination pill, taken as needed, may be helpful. If persistent symptoms are present, particularly nasal congestion, an INS given regularly is usually most effective.

Patients with *moderate* to *severe* symptoms should be reevaluated after 2 to 4 weeks to assess their response to therapy. With an excellent response, anticipated exposures should be considered and the patient treated accordingly. With a partial response, residual complaints should be identified and targeted with specific medications. For significant eye symptoms, an intraocular antihistamine can be taken as needed. If significant redness of the eye persists, referral to an ophthalmologist should be considered. For residual nasal congestion, the addition of an intranasal antihistamine may be the most useful of all options. If rhinorrhea persists as a primary problem, ipratropium bromide may provide additional benefit. If the patient does not improve after maximal medical therapy, the diagnosis should be reconsidered, along with the need for additional diagnostic testing

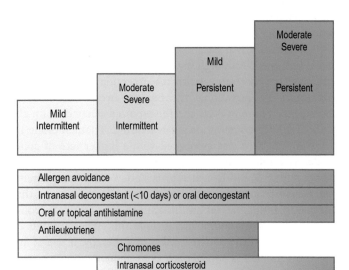

Fig. 8.2 Stepped therapy for allergic rhinitis.

(e.g., CT of the sinuses or nasal endoscopy). For refractory allergic rhinitis that fails to respond to the foregoing treatments, in the absence of obvious complicating factors, consideration for allergen immunotherapy is in order. A stepped-care approach to the treatment of allergic rhinitis is shown in Fig. 8.2.

Non-Allergic Rhinitis

In patients with persistent anterior or posterior discharge associated with any of the forms of non-allergic rhinitis, particularly when it is thick in consistency, nasal irrigation with saline may be very helpful. Nasal saline washes are also extremely important in the management of nasal crusting, as seen in atrophic rhinitis. Nasal saline may have no effect on nasal congestion, however, and other medications will be important in alleviating this symptom.

In patients with chronic congestion, an INS or intranasal azelastine should be administered as a first-line pharmacologic agent, used on an intermittent basis. As in allergic rhinitis, if either agent alone is not completely effective, the addition of the other drug may be useful.

In patients with intermittent acute, watery rhinorrhea caused by irritant or cold air exposure, exercise, or food, ipratropium bromide used before symptoms occur can be very effective.

For patients using medications for systemic diseases, such as antihypertensives, a change in therapy should be considered. If, however, a particular medication is deemed necessary and irreplaceable, the nasal side effects may need to be medicated. This is best accomplished with topical therapy in order to avoid drug interactions and/or additional systemic adverse effects.

Treatment Considerations in Select Populations
Pregnancy

In pregnant women with rhinitis, non-drug therapies should be tried first. Nasal rinsing with normal saline helps to remove thick nasal secretions, and over-the-counter mechanical nasal dilators[90] may improve nasal congestion and snoring at night in some women. In many women, medications will still be required. Nasal cromolyn, one spray four times daily, should be tried next, because of its excellent safety profile and FDA pregnancy category B rating.[91] If a 2-week course of cromolyn is not helpful, particularly if nasal congestion is present, a trial of an INS is indicated. Although most INS are given an FDA pregnancy category C rating (with the exception of budesonide, in category B), gestational risk has not been confirmed in observational human data, and the reported safety data on all of the available compounds are reassuring. Triamcinolone is an exception, as it was associated with a higher rate of congenital respiratory defects in a large Canadian prospective cohort study.[92] When INS therapy is started during pregnancy, budesonide frequently is the drug of choice because of the category B rating.[93] Oral antihistamines may be worth considering if primary complaints include rhinorrhea, sneezing, and pruritus and the patient prefers oral therapy. If use of an oral antihistamine is appropriate, both diphenhydramine and chlorpheniramine have a very long record of use in pregnancy and frequently are the drugs of choice for obstetric patients.[94] In a significant subset of women, however, the central nervous system and anticholinergic effects of these agents will prove difficult to tolerate. Loratadine and cetirizine have been extensively studied during pregnancy, and both belong to pregnancy category B. Topical antihistamines, including olopatadine and azelastine, do not have a long history of use in pregnancy and belong to FDA category C. For these reasons, the other medications listed here would be considered more appropriate choices in pregnancy. Oral decongestants should be avoided, if possible, during the first trimester because of conflicting reports of an association of phenylephrine and pseudoephedrine with congenital malformations such as gastroschisis, small intestinal atresia, limb reduction defects, endocardial cushion defects, and pyloric stenosis. Specific allergen immunotherapy for allergic rhinitis may be continued during pregnancy if it is providing significant benefit and has not caused systemic reactions. Allergen extract doses should be maintained and not increased until the completion of the pregnancy. For these same reasons, immunotherapy should not be started during pregnancy.

Elderly

Two of the most important aspects of treating rhinitis in older patients are improving intranasal moisture content and removing dried secretions.[95] Nasal irrigation using buffered saline or a saline nasal spray should be used by most elderly people with chronic rhinitis, particularly those with non-allergic rhinitis. INS, although generally safe, may cause more bleeding than is usually seen in younger patients, owing to the increased fragility of the nasal mucous membranes in this population. In general, older-generation oral antihistamines should be avoided because of their potential to sedate or cause anticholinergic effects. Oral decongestants should be similarly avoided owing to possible adverse effects on blood pressure (hypertension), cardiac rhythm (extrasystoles, arrhythmias), central nervous system (insomnia, agitation), and urinary tract (obstruction).

INDICATIONS FOR REFERRAL

A number of different patient profiles should be considered for referral to an allergist: (1) patients whose rhinitis symptoms have not responded adequately to combination pharmacotherapy; (2) patients with significant adverse side effects due to pharmacotherapy; (3) patients with secondary complications from their rhinitis, including recurrent or chronic sinusitis, nasal polyposis, recurrent or persistent middle ear disease, and poorly controlled asthma; and (4) patients with positive in vitro or skin tests to a perennial allergen in order to consider and implement a program of allergen avoidance. In addition, because of the significant cost savings associated with allergen immunotherapy for allergic rhinitis, any patient requiring year-around, long-term treatment with combination therapy should also be considered for referral to an allergist. Referral to an otolaryngologist is most important when surgical treatment for nasal polyposis, chronic sinusitis, significant adenoidal enlargement, or anatomic obstructions is being considered (Box 8.4).

BOX 8.4 Indications for Referral

To Allergist/Immunologist

1. Poor response to multiple medications for rhinitis
2. Significant drug-related side effects
3. Secondary complications of rhinitis, including:
   a. Chronic sinusitis/nasal polyposis
   b. Persistent middle ear disease
   c. Poorly controlled asthma
4. Consideration of allergen immunotherapy or complex allergen avoidance measures

To Otolaryngologist

Consideration of surgical treatment for chronic sinusitis/nasal polyposis, adenoidal enlargement, or other anatomic obstructions

CONCLUDING REMARKS

During the past 10 to 15 years, prospective studies of large populations have significantly improved our understanding of the epidemiology of chronic rhinitis in both children and adults. Simultaneously, advances in the basic science of allergic mechanisms have provided new and important insights into the pathophysiology of rhinitis. An integrated approach to therapy, including environmental control measures, pharmacotherapy, and allergen immunotherapy, will provide significant relief of symptoms and improvements in quality of life in the vast majority of patients with allergic rhinitis.

REFERENCES

1. Blackley CH. Experimental Researches on the Cause and Nature of *Catarrhus Aestivus*. Oxford: Oxford Historical Books; 1988.
2. Noon L. Prophylactic inoculation against hay fever. Lancet. 1911;1:1572–1573.
3. Frankland AW, Augustin R. Prophylaxis of summer hayfever and asthma: controlled trial comparing crude grass pollen extracts with isolated main protein component. Lancet. 1954;4:1055.
4. *Strachan D, Sibbald B, Weiland S, et al. Worldwide variations in prevalence of symptoms of allergic rhinoconjunctivitis in children: the International Study of Asthma and Allergies in Childhood (ISAAC). Pediatr Allergy Immunol. 1997;8:161–176.
5. Bjorksten B, Clayton T, Ellwodd P. ISAAC Phase III Study Group Worldwide time trends for symptoms of rhinitis and conjunctivitis: Phase III of the International Study of Asthma and Allergies in Childhood. Pediatr Allergy Immunol. 2008;19:110–124.
6. Kellberger J, Dressel H, Vogelberg C, et al. Prediction of the incidence and persistence of allergic rhinitis in adolescence: a prospective cohort study. J Allergy Clin Immunol. 2012;129: 397–402.
7. Bousquet PJ, Leynaert B, Neukirch F, et al. Geographical distribution of atopic rhinitis in the European Community Respiratory Health Survey I. Allergy. 2008;63:1301–1309.
8. Salo PM, Calatroni A, Gergen PJ, et al. Allergy-related outcomes in relation to serum IgE: results from the National Health and Nutrition Examination Survey 2005–2006. J Allergy Clin Immunol. 2011;127:1226–1235.
9. *Bousquet J, Bullinger M, Fayol C, et al. Assessment of quality of life in patients with perennial allergic rhinitis with the French version of the SF-36 Health Status Questionnaire. J Allergy Clin Immunol. 1994;94(2 Pt 1):182–188.
10. Simons FE. Learning impairment and allergic rhinitis. Allergy Asthma Proc. 1996;17:185–189.
11. Marshall PS, Colon EA. Effects of allergy season on mood and cognitive function. Ann Allergy. 1993;71:251–258.
12. Bousquet J, Van Cauwenberge P, Khaltaev N. Allergic rhinitis and its impact on asthma. J Allergy Clin Immunol. 2001;108 (5 Suppl.):S147–S334.
13. Laynaert B, Neukirch C, Kony S, et al. Association between asthma and rhinitis according to atopic sensitization in a population-based study. J Allergy Clin Immunol. 2004;113:86–93.
14. Bousquet J, Gaugris S, Kocevar VS, et al. Increased risk of asthma attacks and emergency visits among asthma patients with allergic rhinitis: a subgroup analysis of the investigation of montelukast as a partner agent for complementary therapy [corrected]. Clin Exp Allergy. 2005;35:723–727.
15. Fokkens W, Lund V, Mullol J, European Position Paper on Rhinosinusitis and Nasal Polyps Group European position paper on rhinosinusitis and nasal polyps 2007. Rhinol Suppl. 2007;20: 1–136.
16. Van Crombruggen K, Zhang N, Gevaert P, et al. Pathogenesis of chronic rhinosinusitis: inflammation. J Allergy Clin Immunol. 2011;128:728–732.
17. Tewfik TL, Mazer B. The links between allergy and otitis media with effusion. Curr Opin Otolaryngol Head Neck Surg. 2006;14:187–190.
18. Hurst DS. The role of allergy in otitis media with effusion. Otolaryngol Clin North Am. 2011;44:637–654.
19. Lund M, Craig T. Rhinitis and sleep. Sleep Med Rev. 2011;15: 293–299.
20. Hannuksela A, Väänänen A. Predisposing factors for malocclusion in 7-year-old children with special reference to atopic diseases. Am J Orthod Dentofacial Orthop. 1987;92: 299–303.
21. *Sin B, Togias A. Pathophysiology of allergic and non-allergic rhinitis. Proc Am Thorac Soc. 2011;8:106–114.
22. Eccles R. A role for the nasal cycle in respiratory defence. Eur Respir J. 1996;9:371–376.
23. Singh K, Axelrod S, Bielory L. The epidemiology of ocular and nasal allergy in the United States, 1988–1994. J Allergy Clin Immunol. 2010;126:778–783.
24. Pinto JM. Olfaction. Proc Am Thorac Soc. 2011;8:46–52.
25. Smolensky MH, Lemmer B, Reinberg AE. Chronobiology and chronotherapy of allergic rhinitis and bronchial asthma. Adv Drug Deliv Rev. 2007;59:852–882.
26. Billionnet C, Gay E, Kirchner S, et al. Quantitative assessments of indoor air pollution and respiratory health in a population-based sample of French dwellings. Environ Res. 2011;111:425–434.
27. Jacobs R, Lieberman P, Kent E, et al. Weather/temperature-sensitive vasomotor rhinitis may be refractory to intranasal corticosteroid treatment. Allergy Asthma Proc. 2009;30:120–127.
28. Weider DJ, Baker GL, Salvatoriello FW. Dental malocclusion and upper airway obstruction, an otolaryngologist's perspective. Int J Pediatr Otorhinolaryngol. 2003;67:323–331.
29. Marks MB. Allergic shiners: dark circles under the eyes in children. Clin Pediatr. 1966;5:655–658.
30. Castellanos J, Axelrod D. Flexible fiberoptic rhinoscopy in the diagnosis of sinusitis. J Allergy Clin Immunol. 1989;83:91–94.
31. Wood RA, Phipatanakul W, Hamilton RG, et al. A comparison of skin prick tests, intradermal skin tests, and RASTs in the diagnosis of cat allergy. J Allergy Clin Immunol. 1999;103:773.

32. Rondon C, Romero JJ, Lopez S, et al. Local IgE production and positive nasal provocation test in patients with persistent non-allergic rhinitis. J Allergy Clin Immunol. 2007;119:899–905.

33. Demirjian M, Rumbyrt JS, Gowda VC, et al. Serum IgE and eosinophil count in allergic rhinitis—analysis using a modified Bayes' theorem. Allergol Immunopathol (Madr). 2012;40: 281–287.

34. McAfee MF. Imaging of paranasal sinuses and rhinosinusitis. Clin Allergy Immunol. 2007;20:185–226.

35. Bonifazi F, Bilò MB, Antonicelli L, et al. Rhinopharyngoscopy, computed tomography, and magnetic resonance imaging. Allergy. 1997;52(33 Suppl.):28–31.

36. Varonen H, Mäkelä M, Savolainen S, et al. Comparison of ultrasound, radiography, and clinical examination in the diagnosis of acute maxillary sinusitis: a systematic review. J Clin Epidemiol. 2000;53(9):940–948.

37. Sublett JW, Bernstein DI. Occupational rhinitis. Immunol Allergy Clin North Am. 2011;31(787–96):38.

38. Meltzer EO, Hamilos DL, Hadley JA, et al. American Academy of Allergy, Asthma and Immunology (AAAAI), American Academy of Otolaryngic Allergy (AAOA), American Academy of Otolaryngology–Head and Neck Surgery (AAO-HNS), American College of Allergy, Asthma and Immunology (ACAAI), American Rhinologic Society (ARS). Rhinosinusitis: establishing definitions for clinical research and patient care. J Allergy Clin Immunol. 2004;114(6 Suppl.):155.

39. Hamilos DL. Chronic rhinosinusitis patterns of illness. Clin Allergy Immunol. 2007;20:1.

40. Lindberg S, Malm L. Comparison of allergic rhinitis and vasomotor rhinitis patients on the basis of a computer questionnaire. Allergy. 1993;48:602–607.

41. Ellis AK, Keith PK. Non-allergic rhinitis with eosinophilia syndrome. Curr Allergy Asthma Rep. 2006;6:215–220.

42. Chhabra N, Houser SM. The diagnosis and management of empty nose syndrome. Otolaryngol Clin North Am. 2009;42: 311–330.

43. Graf PM. Rhinitis medicamentosa. Clin Allergy Immunol. 2007;19:295–304.

44. *Varghese M, Glaum MC, Lockey RF. Drug-induced rhinitis. Clin Exp Allergy. 2010;40:381–384.

45. Ellegård E, Hellgren M, Torén K, et al. The incidence of pregnancy rhinitis. Gynecol Obstet Invest. 2000;49:98.

46. Franklin KA, Holmgren PA, Jönsson F, et al. Snoring, pregnancy-induced hypertension, and growth retardation of the fetus. Chest. 2000;117:137.

47. Smith K, Edwards PC, Saini TS, et al. The prevalence of concha bullosa and nasal septal deviation and their relationship to maxillary sinusitis by volumetric tomography. Int J Dent. 2010;2010:404982.

48. Santos RS, Cipolotti R, D'Avila FS, et al. Schoolchildren submitted to fiberoptic examination at school: findings and tolerance. J Pediatr (Rio J). 2005;81:443–446.

49. Persky MS, Tabaee A. Cancer of the nasal vestibule and paranasal sinus: surgical management. In: Harrison LB, Sessions RB, Hong WK, eds. Head and neck cancer. 3rd ed. Philadelphia: Lippincott Williams & Wilkins; 2009:454.

50. *Kumar S. Vernal keratoconjunctivitis: a major review. Acta Ophthalmol. 2009;87:133.

51. Elhers WH, Donshik PC. Giant papillary conjunctivitis. Curr Opin Allergy Clin Immunol. 2008;8:445.

52. Tuft SJ, Kemeny DM, Dart JK, et al. Clinical features of atopic keratoconjunctivitis. Ophthalmology. 1991;98:150.

53. Weiss A, Brinser JH, Nazar-Stewart V. Acute conjunctivitis in childhood. J Pediatr. 1993;122:10.

54. Latkany R. Dry eyes: etiology and management. Curr Opin Ophthalmol. 2008;19:287.

55. Nichols KK, Foulks GN, Bron AJ, et al. The international workshop on meibomian gland dysfunction: executive summary. Invest Ophthalmol Vis Sci. 2011;52:1922.

56. Noecker R. Effects of common ophthalmic preservatives on ocular health. Adv Ther. 2001;18:205.

57. Oltz M, Check J. Rosacea and its ocular manifestations. Optometry. 2011;82:92.

58. Leibowitz HM. The red eye. N Engl J Med. 2000;343:345.

59. Congdon NG, Friedman DS. Angle-closure glaucoma: impact, etiology, diagnosis, and treatment. Curr Opin Ophthalmol. 2003;14:70.

60. Sheikh A, Hurwitz B, Shehata Y. House dust mite avoidance measures for perennial allergic rhinitis. Cochrane Database Syst Rev. 2007;1:CD001563.

61. *Sheikh A, Hurwitz B, Nurmatov U, et al. House dust mite avoidance measures for perennial allergic rhinitis. Cochrane Database Syst Rev. 2010;7:CD001563.

62. Bjornsdottir US, Jakobinudottir S, Runarsdottir V, et al. The effect of reducing levels of cat allergen (Fel d 1) on clinical symptoms in patients with cat allergy. Ann Allergy Asthma Immunol. 2003;91:189–194.

63. Wood RA, Johnson EF, Van-Natta ML, et al. A placebo-controlled trial of a HEPA air cleaner in the treatment of cat allergy. Am J Respir Crit Care Med. 1998;158:115–120.

64. Simons FE, Simons KJ. Histamine and H1-antihistamines: celebrating a century of progress. J Allergy Clin Immunol. 2011;128:1139–1150, e1134.

65. *Simons FE. Advances in H_1-antihistamines. N Engl J Med. 2004;351:2203–2217.

66. de Blic J, Wahn U, Billard E, et al. Levocetirizine in children: evidenced efficacy and safety in a 6-week randomized seasonal allergic rhinitis trial. Pediatr Allergy Immunol. 2005;16:267–275.

67. Dykewicz MA, Wallace DV, Amrol DJ, Baroody FM, Bernstein JA, Craig TJ, et al. Rhinitis 2020: A practice parameter update. J Allergy Clin Immunol. 2020;146:721–767.

68. Gray SL, Anderson ML, Dublin S, Hanlon JT, Hubbard R, Walker R, et al. Cumulative use of strong anticholinergics and incident dementia: a prospective cohort study. JAMA Intern Med. 2015;175:401–407.

69. LaForce C, Dockhorn RJ, Prenner BM, et al. Safety and efficacy of azelastine nasal spray (Astelin NS) for seasonal allergic rhinitis: a 4-week comparative multicenter trial. Ann Allergy Asthma Immunol. 1996;76:181.

70. Fairchild CJ, Meltzer EO, Roland PS, et al. Comprehensive report of the efficacy, safety, quality of life, and work impact of Olopatadine 0.6% and Olopatadine 0.4% treatment in patients with seasonal allergic rhinitis. Allergy Asthma Proc. 2007;28: 716–723.

71. Hatton RC, Winterstein AG, McKelvey RP, Shuster J, Hendeles L. Efficacy and safety of oral phenylephrine: systematic review and meta-analysis. Ann Pharmacother. 2007;41:381–390.

72. *Weiner JM, Abramson MJ, Puy RM. Intranasal corticosteroids versus oral H1 receptor antagonists in allergic rhinitis: systematic review of randomized controlled trials. BMJ. 1998;317:1624–1629.

73. *Wilson AM, O'Byrne PM, Parameswaran K. Leukotriene receptor antagonists for allergic rhinitis: a systematic review and meta-analysis. Am J Med. 2004;116:338–344.

74. Bernstein DI, Levy AL, Hampel FC, et al. Treatment with intranasal fluticasone propionate significantly improves ocular symptoms in patients with seasonal allergic rhinitis. Clin Exp Allergy. 2004;34:952–957.

75. Selner JC, Weber RW, Richmond GW, et al. Onset of action of aqueous beclomethasone dipropionate nasal spray in seasonal allergic rhinitis. Clin Ther. 1995;17:1099–1109.

76. Jen A, Baroody F, de Tineo M, et al. As-needed use of fluticasone propionate nasal spray reduces symptoms of seasonal allergic rhinitis. J Allergy Clin Immunol. 2000;105:732–738.

77. Holm AF, Fokkens WJ, Godthelp T, et al. A 1-year placebo-controlled study of intranasal fluticasone propionate aqueous nasal spray in patients with perennial allergic rhinitis: a safety and biopsy study. Clin Otolaryngol. 1998;23:69–73.

78. Schenkel EJ, Skoner DP, Bronsky EA, et al. Absence of growth retardation in children with perennial allergic rhinitis after one year of treatment with mometasone furoate aqueous nasal spray. Pediatrics. 2000;105:E22.

79. Philip G, Malmstrom K, Hampel FC, et al. Montelukast for treating seasonal allergic rhinitis: a randomized, double-blind, placebo-controlled trial performed in the spring. Clin Exp Allergy. 2002;32:1020–1028.

80. Law SWY, Wong AYS, Anand S, Wong ICK, Chan EW. Neuropsychiatric events associated with leukotriene-modifying agents: a systematic review. Drug Saf. 2018;41:253–265.

81. Borum P, Mygind N, Schultz LF. Intranasal ipratropium, a new treatment for perennial rhinitis. Clin Otolaryngol. 1979;4:407.

82. Bronsky EA, Druce H, Findlay SR, et al. A clinical trial of ipratropium bromide nasal spray in patients with perennial non-allergic rhinitis. J Allergy Clin Immunol. 1995;95:1117–1122.

83. Silvers WS. The skier's nose: a model of cold-induced rhinorrhea. Ann Allergy Asthma Immunol. 1991;67:32–36.

84. Katelaris CH, Ciprandi G, Missotten L, et al. A comparison of the efficacy and tolerability of olopatadine hydrochloride 0.1% ophthalmic solution and cromolyn sodium 2% ophthalmic solution in seasonal allergic conjunctivitis. Clin Ther. 2002;24:1561–1575.

85. Hampel FC, Ratner PH, van Bavel J, et al. Double-blind, placebo-controlled study of azelastine and fluticasone in a single nasal spray delivery device. Ann Allergy Asthma Immunol. 2010;105:168–173.

86. Ratner PH, van Bavel JH, Martin BG, et al. A comparison of the efficacy of fluticasone propionate aqueous nasal spray and loratadine, alone and in combination, for the treatment of seasonal allergic rhinitis. J Fam Pract. 1998;47:118–125.

87. Lanier BQ, Abelson MB, Berger WE, et al. Comparison of the efficacy of combined fluticasone propionate and olopatadine versus combined fluticasone propionate and fexofenadine for the treatment of allergic rhinoconjunctivitis induced by conjunctival allergen challenge. Clin Ther. 2002;24:1161–1174.

88. James LK, Shamji MH, Walker SM, et al. Long-term tolerance after allergen immunotherapy is accompanied by selective persistence of blocking antibodies. J Allergy Clin Immunol. 2011;127:509–516.

89. *Brüggenjürgen B, Reinhold T, Brehler R, et al. Cost-effectiveness of specific subcutaneous immunotherapy in patients with allergic rhinitis and allergic asthma. Ann Allergy Asthma Immunol. 2008;101:316–324.

90. Turnbull GL, Rundell OH, Rayburn WF, et al. Managing pregnancy-related nocturnal nasal congestion. The external nasal dilator. J Reprod Med. 1996;41:897.

91. Wilson J. Use of sodium cromoglycate during pregnancy. J Pharm Med. 1982;8:45.

92. Berard A, Sheehy O, Kurzinger ML, Juhaeri J. Intranasal triamcinolone use during pregnancy and the risk of adverse pregnancy outcomes. J Allergy Clin Immunol. 2016;138:97–104, e7.

93. Gluck PA, Gluck JC. A review of pregnancy outcomes after exposure to orally inhaled or intranasal budesonide. Curr Med Res Opin. 2005;21:1075–1084.

94. Seto A, Einarson T, Koren G. Pregnancy outcome following first trimester exposure to antihistamines: meta-analysis. Am J Perinatol. 1997;14:119–124.

95. Tan R, Corren J. Optimum treatment of rhinitis in the elderly. Drugs Aging. 1995;7:168–175.

Key references are preceded by an asterisk.

9

Drug Allergy

Oliver V. Hausmann and Lukas Joerg

CHAPTER OUTLINE

SUMMARY OF IMPORTANT CONCEPTS

- The history and clinical presentation can aid the distinction between immediate- and delayed-type reactions, which have a different diagnostic and therapeutic approach.
- During the acute reaction phase, laboratory tests are advisable: in immediate-type reactions serum tryptase to prove mast cell involvement and in delayed-type reactions eosinophil count, c-reactive protein (CRP), creatinine, and liver enzymes to define organ involvement and severity.
- The most common drug classes involved in hypersensitivity (immediate and delayed) reactions are antibiotics, nonsteroidal antiinflammatory drugs (NSAIDs), and anticonvulsants.
- Some drugs induce severe systemic forms of delayed-type drug hypersensitivities in patients with a certain human leukocyte antigen (HLA) class I allele, for example, abacavir associated with HLA B*57:01. Here, HLA testing is recommended before use.
- Risk for drug hypersensitivity is increased in patients with viral infections (e.g., Epstein–Barr virus [EBV], HIV), during or shortly after a severe drug hypersensitivity reaction ("flare-up") or if high doses, prolonged or repetitive treatment courses are needed (e.g., cystic fibrosis).
- Supporting national pharmacovigilance programs is an important contribution for general drug safety.

INTRODUCTION

Adverse drug reactions (ADRs) are common and inherent to all pharmacologic therapy. Sooner or later, every practicing physician will be confronted with this phenomenon. ADRs in general have been reported to affect 10% to 20% of hospitalized patients and up to 25% of outpatients.[1] Drug allergy is one important subgroup of ADR. Typically, allergic reactions affect the skin, but organ involvement (hepatitis, nephritis) and blood eosinophilia are also common in systemic forms of drug hypersensitivity and may serve as "red flags" for a more severe course. Fortunately, the majority of drug allergic patients have only mild symptoms limited to the skin and do not progress to life-threatening organ involvement and/or anaphylaxis.

Although different classifications have been proposed, ADRs are usually classified into two subtypes (Fig. 9.1): type A reactions, which are predictable from known pharmacologic properties, for example, sleepiness caused by first-generation antihistamines or gastrointestinal toxicity of nonsteroidal antiinflammatory drugs (NSAIDs); and type B reactions, which are unpredictable or unexpected and restricted to a vulnerable subpopulation. The majority of these unexpected type B reactions are hypersensitivity reactions. They are responsible for about one-sixth of all ADRs and comprise (1) allergic (immune-mediated) reactions: the drug is able to form an antigen;

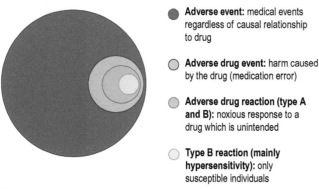

● **Adverse event:** medical events regardless of causal relationship to drug

● **Adverse drug event:** harm caused by the drug (medication error)

● **Adverse drug reaction (type A and B):** noxious response to a drug which is unintended

○ **Type B reaction (mainly hypersensitivity):** only susceptible individuals

Fig. 9.1 Nomenclature for drug reaction.

(2) pharmacological (direct interaction with specific immune receptors (HLA, T cell receptor [TCR]), briefly termed *pharmacological interaction with immune receptors [p-i] concept)* reactions: the drug has an off target activity on immune receptors; and (3) non-allergic intolerance (also called "pseudo-allergic") reactions without involvement of the adaptive immune system.

The term *idiosyncrasy* was previously used synonymously for all type B reactions, but is nowadays limited to non-allergic hypersensitivity reactions with a genetic background, for example, an enzyme defect like glucose-6-phosphate dehydrogenase (G6PD) deficiency, also known as favism. This deficiency leads to hemolytic anemia upon intake of metamizol or one of the other >20 G6PD-dependent drugs.[2]

The use of the terms immediate- or delayed-type reaction to qualify the onset of symptoms has been recommended because they indicate the probable underlying immune mechanism.[3] They refer to the onset of symptoms within or later than 1 hour after dosing, even if this time point is set rather arbitrarily and solid data supporting it are still lacking. Already during the initial evaluation and together with other clinical features, the timing of the reaction might help in distinguishing whether the probable immunologic mechanism is an antibody-mediated (mostly immunoglobulin E [IgE]), immediate-type or a T cell–mediated, delayed-type reaction. However, some IgE-mediated immediate reactions may start later than 1 hour after exposure, and very strong T cell-mediated delayed-type reactions, especially on repetitive exposure, may start rapidly, within hours and may even mimic anaphylaxis; such examples defy the original definition of

these terms. In general, delayed-type reactions are much more frequent than immediate-type reactions.

The risk of sensitization or immune stimulation and sometimes also the consecutive clinical severity depend on different factors, which may be drug- and/or patient-specific (Table 9.1). Of note, an atopic genetic background with an IgE-mediated response to ingested or inhaled proteins, e.g., hay fever, is not associated with an increased risk for drug hypersensitivity.[4]

The aim of this chapter is to stress the significance and importance of drug hypersensitivity in the context of general medicine and ambulatory care. It will therefore only provide a very concise review of the basic pathogenetic concepts of drug hypersensitivity. The focus will be on a detailed clinical description including the warning signs ("red flags") for a potentially severe course on initial evaluation of the patient considering common diagnostic errors and specific pediatric aspects. The management of the acute phase of drug allergy and the necessity and optimal timing for referral to a specialist will be discussed. The specialist's task is then to define the elicitor(s), the underlying mechanism, and the safety of re-administration of the same drug as well as to provide information on safe alternative(s) for further treatment of the patient.

For general safety, most countries run their own pharmacovigilance program for the monitoring of ADRs. Electronic reporting systems like MedWatch (www.fda.gov/Safety/MedWatch) are available and easily accessible. It is the responsibility and an important contribution of the treating physician to inform the regulatory agencies about any relevant ADR that might have been missed during the licensing process. This postmarketing surveillance has led to the drug withdrawal in several cases (Table 9.2).

HISTORICAL PERSPECTIVE

Drug allergy, as is the case with modern pharmacotherapy itself, is a rather young field of medicine. The German dermatologist Heinrich Koebner (1838–1904) was the first to coin the term "drug exanthema" in 1877, describing a quinine-specific skin reaction in two patients, which he clearly separated from the known toxic side effects. In the following years, researchers and clinicians from different countries contributed their observations, highlighting the fact that different drugs may cause the same clinical presentation as well as the same drug may elicit

TABLE 9.1 Factors Conveying a Risk of Sensitization or Immune Stimulation by a Certain Drug and a Risk for Severe Clinical Symptoms	
Patient	**Drug**
Immunogenetic predisposition (particularly the HLA alleles)	Protein binding
	Structure (LMW v HMW)
Pre-activated immune system (particularly chronic viral infection, e.g., EBV, HIV, ongoing drug allergy)	Cross-reactivity
	Dosage
	Route of administration
Underlying disease	Duration of treatment

EBV, Epstein-Barr virus, *HLA,* human leukocyte antigen; *HMW,* high molecular weight; *LMW,* low molecular weight.

TABLE 9.2   List of Drugs Withdrawn for Safety Reasons in all EU Member States Between 2002 and 2011 Grouped by Adverse Drug Reaction or Safety Concern

Drug Name	Drug Class or Use	Year First Marketed	Year of Withdrawal	Length of Time on Market (Years)	Adverse Reaction or Safety Concern
Rofecoxib	NSAID (COX-2 inhibitor)	1999	2004	5	Thrombotic events
Thioridazine	Neuroleptic (α-adrenergic and dopaminergic receptor antagonist)	1958	2005	47	Cardiac disorders
Valdecoxib	NSAID (COX-2 inhibitor)	2003	2005	2	Cardiovascular and cutaneous disorders
Rosiglitazone	Antidiabetic treatment (PPAR agonist)	2000	2010	10	Cardiovascular disorders
Sibutramine	Treatment of obesity (serotonin-noradrenaline reuptake inhibitor)	1999	2010	11	Cardiovascular disorders
Orciprenaline	Sympathomimetic (non-specific β-agonist)	1961	2010	49	Cardiac disorders
Benfluorex	Anorectic and hypolipidemic	1974	2009	35	Heart valve disease—pulmonary hypertension
Clobutinol	Cough suppressant (centrally acting)	1961	2007	46	QT prolongation
Buflomedil	Vasodilator (α1 and α2 receptor antagonist)	1974	2011	37	Neurologic and cardiac disorders (sometimes fatal)
Veralipride	Neuroleptic (and dopaminergic receptor antagonist)	1979	2007	28	Neurologic and psychiatric disorders
Rimonabant	Treatment of obesity (cannabinoid receptor antagonist)	2006	2008	2	Psychiatric disorders
Carisoprodol	Muscle relaxant	1959	2007	48	Intoxication—psychomotor impairment—addiction—misuse
Aceprometazine + Acepromazine + Clorazepate	Hypnotic	1988	2011	23	Cumulative adverse effects—misuse—fatal side effect
Dextropropoxyphene	Opioid painkiller	~1960	2009	49	Fatal overdose
Nefazodone	Antidepressant	1994	2003	9	Hepatotoxicity
Ximelagatran/melagatran	Anticoagulant (thrombin inhibitor)	2003	2006	3	Hepatotoxicity
Lumiracoxib	NSAID (COX-2 inhibitor)	2003	2007	4	Hepatotoxicity
Sitaxentan	Antihypertensive (endothelin receptor antagonist)	2006	2010	4	Hepatotoxicity
Bufexamac	NSAID	~1970	2010	40	Contact allergic reactions

COX, Cyclooxygenase; *EU*, European Union; *NSAID*, nonsteroidal antiinflammatory drug; *PPAR*, peroxisome proliferator-activated receptor.
McNaughton R, Huet G, Shakir S. An investigation into drug products withdrawn from the EU market between 2002 and 2011 for safety reasons and the evidence used to support the decision-making. BMJ Open 2014;4:e004221.

different forms of drug hypersensitivity. They could already define several distinct syndromes, which still apply today. Only with the advent of modern immunology have the underlying mechanisms became apparent, sometimes more than 50 years after their first clinical description. Many aspects of drug hypersensitivity are still unclear and this therefore remains a very active field of applied immunology.

Nowadays, regulatory agencies and a strict jurisdiction control the development and licensing process of new drugs. Protein binding properties and immunogenicity play an important role here. Most of the drugs in use are still low molecular weight (LMW) compounds and should actually not be recognized by our immune system. Only after binding to an endogenous carrier protein (haptenization), immunogenic complexes arise and can elicit a complex immune response with B and T cell reactions.[5] Therefore, strong protein binding properties (leading to hapten formation) of a drug usually lead to termination in the early stages of drug development due to the risk of immune reactions in later clinical use. The highly effective beta-lactam class of antibiotics (penicillins, cephalosporins) with their strong binding to albumin would most probably not have reached the market if invented today or would at least struggle with restrictive licensing requirements. In spite of these restrictions and avoidance of drugs with the potential to bind via covalent bonds to proteins, hypersensitivity reactions still persist. Most of these reactions are due to T cell stimulations and are caused by direct binding of the drug to a human leukocyte antigen (HLA) or a TCR molecule.[5] This process of direct drug binding is summarized under the term *p*harmacological interaction with *i*mmune receptors (p-i) concept.

Therapeutically applied high molecular weight (HMW) proteins, the so-called biologicals or biopharmaceuticals (e.g., antibodies, receptors, cytokines), are still small in number compared to LMW classical drugs, but they represent the future of drug therapy. Most of the drugs in development or in the licensing process belong to this new drug class. They are immunogenic per se and immediate type, antibody mediated, reactions dominate the clinical picture.[5]

EPIDEMIOLOGY

Sound epidemiologic data on drug hypersensitivity reactions are still lacking. The most common drug classes causing hypersensitivity reactions are beta-lactam antibiotics and NSAIDs. Epidemiologic studies indicate that cutaneous reactions, such as maculopapular eruptions and urticaria, are the most common clinical manifestations of drug allergy. Rarely, drugs induce more severe and potentially life-threatening reactions such as toxic epidermal necrolysis (TEN), Stevens-Johnson syndrome (SJS), immune hepatitis or drug reaction with eosinophilia and systemic symptoms (DRESS) for delayed-type reactions, or anaphylaxis for immediate-type reactions. In the US, about 1 in 300 hospitalized patients dies from an ADR, and 6% to 10% of these reactions are most probably allergic in origin.[6]

In the age of personalized medicine based on "next-generation" deoxyribonucleic acid (DNA) sequencing technologies, new aspects in epidemiology of drug allergy arose: immunogenetic studies showed a strong genetic association between certain (HLA) alleles and severe forms of drug hypersensitivity (Table 9.3) and, in this respect, the previously postulated unpredictability of type B reactions no longer holds true. HLA screening before prescribing the drug to avoid these serious conditions is currently only recommended for abacavir with HLA B*57:01 being the risk transferring allele, which is common in White European origin populations and for carbamazepine with HLA B*15:02, the risk allele for South-East Asians.[7] This form of primary prevention of drug hypersensitivity is one of the first great successes of personalized medicine.

Limited data are available on the cost of drug allergy. A study in a hospital setting showed that penicillin-allergic patients had higher medical costs related to the use of alternative antibiotics.[8]

Alternative treatments for drug-allergic patients are commonly more expensive, often more toxic than first-line drugs and less effective. Especially in cases of patients labeled as penicillin allergic, the overuse of alternative antibiotics contributes to the development of bacterial resistance.[9]

PATHOGENESIS AND ETIOLOGY

Drug allergy syndromes (type B reactions) are recognized by the constellation of signs and symptoms linked to a particular mechanism. The Gell and Coombs classification is conceptually useful even if it is unable to cover all mechanisms involved in drug allergy (Table 9.4).

The time of appearance of the first allergic symptoms is helpful to distinguish different forms of drug hypersensitivity: in an already sensitized individual and not on first contact, IgE-mediated reactions tend to appear rapidly, normally within minutes (with i.v. doses) to 1 hour (after oral intake).[3] However, the sensitization and production of IgE antibodies to the drug or drug metabolite must have occurred earlier and been clinically "silent." For sensitization, LMW compounds need to bind to a carrier protein (haptenization) in order to stimulate the immune system. Thus, a symptomless sensitization phase during the initial treatment is succeeded by a sudden allergic to anaphylactic reaction upon reexposure.[5]

On the other hand, delayed-type hypersensitivity, which is mostly T cell–mediated, appears later in the treatment course but may already manifest during the first treatment cycle, if it lasts long enough. In the beginning, only a few T cells seem to react with the drug and no symptoms appear. An exanthema may only arise after expansion and the migration of the drug-specific effector T cells into the tissue.[5] This explains the typical time interval between the start of treatment and the appearance of clinical symptoms, for example, in amoxicillin-induced exanthema from day 7 to 10 of treatment (Fig. 9.2). One should be aware that upon re-exposure, symptoms of these T cell reactions may appear much faster (within 2–48 hours), dependent on the amount of drug-reactive (primed) T cells and drug dosage.

T cell recognition, a cornerstone for both IgE- and T cell–mediated reactions, depends upon drug presentation by antigen presenting cells (APCs) on their HLA molecule and engagement of the corresponding TCR on CD4+ or CD8+ T lymphocytes. Again, haptenization of the presented peptide may be involved, but it is not a prerequisite here. Drug may also directly bind to the immune receptors, namely the HLA molecule, or to the TCR and stimulate T cells directly without haptenization and processing of a hapten-modified protein.[5] This direct binding capacity is an inherent pharmacologic feature of most of the LMW drugs designed to fit into pockets of enzymes (e.g., angiotensin-converting enzyme [ACE] inhibitors) and block their function. This kind of immune stimulation via *p*harmacological interaction with *i*mmune receptors (p-i concept) bypasses the classical control mechanisms of our immune system and can result in severe forms of hypersensitivity.[5] This mechanism may also explain the sometimes puzzling clinical similarities to graft versus host disease (GvHD) where the same immunological principles of direct activation of the grafted T cells by the patient (host) HLA molecules apply.

TABLE 9.3   Associations of Different Forms of Delayed-type Drug Hypersensitivity and HLA Class I Alleles in Association With a Certain Ethnic Background (modified according to [7])

Causative Drug	HLA Allele	Hypersensitivity Reactions	Ethnicity	Odds Ratio (95% CI)
Abacavir	B*57:01	Abacavir hypersensitivity	Caucasians	117 (29–481)
Allopurinol	B*58:01	SJS/TEN/DRESS	Asians	74.18 (26.95–204.14)
			Non-Asians	101.45 (44.98–228.82)
Carbamazepine	B*15:02	SJS/TEN	Han Chinese	115.32 (18.17–732.13)
			Thai	54.43 (16.28–181.96)
			Malaysians	221.00 (3.85–12 694.65)
			Indians	54.60 (2.25–1326.20)
	B*15:11		Japanese	16.3 (4.76–55.61)
			Koreans	18.0 (2.3–141.2)
			Han Chinese	31.00 (2.74–350.50)
	B*15:18		Japanese	13.58 (nd)
	A*31:01	DRESS	Han Chinese	23.0 (4.2–125)
			Europeans	57.6 (11.0–340)
		SJS/TEN	Europeans	4.4 (1.1–17.3)
			All populations	3.94 (1.4–11.5)
		SJS/TEN	Europeans	25.93 (4.93–116.18)
		DRESS	Europeans	12.41 (1.27–121.03)
		MPE	Europeans	8.33 (3.59–19.36)
		SJS/TEN/DRESS	Japanese	10.8 (5.9–19.6)
	B*57:01	SJS/TEN	Europeans	9.0 (4.2–19.4)
Oxcarbazepine	B*15:02	SJS/TEN	Taiwan Han Chinese	80.7 (3.8–1714.4)
Phenytoin	B*15:02	SJS/TEN	Asians	4.55 (1.44–14.14)
	B*13:01	SJS/TEN	Asians	
	B*51:01	SJS/TEN	Asians	
Dapsone	B*13:01	DRESS	Mainland China Han Chinese	20.53 (11.55–36.48)
Lamotrigine	B*15:02	SJS/TEN	Han Chinese	3.59 (1.15–11.22)
Nevirapine	B*35:05	DRESS/MPE	Thai	18.96 (4.87–73.44)
	DRB1*0101	DRESS		4.8, p = 0.01
Beta-lactam antibiotics	C*04:06	SJS/DRESS/MPE	Chinese	13.1 (1.3–137.7)
	C*08:01 DRB1*04:06	Immediate hypersensitivity		4.83 (1.9–16.7)
	B*48:01			55.0 (2.4–1241.2)
				37.4 (1.7–824.6)
Flucloxacillin	B*57:01	Hepatitis	Europeans/Caucasians	80.6 (22.8–284.9)
Flucloxacillin	B*57:03	Hepatitis	Europeans/Caucasians	79.2 (13.6–462.4)
Amoxicillin/clavulanate	DRB1*15:01DRB5*01:01 DQB1*06:02	Hepatitis	Europeans/Caucasians	n/a
Vancomycin	A*32:01	DRESS	Europeans/Caucasians	n/a

CI, Confidence interval; DRESS, drug reaction with eosinophilia and systemic symptoms; HLA, human leukocyte antigen; MPE, maculopapular exanthema; n/a, not applicable; SJS, Stevens-Johnson syndrome; TEN, toxic epidermal necrolysis.

In addition, a "pre-activated" immune system is prone to mounting a drug hypersensitivity reaction, for example, a generalized viral infection (EBV or HIV) with its associated strong T-cell response predisposes to delayed-type drug hypersensitivity. During or shortly after a severe drug hypersensitivity reaction, especially in DHS/DRESS (see later), T cells are highly susceptible to otherwise subthreshold stimuli, a so-called "flare up" reaction may arise or even multiple drug hypersensitivity

(MDH).[10] Under all of these highly stimulatory circumstances, even structurally unrelated drugs taken regularly may elicit allergic reactions, especially when administered in high doses.[10]

On the other hand, a state of "organ predisposition" (e.g., chronic urticaria, asthma, rhinosinusitis) with a lower local reaction threshold may also lead to clinical symptoms even without a compound specific sensitization. A typical example is the non-allergic NSAID intolerance with either skin reactions (exacerbation of chronic urticaria) or reactions in the airways related to the intensity of eosinophilic inflammation in the upper and lower respiratory tract.[11] They occur rapidly, namely

TABLE 9.4 Immunopathologic Penicillin Reactions

Gell-Coombs Classification	Mechanism	Examples of Adverse Penicillin Reactions
I	Anaphylactic (IgE-mediated)	Acute anaphylaxis Urticaria
II	Complement-dependent cytolysis (IgG/IgM)	Hemolytic anemias Thrombocytopenia
III	Immune complex damage	Serum sickness Drug fever Some cutaneous eruptions and vasculitis
IV	Delayed or cellular hypersensitivity	Contact dermatitis maculopapular rash SJS/TEN Hepatitis

The Gell and Coombs classification: IgE-mediated type I drug reactions may involve acute anaphylaxis or urticaria. Cytolytic type II reactions usually are confined to drugs that bind to cell surface structures. Drug-specific immune complexes result from high-dose, prolonged therapy and may produce drug fever, a classic type III serum sickness syndrome, as well as various forms of vasculitis. Contact dermatitis from topically applied drugs as well as maculopapular rashes involves T cell–mediated type IV reactions. Severe blistering skin reactions, such as SJS and TEN, belong to the same reaction type with involvement of drug-specific cytotoxic CD8+ T cells and possibly natural killer (NK) leading to keratinocyte death and the resulting widespread skin damage. *Ig*, Immunoglobulin; *SJS*, Stevens-Johnson syndrome; *TEN*, toxic epidermal necrolysis.

as early as 15 minutes after oral intake, are highly dose-dependent, and do not require a sensitization phase. They are based on the mode of action of all NSAIDs interfering with the arachidonic acid metabolism and ultimately leading to a prostaglandin-leukotriene imbalance. Non-allergic intolerance to radio contrast media (RCM) relies on their capacity of direct mast cell activation, most probably due to their high concentration and rapid infusion rate that is needed for their optimal radiographic characteristics. Again, no sensitization phase is needed here.

The decade-long search for a specific mechanism in non-allergic drug intolerance reactions lately revealed a single receptor, known as Mas-related G-protein coupled receptor member X2 (MRGPRX2) in humans and Mas-related G-protein coupled receptor member B2 (Mrgprb2) in mice, to be crucial for IgE-independent, direct mast cell stimulation by certain drugs associated with systemic non-allergic ("pseudo-allergic," "anaphylactoid") reactions like fluoroquinolone antibiotics and neuromuscular blocking agents (NMBAs).[12] These drugs share a common chemical motif, which might help to predict side effects of future compounds. The fact that the different drugs all triggered a single receptor makes it an attractive drug target to prevent non-allergic drug intolerance reactions. True IgE-mediated allergic reactions are independent of this mechanism and remain unaffected.

CLINICAL FEATURES (PHENOTYPES)

Skin rashes are a frequent phenomenon in daily clinical practice. They may be reactive, for example, due to an underlying infection, drug induced or disease specific. History and presentation alone probably overestimate the role of drug allergies in cutaneous reactions and a thorough allergological workup to prove an allergic mechanism is advisable. Most of the drug

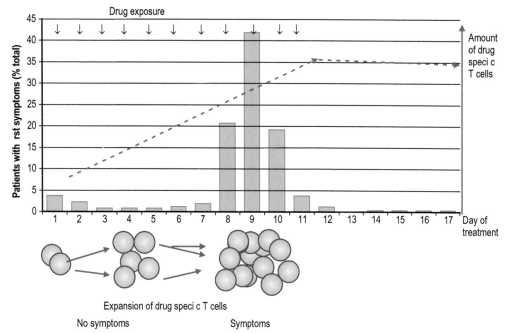

Fig. 9.2 Appearance of first symptoms in delayed type drug hypersensitivity to quinolones (gemifloxacin-treated women, mainly skin rashes, n = 270; Schmid DA, Campi P, Pichler WJ. Hypersensitivity reactions to quinolones. Curr Pharm Des. 2006;12(26):3313–3326.)

allergic patients (>80%) suffer from skin symptoms, mostly maculopapular rashes.[3] Acute urticaria is also common. The latter may quickly progress to anaphylaxis and needs special attention. An intense palmar and plantar itch, anxiety, and a rapid progression of symptoms from skin involvement to circulatory symptoms are warning signs for a severe, potentially lethal course.[13] Immediate treatment with intramuscular epinephrine (0.3–0.5 mg i.m., lateral thigh) with the patient in supine position is the therapeutic cornerstone (see Chapter 13 on anaphylaxis).

One major concern of general internists is the distinction of immediate- and delayed-type drug hypersensitivity on initial clinical investigation. Besides the aforementioned timing of the first symptoms, the morphology of the skin changes is very helpful in this respect: erythema, urticarial, and angioedema (AE) as typical signs of an immediate-type reaction are non-fixed and without involvement of the epidermal structures (no scaling, no blistering). They may quickly change their appearance (confluence, borders) due to the underlying pathomechanism of vasodilation with or without tissue edema. In contrast, the T-cell–mediated inflammation of delayed-type reactions, for example, in maculopapular exanthema (MPE), leads to less transient skin rashes involving the epidermis with either scaling or blister formation as well as to additional sensations like warmth or pain besides itch depending on the extent of tissue infiltration.

In delayed-type reaction involving effector T cells, the skin rash may only be the tip of the iceberg and the involvement of internal organs (liver, lungs, kidney) and the extent of blood eosinophilia (>1.0 G/L is a good indicator of tissue infiltration) should be checked for at least once. In rare cases, drug allergic reactions are limited to the internal organs, for example, drug-induced liver injury (DILI). Because recruitment and expansion of the drug-reactive T cells take several days, symptoms may start as late as 7 to 10 days into therapy or even after cessation of the causative drug(s).[3] In severe forms of drug allergy, for example, DRESS or SJS, it may even take more than 2 weeks until the first symptoms appear.[3] The warning signs (red flags) on initial evaluation of a putative delayed-type hypersensitivity reaction are summarized in Table 9.5.

Every drug may potentially be involved in a hypersensitivity reaction, but there is a fairly consistent "hit list" of common culprits with considerable differences according to the reaction type (Table 9.6). If one of these drugs is involved, it should be stopped immediately.

URTICARIA AND ANGIOEDEMA (IMMEDIATE TYPE)

IgE-mediated drug reactions may involve acute anaphylaxis or urticaria with or without accompanying AE, the latter being a deeper seated variant of urticaria mostly affecting soft tissues like eyelids, lips, tongue, pharyngeal, or genital tissue. Urticaria and AE are mostly histamine-dependent and usually accompanied by an intense itch, but are transient in nature and typically change their location as well as the extent of their skin

TABLE 9.5 Warning Signs (Red Flags) for Progression to a Severe Form of Delayed Type Drug Hypersensitivity, for Example, DRESS, SJS/TEN

Signs and Symptoms	Lab Tests
Confluent infiltrative exanthema with progression to erythroderma	Blood eosinophilia (>10% and/or >1 G/L)
Facial swelling	Presence of lymphoblasts in the peripheral blood
Bullous or pustulous lesions	Hepatitis (elevated liver enzymes)
Painful skin lesions	
Mucosal involvement	
Positive Nikolsky sign (epidermal detachment upon lateral traction of the skin)	Nephritis (creatinine, urine sediment)
"B symptoms" (lymphadenopathy, fever, malaise)	Acute phase protein (elevated CRP, but usually <100 mg/L)

CRP, C-reactive protein; DRESS, drug reaction with eosinophilia and systemic symptoms; SJS, Stevens-Johnson syndrome; TEN, toxic epidermal necrolysis.

TABLE 9.6 Common Elicitors of Drug Hypersensitivity Reactions Corresponding to Their Clinical Presentation

Immediate Type (IgE, Non-allergic Intolerance) <1 h, Mostly <15 min	Delayed Type (T Cell Involvement) >6 h, Mostly 7–14 days
Beta-lactam antibiotics (penicillins, cephalosporins)	Antibiotics (penicillins, cephalosporins, sulfonamides, quinolones, minocycline, vancomycin)
Vancomycin	
Quinolones	
NSAID (aspirin, diclofenac, ibuprofen)	Antiepileptics (carbamazepine, phenytoin, lamotrigine)
Neuromuscular blocking agents (NMBA)	Allopurinol
Therapeutic proteins/peptides (monoclonal antibodies)	Sulfasalazine
	HIV drugs (nevirapine, abacavir)

Ig, Immunoglobulin; NSAID, nonsteroidal antiinflammatory drug.

involvement quickly. It can occur early or late in a course of drug therapy and readily responds to antihistamines (Fig. 9.3A–C).

MACULOPAPULAR EXANTHEM (DELAYED TYPE)

MPE is the most frequent manifestation of drug hypersensitivity and is usually based on a T cell–mediated delayed-type hypersensitivity.[3] A considerable proportion of MPE cases will be reactive due to an underlying infection and not or not only drug-induced. Especially in children, the interaction between virus-induced and drug-induced immune stimulation seems to play an important role,[14] illustrated by the pathognomonic maculopapular skin rash after intake of aminopenicillins in an EBV infection. However, aminopenicillins (and other antibiotics) administered during an EBV episode may result in a persistent drug hypersensitivity[15] (Fig. 9.4).

Of interest for daily clinical practice, there are indications that cutaneous eruptions due to a drug hypersensitivity differ from

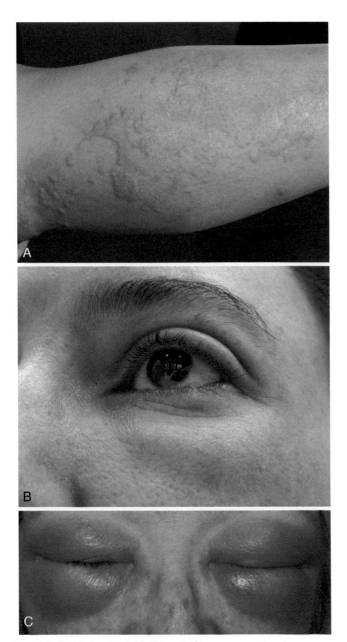

Fig. 9.3 (A) Urticaria. (B) Mild and (C) severe angioedema.

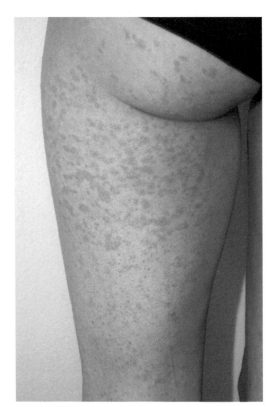

Fig. 9.4 Maculopapular exanthema.

reactive forms in their distribution pattern. In drug allergic skin rashes, the flexural aspects of the proximal extremities are affected first and most, whereas they are typically spared in reactive rashes. This might be consistent with an immunological interaction of drugs or drug metabolites as well as T cell skin homing mechanisms and local factors such as friction, local skin temperature, and possibly eccrine gland distribution. This would explain the typical distribution of drug allergic eruptions in the axillae, genital area, and buttocks, a phenomenon that is still poorly understood and detailed investigations are ongoing. Nevertheless, this typical distribution pattern might be helpful in daily clinical practice, especially for urgent bedside or office decisions (Fig. 9.5A–C).

Extreme forms of this typical flexural distribution of drug allergic skin rashes are the so-called symmetrical drug-related intertriginous and flexural exanthema (SDRIFE, formerly also known as "baboon syndrome") and acute generalized exanthematous

pustulosis (AGEP).[3] SDRIFE is quite strictly limited to the flexural surfaces and buttocks. AGEP shows the same distribution pattern in its early stages but typically spreads over the body later on. They are usually diagnosed on the spot due to their typical and distinctive appearance. In SDRIFE, the flexural skin lesions are of typical maculopapular appearance, whereas in AGEP disseminated sterile pustules are seen and patients may have fever as well as an impressive blood leucocytosis (sometimes with eosinophilia). Often both forms overlap and a clear distinction is sometimes not possible. Mucous membranes are not involved in both. Epicutaneous patch test reactions may cause a similar pustular reaction in AGEP (Fig. 9.6A–C).

FIXED DRUG ERUPTIONS (DELAYED TYPE)

This benign, rather unusual form of drug hypersensitivity is characterized by immune-mediated cutaneous lesions that appear as annular, sometimes blistering, and reddish-brown to dark red macules or plaques.[3] Their diagnostic hallmarks include residual hyperpigmentation after healing and rapid recurrence at the previously affected site on re-exposure. Topical glucocorticoids are advisable, even prophylactically, if repetitive treatment with the same drug is necessary.

EXFOLIATIVE DERMATITIS (STEVENS-JOHNSON SYNDROME AND TOXIC EPIDERMAL NECROLYSIS) (DELAYED TYPE)

The most severe forms of delayed-type drug hypersensitivity reactions involve widespread keratinocyte death and consecutive

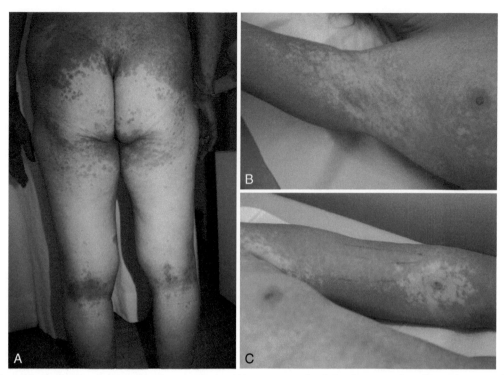

Fig. 9.5 Typical flexural distribution in drug allergic exanthema (A) as opposed to infection-associated reactive exanthema (B) and (C).

skin blistering (Fig. 9.7) and are either called Stevens-Johnson syndrome (SJS) or toxic epidermal necrolysis (TEN) depending on the extent of skin involvement: SJS <10% skin detachment, TEN >30% skin detachment.[3] The intermediate form with 10% to 30% skin detachment is called SJS/TEN overlap syndrome. They are rare (1:100,000 for SJS, 1:1,000,000 for TEN) and according to the European Registry of Severe Cutaneous Adverse Reactions (RegiSCAR) associated with a high mortality (SJS 24%, TEN 43%, SJS/TEN overlap 49%).[16]

SJS/TEN has to be differentiated from erythema multiforme (EM), which may have a central blister as well but is mainly caused by viral infections (especially following a herpes simplex or mycoplasma infection), is often recurrent, and affects younger patients (mean age 24 years).[17] The main causes for SJS/TEN are drugs (Table 9.7), which on a global scale appear to differ in frequency due to the different genetic background (HLA association, see epidemiology section). Most reactions start within the first 5 weeks of treatment (mean onset of symptoms is around day 17). Important risk factors are HIV infection (low CD4/high CD8 counts)[18] and systemic lupus erythematosus.[19]

SJS/TEN can develop from an initial lesion quite rapidly: the initial purple-red maculae may become painful—an ominous sign. Within 12 to 24 hours, the first bullae are seen and the Nikolsky sign becomes positive (epidermal detachment upon lateral traction of the skin; Table 9.5, warning signs). Stopping drug treatment at this stage of SJS might prevent further progression to a more severe form of skin detachment (TEN). Mucous membranes (mouth, genitalia) are involved with blister formation, as well as a purulent keratoconjunctivitis with formation of synechiae, which require intensive ocular care to avoid permanent eye damage.

As a rule of thumb, any drug rash involving mucosal surfaces or blistering warrants immediate drug withdrawal and often require hospitalization (Fig. 9.7A,B).

If no drugs are involved or they are not known to elicit SJS/TEN, paraneoplastic pemphigus (not pemphigus vulgaris) must be considered as well.[20] These forms of cancer-associated skin and mucosal detachment cannot be distinguished from drug-induced SJS/TEN clinically or by standard histology. So whenever doubt prevails, a skin biopsy of the affected area should be examined by direct immunofluorescence (IF) to demonstrate or exclude intercellular immunoglobulin deposition (autoantibodies against desmosomal proteins). If positive, confirmative assays and an extended search for an underlying malignancy must follow and the involvement of an experienced dermatologist is advisable.

SYSTEMIC DRUG REACTIONS—SEVERE DRUG HYPERSENSITIVITY SYNDROMES (DHS/DRESS) (DELAYED TYPE)

Some drugs are known to cause severe systemic disease, with fever, lymphadenopathy, most often hepatitis, and various forms of exanthema associated with the typical facial swelling.[21] Few patients also develop nephritis, colitis, pancreatitis, interstitial lung disease, or cardiac and bone marrow involvement. More than 70% of patients have a marked blood eosinophilia (>1.5 G/L) and atypical lymphocytes are found in differential blood count. During the last decades, this syndrome has had many names, the most frequent ones being drug (induced) hypersensitivity syndrome (DHS or DiHS) and DRESS.

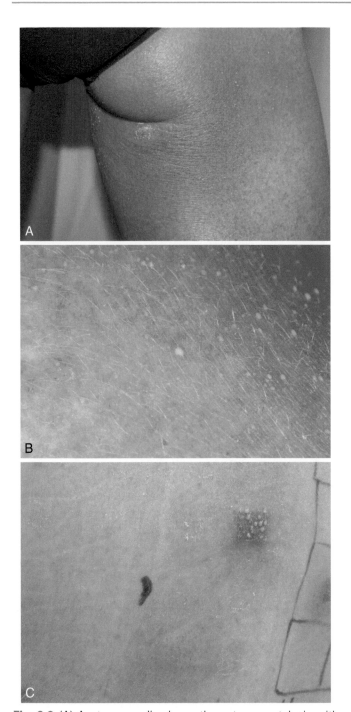

Fig. 9.6 (A) Acute generalized exanthematous pustulosis with typical sterile pustules (B), which can be reproduced in skin testing (C).

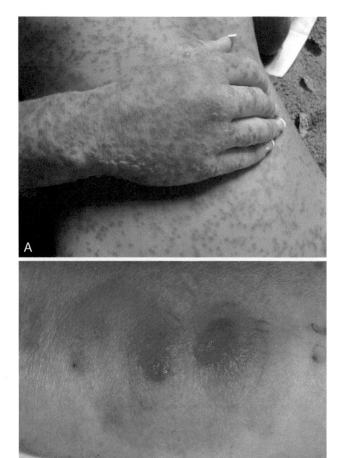

Fig. 9.7 Blistering in the exanthematous skin area (A) as an early sign of Stevens-Johnson syndrome that may progress to toxic epidermal necrolysis, which may again be reproduced in skin testing (B).

Of note, DiHS/DRESS may begin up to 10 weeks after initiation of the treatment, occasionally following an updosing step, and may then persist and recur for many weeks to months, even after cessation of the culprit drug.[22] The clinical picture resembles a generalized viral infection (e.g., acute EBV infection), from which it can usually be distinguished by its prominent blood eosinophilia. Many patients have facial swelling, and some have signs of a capillary leak syndrome. As the clinical picture resembles an infection or an autoimmune disease and the disease tends to persist in spite of stopping all drugs, many patients are not diagnosed correctly or in a timely manner.[23] There may also be persistent intolerance to other, chemically distinct drugs leading to a recurrence of clinical symptoms, so-called flare-up reactions (e.g., acetaminophen) weeks to months after stopping the initial drug therapy, further adding to the confusion.[10,23,24] Treatment often requires high doses of corticosteroids, especially in severe organ involvement. Stopping of all drugs is the most important therapeutic step and requires some courage in critically ill patients, who are frequently treated in an intensive care unit. The mortality is around 10%, and some patients may even require life-saving emergency liver transplantation.

It has been shown that in many patients with this syndrome, circulating human herpes virus (HHV6, HHV 7, CMV, EBV) can be found within a 2- to 4-month course.[25] Especially, the reactivation of CMV seems to be associated with more complications.[26]

Thus, similar to HIV, where T cell activation can also enhance virus production, a massive drug-induced immune stimulation like in DHS/DRESS may somehow reactivate these latent lymphotropic herpes viruses, which subsequently replicate and possibly contribute to the chronic course and persistent drug intolerance in affected patients. Physicians using anticonvulsants should be familiar with this syndrome, as it occurs in

TABLE 9.7 Drugs Eliciting Severe Cutaneous or Systemic Delayed-Type Reactions

Acute Generalized Exanthematous Pustulosis (AGEP)	Stevens-Johnson Syndrome (SJS) and Toxic Epidermal Necrolysis (TEN)	Drug Reaction With Eosinophilia and Systemic Symptoms (DRESS)[b]
Aminopenicillins	**Allopurinol**[a]	**Carbamazepine**[a]
Cephalosporins	**Phenytoin**	**Phenytoin**
Pristinamycin	**Carbamazepine**[a]	**Lamotrigine**
Celecoxib	Lamotrigine	**Beta-lactam**
Quinolone	Cotrimoxazole (SMX)	**Antibiotics**
Diltiazem	Nevirapine	Minocycline
Terbinafine	Barbiturate	Allopurinol[a]
Macrolides	NSAID (Oxicams)	Dapsone[a]
		Sulfasalazine
		Cotrimoxazole (SMX)
		Vancomycin
		Abacavir[a,b]

[a]The type of reaction might be determined by the presence of a certain HLA-allele.
[b]Abacavir-induced systemic reactions are classified outside of DRESS; they often lack eosinophilia and preferentially affect the respiratory and gastrointestinal tract.
List incomplete: the most frequent elicitors are given in bold.
HLA, human leukocyte antigen; *NSAID,* nonsteroidal antiinflammatory drug.

about 1% to 5% patients exposed to this drug class.[27] Highly dosed, longer applied antibiotics are also common triggers.[28]

ISOLATED DRUG-INDUCED ORGAN DAMAGE (DELAYED TYPE)

Drugs may induce isolated hepatitis (DILI) or an isolated interstitial nephritis, for example, penicillins, proton pump inhibitors, and quinolones.[29] In drug-induced interstitial nephritis, eosinophils can sometimes be detected in the urine, even in the absence of blood eosinophilia. More rarely, interstitial lung diseases (furadantin), pancreatitis, isolated fever, or eosinophilia are encountered as the only symptom of a drug allergy.

PEDIATRIC ASPECTS IN DRUG ALLERGY

Children may also develop a drug hypersensitivity: if the symptoms are acute (urticaria, AE, anaphylaxis), a careful diagnosis and strict avoidance are recommended as IgE-mediated reactions are potentially life threatening. Here, drug sensitization may persist until adulthood.

Far more frequent are delayed-onset urticaria or maculopapular rashes. In this situation, in spite of its typical clinical presentation, provocation studies with, for example, beta-lactam antibiotics could only show a low rate of reproducibility (<10%).[30] Viral infections may be the important (co-)factor in many of these skin rashes. Intradermal skin testing and subsequent provocation testing are in most instances negative, maybe because co-factors are missing. Allergological workup should be

considered in those children who develop more severe symptoms. In mild skin rashes after penicillin treatment without evidence of anaphylaxis, a drug challenge without previous skin testing may be directly attempted, and if tolerated, it may help to reduce the overdiagnosis of "penicillin allergy,"[31] which is frequent and leads to unnecessary use of alternative second-line antibiotics.

PATIENT EVALUATION, DIAGNOSIS, AND DIFFERENTIAL DIAGNOSIS

Appropriate diagnosis of drug hypersensitivity reactions depends largely on careful history taking with special attention to prior drug exposure, route of administration, current treatment duration, and dose (Table 9.8), as well as the chronology and type of reaction that is supplemented by compatible physical and laboratory findings. Especially in anaphylaxis, differential diagnoses like vasovagal reactions, vocal cord dysfunction, or panic reactions need to be considered. Co-factors like infectious disease, heat, alcohol, or exercise may also play a relevant role in these acute reactions.[32]

During the acute phase of a drug hypersensitivity reaction, it is recommended to:

1. measure serum tryptase within 15 minutes up to 3 hours after the start of a reaction suspected to be an IgE-mediated immediate-type reaction to prove mast cell involvement. Tryptase is a stable mast cell specific enzyme and samples may be kept at room temperature for at least two days and at 2 °C to 8 °C for at least 5 days before analysis (long-term storage at −20 °C possible). Tryptase values in the acute event should be compared with a basal value, taken at the earliest after 24 hours. Importantly, an increase within the reference range compared to the basal value also indicates mast cell activation.[33]

2. measure liver enzymes, renal function, CRP, and the differential blood count (presence of eosinophilia, lymphoblasts) to define the severity of a suspected T cell–mediated delayed-type reaction.

In most cases, history and physical examination alone are not sufficient for establishing the diagnosis. Provocation tests from a large series of patients with a history of mostly mild drug allergy

TABLE 9.8 Suggestion for a Chronologic Documentation of Drug Intake

Substance	Daily Dose/ Route	Start	End
Amoxicillin/ clavulanic acid	4 × 2.2 g i.v.	2014/11/10	2014/11/17
Amoxicillin/ clavulanic acid	3 × 2.2 g i.v.	2014/11/18	2014/12/04
Levofloxacine	2 × 500 mg oral	2014/12/05	2014/12/16
Rifampicin	2 × 450 mg oral	2014/12/05	Ongoing
Piperacillin/ tazobactam	3 × 4.5 g i.v.	2014/12/16	Ongoing

have shown that less than 20% are currently allergic to the previously offending drugs.[34] Possible explanations include the presence of co-factors at the time of reaction, such as infections or other comorbid situations, and waning sensitivity to the offending drug over time. For a more accurate assessment of current allergy, subjects with a compatible history of drug allergy should be evaluated by further diagnostic tests for definite diagnosis.

In immediate-type reactions, patients with repetitive anaphylaxis or multiple exposures (surgery with general anesthesia, hospitalized patients), a thorough allergological workup might reveal a common culprit like latex, disinfectants (chlorhexidine), dyes, or excipients of soluble drugs.

Skin tests (e.g., skin prick, intradermal, and epicutaneous/patch test) with the suspected offending agent and if positive with potentially cross-reacting as well as alternative drugs are the mainstay of the allergological workup.[35] Intradermal skin tests should be read at 20 minutes (immediate type) and after 24 hours (delayed type). All skin tests should be postponed for at least 4 weeks (immediate type) to 6 to 12 weeks (delayed type) after the clinical reaction to avoid testing during a refractory period where the involved immune cells have not regained their full reactivity.[36] Unfortunately, sensitivity of the tests begins to fade 6 months after the acute phase of the reaction. T cell–mediated delayed-type reaction might still be detectable more than 20 years after the reaction, especially in severe drug hypersensitivity reaction like DRESS. Unfortunately, even under optimal conditions, skin test sensitivity remains low, but is counterbalanced by a good specificity, that is, positive skin tests are virtually always relevant, whereas negative tests do not exclude an allergic mechanism and need to be interpreted with caution![37] Guidelines for standardization of the skin test procedures and the optimal, nonirritative skin test concentration were published by the drug allergy interest group of the European Academy of Allergy and Clinical Immunology (EAACI) with the intention to harmonize the test procedure[37] (Fig. 9.8).

Besides skin testing, serology (drug-specific IgE) and cellular tests like the basophil activation test (BAT) for immediate-type hypersensitivity and the lymphocyte transformation test (LTT), mostly for delayed-type hypersensitivity, are complementing the diagnostic allergological armamentarium.[38] Again, these tests should not be performed within the first weeks of the reaction due to the possible anergy of the involved cell types. Only in SJS/TEN, LTT performed during or shortly after the acute stage of the disease may be helpful. The combination of all test methods available (skin tests, serology, LTT, BAT) allows for an identification of the culprit drug in a majority of patients (around 70%).

Definite diagnosis of drug allergy sometimes involves drug provocation testing (DPT), during which gradually increasing doses of the offending drug are given.[32] It is standardized only for immediate-type reactions and should only be performed by experienced personnel in an appropriate setting. Informed consent must be obtained from the patient before the procedure. The starting dose should be between 1:10,000 and 1:100 of the therapeutic dose with sequential up-dosing every 30 minutes (i.v.) to 60 minutes (p.o./s.c.). DPT can usually be completed within 1 day with a maximum of three to five incremental doses and

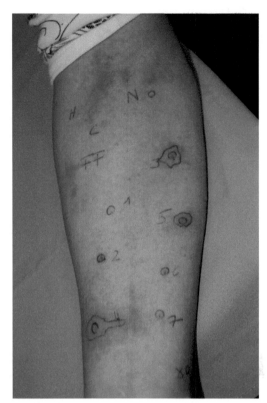

Fig. 9.8 Intradermal skin test.

a 2-hour observation period after the provocation for a patient with history of an immediate-type reaction. Provocation tests should not be performed if an acute reaction occurred within the last 4 to 8 weeks, antihistamines or oral corticosteroids are being used, or there are active signs of underlying disease such as urticaria, uncontrolled asthma (i.e., forced expiratory volume in 1 second [FEV1] of <70% of predicted), or uncontrolled cardiac, renal, hepatic, or infectious disease. Inclusion of a placebo is recommended to eliminate false-positive results for patients with largely subjective reactions, but is rarely performed in clinical practice.

For delayed-type reactions, provocation tests are not standardized and differ significantly between the various centers.[39] Some centers continue treatment after reaching the full dose until the period needed for the initial reaction in delayed-type reactions is covered. They may last days to weeks, namely a full treatment period. Re-challenge, even with incremental dosing, is contraindicated in patients with histories of SJS/TEN, DHS/DRESS, AGEP, or severe organ-specific involvement. Only in patients with penicillin allergy label and unknown or mild delayed cutaneous reaction, a direct rechallenge, similar to the approach in children, may be appropiate.[40]

DRUG CLASSES OF SPECIAL INTEREST

Nonsteroidal Antiinflammatory Drugs (NSAIDs)

NSAIDs are among the most common triggers of hypersensitivity reactions. The anti-inflammatory effect of NSAIDs is linked to the inhibition of cyclooxygenase and thereby reducing the synthesis of prostaglandins, which act as proinflammatory mediators. Cyclooxygenase is present in two isozymes, COX-1 and COX-2 with distinct functions. COX-1 is responsible for house-keeping functions and COX-2 is the inducible form, for example, by tissue damage. Most NSAIDs are isoform-nonspecific cyclooxygenase inhibitors and typical elicitors of acute urticaria and AE, exacerbations of rhinitis and asthma, or blended reactions. Three distinct clinical patterns can be identified: (1) NSAID exacerbated cutaneous disease (NECD): up to 30% of the patients with chronic urticaria (as an underlying disease) experience a "flare-up" reaction after intake of different NSAIDs as a classical dose-dependent, non-allergic intolerance reaction.[41] As soon as the urticaria remits, this intolerance subsides. (2) NSAID exacerbated respiratory disease (NERD): similar to NECD, NSAID can exacerbate a chronic rhinosinusitis with nasal polyposis or asthma in susceptible persons. This is usually a pseudo-allergic mechanism, which is caused by the inhibition of COX-1. This process reduces the formation of prostaglandin E2 and increases the precursor arachidonic acid. This can lead to the formation of new proinflammatory leukotrienes and lipoxygenases by other enzymes. This prostaglandin-leukotriene imbalance is dependent on the dose and the COX-1 inhibitory property of the NSAID.[42] (3) NSAID-induced urticarial angioedema (NIUA): these are mixed reactions, which include skin but also respiratory symptoms up to anaphylaxis. These reactions occur in otherwise asymptomatic individuals without preexisting asthma or urticaria.

The possibility of a truly IgE-mediated drug reaction needs to be considered if there is no cross-sensitivity, that is, only one specific NSAID leads to symptoms and others are well-tolerated. A typical example for a drug causing non-allergic intolerance and true allergic reactions is metamizol. The classical intolerance reaction is strictly dose-dependent and the eliciting NSAID doses should be documented.

Angiotensin-Converting Enzyme Inhibitor (ACE-I)

A special form of AE without itch and accompanying urticarial lesions is ACE-I induced. It affects 0.1% to 0.7% of all ACE-I treated patients and is often seen first in primary care setting.[43] It is a histamine-independent form of AE, attributable to the interference of ACE-I with the metabolism of the vasoactive substance bradykinin. Like with NSAID intolerance, ACE-I intolerance is based on the mode of action and not the chemical structure of the ACE-I molecule. Therefore, once established, it applies for all available ACE-I. Of note, antidiabetics of the gliptin class (inhibitors of dipeptidylpeptidase IV) not only block the metabolism of incretins but also "cross-inhibit" the metabolism of the vasoactive substance P. When used in combination with ACE-I or alone, gliptins may induce AE.[44] The neprilysin inhibitor sacubitril has the same risk for AE as ACE-I and should be avoided in patients with AE to ACE-I.[45]

ACE-I-induced angioedema (AAE) may first manifest after several years of well-tolerated treatment without an obvious cause like updosing or change in medication. AAE has no correlation to the more frequent ACE-I associated cough. Unfortunately, AAE has only mild prodromal symptoms

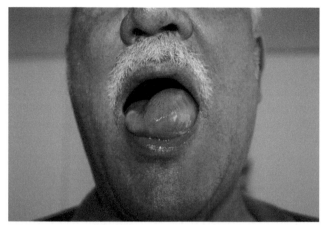

Fig. 9.9 Angioedema of the tongue in angiotensin-converting enzyme inhibitor–induced angioedema (AAE).

compared to the tingling sensations of hereditary AE or the itch of allergic AE. It usually progresses very quickly, which is its most critical and dangerous feature. It mainly affects the tongue, facial, and laryngeal structures, and dysarthria is an early sign indicating laryngeal affection.[46] During the first hours, all patients should be referred to a hospital equipped for emergency intubation and/or tracheotomy until remission is achieved (Fig. 9.9).

Acute treatment relies on immediate withdrawal of all ACE-I and securing patency of the airways. In severe AE, the bradykinin receptor antagonist icatibant, which is only licensed for hereditary AE, may be considered as treatment. Although one randomized trial and several case reports showed efficacy in the treatment of AAE, newer studies did not support these findings.[47] Infusions of C1-Inhibitor and corticosteroids during the acute stage of AAE have also been used in this indication. Emergency treatment with epinephrine (inhalations 1 mg epinephrine in 1 mL NaCl 0.9% using a nebulizer and/or 0.3–0.5 mg-wise i/m, lateral thigh, supine position) has been applied as well.

If antihypertensive therapy interfering with the renin-angiotensin-system is necessary, for example, for nephroprotection in diabetics, a switch-over to an angiotensin II or renin antagonist is usually possible. Both do not interfere with the metabolism of bradykinin and/or substance P.

Beta-Lactams

The beta-lactam antibiotic drug class consists of four major subclasses listed in Fig. 9.10. In the penicillin-allergic patient, the matter of cross-reactivity is a frequent concern of the treating physicians. As a rule of thumb, cross-reactivities are quite frequent within the subclasses mentioned in Fig. 9.9 and are usually based on side chain similarity rather than the beta-lactam ring itself.[31,40] Again, it is very important to distinguish the different reaction types, even if this clear-cut distinction is still inconsequently applied in the literature. In delayed-type reactions cross-reactivities are rare, because T cells recognize larger, more complex structures than IgE molecules. Common clinical examples are the tolerance of cephalosporins in penicillin-allergic subjects. IgE binds to smaller parts of the allergen, for example, a methylated side chain, so the risk of cross-reactivity

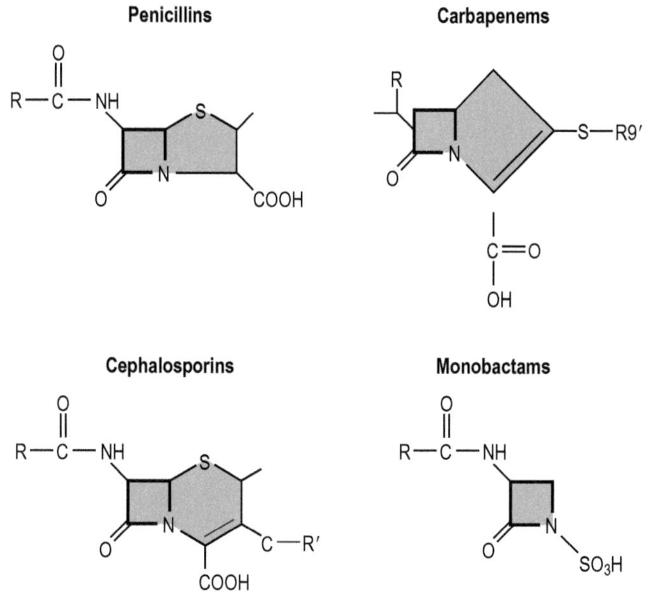

Fig. 9.10 Classes of β-lactam antibiotics.

with cephalosporins is about 1% to 2% in amoxicillin-induced immediate-type reactions with urticaria and/or anaphylaxis.[48] In cases of selective allergy to aminopenicillins, the cross-reactivity rate is higher.[49] The early reports on cross-reactivity rates between penicillins and cephalosporins of up to 10% were likely due to the contamination of cephalosporin antibiotics with trace amounts of penicillin. Therefore, in immediate-type reactions to a penicillin, the use of cephalosporins needs some caution and second line, structurally nonrelated alternative antibiotics have to be considered. The potential to cross react is less than 1% in carbapenems.[50] Monobactams (with the exception of aztreonam in ceftazidime allergic patients) are generally safe in penicillin allergic patients.[50]

In immediate-type reactions, the negative predictive value of intradermal skin testing with a selected set of beta-lactams using non-irritative concentrations (penicillin G, penicilloyl polylysine, minor determinant mixture [MDM], amoxicillin, cefazolin, cefuroxime, and ceftriaxone) is high, and a confirmative provocation test with the beta-lactam in question is safe and recommended.[31]

Fluoroquinolones

Hypersensitivity reactions to quinolone antibiotics can present as both immediate- and delayed-type hypersensitivity reactions. The most common is a MPE. This occurs in about 2% to 3% of patients treated, is usually mild, and subsides spontaneously. An allergy workup by patch test is usually not diagnostic. Cross-reactivity within quinolone antibiotics is usually rare in delayed-type hypersensitivity. Therefore, a provocation test with another quinolone antibiotic is usually helpful.

More problematic are immediate-type reactions. These are partly IgE mediated in the sense of a classical allergy, but much more often quinolones induce a direct mast cell activation by interaction with the mast cell receptor MRGPRX2. The underlying mechanism cannot be distinguished based on clinical characteristics. Skin tests and in vitro tests are not validated and

have a limited sensitivity. Often, a provocation test is necessary for diagnosis. Cross-reactivity among different quinolones is frequent in immediate hypersensitivity.

Antiepileptic Drugs

Hypersensitivity reactions to antiepileptic drugs are less frequent than reactions to antibiotics. They mostly involve delayed drug hypersensitivity reactions. They are a common cause of severe cutaneous drug reactions. In particular, antiepileptic drugs of the aromatic type, namely carbamazepine, oxcarbazepine, lamotrigine, and phenytoin, are most frequently involved. Cross-reactions within the group of aromatic antiepileptic drugs are common. Accordingly, non-aromatic antiepileptic drugs can often be used as an alternative.

Radio Contrast Media (RCM)

Reactions to intravascular RCM are divided into acute, usually during or immediately after the examination, and delayed forms. The latter are typically based on a T cell–based sensitization and intradermal skin testing is helpful for diagnosis and definition of safe alternatives. The acute reactions are also termed "anaphylactoid" because they may have some or all the features of anaphylaxis from upper and lower airway obstruction to hypotensive shock. Concomitant asthma increases the risk for acute reactions to RCM. Since the introduction of non-ionic agents, which are almost exclusively used today, reactions have become less common. A direct stimulation of histamine-rich effector cells (mast cells, basophils) by the high salt content and its rapid application (in bolus form) is thought to be the underlying pathomechanism. Therefore, non-ionic agents are considered safer than ionic agents, which break down into charged and therefore more stimulatory particles when entering the blood stream. Whether such reactions can be prevented by premedication is a subject of much debate among radiologists as well as the treating physicians. In previously mild hypersensitivity reactions, the occurrence of a severe breakthrough reaction is low (<1%).[51] To what extent premedication with corticosteroids (and antihistamines) can also reduce the occurrence of moderate to severe reactions remains open.

Biologicals

Therapeutically applied peptides and proteins, the so-called biologicals or biopharmaceuticals, are mainly used in anti-inflammatory and cancer treatment today. They represent the future of pharmaceutical medicine as the majority of drugs in development or in the licensing process belong to this new drug class. Biologicals usually directly interfere with the immune system and its signaling process (cytokines, chemokines, receptors). As a result, their side effects differ significantly from synthetic drugs like penicillin and can not only be explained by a substance-specific IgE- or T cell–mediated immune response. A new classification of AE to biologicals was proposed, related but clearly distinct from the classification of side effects observed with synthetic drugs.[52] This classification differentiates five distinct types, namely, clinical reactions because of high cytokine levels (type alpha), hypersensitivity because of an immune reaction against the biological agent (type beta) including the classical IgE- and T cell–mediated reactions, immune or cytokine imbalance syndromes (type gamma), symptoms because of cross-reactivity of the target structures (type delta), and symptoms that are either not immune-mediated or unclear (type epsilon),[52] for example, the retinopathy under interferon treatment. This classification could help to better deal with the diverse clinical features of these AE to biologicals.

ADRs to biologicals differ from ADR to LMW synthetic drugs like penicillin. Acute infusion-related reactions (IRRs) are the most frequently observed AE with varying incidence, depending on the substance administered (mostly 0.1%–3%). There is no clear definition of IRR (timing, symptoms) and re-exposure under slightly modified conditions (infusion rate, premedication) is possible in most of the cases.[53] This does not fit into the picture of IgE-mediated anaphylaxis. On the other hand, sporadic anaphylactic fatalities are reported. While regulatory agencies and the pharmaceutical industry focus on immunogenicity (antidrug antibodies, ADA), other possibly involved mechanisms should also be considered (aggregate formation, complement system, coagulation cascade, cytokine release). These additional pathophysiological mechanisms are inadequately reflected in the Gell and Coombs classification.

Checkpoint Inhibitors

Immune checkpoint inhibitors (ICIs) are biologicals (monoclonal antibodies) that downregulate inhibitory molecules, such as cytotoxic T-lymphocyte–associated protein 4 (CTLA-4) or programmed cell death protein 1 (PD-1) or its ligand (PD-L1). As a consequence, the immune system in proximity of the tumor, which has been dampened by products of the tumor cells, is activated again and the tumor cells are attacked. ICIs have changed the treatment and prognosis of several forms of advanced cancer dramatically. Depending on the type of tumor, even end-stages with distant metastasis became treatable with remission rates up to 50%.[54] This success comes at the cost of autoimmune complications of broad clinical variety ranging from skin rashes to lethal autoimmune myocarditis. Nearly every patient treated with checkpoint inhibitors exhibits some form of autoimmune reaction. Severe autoimmune side effects occur in every fourth patient in monotherapy and in every second patient with combined treatment using two different checkpoint inhibitors.

Unfortunately, not all side effects are recognized as such and the clinical course may progress. Skin reactions develop within 2 to 3 weeks, whereas inner organ involvement (gastrointestinal tract, liver, and lung) usually takes 6 to 7 weeks of treatment. Therefore, skin lesion should prompt surveillance of organ function and co-medication with immunosuppressants, including short courses of high-dose corticosteroids, as well as an intermittent ICI discontinuation should be evaluated. Endocrinological side effects such as autoimmune thyroiditis can be treated with hormone substitution alone. If the autoimmune reaction subsides, a cautious reintroduction of the checkpoint inhibitor can be considered. Only half of the patients relapse with their autoimmune side effect, but unfortunately, the relapsing patients show more lethal courses compared with ICI treatment naïve patients.

TREATMENT

Management of acute allergic drug reactions involves (1) identification by history and presentation and withdrawal of the most probable culprit drugs; (2) introduction of required supportive, suppressive, or remittive therapy; and (3) consideration of whether and how the incriminating drug should be substituted. Severe anaphylactic reactions must be treated with parenteral epinephrine (0.3–0.5 mg i/m, repetitive, lateral thigh, supine position) as the therapeutic cornerstone (see Chapter 13 on anaphylaxis). Exfoliative syndromes, including SJS and TEN, and any drug rash involving mucosal surfaces often require hospitalization.

There are a few exceptions to the rule of immediate drug withdrawal. In patients with life-threatening diseases, for example, enterococcal endocarditis, who require long-term treatment with high-dose treatment to effect a cure, "treating through" isolated episodes of urticarial, generalized pruritus or late occurring MPE may be attempted.[55] Experience suggests that most mild episodes (no blistering, no mucosal or organ involvement, no systemic symptoms) are self-limited and will remit with continuous therapy, provided there is a compelling clinical need to do so. H1 antihistamines and systemic/topical corticosteroids can be used to suppress symptoms while careful monitoring for fever, blood eosinophilia, proteinuria, arthralgia, lymphadenopathy, and hepatitis is warranted. Prompt cessation of therapy is mandatory if new signs or symptoms appear. One should be very careful when continuing treating with drugs known to elicit DRESS (Table 9.7). When continuing treating in those with mild type I reactions, it is obligatory to avoid lapses in treatment because restarting treatment after a lapse may invoke anaphylaxis.

There are three approaches to providing acceptable pharmacotherapy for the underlying condition in confirmed drug allergy: administration of (1) an unrelated alternative drug, (2) a potentially cross-reactive drug, or (3) re-administration of the offending drug.

The most common approach is administration of an unrelated alternative drug that is safe and effective for the disease requiring treatment. For the most common outpatient infections, alternative antibiotics provide a reasonable choice for the penicillin-allergic patient. Careful attention should be given to the risks of second-line therapy, especially treatment failure with antibiotics, and to the side effects/toxicity and cost of alternative regimens. In the case of NSAID intolerance, a selective COX-2 inhibitor like etoricoxib is usually well tolerated.

The second alternative for drug-sensitive patients is to receive a medication not identical to, but potentially cross-reactive with the offending drug. As a rule of thumb, cross-reactivities are quite frequent within the drug class, for example, quinolones, penicillins, but the absolute risk of cross-reactions is small. If beta-lactam reactions involve an immediate-type mechanism, preliminary skin testing with the chosen alternative and slow dose escalation, for example, standard intravenous dose at incremental rates over 4 to 6 hours, under observation can minimize the potential for life-threatening anaphylaxis. Whether gradual dose escalation is advantageous for delayed-type reactions is not properly studied and should definitely be avoided in SJS/TEN or DHS/DRESS patients.

The third alternative for drug-allergic subjects is re-administration of the offending drug by desensitization.[39] If an offending drug is irreplaceable or significantly more effective than the alternatives, the drug may need to be re-administered. Desensitization should only be performed under close supervision of a specialist experienced with this multi-step procedure, ideally in a hospital setting. Progressive doses of the offending drug are administered every 15 to 30 minutes for IgE-mediated reactions until a full therapeutic dose is clinically tolerated.[39] The procedure entails risk of acute allergic reactions, which occur in mild form in 30% to 80% of penicillin-allergic patients. Using recommended procedures, the success rate is high. Nevertheless, the risk benefit ratio needs to be evaluated thoroughly, as in rare cases deaths have occurred during desensitization attempts.

The mechanism by which clinical tolerance is induced during drug desensitization is complex and may involve low-level, subthreshold allergen stimulation rendering the involved cells "areactive" to the offending drug. Desensitization is an active process depending on the continuous presence of the drug. After the full therapeutic dose has been achieved without incident, continuous therapy should start immediately with appropriate monitoring. After drug discontinuation, the desensitized state typically gets lost after 2 to 3 days, and repetitive desensitization is usually required for subsequent treatment courses.[39] Again, it is best studied in IgE-mediated immediate-type reactions as well as in NSAID intolerance, whereas desensitization for delayed-type hypersensitivity reactions is still experimental. Especially in patients with HIV and cystic fibrosis, desensitization can be tried if a mild delayed-type drug hypersensitivity has occurred.

Premedication with antihistamines and corticosteroids has not been systematically studied for the prevention of IgE-mediated anaphylaxis. Numerous anecdotal reports attest their failure to prevent serious anaphylactic episodes. Premedication may mask early cutaneous symptoms and allow for a quicker updosing than advisable. Drugs reinstituted under the cover of corticosteroids may still be problematic when steroids are withdrawn. For these reasons, the regular use of premedication when undertaking drug desensitization is not recommended. In mild forms of NSAID hypersensitivity, especially NERD and NECD, a co-medication with a leukotriene antagonist is worth considering.

Some individuals are more vulnerable to mainly delayed-type hypersensitivity reactions as a result of genetic or metabolic abnormalities, frequent and recurrent drug exposure (e.g., antibiotics in cystic fibrosis), or certain disease states related to immune dysfunction (e.g., HIV infection). Such patients are prone to develop a drug allergy and are likely to benefit from a thorough and proactive evaluation that documents sensitizations. Ongoing reevaluation helps to keep the list of usable drugs from becoming unacceptably limited. Prevention of recurrent infections including vaccination is a primary objective in patients with multiple antibiotic sensitivities.

REFERRAL

When ambiguity surrounds which drug induced a severe immunologic reaction, plans should be made to pursue a definitive diagnosis after the patient's convalescence. Involving an allergologist minimizes the risk for another drug reaction without unnecessary limitations for further treatment and is especially important:

1. in severe forms of drug hypersensitivity, for example, anaphylaxis, DRESS, SJS/TEN, etc.;
2. if multiple and/or irreplaceable drugs were involved;
3. to clarify cross-reactivity patterns and define safe alternatives if re-exposure is expected (RCM, NMBA, antibiotics, etc.);
4. in repetitive reactions (e.g., mastocytosis);
5. if the patient needs reassuring.

Experience with the drugs in question, national and international databases, as well as specialized internet resources (excellent example for drug-induced pulmonary AE: www.pneumotox.com) may be helpful in identifying the correct culprit. The allergologist must also consider the significance of the substance for the treatment of the patient as well as the availability of safe alternatives in the individual setting of patient and underlying disease. This needs allergological, a broader medical and pharmacological knowledge as well as an understanding of the individual situation of the patient. This ambitious task can only be addressed by a therapeutic partnership of primary care physician, specialist, and the patient.

If the drug culprit is identified, the use of wallet cards, identification jewelry, and registry services (e.g., MedicAlert) should be recommended for patients with documented severe reactions. The following information should be included and clearly documented:

- culprit drug (non-proprietary name and product name);
- type of reaction (immediate/delayed, organ involvement, severity);
- proof of sensitization (history only, or by skin testing, serology, LTT, BAT);
- cross-reactive substance(s) and safe alternative(s).

Finally, again highlighting the role of the national pharmacovigilance programs, every physician is encouraged to document all relevant ADR encountered. National electronic reporting systems like MedWatch (www.fda.gov/Safety/MedWatch) are usually easily accessible.

CONCLUSIONS

Drug hypersensitivity is an iatrogenic disease and therefore requires special attention! It is a frequent phenomenon, but often presents a frustrating challenge for most practicing physicians. Because immunodiagnostic tests for drug allergy are limited in number and require some sophistication to interpret, many practitioners have concluded that the only reasonable option for drug-reactive patients is permanent and total avoidance of putative offenders. In the extreme, patients with multiple drug hypersensitivity syndromes are sometimes abandoned by their primary care physicians, or they are told to do without all drug therapy.

Armed with an understanding of the distinction between regular side effects, drug allergy and idiosyncrasy, the risk factors for drug allergy, and the pharmacoepidemiology of sensitizing drugs, physicians can safely provide useful drug therapy for a surprisingly large number of drug-allergic patients. For allergy and immunology specialists, the willingness to undertake this task is usually appreciatively obliged by other professionals, who readily refer drug-sensitive patients and are grateful for the assistance received.

Medical progress in understanding and managing drug hypersensitivity states often requires the collaborative efforts of multiple disciplines, including basic immunology, pharmacology, toxicology, genetics, biochemistry, pathology, and epidemiology. The high morbidity rates and costs associated with drug hypersensitivity make this set of disorders a high priority for future research investment.

REFERENCES

1. Cano FG, Rozenfeld S. Adverse drug events in hospitals: a systematic review. Cad Saude Publica. 2009;25(Suppl 3):S360.
2. Youngster I, Arcavi L, Schechmaster R. Medications and glucose6-phosphate dehydrogenase deficiency. Drug Saf. 2010;33:713.
3. Brockow K, Ardern-Jones M, Mockenhaupt M, et al. EAACI position paper on how to classify cutaneous manifestations of drug hypersensitivity. Allergy. 2019;74:14–27.
4. Adkinson NFJr. Risk factors for drug allergy. J Allergy Clin Immunol. 1984;74:567.
5. Pichler WJ. Immune pathomechanism and classification of drug hypersensitivity. Allergy. 2019;74(8):1457–1471.
6. Lazarou J, Pomeranz BH, Corey PN. Incidence of adverse drug reactions in hospitalized patients: a meta-analysis of prospective studies. JAMA. 1998;279:1200.
7. Chang CJ, Chen CB, Hung SI, Ji C, Chung WH. Pharmacogenetic testing for prevention of severe cutaneous adverse drug reactions. Front Pharmacol. 2020;11:969.
8. Macy E. Elective penicillin skin testing and amoxicillin challenge: effect on outpatient antibiotic use, cost, and clinical outcomes. J Allergy Clin Immunol. 1998;102:281–285.
9. Charneski L, Deshpande G, Smith SW. Impact of an antimicrobial allergy label in the medical record on clinical outcomes in hospitalized patients. Pharmacotherapy. 2011;3:742–747.
10. Jörg L, Yerly D, Helbling A, et al. The role of drug, dose, and the tolerance/intolerance of new drugs in multiple drug hypersensitivity syndrome. Allergy. 2019;75:1178–1187.
11. Blanca-Lopez N, Soriano V, Garcia-Martin E, et al. NSAID-induced reactions: classification, prevalence, impact, and management strategies. J Asthma Allergy. 2019;12:217–233.
12. Liu R, Hu S, Zhang Y, et al. Mast cell-mediated hypersensitivity to fluoroquinolone is MRGPRX2 dependent. Int Immunopharmacol. 2019;70:417.
13. Simons FE. 9. Anaphylaxis. J Allergy Clin Immunol. 2008;2(Suppl):S402–S407.
14. Gomes ER, Brockow K, Kuyucu S, et al. Terreehorst I; drug hypersensitivity in children: report from the pediatric task force of the EAACI Drug Allergy Interest Group. Allergy. 2016;71(2):149–161.
15. Dibek Misirlioglu E, Guvenir H, Ozkaya Parlakay A, et al. Incidence of antibiotic-related rash in children with Epstein-Barr virus infection and evaluation of the frequency of confirmed antibiotic hypersensitivity. Int Arch Allergy Immunol. 2018;176(1):33–38.
16. Sekula P, Dunant A, Mockenhaupt M, et al. Comprehensive survival analysis of a cohort of patients with Stevens-Johnson syndrome and toxic epidermal necrolysis. J Invest Dermatol. 2013;133(5):1197–1204.
17. Assier H, Bastuji-Garin S, Revuz J, et al. Erythema multiforme with mucous membrane involvement and Stevens-Johnson syndrome are clinically different disorders with distinct causes. Arch Dermatol. 1995;131:539.
18. Mittmann N, Knowles SR, Koo M, et al. Incidence of toxic epidermal necrolysis and Stevens-Johnson syndrome in an HIV cohort: an observational, retrospective case series study. Am J Clin Dermatol. 2012;13:49.
19. Horne NS, Narayan AR, Young RM, et al. Toxic epidermal necrolysis in systemic lupus erythematosus. Autoimmun Rev. 2006;5:160.
20. Anhalt GJ, Kim SC, Stanley JR, et al. Paraneoplastic pemphigus. An autoimmune mucocutaneous disease associated with neoplasia. N Engl J Med. 1990;323:1729–1735.
21. Husain Z, Reddy BY, Schwartz RA. DRESS syndrome: part I. Clinical perspectives. J Am Acad Dermatol. 2013;68(693):e1–e14.
22. Kardaun SH, Sekula P, Valeyrie-Allanore L, et al. Drug reaction with eosinophilia and systemic symptoms (DRESS): an original multisystem adverse drug reaction. Results from the prospective RegiSCAR study. Br J Dermatol. 2013;169:1071.
23. Jörg L, Helbling A, Yerly D, Pichler WJ. Drug-related relapses in drug reaction with eosinophilia and systemic symptoms (DRESS). Clin Transl Allergy. 2020;10(1):52.
24. Pichler WJ, Daubner B, Kawabata T. Drug hypersensitivity: flare-up reactions, cross-reactivity and multiple drug hypersensitivity. J Dermatol. 2011;38:216–221.
25. Kano Y, Hiraharas K, Sakuma K, Shiohara T. Several herpesviruses can reactivate in a severe drug-induced multiorgan reaction in the same sequential order as in graft-versus-host disease. Br J Dermatol. 2006;155:301.
26. Mizukawa Y, Hirahara K, Kano Y, Shiohara T. Drug-induced hypersensitivity syndrome/drug reaction with eosinophilia and systemic symptoms severity score: useful tool for assessing disease severity and predicting fatal cytomegalovirus disease. J Am Acad Dermatol. 2019;80(3):670–678, e2.
27. Tennis P, Stern RS. Risk of serious cutaneous disorders after initiation of use of phenytoin, carbamazepine, or sodium valproate: a record linkage study. Neurology. 1997;49:542.
28. Santiago LG, Morgado FJ, Baptista MS, Gonçalo M. Hypersensitivity to antibiotics in drug reaction with eosinophilia and systemic symptoms (DRESS) from other culprits. Contact Dermatitis. 2020;82:290–296.
29. Stirnimann G, Kessebohm K, Lauterburg B. Liver injury caused by drugs: an update. Swiss Med Wkly. 2010;140:w13080.
30. Fox S, Park M. Penicillin skin testing is a safe and effective tool for evaluating penicillin allergy in the pediatric population. J Allergy Clin Immunol Pract. 2014;2:439–444.
31. Romano A, Atanaskovic-Markovic M, Barbaud A, et al. Towards a more precise diagnosis of hypersensitivity to beta-lactams: an EAACI position paper. Allergy. 2019;75:1300–1315.
32. Aberer W, Bircher A, Romano A, et al. Drug provocation testing in the diagnosis of drug hypersensitivity reactions: general considerations. Allergy. 2003;58:854.
33. Valent P, Akin C, Bonadonna P, et al. Proposed diagnostic algorithm for patients with suspected mast cell activation syndrome. J Allergy Clin Immunol Pract. 2019;7:1125.
34. Lammintausta K, Kortekangas-Savolainen O. Oral challenge in patients with suspected cutaneous adverse drug reactions: findings in 784 patients during a 25-year-period. Acta Derm Venereol. 2005;85(6):491–496.
35. Brockow K, Romano A, Blanca M, et al. General considerations for skin test procedures in the diagnosis of drug hypersensitivity. Allergy. 2002;57:45–51.

36. Barbaud A, Gonçalo M, Bruynzeel D, Bircher A. Guidelines for performing skin tests with drugs in the investigation of cutaneous adverse drug reactions. Contact Dermatitis. 2001;45(6):321–328.

37. Brockow K, Garvey LH, Aberer W, et al. Skin test concentrations for systemically administered drugs—an ENDA/EAACI Drug Allergy Interest Group position paper. Allergy. 2013;68:702–712.

38. Mayorga C, Celik G, Rouzaire P, et al. In vitro tests for drug hypersensitivity reactions: an ENDA/EAACI Drug Allergy Interest Group position paper. Allergy. 2016;71(8):1103–1134.

39. Scherer K, Brockow K, Aberer W, et al. Desensitization in delayed drug hypersensitivity reactions: an EAACI position paper of the Drug Allergy Interest Group. Allergy. 2013;68:844.

40. Castells M, Khan DA, Phillips EJ. Penicillin allergy. N Engl J Med. 2019;381(24):2338–2351.

41. Setkowicz M, Mastalerz L, Podolec-Rubis M, et al. Clinical course and urinary eicosanoids in patients with aspirin-induced urticaria followed up for 4 years. J Allergy Clin Immunol. 2009;123:174.

42. Stevenson DD, Sanchez-Borges M, Szczeklik A. Classification of allergic and pseudoallergic reactions to drugs that inhibit cyclooxygenase enzymes. Ann Allergy Asthma Immunol. 2001;87:177.

43. Banerji A, Blumenthal KG, Lai KH, Zhou L. Epidemiology of ACE inhibitor angioedema utilizing a large electronic health record. J Allergy Clin Immunol Pract. 2017;5(3):744–749.

44. Scott SI, Andersen MF, Aagaard L, et al. Dipeptidyl peptidase-4 inhibitor induced angioedema-an overlooked adverse drug reaction? Curr Diabetes Rev. 2018;14:327.

45. McMurray JJ, Packer M, Desai AS, et al. Dual angiotensin receptor and neprilysin inhibition as an alternative to angiotensin-converting enzyme inhibition in patients with chronic systolic heart failure: rationale for and design of the Prospective comparison of ARNI with ACEI to Determine Impact on Global Mortality and morbidity in Heart Failure trial (PARADIGM-HF). Eur J Heart Fail. 2013;15:1062.

46. Banerji A, Clark S, Blanda M, et al. Multicenter study of patients with angiotensin-converting enzyme inhibitor-induced angioedema who present to the emergency department. Ann Allergy Asthma Immunol. 2008;100:327.

47. Straka BT, Ramirez CE, Byrd JB, et al. Effect of bradykinin receptor antagonism on ACE inhibitor-associated angioedema. J Allergy Clin Immunol. 2017;140:242.

48. Trubiano JA, Stone CA, Grayson ML, et al. The 3 Cs of antibiotic allergy—classification, cross-reactivity, and collaboration. J Allergy Clin Immunol Pract. 2017;5:1532–1542.

49. Romano A, Valluzzi RL, Caruso C, et al. Cross-reactivity and tolerability of cephalosporins in patients with IgE-mediated hypersensitivity to penicillins. J Allergy Clin Immunol Pract. 2018;6:1662–1672.

50. Gaeta F, Valluzzi RL, Alonzi C, et al. Tolerability of aztreonam and carbapenems in patients with IgE-mediated hypersensitivity to penicillins. J Allergy Clin Immunol. 2015;135:972–976.

51. Davenport MS, Cohan RH, Caoili EM, Ellis JH. Repeat contrast medium reactions in premedicated patients: frequency and severity. Radiology. 2009;253:372.

52. Hausmann OV, Seitz M, Villiger PM, et al. The complex clinical picture of side effects to biologicals. Med Clin North Am. 2010;94:791–804.

53. Boyman O, et al. Adverse reactions to biologic agents and their medical management. Nat Rev Rheumatol. 2014;10:612–627.

54. Chan KK, Bass AR. Autoimmune complications of immunotherapy: pathophysiology and management. BMJ. 2020;369:m736.

55. Lin D, Li WK, Rieder MJ. Cotrimoxazole for prophylaxis or treatment of opportunistic infections of HIV/AIDS in patients with previous history of hypersensitivity to cotrimoxazole. Cochrane Database Syst Rev. 2007;2007:CD005646.

56. Picard D, Vellar M, Janela B, et al. Recurrence of drug-induced reactions in DRESS patients. J Eur Acad Dermatol Venereol. 2015:801–804.

57. Landry Q, Zhang S, Ferrando L, et al. Multiple Drug Hypersensitivity Syndrome in a Large Database. J Allergy Clin Immunol Pract. 2020;8(1):258–266. e1. https://doi.org/10.1016/j.jaip.2019.06.009.

10

Urticaria

Clive E.H. Grattan and Sarbjit S. Saini

CHAPTER OUTLINE

SUMMARY OF IMPORTANT CONCEPTS

- Urticaria is an illness characterized by itchy wheals (hives), angioedema, or both. It may be acute or chronic, depending on the duration of the whole episode.
- Acute urticaria (AU) occurs in up to 20% of the population and may be associated with a drug or food allergy, or with infection but the cause is often unknown. It is, by definition, self-limiting and usually resolves over 2 to 3 weeks.
- Chronic urticaria (CU) occurs in up to 1% of the population. It is defined by continuous disease for ≥6 weeks. All cases go through an acute phase. Most have chronic spontaneous urticaria (CSU). The cause of this is often difficult to identify in the clinic but research studies indicate that up to one-third of patients have functional autoantibodies that release histamine from basophils and mast cells in the laboratory (autoimmune urticaria). There is also emerging evidence that immunoglobulin E (IgE) against self-antigens is expressed more often in CU (autoallergic urticaria) but their pathogenic role is under study. A small number may relate to underlying infection.

- Approximately 25% of patients with CU have a reproducible external trigger for their skin lesions, although the cause of their illness remains unknown. These patients are said to have an inducible urticaria.
- Urticaria should be managed by treatment of the cause (if one can be found), minimizing of aggravating factors that worsen spontaneous disease, avoidance of inducing triggers, and control of symptoms with nonsedating H_1-antihistamines, until natural disease remission occurs.
- In patients in whom antihistamines are ineffective, or in those who have been dependent on oral corticosteroids for relief, several antiinflammatory or immunsuppresive approaches can be tried, with careful monitoring for toxicity. The monoclonal antibody omalizumab (anti-IgE) can be highly effective for CSU and other treatment-refractory inducible urticarias.
- When recurrent angioedema occurs without wheals, the possibility of C1 esterase inhibitor deficiency or other types of bradykininergic angioedema should be excluded.

INTRODUCTION AND HISTORICAL PERSPECTIVE

Urticaria affects people of all ages and is common. For the purposes of this chapter, the terms *chronic idiopathic urticaria (CIU)* and *chronic spontaneous urticaria (CSU)* are used as being directly equivalent and the term "CSU" has been used throughout in line with recent international guidelines.[1] Nearly one in five persons will experience an episode of urticaria in their lifetime; the chronic spontaneous form of disease affects up to 1% of the general population at any one time[2] but the prevalence of all types of chronic urticaria (CU) will be higher. Because of the similarity of CU symptoms to those seen in patients suffering allergic reactions to drugs or foods, the condition often leads to a search for an environmental (and avoidable) cause. In most cases, no identifiable cause can be identified, and the disease is managed by controlling symptoms and avoidance of triggers.

DEFINITIONS AND CLASSIFICATIONS

Urticaria

The condition is characterized by the appearance of short-lived, pruritic, pink wheals (hives) that fade rapidly without a mark. Wheals are superficial swellings of the dermis. Angioedema is a deeper swelling of the dermis or subcutaneous tissue that may occur on its own or with wheals. Angioedema swellings are pale, poorly defined, painful rather than itchy, and usually take more than a day to fade. They affect skin and submucosal tissues. *Acute* urticaria (AU) is defined by a disease duration of less than 6 weeks, whereas *chronic* urticaria (CU) is generally defined by the presence of urticaria on most days of the week, for a period of 6 weeks or more. Approximately 50% of patients with CU have accompanying episodes of angioedema, whereas 10% have angioedema as their main manifestation.

CU can be further classified using various criteria. Approximately 25% of patients with CU have a reproducible external trigger for their skin lesions, rather than spontaneous swellings; this form of the disorder used to be termed "physical urticaria," but the term *inducible urticaria* is now preferred.[1] Inducible urticarias include physical, cholinergic, and contact urticaria subtypes. These cases are labeled according to the nature of the inciting stimulus (Table 10.1). In the remaining 75% of cases, no external cause or physical trigger can be identified; accordingly, the condition has historically been called "chronic idiopathic urticaria" (CIU), implying that an etiology cannot be found. However, the clinical term *chronic spontaneous urticaria* (CSU) is now preferred because it carries no inference about etiology but serves to separate those patients with the ordinary presentation of CU from those with inducible urticarias. Some guidelines and experts identify a subset of CSU patients with an autoimmune etiology on the basis of serological evidence of functional autoantibodies targeting immunoglobulin E (IgE) or the high affinity IgE receptor (observed in 30%–40% of these patients) and strong circumstantial evidence for having an autoimmune illness chronic autoimmune urticaria (CAU). Those CSU patients without evidence of an

TABLE 10.1 Physical Urticaria: Subtypes, Triggers, and Testing Procedures.

Disorder	Triggering Factor	Test Description
Symptomatic dermographism (urticaria factitia)	Stroking, scratching, friction	Mild stroking of skin with tip of pen or tongue blade or dermographometer at ≤36 g/mm²
Delayed pressure urticaria (DPU)	Application of pressure 30 min to 12 h before onset	Shoulder sling with weight of 7 kg placed for 15 min; patient records symptoms over 24 h or a dermographometer held at 100 g/mm² on the shoulder for 70 s
Cholinergic urticaria	Elevation of body temperature with exercise, hot water, strong emotion, or spicy food	Exercise with a stationary bike for 15 min beyond onset of sweating; or passive heating of one arm to 42 °C with water bath or whole body immersion Evidence of reaction to sweat antigen
Cold urticaria	Exposure of skin to cold air, cold objects, or cold liquids	Ice cube test for 5 min on arm Temperature "threshold" test if available (TempTest)
Heat urticaria	Warm object in direct contact with skin	Application of test-tube containing warm water at 44 °C or use of TempTest
Exercise-induced urticaria	Exercise activity	Treadmill testing or exercise bicycle
Aquagenic urticaria	Skin contact with water at any temperature	Application of water compress at 35 °C to the trunk or water immersion for 10 min
Solar urticaria	Exposure of skin to sunlight of specific wavelength	Exposure of skin to UVA, UVB, or visible light
Vibratory urticaria	Lawn mowing, riding a bike, exposure to vibrating machinery	Vortex platform held to forearm skin for 10 min

UVA, Ultraviolet A; *UVB*, ultraviolet B.

autoimmune or infectious etiology remain idiopathic where the etiology is likely to be multifactorial to endogenous and environmental factors.

EPIDEMIOLOGY

Both children and adults can acquire CU, although it appears to be more common in adults, with women with CSU being affected twice as often as men. The average age of patients suggests that the condition typically begins in the third to fifth decades of life. The coexpression of atopic disease diagnosis in patients with CU appears to be only slightly higher than in the general population.

NATURAL HISTORY AND PROGNOSIS

CU is a self-limited disorder in nearly all patients, although it not infrequently persists for years. Estimates of disease duration vary, but one study indicated that 50% of patients are better in 6 months, another 20% by 3 years, and a further 20% by 5 years, with just 8% persisting for more than 10 years.[3]

Angioedema, thyroid autoimmunity, hypertension,[4] and increased disease severity have been identified as factors associated with longer disease duration.[5]

DISEASE ASSOCIATIONS

Autoimmunity

An association of CSU with autoimmune thyroid disease has been confirmed in multiple publications since it was first reported in 1983. The association is particularly strong (30%) in patients with histamine-releasing autoantibodies in their blood. Other autoimmune disorders are also more prevalent in CSU than in the general population.[6] Furthermore, increased human leukocyte antigen (HLA) class II DR antigen expression is noted in subjects with CSU and, in particular, those with evidence of functional autoantibodies in their serum.[7]

Infections

The topic of infections and CU has been reviewed.[8] A link between infections and CU onset has often been proposed but is difficult to prove. *Helicobacter pylori* infection of the stomach has been widely studied, but the data are conflicting. Upper respiratory viral and pyogenic bacterial infections are associated with AU, especially in children. Some pediatric series suggest that an infection is associated with disease or possibly is related to the antibiotic used to treat the illness, although it is usually the former. AU can be observed in the early stages of hepatitis A, B, and C infection, but little evidence exists for a causative association with CU.

In the past, exhaustive stool studies to exclude parasites as a cause of urticaria have been recommended. Pathogens such as *Ancylostoma*, *Strongyloides*, *Filaria*, *Echinococcus*, *Trichinella*, *Fasciola*, *Schistosoma mansoni*, and *Blastocystis hominis* have all been associated with CSU. Stool studies for parasites probably are relevant only in persons with a history of recent travel to endemic areas and often with peripheral eosinophilia. Ingestion of fish contaminated with *Anisakis simplex* also can lead to urticaria in presensitized patients.

Allergen-Triggered Urticaria

Patients experiencing anaphylaxis triggered by foods, drugs, and other agents or conditions frequently demonstrate skin symptoms within 30 minutes, and such allergens may be viewed as a direct cause of urticaria (see Chapters 9 and 12). Certain foods such as strawberries and tomatoes may cause skin eruptions without a clear allergic basis (histamine liberators or high histamine content). Skin contact with raw fruits, certain foods, and aeroallergens in an allergic host can elicit immunological contact urticaria.

Nonsteroidal Antiinflammatory Drugs (NSAIDs)

NSAIDs, which include aspirin, ibuprofen, and naproxen, are in common use and can trigger urticaria acutely or aggravate preexisting CSU. This reaction is related to inhibition of cyclooxygenase by these agents. The reported frequency of NSAID-induced exacerbations of skin disease ranges from 25% to 50%. In some affected patients, the period of aspirin sensitivity ends after the urticaria resolves. Genetic variability of prostaglandin E_2 receptor subtype EP4 gene in aspirin-intolerant CSU has also been described.

Malignancy

Older studies raised concern that CU may be due to an underlying malignancy. The question of whether patients with CU are at higher risk for malignancies has not been conclusively answered. Two large studies have addressed this question and reached opposite conclusions. In the first study, 1155 Swedish patients with CU were followed in an academic dermatology department for an average of 8.2 years. The incidence of malignant cancer during the observation period was compared with the expected number of cancers from the Swedish Cancer Registry, yielding a relative risk of 0.88 (95% confidence interval, 0.61–1.12).[9] In the second study, a cohort of 12,720 Taiwanese patients were identified as having CU from a National Cancer Registry. The rate of malignancies diagnosed in this cohort over an average follow-up period of 5 years was compared with expected rates. The standardized incidence ratio for patients with CU was 2.2 (95% CI, 2.0–2.4).[10] Younger patients appeared to be at higher risk for hematologic malignancies, including lymphoma.

PATHOGENESIS AND ETIOLOGY

Skin Histopathologic Features

Histopathologic examination of an urticarial lesion will show skin mast cells that have degranulated in the dermis, as well as a perivascular leukocyte infiltrate composed of lymphocytes, eosinophils, neutrophils, and also basophils that have migrated to the skin lesion. Both mast cells and basophils release histamine and other inflammatory mediators (e.g., prostaglandins, leukotrienes, cytokines, and kinins) on activation, which are capable of causing local vasodilation, itch, and swelling in the skin. Histamine appears to be a central mediator, as suggested by the prominent clinical symptom of pruritus and the beneficial response to H_1-antihistamines.

Current understanding of the roles for eosinophils, lymphocytes, and neutrophils in disease pathology is limited. A predominance of neutrophils in the skin lesion biopsy, the definitive feature of *neutrophilic urticarial dermatosis*, should lead to a search for associated systemic diseases such as Schnitzler syndrome, adult-onset Still disease, systemic lupus erythematosus (SLE), and the hereditary autoinflammatory fever syndromes. Studies of other immune pathways involved in CSU have focused mainly on T lymphocytes and circulating serum cytokines. Increased IL-6 and C-reactive protein (CRP) levels are noted in the serum of subjects with CU plus NSAIDs sensitivity demonstrated on aspirin challenge, lending support to the concept that increased inflammatory markers reflect the urticarial disease. Immune features in patients with CSU resistant to high-dose antihistamine therapy relative to antihistamine responders include greater basopenia, eosinopenia, higher mean platelet volume, higher levels of CRP, and higher levels of serum complement component, C3, which are features of low-grade inflammation and platelet activation.[5] A series of studies suggest that the extrinsic coagulation pathway is activated in CU associated with increased levels of the fibrin degradation product, D-dimer, and prothrombin fragments.

Pathogenesis

Of the several theories regarding the pathogenesis of CSU, none has been conclusively established. Most studies have examined the autoimmune theory of disease and the serologic tests to establish autoimmunity. Other theories involve abnormalities in skin mast cells and basophils. Limited data on other causes, such as chronic infections, provide some support for additional pathogenesis mechanisms.

Autoimmune Hypothesis

It is thought that 30% to 40% of patients with CSU have an autoimmune disease driven by pathogenic immunoglobulin G (IgG) autoantibodies to either IgE or the α-subunit of the high-affinity IgE receptor that activates mast cells and basophils immunologically (Fig. 10.1). The evolution of the autoimmune theory (Fig. 10.2) dates back to the 1980s when a serum factor that could elicit an immediate red wheal response on intradermal reinjection was described in over 50% of patients with CSU. This became known as the autologous serum skin test (ASST). However, a positive ASST reaction has also been described in persons with allergic airway disease and in healthy control subjects, raising issues about its specificity in CSU disease.

In parallel with early studies of ASST, nonfunctional IgG antibodies targeting the Fc region of IgE were found by an immunoassay, followed by a study that demonstrated IgG antibodies with properties of anti-IgE in CSU sera could release histamine from basophils of healthy donors. Subsequently, IgG autoantibodies with specificity against the alpha-chain of the high-affinity IgE receptor (anti-Fc$_\varepsilon$RI$_\alpha$) were identified as the main serum factor responsible for histamine-releasing activity (HRA) on basophils.[11] Early reports suggested that basophil HRA and ASST reactions decreased in disease remission. Subsequent studies showed that IgG from CSU sera could also release histamine from neonatal foreskin slices containing mast cells, which are thought to be the primary effector cell of CU. Immunoassays that detect functional and nonfunctional autoantibodies have demonstrated anti-Fc$_\varepsilon$RI$_\alpha$ in other diseases and healthy controls. As yet, no simple and reproducible assay for functional autoantibodies in CSU has been developed for use in routine clinical practice. This has hampered studies on epidemiology, disease associations, and establishing therapeutic relevance of histamine release autoantibodies in CSU. Low total

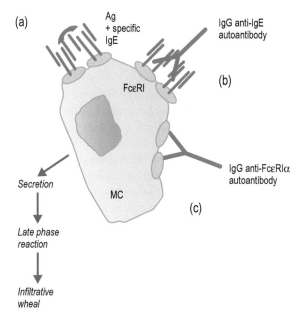

Fig. 10.1 Diagrammatic representation of different modes of mast cell (MC) activation in the pathogenesis of urticaria. (a) An antigen cross-linking IgE; (b) IgG anti-IgE antibody, as seen in 5%–10% of patients with chronic spontaneous urticaria (CSU). (c) IgG anti-IgE receptor antibody directed to the α-subunit (FcεRIα), as seen in 40% of patients with CSU. IgE, IgG, Immunoglobulins E and G. Modified from Kaplan AP, Greaves M. Pathogenesis of chronic urticaria. Clin Exp Allergy 2009; 39:777–787.

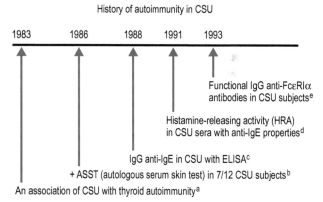

Fig. 10.2 Timeline of recognition of autoimmune theory in chronic spontaneous urticaria (CSU). IgG, Immunoglobulins E and G. Modified from [a] Leznoff A, Josse RG, Denburg J, et al. Association of chronic urticaria and angioedema with thyroid autoimmunity. Arch Dermatol 1983;119:636–40. [b] Grattan CEH, Wallington TB, Warin RP, Kennedy CTC, Bradfield JW. A serological mediator in chronic idiopathic urticaria: a clinical, immunologic and histological evaluation. Br J Dermatol 1986;114:583–90. [c] Gruber BL, Baeza ML, Marchese MJ, et al. Prevalence and functional role of anti-IgE autoantibodies in urticarial syndromes. J Invest Dermatol 1988;90:213–7. [d] Grattan CE, Francis DM, Hide M, et al. Detection of circulating histamine-releasing autoantibodies with functional properties of anti-IgE in chronic urticaria. Clin Exp Allergy 1991;21:695–704. [e] Hide M, Francis DM, Grattan CE, et al. Autoantibodies against the high-affinity IgE receptor as a cause of histamine release in chronic urticaria. N Engl J Med 1993;328:1599–604.

IgE and positive thyroid autoantibodies may be a useful marker of autoimmune urticaria.[12] Conversely, elevated IgE is a potential marker of autoallergic urticaria.[13]

Skin Mast Cells

Mast cell degranulation is a central event in the development of the lesions in urticaria, and histamine levels may be elevated in biopsied skin. A three fold increase in mast cell numbers was found in CSU compared with controls, but no difference was observed between lesional and uninvolved skin.[14] Total serum tryptase level, an indirect measure of total body mast cell numbers, is only slightly elevated in subjects with CU in comparison with healthy and atopic subjects but is still within the normal range.

Blood Basophils

A role for blood basophils in the pathogenesis of CU has emerged. Since the 1960s, it has been known that the number of circulating basophils in CSU is reduced. This basopenia is linked to the presence of serum HRA. In the 1970s, two groups of investigators demonstrated that blood basophils of patients with CU were reduced in their ability to release histamine after IgE receptor activation. Blood basophil IgE receptor responses of patients with CIU have been segregated into two basophil phenotypes: CSU responders and CSU nonresponders to anti-IgE, a standard laboratory stimulus. These two functional phenotypes are stable in active disease, are independent of the presence of autoimmune serum factors, and also reflect differences in some clinical features. Furthermore, hyporeleasability of basophil response becomes less so in disease remission. Skin biopsy studies using basophil-specific stains have provided evidence for basophil presence in both lesional sites and nonlesional skin tissues, a finding not seen in healthy skin. The degree of basopenia is correlated with disease severity and may reflect blood basophil recruitment to the skin lesions, whereas with CIU remission, basopenia remits. Collectively, this evidence suggests that altered basophil IgE receptor function and trafficking are present in CU.

DIAGNOSTIC APPROACH

Evidence-based guidelines have been published on the approach to diagnosis and the treatment of CU.[1]

History

The duration of the skin symptoms should be sought for classification of the urticaria as either acute or chronic, as well as the details of the characteristic and other lesions. Wheals are typically pruritic, and the discomfort can be severe enough to disrupt work, school, or sleep, with significant impairment of quality of life. Any area of the body may be affected, and areas in which clothing compresses the skin (e.g., waistbands) or areas of skin friction are more often affected. Patients whose symptoms have resolved can have difficulty describing urticarial lesions in a detailed manner, and in such cases, reviewing any photographs of the urticarial lesions can be helpful. The duration of an individual lesion can be useful to distinguish

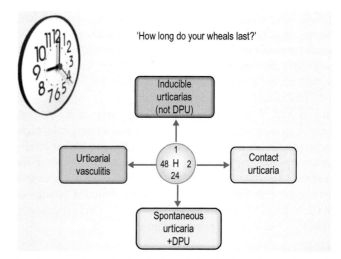

Fig. 10.3 Timing of wheals is helpful in the diagnosis of the different patterns of chronic urticaria ("the urticaria clock"). *DPU,* Delayed pressure urticaria.

CU from urticarial vasculitis. In CSU, wheals typically last less than 24 hours without residual change to the skin area, whereas lesions in urticarial vasculitis generally last for days and may bruise. By contrast, the wheals of inducible urticaria (with the exception of delayed pressure urticaria [DPU] that lasts up to a day) fade within an hour, and this can be a very helpful part of the history (Fig. 10.3).

The pruritus of CU is often most noticeable at night. Patients also may report more severe symptoms during periods of stress and may suffer from other emotional issues. Food allergies often are suspected by patients but are rarely substantiated. Pseudoallergens, or chemicals in foods (histamine, natural salicylates, additives, spices, and alcohol), have been linked to CSU but appear to aggravate established disease rather than cause it. Restricted diets over a 3-week trial initially followed by stepwise reintroduction may assist patients so affected. Aspirin or other NSAIDs may exacerbate CSU in up to 30% of patients and should generally be avoided unless there is a specific indication, such as low-dose aspirin for cardiovascular prophylaxis, or severe pain. Patterns of skin symptoms such as an association with menstrual cycles should be ascertained and may suggest other diseases such as progesterone dermatitis. Physical factors such as pressure, friction, and heat can exacerbate skin manifestations. The presence (both recent and remote) of systemic signs and symptoms such as fever, weight loss, and arthralgias should lead to further investigation for an underlying disorder, such as systemic lupus or other autoinflammatory disease.

Physical Examination

The typical hive is pruritic, raised, and erythematous and may exhibit central pallor due to intense edema as it first comes up. The lesion can take several forms in CSU and may appear round, oval, or serpiginous, and multiple lesions may become confluent (Fig. 10.4). Wheals of symptomatic dermographism and cholinergic urticaria have a distinctive morphology: dermographic wheals are typically linear but may form large plaques where the skin has been scratched (Fig. 10.5), whereas

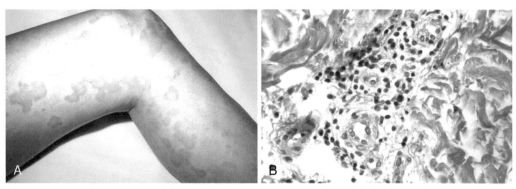

Fig. 10.4 (A) Typical skin lesions in a patient with chronic spontaneous urticaria (CSU). (B) Skin biopsy findings from a patient with CSU (hematoxylin-eosin stain).

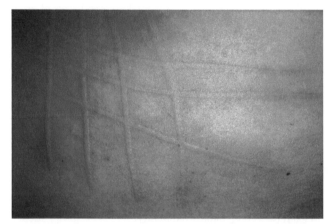

Fig. 10.5 Symptomatic dermographism. Onset was within minutes of scratching. (From Bolognia JL, Jorizzo JL, Schaffeer JV, eds. Dermatology. 3rd ed. London: Saunders; 2012. Courtesy Jean L. Bolognia, MD.)

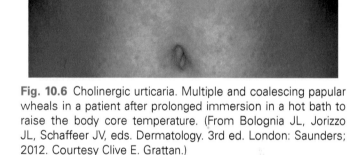

Fig. 10.6 Cholinergic urticaria. Multiple and coalescing papular wheals in a patient after prolonged immersion in a hot bath to raise the body core temperature. (From Bolognia JL, Jorizzo JL, Schaffeer JV, eds. Dermatology. 3rd ed. London: Saunders; 2012. Courtesy Clive E. Grattan.)

wheals of cholinergic urticaria are small, with a pale papular center initially surrounded by a red flare, and often become confluent (Fig. 10.6). Coexistence of different patterns of CU is relatively common, such as DPU or dermographism with CSU or cholinergic and cold urticaria. If the patient is currently taking H_1-antihistamines, the lesions may not be itchy or raised. Wheals can range in diameter from a few millimeters to several centimeters across.

Angioedema involving the face, lips, tongue, extremities, or genitalia may occur with or without wheals at different times in the same patient (Fig. 10.7). Angioedema without wheals should prompt an investigation for underlying hereditary angioedema or acquired C1 esterase inhibitor deficiency with appropriate laboratory testing, or for drug-induced angioedema (such as that related to angiotensin-converting enzyme [ACE] inhibitors). However, recurrent angioedema presenting without wheals most commonly represents a type of idiopathic angioedema due to mast cell mediator release, rather than due to bradykinin-induced angioedema.

Laboratory Assessments

The diagnosis of CU is made clinically, on the basis of findings on the history and physical examination. No cause can be identified by routine laboratory tests in most adults and children with CU, although up to one-third of patients with CSU will be found to have a positive serum basophil histamine release assay, where this assay is available, and around 50% of children and adults will have a positive ASST. Current guidelines do not recommend the ASST as a routine investigation because its clinical significance is uncertain.[1,15] Although results on laboratory testing are rarely abnormal, consensus statements recommend limited testing: a complete blood count with differential to assess for eosinophilia associated with parasitic infection, CRP or erythrocyte sedimentation rate (ESR) determination to screen for an underlying rheumatic disease or an autoinflammatory syndrome, and measurement of thyroid autoantibodies with thyroid-stimulating hormone (TSH) level in view of the known association between CSU and autoimmune thyroiditis are suggested. Results of these laboratory studies are normal in most patients who lack signs and symptoms of systemic disease. A meta-analysis of the workup findings in patients with CU involving 29 clinical studies and more than 6000 cases found no association between the number of tests ordered and the diagnosis reached. An underlying disease was found in 1.6% of cases tested (105 of 6462) and included, in rank order: cutaneous vasculitis (60 cases); thyroid disease (17 cases); SLE (7 cases); connective tissue disease

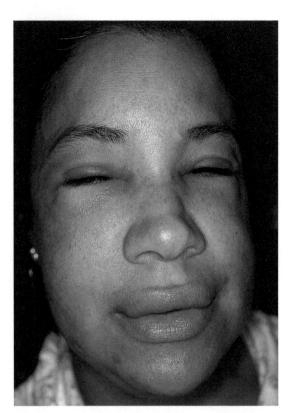

Fig. 10.7 The swelling is deeper than that with typical wheals and may affect mucosal surfaces. Note the swelling of the lips and periorbital region and the lack of erythema. (From Bolognia JL, Jorizzo JL, Schaffeer JV, eds. Dermatology. 3rd ed. London: Saunders; 2012.)

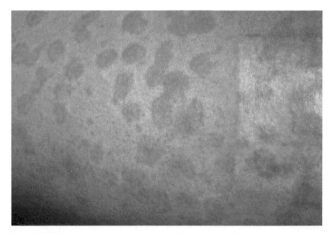

Fig. 10.8 Urticarial vasculitis. Lesions look like those of spontaneous urticaria but last longer and may bruise. An incidental finding in a skin graft donor site. (From Bolognia JL, Jorizzo JL, Schaffeer JV, eds. Dermatology. 3rd ed. London: Saunders; 2012. Courtesy Jean L. Bolognia, MD.)

(16 cases); and paraproteinemia (3 cases).[16] Rarely of any value is testing for chronic infections such as those caused by viral hepatitis or *H. pylori*, although this may be more relevant in parts of the world where these diseases are prevalent. Removal of suspected offending drugs can be attempted (such as NSAIDs), or replacement with another class of compound can be tried.

The value of testing for thyroid autoantibodies is linked to the idea of identifying an underlying association with an autoimmune etiology for CSU. Patients with a positive result, however, can be given forewarning that they may be at risk of hypo- or hyperthyroidism developing over their lives. In the case of specific physical urticarias, provocation testing such as with a melting ice cube in thin polythene applied to the forearm for 5 minutes or TempTest (Courage, Khazaka Electronic GmbH) for cold contact urticaria, or exercise testing for cholinergic urticaria, may be helpful to confirm diagnostic suspicions (Table 10.1). Provocation tests for inducible urticarias are relatively simple to perform in the outpatient setting, but some experience and skill are required to interpret the outcomes, and there is a small but important risk of inducing anaphylaxis with exercise testing for cholinergic urticaria or exercise-induced anaphylaxis. Allergen skin-prick testing is of little value in CSU except in rare cases where there is a strongly suggestive history of allergic triggers, or in very young children suspected of having food allergies, and it is of no value for inducible urticarias elicited by physical triggers. A high rate of false-positive results may be expected when

dermographism is also present. Allergen testing for specific IgE may be important in AU suspected of being caused by a food allergen, immunologic contact urticaria (e.g., due to animal or vegetable protein contact), and food and exercise-induced anaphylaxis where preexercise ingestion of a food to which the individual is presensitized; for instance, omega-5 gliadin (a gluten in wheat, barley, oats, and rye) or shrimp may act as a co-factor with exercise to precipitate anaphylaxis.

A *skin biopsy* should be performed if urticarial vasculitis is suspected or the patient fails to respond to usual treatments. SLE is an important differential diagnosis because urticaria and urticarial vasculitis are among the reported cutaneous manifestations of SLE. Urticarial vasculitis should be considered when the hives are painful rather than pruritic, last longer than 48 hours, or leave residual pigmentation changes (Fig. 10.8). Neutrophil-rich biopsies involving skin appendages without vasculitis point to a possible autoinflammatory disease, such as Schnitzler syndrome, a rare disease characterized by CU rash and periodic fever, high ESR, IgM gammopathy, leukocytosis, bone pain, and joint pain (sometimes with joint inflammation). It may also be associated less commonly with weight loss, malaise, fatigue, pruritus, swollen lymph glands, and enlarged spleen and liver.

Inducible Urticarias

The inducible urticarias merit classification as a separate group on the basis of their unique eliciting trigger and short attack duration, which is usually less than an hour, except in DPU, where swellings can last a day or more (Table 10.1). Available evidence regarding underlying mechanisms suggests that certain physical urticarias have a basis in IgE and can be passively transferred to a nonaffected individual, such as in cold contact urticaria, solar urticaria, and symptomatic dermographism.

Cold-Induced Urticarias. In *cold urticaria*, exposure to cold will rapidly generate symptoms of pruritus, erythema, and swelling at the site of exposure. Symptoms may only appear after rewarming. Cold drinks may trigger pharyngeal symptoms.

Hypotension and fatalities have been reported after whole body cold water immersion, although this is fortunately a very rare event. Alternative diagnoses, such as secondary cold contact urticaria presenting with cryoglobulinemia, must be considered, as well as familial cold inherited syndromes, which typically also manifest with systemic signs along with nonitchy wheals. Hepatitis B and C infections should be excluded in patients with cryoglobulinemia.

Cholinergic urticaria typically is related to elevation of core body temperature after active or passive overheating and is associated with the appearance of numerous intensely pruritic papular wheals that may coalesce, with or without angioedema, after hot bath challenge testing (Fig. 10.6). Recent data suggest that some cases may result from an autoantibody to a sweat antigen that consists of a protein that induces degranulation of basophils and mast cells via antigen-specific IgE.

Mechanically Induced Urticaria. Very itchy linear wheals that come up rapidly after gentle skin stroking or light scratching are known as "symptomatic dermographism"; a nonitchy variant occurs in around 5% of the general population after skin scratching, known as simple dermographism. DPU, by contrast, appears several hours after a sustained pressure stimulus, with deep urticarial lesions that may resemble angioedema (e.g., under a shoulder strap or tight boots). In biopsied skin samples from patients with DPU, evidence of neutrophils and eosinophils can be seen.

Other Inducible Urticarias. *Solar urticaria* is defined by mast cell activation by certain wavelengths of solar radiation. Classification of this form of urticaria into six different forms is based on the wavelengths of solar radiation that are implicated, or on identification of an underlying metabolic disease such as protoporphyria. Repeated exposure to the eliciting wavelength has been attempted to desensitize patients with solar urticaria.

Aquagenic urticaria is a rare form of disease that results in lesions when contact is made with any water, regardless of temperature.

Diseases Resembling Urticaria

Differential Diagnosis

A number of conditions can manifest with urticarial rash that are clinically and pathogenetically different to urticaria. Among the possibilities are a drug- or food-based reaction; unrecognized infections such as hepatitis or mononucleosis; insect bites leading to papular urticaria; the whealing response seen after rubbing urticaria pigmentosa (Darier's sign); urticarial vasculitis; familial cold autoinflammatory syndrome (FCAS); hereditary and acquired angioedemas (nonhistaminergic); and rare syndromes such as Muckle–Wells syndrome (MWS; periodic fever, chills, and painful joints caused by a defect in the *NLRP3* gene, which creates the protein cryopyrin). MWS is closely related to two other syndromes, familial cold urticaria and neonatal-onset multisystem inflammatory disease (NOMID), which are related to mutations in the same gene and designated as cryopyrin-associated periodic syndromes (CAPS), Schnitzler syndrome, Gleich syndrome (episodic angioedema with eosinophilia), and Wells syndrome (eosinophilic dermatitis). Some of

the more commonly encountered entities are discussed next, by etiologic category.

Systemic Diseases

Systemic diseases may also be associated with urticarial eruptions. Accompanying signs and symptoms may include fever, arthralgias, arthritis, weight change, bone pain, and lymphadenopathy. Urticarial vasculitis is usually normocomplementemic, in which case it is usually skin-limited, or hypocomplementemic, in which case it is a multisystem disorder and may be associated with anti-C1q antibodies. Urticarial vasculitis may occur in patients with other systemic inflammatory diseases, such as Sjögren syndrome, in addition to SLE, and warrants testing for other autoimmune conditions. Anti–nuclear antibody testing and rheumatoid factor assay should be considered in this setting.

Schnitzler syndrome is a rare condition characterized by periodic fever, urticaria, and IgM monoclonal gammopathy. This syndrome has been described in patients with a monoclonal IgM or, very rarely, an IgG component (monoclonal gammopathy), who have associated fever, leukocytosis, weight loss, bone pain, adenopathy, and urticarial rash. The striking and consistent response to an interleukin 1 receptor antagonist, anakinra, implicates the inflammasome (a multiprotein complex expressed in myeloid cells and a component of the innate immune system) in its etiology.

Hypereosinophilic syndrome refers to a group of disorders characterized by persistent overproduction of eosinophils that infiltrate and damage tissues. Cutaneous symptoms include recurrent urticarial rash and angioedema.

The CAPS embraces FCAS, MWS, and NOMID. These are rare genetic disorders characterized by mutations in the *NLRP3* gene. *FCAS* manifests with periodic fever, urticaria, leukocytosis, conjunctivitis, and muscle and skin tenderness after exposure to cold. The onset of symptoms occurs during infancy in most cases and varies in severity between individuals and at different times of the disease. *MWS* involves periodic urticarial eruptions without obvious cold exacerbations, sensorineural deafness, and amyloidosis that may lead to renal failure if the disease is not recognized and treated. NOMID represents the most severe form of the CAPS spectrum and often presents early in life with neurological impairment, in addition to the other features.

TREATMENT OF URTICARIA

General Principles

Recent evidence-based guidelines support that the most effective, first-line therapy for CU is the use of nonsedating, newer-generation H_1-antihistamines such as fexofenadine, loratadine, desloratadine, cetirizine, and levocetirizine. These agents alleviate the main symptom of pruritus and reduce the occurrence of wheals. Another important measure is reduction of aggravating factors (e.g., overheating, clothing pressure, and, possibly, stress). In addition, avoidance of aspirin and other NSAIDs is advisable, in view of the fact that up to one-third of patients will suffer skin exacerbations with use of this class of compounds.

First-Line Treatments

Nonsedating H_1-antihistamines are effective at controlling the symptoms of urticaria in up to 50% of CU patients. They should be taken prophylactically while symptoms are active, rather than after an eruption of wheals, since peak absorption after a single dose in healthy volunteers ranges from 45 minutes to 3 hours (fastest is rupatadine; longest is desloratadine). It has been common practice to offer "classical" sedating antihistamines (e.g., chlorphenamine, diphenhydramine, hydroxyzine) at night to aid sleep because they often cause sedation, but there is no pharmacologic advantage in updosing second-generation nonsedating H_1-antihistamines. Rapid eye movement (REM) sleep is suppressed, leading to poor-quality sleep and "hangover" effects the following day. Avoiding sedating antihistamines for CU is now a strong recommendation of recent international guidelines.[1] A possible link between using classical antihistamines with additional anticholinergic properties and increased incidence of dementia has also been highlighted recently.

If nonsedating antihistamines are only partially effective at their licensed doses, as may be the case in up to 50% of these patients, the dose of the nonsedating H_1-antihistamines can be increased up to four fold, in line with current guidelines, followed by the addition of an H_2-antihistamine. Although the evidence for doing so is very limited due to lack of well-controlled published studies, clinical experience with this combination indicates that it can improve disease control in some patients and be effective for the hyperacidity that may occur in severe CSU.

Evidence of the benefits of escalating doses of selective, nonsedating antihistamines has been recently demonstrated in CSU and cold urticaria. Combination therapy approaches of various classes have limited evidence in the literature. The possibility of sedation after updosing minimally sedating H_1-antihistamines (cetirizine and levocetirizine) should be explained to patients, and caution should be exercised when updosing H_1-antihistamines with potential to prolong the electrocardiogram (ECG) QTc interval, including mizolastine.

Second-Line (Targeted) Treatments

Leukotriene Pathway Inhibitors

Controlled studies have shown mixed results with the use of leukotriene pathway inhibitors in CU, but these agents are often tried because of their favorable safety profile. In patients with CSU in association with aspirin sensitivity, montelukast was found to be superior to placebo and to cetirizine and also offered protection in aspirin challenges. In a second study in patients with CSU, no benefit was identified for montelukast as an add-on to desloratadine. In a third trial, only subjects with ASST positivity were found to benefit from the addition of zafirlukast to cetirizine, whereas monotherapy with zafirlukast offered no benefit over placebo. Studies of montelukast in combination with loratadine or desloratadine showed benefit over antihistamine therapy alone for DPU.

Oral Corticosteroids

Short courses of oral corticosteroids are widely used and nearly always effective in terms of rescue therapy if the aforementioned second-line agents fail to provide relief. However, the optimal dose and duration of such rescue corticosteroid therapy are not well studied. The adverse effects of repeated courses of oral corticosteroids should prompt consideration of an alternative treatment agent such as an immunomodulator and possibly a skin biopsy to confirm the diagnosis of CU if there is clinical uncertainty.

Other Second-Line Therapies

Several agents have been demonstrated to offer benefit as alternatives to corticosteroids in antihistamine-refractory cases of CU and include *sulfasalazine*, *dapsone*, and *hydroxychloroquine*. The mechanism of action of these alternative agents in CU is unknown but may be antiinflammatory in part. Patients should be screened for glucose-6-phosphatase deficiency before starting any of the three drugs. *Sulphasalazine* can be especially valuable for DPU but should be avoided in NSAID-sensitive patients because its aminosalicylate component may aggravate associated CSU. The most frequent side effects are gastrointestinal intolerance and headache, but Stevens–Johnson syndrome (with or without toxic epidermal necrolysis) has also been reported.

Although evidence on the use of *dapsone* in CU, especially in neutrophilic urticaria, is limited, it is preferred in urticarial vasculitis and in DPU and angioedema. Monitoring for dapsone toxicity including anemia, neuropathy, and methemoglobinemia is required. Dapsone hypersensitivity syndrome may start within a month of drug initiation, and patients should be warned of the presenting symptoms.

Doxepin has a long history of use in antihistamine-refractory CU and is positioned as a fourth-line therapy in the latest US Practice Parameter.[15] It is a tricyclic antidepressant with potent properties of an H_1- and H_2-antihistamine. It is generally given at doses considerably lower than used for its licensed indication of depression (i.e., 25–75 mg at night rather than up to 300 mg daily), but nevertheless may not be tolerated due to sedation and its anticholinergic properties (blurred vision and dry mouth).

Other targeted drugs used for H_1-antihistamine–unresponsive CU include *danazol* (a derivative of the synthetic steroid ethisterone that suppresses the production of gonadotrophins and has some weak androgenic effects) for cholinergic urticaria, anticoagulants and calcium channel blockers for CSU, *cyclophosphamide* for severe steroid-dependent CSU, and *thyroxine* in euthyroid CSU patients with positive thyroid autoantibodies.

Third-Line (Immunosuppresive) Drugs

Immunosuppressive drugs have been used effectively for over 25 years to treat H_1-antihistamine–unresponsive CSU on the basis that severely affected patients may have an autoimmune etiology with relatively little evidence from clinical trials to support the practice. A small but controlled study supported an effect of *ciclosporin* in patients with ASST-positive CSU at 4 mg/kg per day for 1 to 2 months, with reduction of serological HRA on basophils; reduction in size of the ASST; and control of symptoms for up to 6 months after stopping an H_1-antihistamine in 25% of patients, suggesting a possible disease-modifying effect in these patients.[17] Other studies have shown a sustained benefit from cyclosporine at much lower doses. Patients with a positive basophil histamine release assay generally respond quicker and more completely than those with a negative assay. The latter often need long-term treatment with attendant risks of adverse effects, including hypertension and renal impairment. Evidence from a small open series has shown benefits from a range of immunomodulatory approaches, including intravenous immunoglobulins, plasmapheresis, tacrolimus, methotrexate, and mycophenolate mofetil, but properly powered randomized controlled studies need to be done, with adequate follow-up information, to determine whether or not these interventions have a disease-modifying effect on CU.

The most recently licensed treatment for antihistamine-unresponsive CSU is the anti-IgE monoclonal antibody, *omalizumab*. Following a single-dose study demonstrating dose-related control of CSU symptoms,[18] further double-blind, placebo-controlled phase III licensing studies were conducted that demonstrated efficacy[19] and safety.[20] The X-ACT study showed that omalizumab treatment reduces angioedema-burdened days per week three fold compared to placebo in patients with CSU and recurrent angioedema.[21] What has emerged from these studies is a novel treatment with rapid onset (often within 1 week) and a slower relapse (usually 5–8 weeks after the last dose) that controls symptoms effectively but does not appear to modify the course of the illness. Small studies indicate that omalizumab can also be effective for inducible urticarias, including DPU. It is likely that the landscape for treating CU patients in the near future will be based on stronger evidence with more effective therapies than in the past but, to date, no cure has emerged.

Special Considerations
Urticaria and Angioedema in Children

Most clinicians prefer to manage CU in children with nonsedating H_1-antihistamines at approved doses over older-generation compounds, out of concerns of sedation. No clear difference in total IgE levels or in specific IgE levels between children with acute and those with the chronic form of urticaria has been noted.

Urticaria in Pregnancy

Treatment of urticarial disease in pregnancy raises concerns regarding drug safety. Safety data are limited, and only loratadine and cetirizine (both Food and Drug Administration [FDA] category B) are currently recommended for use in pregnancy.

Urticaria is a multifaceted illness with different clinical presentations and etiologies. Management strategies include removing the cause, where one can be identified, minimizing aggravating factors, and alleviating symptoms pending spontaneous remission.

REFERENCES

1. Zuberbier T, Aberer W, Asero R, et al. The EAACI/GA²LEN/EDF/WAO guideline for the definition, classification, diagnosis and management of urticaria. Allergy. 2018;73:1393–1414.
2. *Maurer M, Weller K, Bindslev-Jensen C, et al. Unmet clinical needs in chronic spontaneous urticaria. A GA²LEN task force report. Allergy. 2011;66:317–330.
3. Beltrani VS. An overview of chronic urticaria. Clin Rev Allergy Immunol. 2002;23:147–169.
4. Nebiolo F, Bergia R, Bommarito L, et al. Effect of arterial hypertension on chronic urticaria duration. Ann Allergy Asthma Immunol. 2009;103(5):407–410.
5. Deza G, Ricketti PA, Giménez-Arnau AM, et al. Emerging biomarkers and therapeutic pipelines for chronic spontaneous urticaria. J Allergy Clin Immunol Pract. 2018;6(4):1108–1117.
6. Confino-Cohen R, Chodick G, Shalev V, et al. Chronic urticaria and autoimmunity: associations found in a large population study. J Allergy Clin Immunol. 2012;129(5):1307–1313.
7. O'Donnell BF, O'Neill CM, Francis DM, et al. Human leucocyte antigen class II associations in chronic idiopathic urticaria. Br J Dermatol. 1999;140(5):853–858.
8. Wedi B, Raap U, Kapp A. Chronic urticaria and infections. Curr Opin Allergy Clin Immunol. 2004;4:387–389.
9. Lindelöf B, Sigurgeirsson B, Wahlgren CF, et al. Chronic urticaria and cancer: an epidemiological study of 1155 patients. Br J Dermatol. 1990;123:453–456.
10. Chen YJ, Wu CY, Shen JL, et al. Cancer risk in patients with chronic urticaria: a population-based cohort study. Arch Dermatol. 2012;148:103–108.
11. Hide M, Francis DM, Grattan CE, et al. Autoantibodies against the high-affinity IgE receptor as a cause of histamine release in chronic urticaria. N Engl J Med. 1993;328:1599–1604.
12. Schoepke N, Asero R, Ellrich A, et al. Biomarkers and clinical characteristics of autoimmune chronic spontaneous urticaria: results of the PURIST study. Allergy. 2019;74:2427–2436.
13. Bracken SJ, Abraham S, MacLeod AS. Autoimmune theories of chronic spontaneous urticaria. Front Immunol. 2019;10:627.
14. Kay AB, Ying S, Ardelean E, et al. Elevations in vascular markers and eosinophils in chronic spontaneous urticarial weals with low-level persistence in uninvolved skin. Br J Dermatol. 2014;171:505–511.
15. Bernstein JA, Lang DM, Khan DA, et al. The diagnosis and management of acute and chronic urticaria: 2014 update. J Allergy Clin Immunol. 2014;133:1270–1277.
16. Kozel MM, Bossuyt PM, Mekkes JR, et al. Laboratory tests and identified diagnoses in patients with physical and chronic urticaria and angioedema: a systematic review. J Am Acad Dermatol. 2003;48:409–416.
17. Grattan CE, O'Donnell BF, Francis DM, et al. Randomized double-blind study of cyclosporin in chronic 'idiopathic' urticaria. Br J Dermatol. 2000;143:365–372.
18. Saini S, Rosen KE, Hseih H-J, et al. A randomized, placebo-controlled, dose-ranging study of single-dose omalizumab in patients with H_1-antihistamine-refratory chronic idiopathic urticaria. J Allergy Clin Immunol. 2011;128:567–573.
19. Maurer M, Rosén K, Hsieh HJ, et al. Omalizumab for the treatment of chronic idiopathic or spontaneous urticaria. N Engl J Med. 2013;368:924–935.
20. Kaplan A, Ledford D, Ashby M, et al. Omalizumab in patients with symptomatic chronic idiopathic/spontaneous urticaria despite standard combination therapy. J Allergy Clin Immunol. 2013;132:101–109.
21. Staubach P, Metz M, Chapman-Rothe N, et al. Omalizumab rapidly improves angioedema-related quality of life in adult patients with chronic spontaneous urticaria: X-ACT study data. Allergy. 2018;73:576–584.

Key references are preceded by an asterisk.

11

Atopic Dermatitis and Allergic Contact Dermatitis

Mark Boguniewicz, Luz Fonacier, and Donald Y.M. Leung

CHAPTER OUTLINE

ATOPIC DERMATITIS

Summary of Important Concepts in Atopic Dermatitis

- Atopic dermatitis (AD) is the most common inflammatory skin disease.
- Abnormal skin barrier differentiation and immune response genes play key roles in AD.
- Treatment for most AD includes avoidance of irritants and proven allergens, hydration and moisturizers to maintain a healthy epidermis, antimicrobial therapy for acute infections, and topical antiinflammatory agents.
- Because nonlesional skin in AD patients is associated with skin barrier and immune abnormalities, proactive (maintenance) therapy may be appropriate for a subgroup of patients with relapsing disease.
- Dupilumab, a biologic targeting interleukin-4 (IL-4)/interleukin-13 (IL-13) has been approved for patients 6 years and older with moderate-to-severe AD failing topical therapy.
- A number of studies have reported an increased frequency of allergic contact dermatitis (ACD) in AD.

INTRODUCTION

Atopic dermatitis (AD) is a chronically relapsing inflammatory skin disease usually associated with respiratory allergy.[1] In the 1930s, Hill and Sulzberger[2] suggested the name "AD" to describe both the weeping eczema of early childhood and the chronic xerosis and lichenified lesions more typical of older patients. Before that time, however, a number of other terms were used to describe this disease, with the earliest illustrations consistent with AD dating to the late 1700s and early 1800s (Fig. 11.1).[3] Of note, the term *atopic dermatitis* recognized the close relationship among AD, asthma, and allergic rhinitis. In support of this observation, in the largest cross-sectional study of a cohort of 2270 children with physician-confirmed AD, almost 66% had symptoms of at least one additional form of atopy (particularly

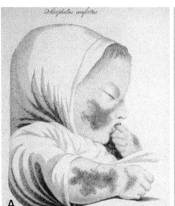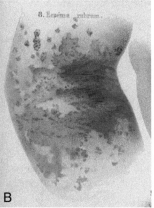

Fig. 11.1 Early historical drawings of atopic dermatitis (AD). (A) Strophulus confertus, 1796; (B) Eczema rubrum, 1835. (From Wallach D, Coste J, Tilles G, Taïeb A. The first images of atopic dermatitis: an attempt at retrospective diagnosis in dermatology. J Am Acad Dermatol 2005;53:684–689.)

asthma or allergic rhinitis) by the third year of life.[4] Although significant progress has been made in the understanding of AD, its cause is still unknown, and much remains to be learned about the complex interrelationship of genetic, environmental, immunologic, and epidermal factors in this disease.[1,5]

HISTORICAL PERSPECTIVE

Descriptions of illness consistent with AD can be found dating back to the ancient Roman empire. In the 1800s, clinical descriptions of skin disorders by Willan and others included terms such as *strophulus confertus, lichen agrius, porrigo larvalis*, and *eczema rubrum* whose images are consistent with the diagnosis of AD on retrospective review. Besnier's *diathetic prurigo* established an association between pruritic skin disease and respiratory as well as gastrointestinal symptoms. The discovery of the concept of allergy in the early 1900s was followed by descriptions of "atopy" in the 1920s, which in turn eventually led to introduction of the term "AD" in the 1930s.[2] The role of allergens in AD was demonstrated by Tuft in the 1940s, while the role of *Staphylococcus aureus* was shown in the 1970s. The 1980s saw important insights into immune abnormalities associated with the disease, including recognition of the role of immunoglobulin E (IgE) molecules on epidermal Langerhans cells (LCs). In the 1990s, Leung et al. demonstrated a role for Th2 cytokines and staphylococcal toxins as novel allergens in AD as well as important immunologic distinctions between uninvolved, acutely involved, and chronically involved skin at the lesional level. In addition, the concept of T cell homing to the skin via a unique skin-selective receptor, cutaneous lymphocyte-associated antigen, was described in AD. The following decade started with the Food and Drug Administration's (FDA) approval in 2000 of tacrolimus ointment, the first topical calcineurin inhibitor (TCI) indicated for AD, described as "a new milestone in the management of AD." The publication of a landmark study in 2006 established a strong association between loss-of-function mutations in the gene encoding *FLG*, a skin barrier protein and risk for AD. Of note, the authors also found that mutations in the *FLG* gene were associated with increased risk for asthma in patients with AD, suggesting a mechanism for the atopic march. Although *FLG* mutations are associated with AD, food allergy, and the atopic march, they are only observed in a minority of subjects undergoing the atopic march. Other factors that can contribute to deficiency in skin filaggrin levels warrant investigation.[1] Further investigation into uninvolved skin in AD pointed to broad terminal differentiation abnormalities along with previously described immune abnormalities. These studies provided a rationale for a paradigm shift in treating AD patients with a relapsing course by changing from reactive to proactive management. Studies addressing both skin barrier and immune abnormalities, utilizing a molecular signature for AD, provide a rationale for the next generation of therapies in this disease.

EPIDEMIOLOGY

A number of studies suggest an increasing prevalence of AD. In Denmark, Schultz Larsen[6] demonstrated a cumulative incidence rate (up to 7 years) of 12% for twins born between 1975 and 1979 versus 3% for twins born from 1960 to 1964. A 1992 cross-sectional questionnaire confirmed this increased prevalence with a frequency of AD of 15.6% in 3000 children age 7 years from Denmark, Germany, and Sweden.[7] Questionnaire data derived from the 2003 National Survey of Children's Health in the US found prevalence ranging by state from 8.7% to 18.1% in a sample of 102,353 children age 17 years and younger.[8] In adults, prevalence of AD was 7% in a recent AD in America study.[9] A Japanese study used skin examinations rather than questionnaires to ascertain the prevalence of childhood and adolescent AD.[10] More than 7000 patients were examined, and AD was documented in 24% of those age 5 to 6 years, 19% of those 7 to 9 years, 15% of those 10 to 12 years, 14% of those 13 to 15 years and 11% of those age 16 to 18 years. Importantly, the prevalence of AD in 9- to 12-year-old children was twice that in children of similar age examined 20 years earlier, and for 18-year-old adolescents, it was five times higher. A subsequent study in 23,719 children age 6 to 7 and 11 to 12 years examined by dermatologists in eight prefectures of Japan randomly selected from urban and rural districts found a point prevalence of AD of 11.2% (7.4% to 15.0%).[11] Of the patients, 74% were classified with mild, 24% with moderate, 1.6% with severe, and 0.3% with severe AD. Prevalence in the younger cohort was slightly higher than in the older patients (11.8% versus 10.5%; $p < 0.01$). No apparent difference was seen in prevalence between urban and rural districts or between boys and girls.

Increased exposure to pollutants and indoor allergens (especially house-dust mites) and a decline in breastfeeding, along with a greater awareness of AD, have been suggested as reasons for the increased frequency of AD.[12] In a prospective study, Zeiger and associates[13] found that restricting the pregnant mother's diet during the third trimester and lactation and the child's diet during the first 2 years of life resulted in decreased prevalence of AD in the prophylaxis group compared with a control group at age 12 months but not at 24 months. Follow-up through 7 years of age showed no difference between the prophylaxis and control groups for AD or respiratory allergy.[14] In a large study of an ethnically and socially diverse group of children in suburban Birmingham, England, Kay and coworkers[15] found that breastfeeding did not affect the lifetime AD prevalence rate of 20%. A study of prevalence of childhood eczema found a correlation with increased socio-economic class that did not result from heightened parental awareness.[16] The National Survey of Children's Health analysis by Shaw and associates[8] also found increased prevalence of eczema to be related to metropolitan living, along with Black race and higher education level.

The effects of genetic and environmental factors on allergic diseases were studied in two Japanese cities with differing climates.[17] The prevalence of allergic diseases and AD in the city with a temperate climate was significantly higher than in the one with a subtropical climate, even after controlling for genetic and environmental factors. In both cities, children from atopic families had a significantly higher risk of contracting respiratory allergies and AD. In a global survey of the prevalence of asthma, allergic rhinoconjunctivitis, and AD, 463,801 children age 13 to 14 years from 155 centers in 56 countries

participated.[18] The highest prevalence of AD was reported from scattered centers, including sites in Scandinavia and Africa, that were not among centers with the highest prevalence of asthma. On the other hand, the lowest prevalence rates for AD occurred in centers with the lowest prevalence of asthma and allergic rhinoconjunctivitis. Thus, the ultimate presentation of an atopic disease may depend on a complex interaction of environmental exposures with end-organ response in a genetically predisposed individual.

Updated data from the International Study of Asthma and Allergies in Childhood (ISAAC phase III) on 385,853 participants age 6 to 7 years from 143 centers in 60 countries showed that the prevalence of current AD ranged from 0.9% in India to 22.5% in Ecuador, with new data showing high values in Asia and Latin America.[19] Prevalence in 663,256 participants age 13 to 14 years from 230 centers in 96 countries ranged from 0.2% in China to 24.6% in Columbia, with the highest occurrence in Africa and Latin America. These data emphasize the importance of AD as a global health problem in both developed and developing countries.

PATHOGENESIS AND ETIOLOGY

Genetics

The genetics of atopic disease is complex and an area of active research.[20] A number of genes are likely involved in the development of AD, but skin barrier/epidermal differentiation genes[21–24] and immune response/host defense genes have been proposed as playing a key role. An important advance in understanding the contribution of skin barrier abnormalities was recognizing loss-of-function mutations of the gene encoding the epidermal barrier protein filaggrin as a major predisposing factor for AD.[25] Patients with *FLG* gene mutations have early onset, severe, and persistent AD,[26] although most appear to outgrow their disease, just more slowly than those without *FLG* mutations.[27] Importantly, AD patients with *FLG* mutations are at increased risk for development of asthma, as well as food and inhalant allergies[25] (see Role of the Epidermal Barrier later). These observations establish a key role for impaired skin barrier function in AD pathogenesis, allowing increased transepidermal water loss and, importantly, increased entry of allergens, antigens, and chemicals from the environment, resulting in skin inflammatory responses (Fig. 11.2).

Atopic Diathesis

Most patients with AD have a genetic predisposition to develop an IgE response to common environmental allergens. Abnormal IgE responses are associated with cellular abnormalities resulting in overproduction of helper T type 2 (Th2)–type cytokines, which also contribute to the eosinophilia seen in these diseases. Early onset of AD is associated with an increased risk for respiratory allergy. The highest incidence of asthma at a given age has been observed in children with onset of AD before 3 months, in those with severe AD and a family history of asthma. An association of increased risk for asthma and/or rhinoconjunctivitis with early onset of AD has been confirmed.[28] Respiratory allergy

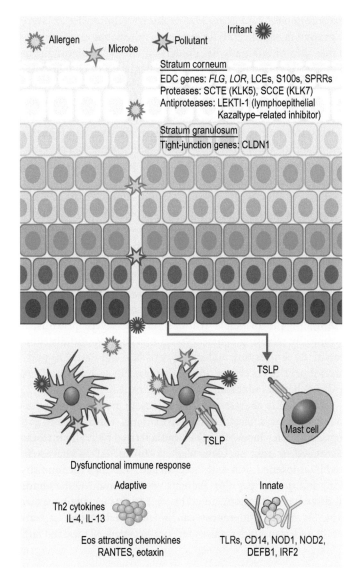

Fig. 11.2 Epidermal barrier abnormalities and immune dysregulation. *SCCE*, Stratum corneum chymotryptic enzyme; *SCTE*, stratum corneum tryptic enzyme; *TLRs*, Toll-like receptors; *TSLP*, thymic stromal lymphopoietin. (From Barnes KC. An update on the genetics of atopic dermatitis: scratching the surface in 2009. J Allergy Clin Immunol 2010;125:16–29, e1–e11.)

TABLE 11.1 Differential Diagnosis in Patients With Atopic Dermatitis

Differential Category	Diagnostic Examples
Congenital disorders	Netherton syndrome
Chronic dermatoses	Seborrheic dermatitis
	Contact dermatitis (allergic or irritant)
	Nummular eczema
	Lichen simplex chronicus
Infections and infestations	Scabies
	Human immunodeficiency virus–associated dermatitis
Malignancy	Cutaneous T cell lymphoma (mycosis fungoides/Sézary syndrome)
Immunodeficiencies	Wiskott–Aldrich syndrome
	Severe combined immunodeficiency
	Immune dysregulation, polyendocrinopathy, enteropathy, X-linked (IPEX) syndrome
	Hyper-IgE syndrome
	DOCK8 mutation associated immunodeficiency
Metabolic disorders	Zinc deficiency
	Pyridoxine (vitamin B_6) and niacin deficiency
	Multiple carboxylase deficiency
	Phenylketonuria
Proliferative disorders	Letterer–Siwe disease

DOCK8, Dedicator of cytokinesis 8 protein.

occurred in 50% of children who had onset of AD during the first 3 months of life and two or more atopic family members, compared with 12% of children who had onset of AD after 3 months of age and no atopic family members.

In addition, children with AD have more severe asthma than asthmatic children without AD, suggesting that epidermal allergen sensitization may predispose to more severe and persistent respiratory disease through effects on the systemic allergic response.

Natural History

AD typically manifests in early childhood, with onset before 5 years of age in approximately 90% of patients. In adults with new-onset dermatitis, especially without a history of childhood eczema, asthma, or allergic rhinitis, other diseases need to be considered (Table 11.1).

Although a 20-year follow-up study suggested that 84% of children outgrow their AD by adolescence,[29] more recent data present less optimistic outcomes. In one study, AD had disappeared in only 18% of children observed from infancy until age 11 to 13 years, although it had become less severe in 65%.[30] In another study, 72% of patients diagnosed during the first 2 years of life continued to have AD 20 years later.[31] In a prospective study from Finland, 77% to 91% of adolescent patients treated for moderate or severe AD had persistent or frequently relapsing dermatitis as adults, although only 6% had severe disease.[32] In addition, more than half the adolescents treated for mild dermatitis experienced a relapse of disease as adults. Often, adults whose childhood AD has been in remission for a number of years present with hand dermatitis, especially if daily activities require repeated hand wetting. A prospective study of children with AD observed through age 7 years found that, although most had milder eczema by 7 years, only approximately one-third had no evidence of disease activity.[33]

The Multicenter Allergy Study, a German birth cohort, followed 1314 children from birth to age 7 years with physical examinations and parental interviews on atopic symptoms and diagnoses, along with determination of specific IgE levels.[34] The cumulative prevalence of AD in the first 2 years of life was 21.5%. Of these children with early AD, 43.2% were in complete remission by age 3 years, 38.3% had an intermittent pattern of disease, and 18.7% had symptoms of AD every year. Severity and atopic sensitization were major determinants of prognosis. Of note, the insights into the genetics of AD previously discussed provide new information regarding risk factors for persistent AD into adulthood.[26]

Role of the Abnormal Epidermal Barrier

AD is associated with abnormalities in skin barrier function that include increased transepidermal water loss, increased levels of endogenous proteolytic enzymes, and reduced ceramide levels. Use of soaps can increase skin pH, increasing activity of endogenous proteases and leading to breakdown of epidermal barrier function.[5] The epidermal barrier may be further damaged by exogenous proteases from house-dust mites and *S. aureus*. This is worsened by the lack of endogenous protease inhibitors in the skin of patients with AD. These epidermal changes likely contribute to increased allergen absorption into the skin and microbial colonization. As previously discussed, mutations in the *FLG* gene, located in the epidermal differentiation complex on chromosome 1q21, have been shown to result in complete or partial decrease of expression of a key epidermal protein, filament-aggregating protein (filaggrin), involved in formation of the epidermal barrier.[21-24] In addition, type 2 cytokines such as interleukins 4 and 13 (IL-4, IL-13), which are upregulated in AD, were shown to downregulate *FLG* expression.[35] In addition, a distinct subpopulation of IL-22–producing Th22 CD4[+] and CD8[+] cells has been reported in the skin of AD patients, and IL-22–regulated genes include those implicated in epidermal barrier abnormalities in AD such as *FLG*, as well as the proteins loricrin and involucrin.[36]

The growing number of mutations reported includes many unique for Caucasians of European ancestry and others for Asian populations.[25] Importantly, *FLG* mutations were a major risk factor for eczema-associated asthma. Importantly, because epicutaneous sensitization to allergens results in a greater immune response than sensitization via the airway, decreased epidermal barrier function could act as a site for allergen sensitization and predispose such children to the development of respiratory allergy later in life.[37] Metaanalyses support the association of *FLG* mutations with increased risk for both asthma[38] and allergies.[39]

DeBenedetto and colleagues[40] pointed to a role of a second barrier defect in AD. Tight junctions (TJs) located directly below the stratum corneum regulate the selective permeability of the paracellular pathway. Reduced expression of the TJ proteins claudin-1 and claudin-23 were observed only in patients with AD, validated at the messenger RNA (mRNA) and protein levels. Claudin-1 expression inversely correlated with Th2 biomarkers. CLDN1 haplotype-tagging single-nucleotide polymorphisms (SNPs) were associated with AD. These data suggest that an impairment in TJs contributes to the barrier dysfunction and immune dysregulation observed in AD patients, which may be mediated in part by reduction in claudin-1 (see Fig. 11.2).

In a novel approach, Broccardo and associates[41] used a noninvasive, semiquantitative profiling method to identify proteins involved in the pathogenesis of AD. Proteins related to the skin barrier (filaggrin-2, corneodesmosin, desmoglein-1, desmocollin-1, transglutaminase-3) and generation of natural moisturizing factor (arginase-1, caspase-14, γ-glutamylcyclotransferase) were expressed at significantly lower levels in lesional versus nonlesional sites of AD patients. Epidermal fatty acid-binding protein was expressed at significantly higher levels in patients with methicillin-resistant *S. aureus* (MRSA). The lower expression of skin barrier proteins and enzymes involved in the generation of natural moisturizing factor could further exacerbate barrier defects and perpetuate water loss from the skin. The greater expression of epidermal fatty acid–binding protein, especially in patients colonized with MRSA, might perpetuate the inflammatory response through eicosanoid signaling.

CLINICAL FEATURES (PHENOTYPE)

AD has no pathognomonic skin lesions or unique laboratory parameters. Therefore, the diagnosis is based on the presence of major and associated clinical features[42] (Box 11.1). Attempts to standardize signs and symptoms of AD include severity scoring of AD (SCORAD) and the eczema area and severity index (EASI).[43,44] The principal features include severe pruritus, a chronically relapsing course, typical morphology and distribution of the skin lesions, and a history of atopic disease. The presence of pruritus is critical to the diagnosis of AD, and patients with AD have a reduced threshold for pruritus.

Acute AD is characterized by intensely pruritic, erythematous papules associated with excoriations, vesiculations, and serous exudate. Subacute AD is characterized by erythematous, excoriated, scaling papules, whereas chronic AD is characterized by thickened skin with accentuated markings (lichenification) and fibrotic papules. Patients with chronic AD may have all three types of lesions. In addition, patients usually have dry skin. Significant differences can be observed in pH, capacitance, and transepidermal water loss between AD lesions and

---

BOX 11.1 Clinical Features of Atopic Dermatitis

Major Features

Pruritus

Facial and extensor involvement in infants and children

Flexural lichenification in adults

Chronic or relapsing dermatitis

Personal or family history of atopic disease

Minor Features

Xerosis

Cutaneous infections

Nonspecific dermatitis of hands or feet Ichthyosis, palmar hyperlinearity, keratosis pilaris

Pityriasis alba

Nipple eczema

White dermatographism and delayed blanch response

Anterior subcapsular cataracts

Elevated serum IgE levels

Positive immediate-type allergy skin tests

Modified from Hanifin JM, Rajka G. Diagnostic features of atopic dermatitis. Acta Derm Venereol (Stockh) 1980;92:44–47.

uninvolved skin in the same patient and on skin of normal controls.

During infancy, AD involves primarily the face, scalp, and extensor surfaces of the extremities. The diaper area is usually spared; if involved, it may be secondarily infected with *Candida* species, in which case the dermatitis does not spare the inguinal folds. In contrast, infragluteal involvement is a common distribution in children. In older patients with long-standing disease, the flexural folds of the extremities are the predominant location of lesions. In the Copenhagen Prospective Study on Asthma in Childhood, arm and joint involvement carried the highest predictive value for the development of AD at age 3 years.[45] Localization of AD to the eyelids may be an isolated manifestation but should be differentiated from allergic contact dermatitis (ACD).

COMPLICATING FEATURES

Ocular Problems

Increased numbers of IgE-bearing LCs are found in the conjunctival epithelium of patients with AD. These cells can capture aeroallergens and present them to infiltrating T cells, thus contributing to ocular inflammation. Ocular complications associated with AD can result in significant morbidity.

Atopic keratoconjunctivitis is always bilateral, and symptoms include itching, burning, tearing, and copious mucoid discharge.[46] It is frequently associated with eyelid dermatitis and chronic blepharitis and may result in visual impairment from corneal scarring. Keratoconus is a conical deformity of the cornea that is believed to result from persistent rubbing of the eyes in patients with AD and allergic rhinitis. Anterior subcapsular cataracts may develop during adolescence or early adult life.

Hand Dermatitis

Patients with AD often have nonspecific hand dermatitis that is frequently irritating and aggravated by repeated wetting, especially in the occupational setting. A history of past or present AD at least doubles the effects of irritant exposure and doubles the risk in occupations where hand eczema is a common problem.

Infections

Patients with AD have an increased susceptibility to infection or colonization with a variety of organisms.[47] These include viral infections with herpes simplex virus (HSV), molluscum contagiosum, and human papillomavirus (HPV). Important insights into our understanding of the unique susceptibility that AD patients have to eczema herpeticum (EH) and eczema vaccinatum (a potentially lethal complication of smallpox vaccine) include the demonstration of an acquired defect in the cutaneous antimicrobial peptide response (see Immunopathologic Features, later).[48] Beck and colleagues[49] showed that AD patients with EH had more severe disease based on scoring systems, body surface area affected, and biomarkers (e.g., circulating eosinophil counts, serum IgE, thymus and activation-regulated chemokine [TARC], cutaneous T cell-attracting chemokine [CTACK]) than AD patients without a history of EH. AD patients

with EH also had more cutaneous infections with *S. aureus* or molluscum contagiosum virus and were also more likely to have a history of asthma and food and inhalant allergies. Leung and associates[50] showed that AD patients with EH have reduced interferon-γ (IFN-γ) production, and that IFN-γ and receptor (IFN-γR1) SNPs are significantly associated with AD and EH and may contribute to an impaired immune response to HSV. In addition, genetic variants in interferon regulatory factor 2 were also shown to be associated with AD and EH and may contribute to abnormal immune responses to HSV.[51]

Superimposed dermatophytosis may cause AD to flare. The opportunistic yeast *Malassezia sympodialis* (formerly *Pityrosporum ovale*) has also been associated with a predominantly head and neck distribution of AD and reported to occur in both extrinsic and intrinsic subtypes of AD.[52]

A number of studies have elucidated the importance of *S. aureus* in AD.[47]

Preferential adherence of *S. aureus* may be related to expression of adhesins such as fibronectin and fibrinogen in inflamed skin.[53] *S. aureus* can be cultured from the skin of more than 90% of patients with AD, compared with only 5% of normal subjects.[54] The higher rate of *S. aureus* colonization in AD lesions compared with lesions from other skin disorders may also be associated with colonization of the nares, with the hands serving as the vector of transmission.[55] Patients without obvious superinfection may have a better response to combined antistaphylococcal and topical corticosteroid therapy than to corticosteroids alone.[56] Recurrent pustulosis has become a significant problem for a number of patients, especially with the emergence of MRSA as an important pathogen in AD.[57]

PATIENT EVALUATION, DIAGNOSIS, AND DIFFERENTIAL DIAGNOSIS

A number of diseases may be confused with AD (see Table 11.1). In infants, immunodeficiency, including immune dysregulation, polyendocrinopathy, enteropathy, and X-linked (IPEX) syndrome, needs to be considered. IPEX is a rare disorder associated with dermatitis, enteropathy, type 1 diabetes, thyroiditis, hemolytic anemia, and thrombocytopenia.[58] IPEX results from mutations of *FOXP3*, a gene located on the X chromosome that encodes the DNA-binding forkhead box P3 protein required for development of regulatory T cells.

Wiskott–Aldrich syndrome is an X-linked recessive disorder characterized by an eczematous rash, associated with thrombocytopenia along with variable abnormalities in humoral and cellular immunity and severe bacterial infections. Hyper-IgE syndrome (HIE) with mutations in the gene encoding signal transducer and activator of transcription 3 (*STAT3*) is a multisystem autosomal dominant disorder characterized by recurrent deep-seated bacterial infections, including cutaneous cold abscesses and pneumonias caused by *S. aureus*.[59] Patients with mutations in the gene encoding dedicator of cytokinesis 8 protein (*DOCK8*) have a unique combined primary immunodeficiency that accounts for most cases of autosomal recessive HIE.[60] These patients have an eczematous dermatitis with recurrent viral skin infections but lack the coarse facies of autosomal dominant HIE.

Scabies can present as a pruritic skin disease. However, distribution in the genital and axillary areas, the presence of linear lesions, and the finding of mites, ova, and scybala in epithelial debris from skin scrapings help distinguish scabies from AD. An adult who has eczematous dermatitis with no history of childhood eczema and without other atopic features may have contact dermatitis, but more importantly, cutaneous T cell lymphoma needs to be ruled out. Ideally, biopsies should be sent from three separate sites to increase the yield in identifying abnormal Sézary cells. In addition, eczematous rash suggestive of AD can be seen in patients with human immunodeficiency virus (HIV) infection.

Contact dermatitis should be considered in patients whose AD does not respond to appropriate therapy (see later). ACDs complicating AD may appear as an acute flare of the underlying disease rather than the more typical vesiculobullous eruption following direct contact with the injurious substance.

Psychosocial Implications

Patients with AD may have high levels of anxiety and problems dealing with anger and hostility.[61] Although not a cause, these emotions can exacerbate AD. Patients often respond to stress or frustration with itching and scratching. Stimulation of the central nervous system may intensify cutaneous vasomotor and sweat responses and contribute to the itch-scratch cycle. In some patients, scratching is associated with significant secondary gain or with a strong component of habit. Severe disease can have a significant impact on patients, leading to problems with social interactions and self-esteem. Importantly, sleep disturbance is common in this chronic disease and significantly impacts the quality of life of patients and family members.

Role of Allergens

Although elevated serum IgE levels can be demonstrated in 80% to 85% of patients with AD, particularly those seen in tertiary care/specialist centers, and a similar number have immediate skin test response or positive in vitro tests to food and inhalant allergens, the relationship between the course of AD and implicated allergens has been difficult to establish. Nevertheless, well-controlled studies suggest that allergens can impact the course of this disease.[62]

Foods

May[63] first recognized that patients with AD and positive food allergen skin tests could have negative food challenges to the implicated allergen, distinguishing between symptomatic and asymptomatic hypersensitivity. Thus, triggers for clinical disease cannot be predicted simply by performing allergy testing. However, double-blind placebo-controlled food challenges have demonstrated that food allergens can cause exacerbations in a subset of patients with AD.[64] Approximately 33% of infants and young children with AD will show clinically relevant reactivity to a food allergen.[65]

Although lesions induced by single positive challenges are usually transient, repeated challenges, more typical of real-life exposure, can result in eczematous lesions. Food-specific T cells have been cloned from lesional skin and peripheral blood of patients with AD.[66,67] Furthermore, elimination of food allergens results in amelioration of skin disease and a decrease in spontaneous basophil histamine release.[68]

Aeroallergens

The evidence supporting a role for aeroallergens in AD includes the finding of both allergen-specific IgE antibodies and allergen-specific T cells.[69] Exacerbation of AD can occur with exposure to allergens such as house-dust mites, animal danders, and pollens. In the 1940s, Tuft[70] demonstrated that introduction of aeroallergens intranasally could exacerbate AD. Subsequently, in a double-blind randomized placebo-controlled trial (RCT), a subgroup of patients with AD who underwent bronchoprovocation with a standardized house-dust mite extract developed unequivocal cutaneous lesions after inhalation of dust mite.[71] All the patients with dust mite–induced dermatitis had a history of asthma, and in eight of these nine patients, the skin reaction was preceded by an early bronchial reaction. Therefore, the respiratory route may be important in the induction and exacerbation of AD. Direct contact with inhalant allergens can also result in eczematous skin eruptions.[72] Using the atopy patch test, Langeveld-Wildschut and coworkers[73] showed that positive reactions to house-dust mite were associated with IgE+ LCs in the epidermis of AD patients.

In addition, the severity of AD has been correlated with the degree of sensitization to aeroallergens.[74] Most importantly, environmental control measures aimed at reducing dust mite allergen have been shown to result in clinical improvement in AD patients.[75,76] These studies suggest that inhalation or contact with aeroallergens may be involved in the pathogenesis of AD.

Microbial Agents

In addition to their role as infectious agents, both the lipophilic yeast M. sympodialis[52] and the superficial dermatophyte Trichophyton rubrum have been associated with elevated specific-IgE levels. Patients with AD predominantly of the head and neck, compared with a group without this distribution and with a group of normal controls, more often demonstrated IgE testing, and specific histamine release to M. sympodialis. These findings are of clinical significance because patients improve after antifungal therapy.

Leung and colleagues[77] showed that exotoxins secreted by S. aureus are superantigens that can contribute to persistent inflammation or exacerbations of AD. More than half of the AD patients studied had S. aureus cultured from their skin; the organisms secreted primarily enterotoxins A and B and toxic shock syndrome toxin-1. In addition, almost half of the patients had specific IgE antibodies directed against the staphylococcal toxins found on their skin. AD patients are unique in that they can be colonized by S. aureus bacteria that secrete more than one superantigen compared to patients with other superantigen-mediated disease such as toxic shock syndrome.[57] Basophils from patients with antitoxin IgE released histamine on exposure to the relevant toxin but not in response to toxins to which they had no specific IgE. Other investigators have confirmed these observations.[78,79] In addition, analysis of the peripheral blood skin-homing (CLA+) T cells of superantigen-positive patients as well as their skin lesions revealed that they had undergone expansion of the T cell receptor variable-domain β chain, consistent with superantigenic stimulation.[80,81] A correlation also has been found between the presence of IgE against superantigens and severity of AD.[78] Furthermore, superantigens have an additive effect with conventional allergens in inducing cutaneous inflammation.[82] Superantigens can also augment allergen-specific IgE synthesis,[83] subvert T regulatory (Treg) cell function,[84] and induce corticosteroid resistance,[85] suggesting several mechanisms by which superantigens could aggravate the severity of AD. In addition, staphylococcal enterotoxin B applied to the skin induced erythema and induration, with the infiltrating T cells selectively expanded in response to the specific superantigen.[86,87]

Autoantigens

Several groups have suggested a role for autoantigens in chronic AD showing that the majority of sera from patients with severe AD contain IgE antibodies directed against human proteins.[88] One of these IgE-reactive autoantigens, a 55-kD cytoplasmic protein in skin keratinocytes, has been cloned from a human epithelial complementary DNA expression library and designated Hom s 1.[89] Although the autoallergens characterized to date have mainly been intracellular proteins, they have been detected in IgE immune complexes of AD sera, suggesting that release of these autoallergens from damaged tissues could trigger IgE or T cell–mediated responses. These data suggest that skin inflammation in AD, especially in severe cases, could be maintained by endogenous human antigens. Because these autoantigens are primarily nuclear or microsomal in origin, damage to the skin by infectious organisms or scratching could release intracellular antigens that in turn could elicit and perpetuate IgE and T cell responses in AD. Of interest, human manganese superoxide dismutase (MnSOD) may play a role as an autoallergen in a subset of patients with AD.[90] By molecular mimicry leading to cross-reactivity, such sensitization might be induced primarily by exposure to MnSOD of the skin-colonizing yeast *M. sympodialis* (see Complicating Features earlier).

Immunology

A number of immunoregulatory abnormalities have been described in AD[91] (Box 11.2). B cells from patients with AD synthesize high levels of IgE. T cells from these patients produce increased amounts of IL-4 and express abnormally high levels of IL-4 receptor. Peripheral blood mononuclear cells (PBMCs) isolated from patients with AD have a decreased capacity to make IFN-γ, which is inversely correlated with serum IgE levels. Among differences noted between the intrinsic and extrinsic forms of AD, skin-derived T cells from extrinsic AD interacted with B cells to support IgE synthesis, whereas T cells from the intrinsic form of AD did not.[92]

Studies have shown an increased frequency of both circulating[93,94] and lesional allergen-specific Th2 cells secreting IL-4, IL-5, and IL-13 in patients with AD.[92,95] Furthermore, an increased frequency of circulating skin-homing (CLA+) type 2

> ### BOX 11.2 Immunoregulatory Abnormalities in Atopic Dermatitis
>
> Increased synthesis of IgE
> Increased levels of specific IgE to multiple allergens, including foods, aeroallergens, microorganisms, and enterotoxins
> Increased expression of CD23 on B cells and monocytes
> Increased surface expression of FcεRI on antigen-presenting cells in the skin
> Increased levels of cutaneous T cell–attracting chemokine (CTACK) and thymus- and activation-regulated chemokine (TARC)
> Increased secretion of interleukin-4 (IL-4), IL-5, and IL-13 by T helper type 2 (Th2) cells
> Decreased secretion of interferon-γ by Th1 cells
> Decreased CD4+/CD25+ regulatory T (Treg) cell immunosuppressive activity after superantigen stimulation
> Decreased secretion of antimicrobial peptides by keratinocytes
> Increased levels of monocyte cyclic adenosine monophosphate phosphodiesterase, with increased IL-10 and prostaglandin E2

cytokine-producing cells and decreased frequency of CLA+ type 1 cytokine-producing cells have been reported in the peripheral blood of AD patients.[96] In addition to acting as an IgE isotype–specific switch, IL-4 also inhibits the production of IFN-γ and downregulates the differentiation of Th1 cells.[97] The importance of Th2 cytokines in driving AD skin inflammation is strongly supported by the observation that a fully human monoclonal antibody that blocks the action of IL-4 and IL-13 was found to reduce the skin severity of AD.[98]

Immunopathologic Features

Routine histologic examination of clinically normal-appearing skin in AD reveals mild epidermal hyperplasia and a sparse, predominantly lymphocytic infiltrate in the dermis.[91] Acute eczematous lesions are characterized by both intercellular edema of the epidermis (spongiosis) and intracellular edema. A sparse lymphocytic infiltrate may be observed in the epidermis, whereas a marked perivenular infiltrate consisting of lymphocytes and some monocytes with rare eosinophils, basophils, and neutrophils is seen in the dermis. In chronic lichenified lesions, the epidermis has prominent hyperkeratosis with increased numbers of epidermal LCs and predominantly monocytes/macrophages in the dermal infiltrate.

Immunohistochemical staining of acute and chronic skin lesions in AD shows that the lymphocytes are predominantly CD3, CD4, and CD45RO memory T cells; that is, the lymphocytes previously encountered antigen[99] (Fig. 11.3). These cells also express CD25 and human leukocyte antigen (HLA)–DR on their surface, indicative of intralesional activation. In addition, almost all the T cells infiltrating into atopic skin lesions express high levels of the skin lymphocyte–homing receptor cutaneous lymphocyte antigen (CLA).

The role of keratinocytes in skin inflammation in AD has been increasingly recognized.[99] Keratinocytes are an important source of thymic stromal lymphopoietin (TSLP), which activates dendritic cells to prime naïve T cells to produce IL-4 and IL-13 (Th2 cell differentiation). In addition, *S. aureus* membrane–derived lipopeptides were shown to induce TSLP in keratinocytes through the Toll-like receptor 2 (TLR2)–TLR6 pathway.[100]

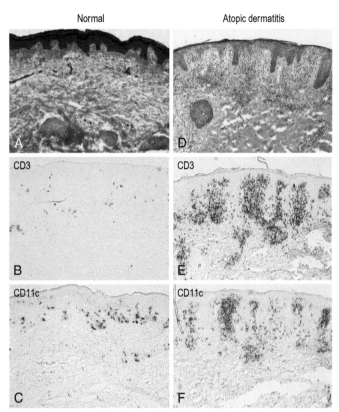

Normal   Atopic dermatitis

Fig. 11.3 Immunohistology of atopic dermatitis versus normal skin showing epidermal hyperplasia with T cells (CD3) and dendritic cells (CD11c) in the superficial dermis. (From Guttman-Yassky E, Nograles KE, Krueger JG. Contrasting pathogenesis of atopic dermatitis and psoriasis. Part I. Clinical and pathologic concepts. J Allergy Clin Immunol 2011;127:1110–1118.)

Besides producing proinflammatory cytokines, keratinocytes also play a vital role in the cutaneous innate immune responses by secreting antimicrobial peptides, including human β-defensins and β-cathelicidins, in response to microbial insult or tissue injury. Their keratinocytes produce reduced amounts of antimicrobial peptides, which may predispose AD patients to their frequent colonization and infection by S. aureus, viruses, and fungi.[101] Vitamin D has been found to be involved in the regulation of antimicrobial peptides in keratinocytes,[102] and the treatment with oral vitamin D in AD patients supports this hypothesis.[103] Patients with AD receiving oral vitamin D supplementation showed prevention of winter time exacerbation of eczema.[104]

Cytokine Expression

Cytokine expression in AD lesions reflects the nature of the underlying inflammation (Fig. 11.4). Hamid and associates[105] used in situ hybridization to study IL-4, IL-5, and IFN-γ mRNA expression in acute and chronic skin lesions as well as uninvolved skin of patients with AD. Biopsies from uninvolved atopic skin showed a significant increase in the number of cells expressing IL-4 mRNA, but not IL-5 or IFN-γ mRNA. Both acute and chronic lesions had significantly greater numbers of cells positive for IL-4 and IL-5 than did uninvolved or

normal skin. Neither acutely involved nor uninvolved atopic skin showed significant numbers of IFN-γ mRNA–expressing cells. In contrast, chronic AD skin lesions had significantly fewer IL-4 mRNA–expressing cells and significantly more IL-5 mRNA–expressing cells than acute lesions. T cells made up the majority of IL-5–expressing cells in both acute and chronic lesions. Activated eosinophils were found in significantly greater numbers in chronic than in acute lesions. These data suggest that although both acute and chronic lesions in AD are associated with increased IL-4 and IL-5 gene activation, acute skin inflammation is associated with predominantly IL-4 expression, whereas chronic inflammation is associated with IL-5 expression and eosinophil infiltration.

IL-13 expression was also found to be higher in acute AD lesions than in chronic AD or psoriatic lesions.[106] These data suggest that IL-13 may be involved in the pathogenesis of AD and further support the hypothesis that acute inflammation in AD is mediated by Th2-type cytokines. Chronic lesions had increased numbers of IL-12 mRNA–positive cells compared with acute or uninvolved skin. IL-12 is a potent inducer of IFN-γ synthesis, and consistent with this observation, increased IFN-γ expression has been reported in chronic AD lesions.[107] At a clonal level, T cells from AD patients with cow's milk allergy showed significantly greater production of IL-4, whereas IFN-γ production was greater in the milk-tolerant patients.[67] IL-5 and IL-13 cytokine production strongly correlated with IL-4 production.

Pruritus is a hallmark of AD, and the underlying processes involved are complex.[108] Mice that overexpress the T cell–derived cytokine IL-31 develop intense pruritus and dermatitis, and patients with AD have CLA+ T cells that produce higher levels of IL-31.[109] In patients with AD as well as in those with ACD (another pruritic dermatosis), expression of IL-31 is associated with expression of IL-4 and IL-13, which are Th2 cytokines that characterize the atopic phenotype.[110] In addition, S. aureus superantigen rapidly induces IL-31 expression in atopic individuals, and because patients with AD are heavily colonized with toxin-producing S. aureus, this can further contribute to their pruritus.[111] Calcineurin inhibitors and other agents that target T cells are effective at reducing pruritus in AD patients, and new insights into the role of IL-31 in AD may reveal new targets for antipruritic therapy. Of note, a biologic targeting IL-31 receptor A has been shown to improve both pruritus and AD lesions.[112]

Increasingly, as previously discussed, the keratinocyte-derived cytokine TSLP has been recognized as the "master switch" for allergic inflammation.[113] In AD the TSLP-induced Th2 cytokine milieu can participate in a vicious cycle impacting the skin barrier and microbial colonization.[100] Genetic variants in TSLP have been shown to be associated with AD and EH.[114]

Role of IgE in Cutaneous Inflammation

In AD patients, IgE may play an important role in allergen-induced, cell-mediated reactions involving Th2-type cells that are distinct from conventional delayed-type hypersensitivity reactions mediated by Th1-type cells.[115] IgE-dependent biphasic reactions are frequently associated with clinically significant

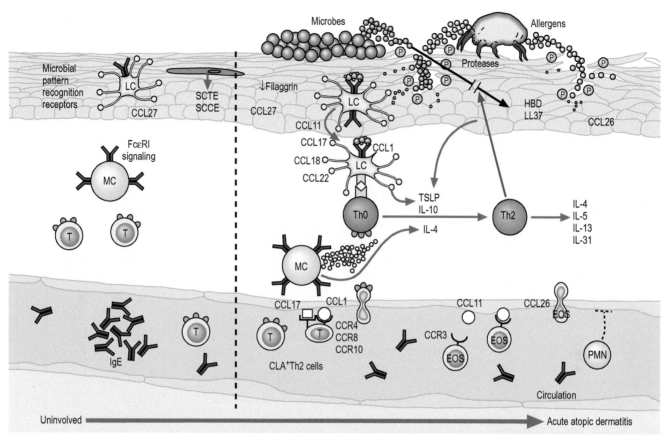

Fig. 11.4 Immunologic abnormalities in the progression of atopic dermatitis. *MC*, Mast cell; *PMN*, polymorphonuclear neutrophil; *T*, T lymphocyte; *Th*, helper T cell. (Reproduced from J Allergy Clin Immunol 2006;118:cover.)

allergic reactions and may contribute to the inflammatory process of AD. Immediate-type reactions related to mediator release by mast cells bearing allergen-specific IgE may result in the pruritus and erythema that occur after exposure to relevant allergens. IgE-dependent late-phase reactions can then lead to more persistent symptoms. The T cell infiltrate in cutaneous allergen-induced late-phase reactions has increased mRNA for IL-3, IL-4, IL-5, and granulocyte-macrophage colony-stimulating factor (GM-CSF), but not for IFN-γ. These cells are therefore similar to the Th2-type cells found in AD lesions. In addition, the cutaneous late-phase reaction is associated with a pattern of cell adhesion molecule (CAM) expression similar to that in AD. Therefore, a sustained IgE-dependent late-phase reaction may be part of the chronic inflammatory process in AD patients.

Furthermore, epidermal LCs in AD skin express IgE on their cell surface and are significantly more efficient than IgE-negative LCs at presenting allergen to T cells.[116] In addition, LCs from atopic individuals have a much higher level of FcεRI expression.[117] Efficient allergen capture and presentation to Th2 cells in atopic skin may be an important mechanism for sustaining local T cell activation.

Skin-directed Th2-like Cell Response

A number of studies have demonstrated important similarities between the allergic inflammation of asthma and AD. Common features include local infiltration of Th2-type cells in response to allergens, development of specific IgE to allergens, a chronic inflammatory process, and organ-specific hyperreactivity. In both diseases, IL-4– and IL-5–secreting memory Th2-type cells have a central role in the induction of local IgE responses and recruitment of eosinophils.[105] The recognition of T cell heterogeneity based on expression of tissue-selective homing receptors suggests that an individual's propensity for specific allergic disease may be a function of end-organ targeting by effector T cells. In this respect, T cells migrating to the skin express CLA, whereas most memory/effector T cells isolated from asthmatic airways do not.

In a study of patients with milk-induced AD, casein-reactive T cells expressed significantly higher levels of CLA than did *Candida albicans*–reactive T cells from these patients or casein-reactive T cells from patients with milk-induced enterocolitis or eosinophilic gasteroenteritis.[118] As further evidence for selective end-organ targeting by T cell subsets in allergic inflammation, data show that dust mite–specific T cell proliferation in mite-sensitized patients with AD was localized to the CLA-expressing fraction of T cells.[119] In contrast, T cells isolated from mite-allergic asthmatic patients that proliferated on exposure to the relevant allergen were CLA⁻. Furthermore, CLA-expressing T cells isolated from patients with AD, but not from normal controls, showed evidence of activation (HLA-DR expression) and also spontaneously produced IL-4 but not IFN-γ. This suggests that T cell effector function in AD is closely linked to CLA expression.

TREATMENT

Conventional Therapy

Current understanding of the pathophysiology of AD supports the concept that assessing the role of allergens, infectious agents, irritants, physical environment, and emotional stressors is as important as initiating therapy with first-line agents. The acute and chronic aspects of AD need to be considered when designing an individualized treatment plan. Patients should understand that therapy is not curative, but that avoidance of exacerbating factors together with proper daily skin care can control symptoms and improve the long-term outcome. Management of patients with AD has been comprehensively reviewed (Fig. 11.5).[120–122]

Irritants

Patients with AD have a lowered threshold of irritant responsiveness. Therefore, recognition and avoidance of irritants are integral to successful management of this disease. Irritants include detergents, soaps, chemicals, pollutants, and abrasive materials, as well as extremes of temperature and humidity. Cleansers with minimal defatting activity and a neutral pH should be used rather than soaps. A number of mild cleansers are available in sensitive skin formulations. New clothing should be laundered before it is worn, to reduce the content of formaldehyde and other chemicals. Residual laundry detergent in clothing may be irritating, and although changing to a milder detergent can be helpful, using liquid rather than powder detergent and adding an extra rinse cycle are more beneficial. Occlusive clothing should be avoided, and cotton or cotton blends should be used.

Ideally, the temperature in the home and work environments should be temperate to minimize sweating. Swimming is usually well tolerated; however, because swimming pools are treated with chlorine or bromine, it is important for patients to shower and use a mild soap immediately afterward, to remove these potentially irritating chemicals, and then to apply moisturizers or occlusives. Although sunlight may be beneficial to some patients with AD, nonsensitizing sunscreens should be used to avoid sunburn. Products developed for use on the face are often best tolerated by patients with AD. Prolonged sun exposure can cause evaporative losses, overheating, and sweating, which can be irritating.

Allergens

Identification of allergens involves taking a careful history and doing selective immediate-hypersensitivity skin tests or in vitro tests when appropriate. Negative skin tests with proper controls have a high predictive value for ruling out a suspected allergen. Positive skin tests have a lower correlation with clinical symptoms in suspected food allergen–induced AD and should be confirmed with double-blind placebo-controlled food challenge, unless the patient has a history of anaphylaxis to the suspected food (see Chapter 12). In children who have undergone such a challenge, milk, egg, peanut, soy, wheat, and fish account for approximately 90% of the food allergens found to exacerbate AD. More importantly, avoidance of foods implicated in controlled challenges results in clinical improvement.[64,68]

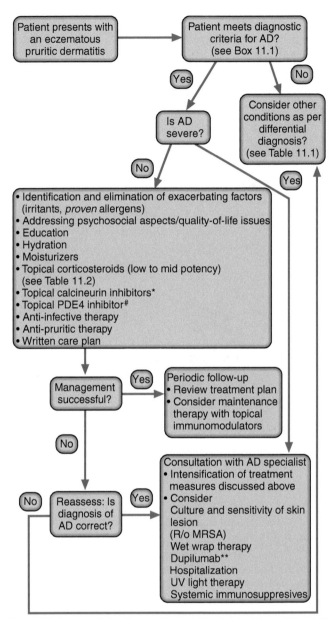

Fig. 11.5 Approach to the patient with atopic dermatitis (AD). *R/o MRSA*, Rule out methicillin-resistant *Staphylococcus aureus*; *UV*, ultraviolet. *Per boxed warning: second-line, intermittent therapy for patients ≥2 years of age. #Approved for mild-moderate AD down to 3 months of age. **Approved for moderate-severe AD down to 6 years of age.

Extensive elimination diets, which may be both extremely burdensome and at times nutritionally unsound, are almost never warranted. In addition, elimination of foods without a convincing history of clinical allergy may result in an immediate type reaction at later reintroduction.[123] It is important to recognize that specific IgE levels address probability of a reaction, not severity or type of reaction and that the in vitro assay does not perform well when total serum IgE levels are in the thousand IU/mL or greater.

Environmental control measures aimed at reducing dust mite load may improve AD in patients who demonstrate specific IgE to dust mite allergen.[75] These measures include using dust mite–proof encasings on pillows, mattresses, and box springs; washing linens in hot water weekly; removing bedroom carpeting; and decreasing indoor humidity levels. Adult AD patients not sensitized to house-dust mite benefited from allergy-proof covers as much as sensitized patients, suggesting that impermeable covers may reduce exposure to other allergens, irritants, or infectious organisms.[76]

Psychosocial Factors

Recognizing and addressing sleep disturbance problems in both patients and caregivers are critical in a chronic, relapsing disease such as AD. Counseling is often helpful in dealing with the frustrations associated with AD. Relaxation, behavioral modification, and biofeedback may all be of benefit, especially for patients with habitual scratching.[61]

Patient Education

Learning about the chronic nature of AD, exacerbating factors, and appropriate treatment options is important for both patients and caregivers.[124] In addition, patients and their families should be counseled about the natural history and prognosis and receive appropriate vocational counseling. The International Study of Life with Atopic Eczema (ISOLATE) found that patients and caregivers often delay initiation of treatment for AD flares and have concerns about their prescribed medications.[125] Clinicians should provide patients and their families with detailed written skin care recommendations and should review this information on follow-up. Educational materials may be obtained from the National Eczema Association (www.nationaleczema.org), a national not-for-profit, patient-oriented organization. In addition, written information and a DVD on skin care are available from the Office of Professional Education, National Jewish Health (800–844-2305).

Hydration

Atopic dry skin shows enhanced transepidermal water loss and reduced water-binding capacity. Patients may also have decreased ceramide levels in their skin, resulting in reduced water-binding capacity, higher transepidermal water loss, and decreased water content.[126] Therefore, skin hydration is an essential component of therapy. The best way to reestablish the skin's barrier function is to soak the affected area or bathe for approximately 10 minutes in warm (not lukewarm) water and then apply an occlusive agent to retain the absorbed water. Substances such as oatmeal or baking soda added to the bathwater may feel soothing to certain patients but do not affect water absorption. Hydration of the face or neck can be achieved by applying a wet facecloth or towel to the involved area. A wet washcloth may be more readily accepted if holes are cut out for the eyes and mouth, allowing the patient to remain functional. Hand or foot dermatitis can be treated by soaking the limb in a basin. Baths may need to be taken several times a day during flares of AD, whereas showers may be adequate for patients with mild disease. It is essential to use an occlusive preparation within a few minutes after hydrating the skin to prevent evaporation, which is damaging to the epidermis. Of note, a recent randomized, single-blind cross-over trial found that twice daily bathing was superior to twice weekly bathing when combined with moisturizer and the same low-potency topical steroid for treatment of acute AD.[127]

Patients and their families need to understand proper hydration techniques. Bathing may also remove allergens from the skin surface and reduce colonization by *S. aureus*. Bleach baths with dilute sodium hypochlorite have been recommended to reduce skin infections (¼ to ½ cup of household bleach per full tub of water), but this approach may lead to skin irritation and should be used with caution. A metaanalysis concluded that dilute bleach baths were no more effective than plain water baths.[128]

Moisturizers and Occlusives

The use of an effective emollient, especially when combined with hydration therapy, helps to restore and preserve the stratum corneum barrier and can decrease the need for topical corticosteroids (TCS).[129] Moisturizers are available as lotions, creams, and ointments. Lotions contain more water than creams and may be more drying because of an evaporative effect. Both lotions and creams can cause skin irritation secondary to added preservatives and fragrances. Because moisturizers usually need to be applied several times daily on a long-term basis, they should be obtained in 1-pound (0.45-kg) jars if available. Vegetable-oil shortening (e.g., Crisco) can be used if an inexpensive moisturizer is needed. Petroleum jelly (e.g., Vaseline) is an effective occlusive when used to seal in water after bathing.

Alpha-hydroxy acids affect keratinization through corneocyte cohesion and stratum corneum formation and increase dermal mucopolysaccharides and collagen formation. Assessment of 12% ammonium lactate emulsion by clinical criteria and by noninvasive methods showed a significant increase in electrical capacitance, skin surface lipids, dermal extensibility and firmness, and improvement in the skin barrier function and skin surface topography in all patients.[130] Ammonium lactate mitigated the epidermal and dermal atrophy associated with topical corticosteroid use.[131]

In contrast to changes in sphingolipid metabolism caused by aging, the enzyme SM deacylase is highly expressed in the epidermis of AD patients and competes with sphingomyelinase or β-glucocerebrosidase for the common substrate SM or glucosylceramide.[132] This in turn leads to ceramide deficiency of the stratum corneum in AD. Whereas an equimolar ratio of ceramides, cholesterol, and either the essential fatty acid linoleic acid or the nonessential palmitic or stearic fatty acids allows normal repair of damaged human skin, further acceleration of barrier repair occurs as the ratio of any of these ingredients is increased up to three-fold.[133] Nonsteroidal creams (e.g., Atopiclair, EpiCeram, MimyX) marketed as "medical devices" have unique formulations and have not been compared; although not regulated by the US FDA, these creams do require a prescription.[134]

Corticosteroids

Corticosteroids reduce inflammation and pruritus and are effective for both the acute and chronic components of AD. They affect multiple resident and infiltrating cells primarily through suppression of inflammatory genes, reducing inflammation and pruritus. TCS are available in a wide variety of formulations,

TABLE 11.2 Select Topical Corticosteroid Preparations[a]

Group	Preparations
1	Clobetasol propionate (Temovate) 0.05% ointment/cream
	Betamethasone dipropionate (Diprolene) 0.05% ointment/cream
2	Mometasone furoate (Elocon) 0.1% ointment
	Halcinonide (Halog) 0.1% cream
	Fluocinonide (Lidex) 0.05% ointment/cream
	Desoximetasone (Topicort) 0.25% ointment/cream
3	Fluticasone propionate (Cutivate) 0.005% ointment
	Halcinonide (Halog) 0.1% ointment
	Betamethasone valerate (Valisone) 0.1% ointment
4	Mometasone furoate (Elocon) 0.1% cream
	Triamcinolone acetonide (Kenalog) 0.1% ointment/cream
	Fluocinolone acetonide (Synalar) 0.025% ointment
5	Fluocinolone acetonide (Synalar) 0.025% cream
	Hydrocortisone valerate (Westcort) 0.2% ointment
6	Desonide (DesOwen) 0.05% ointment/cream/lotion/gel
	Alclometasone dipropionate (Aclovate) 0.05% ointment/cream
7	Hydrocortisone (Hytone) 2.5% and 1% ointment/cream

[a]Representative corticosteroids are listed by group from 1 (superpotent) through 7 (least potent).
Modified from Stoughton RB. Vasoconstrictor assay-specific applications. In: Maibach HI, Surber C, editors. Topical corticosteroids. Basel, Switzerland: Karger; 1992, pp. 42–53.

ranging from extremely high-potency (group 1) to low-potency (group 7) preparations (Table 11.2). The vehicle in which the product is formulated can alter the potency of the corticosteroid and move it up or down in this classification. Generic formulations of TCS are required to have the same active ingredient and the same concentration as the original product. However, many generics do not have the same vehicle formulation, and the bioequivalence of the product can vary significantly.

Choice of a particular product depends on the severity and distribution of skin lesions. In general, an effective topical corticosteroid of the lowest potency should be used. However, choosing a preparation that is too weak may result in persistent or worsening AD. Resistant lesions may respond to a potent topical corticosteroid under occlusion, although this needs to be used cautiously to prevent irreversible atrophic changes. When treating pediatric patients, clinicians should be aware of age-appropriate indications (e.g., fluticasone 0.05% cream, up to 28 days in children age ≥3 months; fluticasone lotion, ≥12 months of age; mometasone cream/ointment, ≥2 years of age).

With appropriately used low- to medium-potency TCS, side effects are infrequent. Thinning of the skin with telangiectasias, bruising, hypopigmentation, acne, striae, and secondary infections may occur. The face, particularly the eyelids, and the intertriginous areas are especially sensitive to these adverse effects, and only low-potency preparations should be used routinely on these areas. Perioral dermatitis, characterized by erythema, scaling, and follicular papules and pustules that occur around the mouth, in the alar creases, and sometimes on the upper lateral eyelids, can occur with the use of TCS on the face. "Steroid addiction" describes an adverse effect primarily of the face of adult women treated with TCS, who complain of a burning sensation. Patients improve with total discontinuation of the corticosteroid therapy.[135] High-potency TCS must be used cautiously, especially under occlusion, because they may lead to significant atrophic changes and systemic side effects.

TCS are available in a variety of bases, including ointments, creams, lotions, solutions, gels, sprays, oil, and even tape (see Table 11.2). Therefore, no need exists to compound these medications. Ointments are most occlusive and as a rule provide better delivery of the medication while preventing evaporative losses. In addition, ointments spread more evenly than other creams or solutions. In a humid environment, creams may be better tolerated than ointments because the increased occlusion can cause itching or even folliculitis. In general, however, creams and lotions, although easier to spread, are less effective and can contribute to skin dryness and irritation. Solutions can be used on the scalp and hirsute areas, although the alcohol content can be irritating, especially if used on inflamed or open lesions, and additives used to formulate the different bases can cause sensitization. Furthermore, ACD to the corticosteroid molecule is being recognized with increasing frequency.[136] This diagnosis is often difficult to establish clinically because it can present as acute or chronic eczema. Patch testing has been done primarily with tixocortol pivalate and budesonide. Expanded testing has been associated with both false-positive and false-negative reactions.

An inadequate prescription size often contributes to suboptimally controlled AD, especially when patients have widespread, chronic disease. Approximately 30 g of medication is needed to cover the entire body of an average adult. The *fingertip unit* (FTU) has been proposed as a measure for applying TCS and has been studied in children with AD.[137] This is the amount of topical medication that extends from the tip to the first joint on the palmar aspect of the index finger. It takes approximately 1 FTU to cover the hand or groin, 2 FTUs for the face or foot, 3 FTUs for an arm, 6 FTUs for the leg, and 14 FTUs for the trunk.

Patients need to be instructed in the proper use of TCS. Application of an emollient immediately before or over a topical corticosteroid preparation may decrease the effectiveness of the corticosteroid. Patients often assume that the potency of their prescribed corticosteroid is based solely on the percentage noted after the compound name (e.g., they believe that hydrocortisone 2.5% is more potent than clobetasol 0.05%) and therefore may apply the preparations incorrectly. In addition, patients are often given a high-potency corticosteroid and told to discontinue it after a time without being given a lower-potency corticosteroid; this can result in rebound flaring of the AD, similar to that often seen with oral corticosteroid therapy for AD. A stepwise care approach with a midrange or high-potency preparation (although usually not to face, axillae, or groin) followed by low-potency preparations may be more successful.

Once-daily treatment may help with patient adherence to the regimen and has been effective for fluticasone propionate, a molecule with an increased binding affinity for the corticosteroid receptor.[138] Topical mometasone has been studied in children with AD and is also approved for once-daily use.[139] TCS usually have been discontinued after the inflammation resolves, while hydration and moisturizers are continued. An important concept to recognize is that normal-appearing skin in AD shows evidence of immunologic dysregulation,[105] and more recently, skin barrier abnormalities have been demonstrated in nonlesional skin.[140] These data provide a rationale for the use of TCS as "proactive" or maintenance therapy.[141]

In several studies with fluticasone, after control of AD with a once-daily regimen was achieved, long-term control could be maintained with twice-weekly applications of the topical corticosteroid to areas that had previously been involved but now appeared normal. This approach has resulted in fewer relapses and less need for TCS than has "reactive" eczema therapy.

In addition to their antiinflammatory properties, TCS can decrease *S. aureus* colonization in patients with AD. In a double-blind randomized 1-week trial of desonide compared with a vehicle in children with AD, clinical scores improved and *S. aureus* density significantly decreased within the desonide group but not in the vehicle group.[142]

A number of AD patients may not show clinical improvement with TCS, perhaps the result of superinfection complication or inadequate drug potency. In addition, allergen-induced immune activation can alter the T cell response to glucocorticoids by inducing cytokine-dependent abnormalities in glucocorticoid receptor–binding affinity.[143] PBMCs from patients with chronic AD have reduced glucocorticoid receptor–binding affinity, which can be sustained with the combination of IL-2 and IL-4 in vitro. In addition, corticosteroid unresponsiveness may contribute to treatment failure in some patients.[119] Endogenous cortisol levels have been found to control the magnitude of cutaneous allergic inflammatory responses, suggesting that an impaired response to corticosteroids could contribute to chronic AD.[144]

Alternatively, chronic corticosteroid therapy can have deleterious but insidious immunologic effects in allergic patients.[145] These results are based on in vitro data that may not recreate the complex milieu in allergic inflammation. A much more common reason for failure of corticosteroid therapy is nonadherence to the treatment regimen. Patients or parents often expect a quick and permanent resolution of the AD and become disillusioned by the lack of cure with current therapy. A significant number of patients and caregivers also admit to nonadherence to prescribed topical corticosteroid therapy because of fear of using this class of medications.[125,146] These findings emphasize the need for both education and alternative therapies.

Systemic corticosteroids, including oral prednisone, should be avoided in the management of a chronic, relapsing disorder such as AD.[121] Often, patients or parents demand immediate improvement of the disease and find systemic corticosteroids more convenient to use than topical therapy. However, the dramatic improvement observed with systemic corticosteroids may be associated with an equally dramatic flaring of AD after discontinuation. If a short course of *oral* corticosteroids is given, topical skin care should be intensified during the taper to suppress rebound flaring of AD.

Topical Calcineurin Inhibitors

The approval of the topical calcineurin inhibitors (TCIs) tacrolimus ointment 0.03% and 0.1% and pimecrolimus cream 1% represented a milestone in AD management. Both nonsteroidal drugs have proved effective, with a good safety profile for treatment up to 4 years with tacrolimus ointment[147] and up to 2 years with pimecrolimus cream.[148] A fairly common side effect with TCIs is a transient burning sensation of the skin, although a few patients may complain of more prolonged burning or stinging. TCIs are not associated with skin atrophy and thus are particularly useful on the face and intertriginous regions. TCIs may be particularly useful in the treatment of steroid-insensitive patients.[149] Ongoing surveillance and recent reports have shown no trend for increased frequency of viral superinfections, especially EH, and no problems with response to childhood vaccinations.[150]

Currently, tacrolimus ointment 0.03% is approved for intermittent treatment of moderate-severe AD in children 2 years and older, tacrolimus ointment 0.1% for intermittent treatment of moderate-severe AD in adults, and pimecrolimus cream 1% for intermittent therapy of patients 2 years and older with mild-moderate AD.

Although there is no evidence of a causal link between cancer and TCIs, the FDA has issued a boxed warning for tacrolimus ointment 0.03% and 0.1% (Protopic, Astellas) and pimecrolimus cream 1% (Elidel, Novartis) because of a lack of long-term safety data (see US package inserts for Protopic, Astellas; and Elidel, Novartis). Further, the new labeling states that these drugs are recommended as second-line treatments and that their use in children under age 2 years is currently not recommended. Long-term safety studies with TCIs in patients with AD, including infants and children, are ongoing. A joint task force of the American College of Allergy, Asthma and Immunology and the American Academy of Allergy, Asthma and Immunology reviewed the available data and concluded that the risk/benefit ratios of tacrolimus ointment 0.03% and 0.1% and pimecrolimus cream 1% are similar to those of most conventional therapies for the treatment of chronic relapsing eczema.[151] In addition, a nested case-control study of a large database ($n=293,253$) did not find an increased risk of lymphoma in AD patients treated with TCIs.[152]

Studies with TCIs have shown that pimecrolimus cream 1% is well tolerated and effective in infants 3 to 23 months of age with AD.[153,154] Given the chronic and relapsing nature of AD, the question of whether TCI therapy for early signs or symptoms of disease could influence long-term outcomes was addressed in clinical trials up to 1 year in duration with pimecrolimus cream 1%.[155] The primary efficacy parameter was the incidence of flares and need for topical corticosteroid rescue. In the infant study, 64% of the pimecrolimus group versus 35% of the vehicle group did not require TCS during the study.[154] Subgroup analysis showed significantly fewer flares in the pimecrolimus-treated children of all degrees of clinical severity, including severe AD. These studies suggest that earlier use of a TCI can lead to better long-term disease control with fewer flares and significantly less need for topical corticosteroid rescue therapy. Similar to the proactive use of TCS, several studies of tacrolimus ointment in both adults and children have shown efficacy with this approach.[141] Proactive therapy with tacrolimus ointment has been approved for use in Europe for up to 12 months in patients 2 years or older.

Topical Phosphodiesterase 4 Inhibitor

Crisaborole is a phosphodiesterase 4 (PDE4) inhibitor, which increases cyclic adenosine monophosphate (cAMP) levels and reduces inflammation. In vitro, crisaborole inhibits cytokine production by PBMCs distinct from corticosteroids.[156] It has been studied and found to be safe and effective when applied twice daily in both children and adults with mild to moderate AD.[157] It has been approved by the FDA as a 2% topical ointment in patients with mild to moderate AD down to 3 months of age.[158]

Tar Preparations

Crude coal tar extracts have antiinflammatory properties that are not as pronounced as those of TCS. Nevertheless, in a study using the atopy patch test, tar performed similar to a topical corticosteroid in its ability to inhibit the influx of proinflammatory cells and in the expression of CAMs in response to epicutaneous allergen challenge.[159] Tar preparations used with TCS in chronic AD may reduce the need for more potent corticosteroid preparations. Tar shampoos are often beneficial for scalp involvement. The use of tar preparations on acutely inflamed skin should be avoided because it may result in skin irritation. Other than dryness or irritation, side effects associated with tar products are rare but include photosensitivity reactions and a pustular folliculitis.

Antiinfective Therapy

Systemic antibiotics may be necessary to treat AD when a secondary infection with *S. aureus* is present.[120] Therapy with semisynthetic penicillins or first- or second-generation cephalosporins for 7 to 10 days is usually effective. Erythromycin-resistant organisms are fairly common, making macrolides less useful alternatives. Unfortunately, recolonization after a course of antistaphylococcal therapy occurs rapidly.[160] Maintenance antibiotic therapy should be avoided, however, because it may result in colonization by methicillin-resistant organisms. The topical antistaphylococcal antibiotic mupirocin (Bactroban), applied three times daily to affected areas for 7 to 10 days, may be effective for treating localized areas of involvement. Twice-daily treatment for 5 days with a nasal preparation of mupirocin may reduce nasal carriage of *S. aureus*, which may result in clinical benefit in AD patients. Although effective in reducing bacterial skin flora, antibacterial cleansers can cause significant skin irritation.

Patients with disseminated EH, also called Kaposi varicelliform eruption, usually require treatment with systemic acyclovir.[47] Recurrent cutaneous herpetic infections can be controlled with daily prophylactic oral acyclovir. Superficial dermatophytosis and *M. sympodialis* infections can be treated with topical (or rarely with systemic) antifungal drugs.[47]

Antipruritic Agents

Pruritus is the most common and usually the worst-tolerated symptom of AD. Even partial reduction of pruritus can significantly improve quality of life for patients with severe AD. The participation of histamine in the pruritus of AD has been questioned, and a dermal microdialysis study of mast cell degranulation concluded that mediators other than histamine cause pruritus.[161] Neuropeptides or cytokines may be important mediators because centrally acting agents such as opioid receptor antagonists have been effective against the itch of AD.[162] Use of cyclosporin A, which results in decreased transcription of several proinflammatory cytokines, leads to rapid improvement in pruritus for many AD patients.[163]

Systemic antihistamines and anxiolytics may be most useful through their tranquilizing and sedative effects and can be used primarily in the evening to avoid daytime drowsiness. The tricyclic antidepressant doxepin, which has both histamine H1 and H2 receptor-binding affinity as well as a long half-life, may be given as a single 10- to 50-mg dose in the evening in adults. If nocturnal pruritus remains severe, short-term use of a sedative to allow adequate rest may be appropriate. Although reportedly ineffective in treating the pruritus associated with AD, second-generation antihistamines have shown modest clinical benefit in at least some AD patients.[164]

Treatment of AD with topical antihistamines and topical anesthetics should be avoided because of potential sensitization. Although in a 1-week study, topical 5% doxepin cream resulted in significant reduction of pruritus and no sensitization,[165] rechallenge with the drug after the 7-day course of therapy was not evaluated. Later case reports have documented reactions to topical doxepin.[166]

Biologic Therapy

Dupilumab is a fully human monoclonal antibody directed against the IL-4 receptor α subunit that blocks signaling of both IL-4 and IL-13. Treatment of adults with moderate-to-severe AD with dupilumab monotherapy resulted in significant improvement in physician- and patient-reported clinical parameters and patient-reported outcome measures.[167] Of the patients in the dupilumab group, 85% had a 50% reduction in the EASI score compared with 35% in the placebo group; 40% of patients in the dupilumab group had an investigator's global assessment score of 0 to 1 (clear or almost clear) compared with 7% in the placebo group; and pruritus scores decreased by 55.7% in the dupilumab group versus 15.1% in the placebo group. In a 52-week study of dupilumab with concomitant topical steroids, 100% of the patients in the dupilumab group had a 50% improvement in EASI, compared with 50% of those in the placebo group, even though the patients who received dupilumab used less than half the amount of topical steroids compared with those in the placebo group.[167] Adverse events, such as skin infection, occurred more frequently with placebo; nasopharyngitis and headache were the most frequent adverse events with dupilumab. In addition, conjunctivitis was reported in approximately 10% of patients in the phase 3 trials, although this adverse event did not require discontinuation in the majority of patients. Studies in adolescents and children confirmed both safety and efficacy of dupilumab.[168,169] Dupilumab is indicated for the treatment of patients ≥6 years with moderate-to-severe AD whose disease is not adequately controlled with topical prescription therapies or when those therapies are not advisable. Dupilumab can be used with or without TCS. Dosing in adults is 600 mg loading dose subcutaneously followed by 300 mg every other week. In children and adolescents, dosing is weight dependent with patients ≥60 kg receiving adult dosing, patients 30 kg to <60 kg receiving 400 mg loading dose followed by 200 mg every other week, and patients 15 kg to <30 kg 600 mg loading dose followed by 300 mg every 4 weeks. Currently, no laboratory monitoring is required.

RECALCITRANT DISEASE

Hospitalization

Patients with AD who are erythrodermic or who appear toxic may need to be hospitalized. Hospitalization may also be appropriate for patients with severe disseminated AD resistant to first-line therapy. Often, removing the patient from environmental allergens or stressors, together with intense education and assurance of compliance with therapy, results in marked clinical improvement. In this setting, the patient can also undergo appropriately controlled provocative challenges to help identify potential triggering factors. This can be done in a day hospital model.[122]

Wet Dressings

Wet-wrap dressings reduce pruritus and inflammation, act as a barrier to trauma associated with scratching, and improve penetration of TCS.[122] In addition, wet-wrap therapy can aid with epidermal barrier recovery that persists even after wrap therapy is discontinued.[170] In one study, children with severe AD showed significant clinical improvement after 1 week of treatment using tubular bandages applied over diluted TCS.[171] No significant differences were demonstrated among several dilutions of a mid-potency corticosteroid, suggesting that clinical benefit can be achieved with this approach in more severely affected patients even with the use of lower-potency corticosteroids. Although long-term studies with wet-wrap therapy are lacking, most of the improvement in the latter study occurred during the first week. An alternative approach employs clothing, using wet pajamas or long underwear, with dry pajamas or a sweatsuit on top.[122] Hands and feet can be covered by wet tube socks under dry tube socks. Alternatively, the face, trunk, or extremities can be covered by wet gauze and then dry gauze and secured in place with an elastic bandage or pieces of tube socks. Dressings may be removed when dry or may be rewetted. Dressings are often best tolerated at bedtime.

Overuse of wet-wrap dressings can result in chilling, maceration of the skin, or infrequently secondary infection. Because this approach can be labor intensive, it is best reserved for acute exacerbations of AD, along with selective use in areas of resistant dermatitis. The package inserts recommend that TCIs not be used under any occlusive dressing.

Systemic Immunosuppressive Agents

Treatment with systemic immunosuppressants should be reserved for patients with severe recalcitrant disease, which should be appropriately documented.[120–122] Other than systemic steroids that are approved for inflammatory conditions, including AD, none of the other drugs, including cyclosporine, methotrexate, mycophenolate, or azathioprine, are approved for AD in the US. Treatment with systemic steroids should be avoided in the management of a chronic relapsing disease disorder such as AD.[172] Often, improvement seen during treatment is quickly followed by rebound flaring when systemic corticosteroids are discontinued. If a short course of oral corticosteroids is given, topical skin care should be intensified during the taper to suppress rebound flaring of AD. Immunosuppressants should be prescribed by clinicians familiar with their adverse event profile with appropriate monitoring.[121,122,172]

Phototherapy and Photochemotherapy

Ultraviolet (UV) light therapy can be a useful treatment for chronic recalcitrant AD, but should be done under the supervision of an experienced dermatologist. The most common phototherapy modalities are narrowband UVB, broadband UVB, and UVA1.[121,172] Short-term adverse effects from phototherapy may include erythema, skin pain, pruritus, and pigmentation. Potential long-term adverse effects include premature skin aging and cutaneous malignancies.

Allergen Immunotherapy

Uncontrolled trials have suggested that desensitization to specific allergens may improve AD. In a double-blind controlled trial of desensitization with tyrosine-adsorbed *Dermatophagoides pteronyssinus* (house-dust mite) extract (Der p 1), children with AD and immediate hypersensitivity to *D. pteronyssinus* failed to demonstrate any clinical benefit from desensitization compared with placebo after an 8-month course of treatment.[173] In a second phase, children to whom *D. pteronyssinus* extract was initially administered were randomly assigned to continue on active treatment or placebo for an additional 6 months. The clinical scores suggested that extended desensitization was more effective than placebo, but the numbers were too small to permit confident conclusions. A high placebo effect may have concealed any additional therapeutic effect from active treatment. In a systematic review of immunotherapy for AD that included four comparable placebo-controlled studies involving a small number of patients, statistical analysis showed significant improvement in symptoms in patients with AD who received subcutaneous immunotherapy.[174]

A multicenter 1-year RCT of dust mite–specific immunotherapy in sensitized AD patients showed a dose-dependent effect on disease symptoms.[175] An open-label study of patients with dust mite allergy and AD treated with subcutaneous dust mite allergoid demonstrated serologic and immunologic changes consistent with tolerance, in addition to significant reductions in objective and subjective SCORAD.[176] One double-blind placebo-controlled study of children with AD treated with dust mite sublingual immunotherapy reported a significant difference from baseline values in visual analog scores, SCORAD, and medication use in the mild to moderate severity group, whereas patients with severe disease had only a marginal benefit.[177] Based on a review of available studies, the most recent practice parameter states that some data indicate immunotherapy can be effective for patients with AD when it is associated with aeroallergen sensitivity.[178] However, a Cochrane review of randomized controlled trials of allergen immunotherapy in AD found that results were confounded by high loss to follow-up and lack of blinding.[179] Subgroup analyses did not identify if a particular allergen, age, or level of disease severity predicted treatment success.

EXPERIMENTAL AND UNPROVEN THERAPIES

Omalizumab

Treatment of patients with AD with omalizumab off label has mainly been reported in case reports and case series, showing both clinical improvement and lack of benefit.[121] No specific markers have been identified that define responders, although a one study suggested that adult patients with AD that responds to treatment have wild-type *FLG* mutations. In addition, patients receiving omalizumab have been shown to have decreased levels of TSLP, OX40L, TARC, and IL-9 and marked increase in IL-10 compared with placebo. A systematic review and meta-analysis of omalizumab in AD found that fewer than 50% of the patients treated with this biologic achieved a significant clinical improvement.[180] In the two randomized controlled trials in that review, patients failed to show any significant clinical improvement with omalizumab or their clinical response was comparable to that of the control group. However, the authors noted that 43% of patients treated with omalizumab had a good response, suggesting that a subset of patients with AD, possibly those with an urticarial component to their disease might still benefit from this therapy. Furthermore, a recent randomized clinical trial in children with severe AD found that omalizumab significantly reduced disease severity and topical steroid use.[181]

Probiotics

Lactobacilli and bifidobacteria are gut microorganisms hypothesized to educate the neonatal immune system by converting the Th2-biased prenatal responses into balanced immune responses.

Clinical trials of probiotics in patients with AD have shown clinical benefit, but also lack of benefit. Probiotic supplementation during the prenatal and the postnatal period in some studies has been reported to reduce the incidence of AD in infants and children. However, the most recent Cochrane review found no benefit for probiotics as a treatment for eczema.[182]

Other experimental and unproven therapies for AD include intravenous immune globulin, recombinant human IFN-γ, systemic antifungals, traditional Chinese herbal therapy, essential fatty acids, and leukotriene receptor antagonists.

Emerging Therapies and Investigational Agents

A number of biologics are currently in trials for moderate-to-severe AD (reviewed in Ref. 24). These include anti–IL-13 (lebrikizumab, tralokinumab), anti–IL-31-receptor A (nemolizumab), anti-TSLP (tezepelumab), anti–IL-22 (fezakinumab), and anti-OX40 (GBR 830). In addition, several Janus kinase inhibitors in both topical (ruxolitinib, delgocitinib) and oral (abrocitinib, baricitinib, upadacitinib) formulations are being

studied in AD.[183] New insights into AD phenotypes and endotypes will likely lead to improved selection of appropriate patients for more targeted therapies.

CONCLUSIONS REGARDING AD

Although the diagnosis of AD continues to be based on the recognition of characteristic signs and symptoms, significant advances have been made in understanding the role of epidermal barrier defects and immune abnormalities in this increasingly prevalent disease. These studies have identified new mutations of key stratum corneum proteins and a deficiency in antimicrobial peptide synthesis by keratinocytes contributing to skin colonization and infection in AD. Other studies have revealed a multifunctional role for IgE in atopic skin inflammation. Furthermore, Th2-type cells with skin-homing capability, Th22 cells, LCs, other dendritic cells, keratinocytes, mast cells, and eosinophils all contribute to the complex inflammatory process in AD. These observations have provided the rationale for development of immunomodulatory and antiinflammatory agents in the treatment of chronic AD. Identification of a specific biochemical or genetic marker could not only improve diagnostic capabilities but also lead to more specific strategies for studying the epidemiology and genetics of AD. Undoubtedly, the new insights into pathogenesis of AD will lead to more specific therapeutic agents and, perhaps eventually, to prevention of this disease.

ALLERGIC CONTACT DERMATITIS

Summary of Important Concepts in Allergic Contact Dermatitis

- Allergic contact dermatitis (ACD) is a common skin disorder caused by contact with an exogenous agent and affects millions of Americans.
- ACD can present as an acute, subacute, or chronic dermatitis.
- Allergens causing ACD are found in daily products, at home, work, and even in foods.
- Diagnosis of ACD is based upon a thorough history, physical exam, and by the use of patch testing.
- Once the allergen is identified, the mainstay of treatment is avoidance.

INTRODUCTION

Contact dermatitis (CD) is a common skin condition caused by contact with an exogenous agent that elicits an inflammatory response. Allergens are found in a wide variety of daily products, occupational exposures, and even foods. CD can be further divided into ACD and irritant contact dermatitis (ICD), with the latter being more common (~80% of CD). ACD can result in considerable morbidity and is the chief complaint of thousands of internist visits a year. Diagnosis is based upon a thorough history, physical exam, and by the use of patch testing. The location of the dermatitis can be very helpful in making the diagnosis but patch testing is the only practical, scientific, and objective method to confirm diagnosis of ACD.

EPIDEMIOLOGY

ACD is common, with some studies demonstrating prevalence rates as high as 20% of the general population.[184] In the US, it is estimated that CD affects approximately 4.17% of the population with the estimated cost associated with this condition as over $1.5 billion in 2013.[185]

Women appear to be at higher risk of developing ACD likely due to exposures; for example, women have higher rates of nickel allergy potentially due to the increased frequency of wearing jewelry. Certain groups are at higher risk of developing ACD, with both genetics and environmental exposures likely playing a role. Individuals sensitized to one allergen are more susceptible to sensitization with another.[186] Patients with a history of AD have higher susceptibility in developing ICD and ACD, likely related to disruptions in the skin barrier and a greater inflammatory response.

CD, both allergic and irritant, is a common cause of occupational skin disorder in the western world.[187] Hairdressers, health care workers, food handlers, building and construction workers, and metal workers have high rates of developing ACD resulting in decreased productivity, increased expenses, prolonged absences from work, alteration of practices at work, or even change to another line of work.

PATHOGENESIS AND ETIOLOGY

ACD is a delayed-type, T cell–mediated response with an afferent limb or sensitization phase and an efferent or elicitation phase. The first phase (sensitization) occurs when a person is first exposed to a low-molecular-weight antigen, that when bound to a larger carrier can elicit an immune response. Initially, LCs or dermal dendritic cells engulf the hapten. The hapten-peptide complexes are brought to the regional lymph nodes of the skin, where they prime hapten-specific T cells (Th1, Th2, Th17, and Treg cells) that proliferate and circulate in the blood. The naïve T cells that specifically recognize allergen-MHC molecule complexes expand and create effector and memory T cells. During the elicitation phase, reexposure to the allergen results in recognition by the now-sensitized, hapten-specific T cells and an inflammatory cascade of cytokines and cellular infiltrates occur producing the clinical picture of ACD.[188]

ICD is caused by the direct toxic effect of an irritant on epidermal keratinocytes, resulting in skin barrier disruption and triggering the innate immune system. An irritant can be directly toxic to epidermal keratinocytes or cause disruption of the epithelial barrier by loss of lipids, thereby increasing permeability of irritants and even allergens.[189] Chronic epithelial injury from repetitive exposure to the irritant triggers the innate immune response with release of several proinflammatory cytokines, including IL-1α, IL-1β, tumor necrosis factor-α (TNF-α), GM-CSF, IL-6, and IL-8 from the keratinocytes.[190] These cytokines activate LCs, dermal dendritic cells, and endothelial cells. Release of chemokines results in the recruitment of neutrophils, lymphocytes, macrophages, and mast cells to the epidermis causing further inflammation (Fig. 11.6).

CLINICAL FEATURES

ACD may present as acute, subacute, or chronic dermatitis. Erythematous papules and vesicles most often characterize acute ACD (Fig. 11.7). Recurrence and persistence of the dermatitis may lead to subacute and chronic lesions. Chronic ACD tends to present as erythematous and pruritic lesions with lichenification, scaling, and fissuring (Fig. 11.8). Subacute ACD is more difficult to characterize, and can display a mixture of features.

Distribution of the dermatitis can serve as an important clue to the source of the offending chemical. The most common areas involved are the hands, scattered generalized, face, and eyelids (Table 11.3).[191] However, multiple factors contribute to the distribution of ACD. Spread from the principal site of exposure to a distant site by inadvertent contact can occur. Areas of the scalp, palms, and soles have thicker skin, whereas the eyelid, face, and genital areas have thinner skin that is more sensitive to contact allergens. Certain distributions, such as on the eyelid, lateral face, central face, neck, or hands, should trigger the consideration of ACD to cosmetics and personal products.

Hands

The hands are the most common primary body site involved in CD.[191] The most common cause of hand dermatitis is ICD and commonly presents as a localized dermatitis without vesicles in the webs of fingers, extending onto the dorsal and ventral surfaces, dorsum of hands, palms, and ball of thumb (Fig. 11.9). In contrast, ACD of the hand usually presents as well-demarcated plaques and vesicles involving the dorsum of the hands, fingers, and wrists and less commonly involves the palms. ICD often precedes ACD, which will cause a progression of the distribution of rash.[192]

Common allergens causing ACD of the hands include preservatives, fragrances, metals, rubber, and topical antibiotics.[193]

Other causes of hand dermatitis are AD (more common in adults), dyshidrotic hand eczema, psoriasis, or as a manifestation of systemic contact dermatitis (SCD).

Dermatitis With Scattered Generalized Distribution

Dermatitis with scattered generalized distribution lacks the characteristic distribution that gives a clue as to the possible etiology of ACD. In such patients, one should consider ACD with diffuse contact such as to textile, SCD, drug-elicited systemic allergic dermatitis and AD. The two most common causes of ACD to textile are textile dyes and formaldehyde resin.

SCD, specifically the "baboon syndrome," is a diffuse eruption involving flexural and intertriginous areas following oral, intravenous, or transcutaneous exposure to the allergen in a contact-sensitized individual. Aside from the baboon syndrome, SCD could also manifest as a recall reaction (reactivation of a previous site of dermatitis or a previous positive patch tests), dyshidrotic hand eczema, flexural dermatitis, exanthematous rash, erythroderma, and even vasculitis-like lesions. Patients with CD to nickel may develop SCD with ingestion of food high in nickel. The most common causes of SCD are (i) metals, such as mercury, nickel, and gold; (ii) medications, including aminoglycoside antibacterial, TCS, and aminophylline; and (iii) plants and herbal products, including Compositae

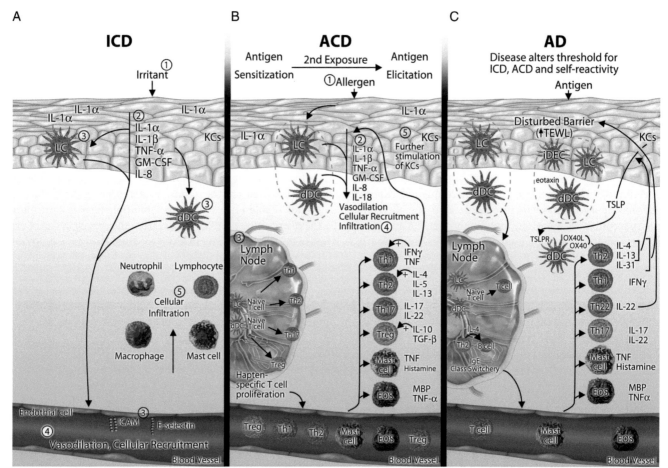

Fig. 11.6 Immune mechanism in the pathogenesis of irritant contact dermatitis *(ICD)*, allergic contact dermatitis *(ACD)*, and atopic dermatitis *(AD)*. Immune mechanism in the pathogenesis of ICD, ACD, and AD. (A) In patients with ICD, exposure to an irritant exerts toxic effects on keratinocytes, activating innate immunity with release of IL-1α, IL-1β, TNF-α, GM-CSF, and IL-8 from epidermal keratinocytes. In turn, these cytokines activate LCs, dDCs, and endothelial cells, all of which contribute to cellular recruitment to the site of keratinocyte damage. Infiltrating cells include neutrophils, lymphocytes, macrophages, and mast cells, which further promote an inflammatory cascade. (B) In the sensitization phase of ACD, similar to ICD, allergens activate innate immunity through keratinocyte release of IL-1α, IL-1β, TNF-α, GM-CSF, IL-8, and IL-18, inducing vasodilation, cellular recruitment, and infiltration. LCs and dDCs encounter the allergen and migrate to the draining LNs, where they activate hapten-specific T cells, which include Th1, Th2, Th17, and regulatory T (Treg) cells. These T cells proliferate and enter the circulation and site of initial exposure, along with mast cells and eosinophils. On reencountering the allergen, the elicitation phase occurs, in which the hapten-specific T cells, along with other inflammatory cells, enter the site of exposure and, through release of cytokines and consequent stimulation of keratinocytes, induce an inflammatory cascade. (C) In patients with AD, a disturbed epidermal barrier leads to increased permeation of antigens, which encounter LCs, inflammatory dendritic epidermal cells (IDECs), and dDCs, activating Th2 T cells to produce IL-4 and IL-13. DCs then travel to LNs, where they activate effector T cells and induce IgE class-switching. IL-4 and IL-13 stimulate keratinocytes to produce TSLP. TSLP activates OX40 ligand–expressing dDCs to induce inflammatory Th2 T cells. Cytokines and chemokines, such as IL-4, IL-5, IL-13, eotaxins, CCL17, CCL18, and CCL22, produced by Th2 T cells and DCs stimulate skin infiltration by DCs, mast cells, and eosinophils. Th2 and Th22 T cells predominate in patients with AD, but Th1 and Th17 T cells also contribute to its pathogenesis. The Th2 and Th22 cytokines (IL-4/IL-13 and IL-22, respectively) were shown to inhibit terminal differentiation and contribute to the barrier defect in patients with AD. Thus, both the barrier defects and immune activation alter the threshold for ICD, ACD, and self-reactivity in patients with AD. *dDC,* Dermal dendritic cells; *EOS,* eosinophil; *KCs,* keratinocytes; *LCs,* Langerhans cells; *LNs,* lymph nodes; *MBP,* major basic protein; *TSLP,* thymic stromal lymphopoietin. (From Gittler JK, Krueger JG, Guttman-Yassky E. Atopic dermatitis results in intrinsic barrier and immune abnormalities: implications for contact dermatitis. J Allergy Clin Immunol 2013;131:300–313, Fig. 2.)

and Anacardiaceae families and Balsam of Peru (also known as *Myroxylon pereirae* resin).

Face

The following are general patterns of facial contact dermatitis:[194]
1. Dermatitis involving the central face (cheeks, nose, chin, and forehead) may be due to ACD to make-up, moisturizers,

wrinkle creams, topical medications, and gold (released from gold jewelry and contaminating titanium-containing foundation).
2. Dermatitis involving the lateral face (preauricular areas, postauricular area, jaw lines, and/or lateral neck) is most commonly due to shampoo and/or conditioner dripping down over these areas (Fig. 11.10).

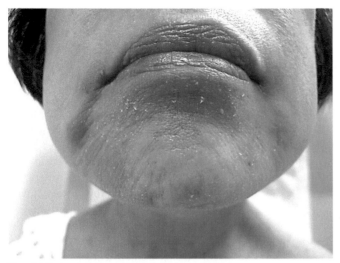

Fig. 11.7 Acute allergic contact dermatitis.

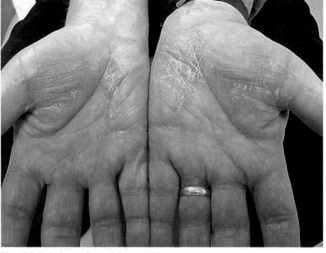

Fig. 11.9 Irritant hand dermatitis.

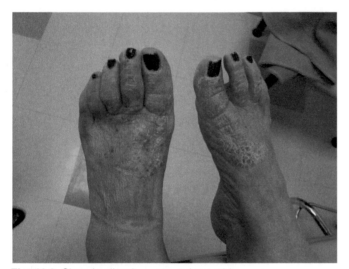

Fig. 11.8 Chronic allergic contact dermatitis.

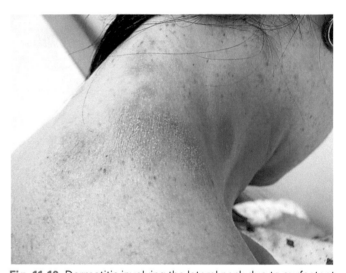

Fig. 11.10 Dermatitis involving the lateral neck due to surfactant from shampoo.

TABLE 11.3 Top Body Sites of Dermatitis Based on the North American Contact Dermatitis Group (NACDG) Patch Test Results[191]		
Dermatitis Site	**n**	**%**
Hand	962	20.2
Scattered/generalized	808	16.6
Face	755	15.5
Eyelids	514	10.5
Trunk	319	6.6
Arm	251	5.2
Leg	224	4.6
Scalp	210	4.3
Lips	187	3.9
Anal/genital	147	3.0
Foot	126	2.6
Total n = 4854		

3. Full facial dermatitis may be due to make-up foundation, facial cleansers, moisturizers, and airborne contactants.
4. Unilateral facial dermatitis may be due to an ectopic transfer from the hands of contact allergens in nail products, fragrances, and topical medication. Connubial or consort CD to products used by the partner or parent may also be transferred predominantly to one side of the face.

Eyelids

The skin of the eyelids is most sensitive and is susceptible to irritants and allergens. ACD of the lids and periorbital area is primarily caused by cosmetics applied to the hair, face, or fingernails. Shellac and pigments in mascara can cause ACD of the eyelids. Allergy to hair dye may manifest as marked edema of the eyelids. Hair products such as dyes, bleaching agents, setting lotions, sprays, gels, and mousses are more likely to involve the scalp or forehead in addition to the eyelid. Ectopic dermatitis from nail polish and acrylic nail dermatitis more commonly affects some combination of the eyelids, face, and neck rather than an isolated eyelid dermatitis. Airborne pollen, dust, and all types of volatile agents may affect the eyelids and manifest as a Type 4 cell–mediated hypersensitivity reaction.

Eyelid dermatitis may also be due to seborrheic dermatitis, AD, or ICD. Common allergens associated with eyelid dermatitis include fragrances, formaldehyde-related preservatives, cocamidopropyl betaine (CAPB) (surfactant in shampoos and soaps), methylisothiazolinone, (preservative in both industrial and consumer products), and gold.[195]

PATIENT EVALUATION, DIAGNOSIS, AND DIFFERENTIAL DIAGNOSIS

Patch testing is the only practical, scientific, and objective method to confirm diagnosis of ACD. Patch tests (PTs) are prepared by placing allergens into individual chambers and are applied on the back for 48 hours. An initial reading is done in 48 hours and a second reading should be done at 72 to 96 hours after placement. Once there is a positive PT result, the allergist or dermatologist should determine the clinical relevance. The clinical relevance depends on the correlation between the patient's history in conjunction with the PT results.

The most frequently positive allergic reactions in the most recent North American Contact Dermatitis Group (NACDG) Series report[191] included two metals, nickel sulfate (17.5%) and cobalt (6.2%); two antibiotics, neomycin (7.0%) and bacitracin (6.9%); three fragrances (fragrance mix I [11.3%], fragrance mix II [5.3%], and *M. pereirae* [7.0%]); and four preservatives (methylisothiazolinone [MI] [13.4%], methylchloroisothiazolinone/methylisothiazolinone [MCI/MI] [7.3%], formaldehyde [1% {6.4%} and 2% {8.4%}], and iodopropynyl butylcarbamate [3.9%]), propylene glycol (4.0%), p-phenylenediamine (PPD) (6.4%), lanolin alcohol (4.1%), and carba mix (4.6%). Table 11.4 lists common selected allergens and their sources of exposure.[196]

TABLE 11.4 Selected Allergens and Common Sources of Exposure	
Allergen	**Common Sources of Exposure**
Fragrances	
Balsam of Peru	Cosmetics, fragrances, dental hygiene products, topical medications, food
Fragrance mix I and II	Fragrances, scented household products
Formaldehyde and Formaldehyde-Releasing Preservatives (FRP)	
Formaldehyde	Fabric finishes, cosmetics
Quaternium-15	Preservative in cosmetics and skin care products
Diazolidinyl urea	Products for personal care, hygiene and hair care, cosmetics, pet shampoos
Imidazolidinyl urea	Products for personal care, hygiene and hair care, cosmetics, liquid soaps, moisturizers
2-Bromo-2-nitropropane-1,3-diol	Topical antibiotic/antifungal creams/ointments, finger paints, kitty litter, detergents, toiletries and cleansers, cleansing lotions, mouthwash, shampoos
1,2-dimethylol-5,6-dimethyl hydantoin (DMDM hydantoin)	Wipes, personal care/hygiene products, cosmetics, baby care products, polishes
Non–Formaldehyde-Releasing Preservatives	
Parabens	Preservative in topical formulations, cosmetics, personal care products
Methylchloroisothiazolinone-methylisothiazolinone (MCI-MI)	Baby products, personal care/hygiene products, cosmetics
Methyldibromoglutaronitrile-phenoxyethanol (MDBGN-PE)	Skin care products, sunscreens, baby care, personal hygiene products (moist toilet paper, shampoos, shower gel)
Iodopropynyl butylcarbamate	Baby care, personal care/hygiene products, cosmetics, hair dye, industry, lip products, paints, yard care
Surfactants	
Cocamidopropyl betaine (CAPB)	Hair and bath products, medicated ointments and creams, cosmetics, oral care
Oleamidopropyl dimethylamine	Cosmetics, conditioners, baby lotions, body lotions, deodorants
Decyl glucoside	Cosmetics, baby shampoo, body washes
Dimethylaminopropylamine (DMAPA)	Personal care/hygiene products, medicated ointments and creams, cosmetics, hair detanglers
Amidoamine	Personal care/hygiene products, medicated ointments and creams, cosmetics, hair detanglers
Acrylates	
2-hydroxyethyl methacrylate (HEMA)	Possible exposure to acrylic compounds include nail polish, artificial finger nails, hair spray, paints, plastics, adhesives
Ethyl acrylate	Crosslink agent in rubber

(Continued)

TABLE 11.4 Selected Allergens and Common Sources of Exposure—cont'd

Allergen	Common Sources of Exposure
Methyl methacrylate	Resin used in dentistry, bone cement, adhesive artificial nails
Metals	
Nickel	Buckles, snaps, jewelry, food
Cobalt	Metal plated utensils, keys, fasteners, paints, cobalt-based pigments, Vit. B12 supplements
Gold sodium thiosulfate	Gold or gold plated jewelry, dental restorations
Chemical Additives Integral to Rubber Manufacturing	
Carba mix	Rubber products, shampoo, disinfectants
Mercaptobenzothiazole	Rubber products, nitrile, neoprene, sports equipment
Thiuram	Rubber products, adhesives
Other Allergens	
Propolis	Homeopathic remedies, food supplements, cosmetics, gum, medicated ointments/creams
Benzophenone-4	Chemical sunblock
Ammonium persulfate	Hair color allergen added to hydrogen peroxide
p-Phenylenediamine (PPD)	Permanent or semipermanent hair dyes, cosmetics, printing ink, black henna tattoo
Propylene glycol	Vehicle in topical medications, personal care/hygiene products, auto care, cosmetics, foods, household cleaners, oral care, industry, sunscreens, wipes, yard care
Lanolin (wool alcohols)	Cosmetics, skin care products, personal hygiene items, facial masks, sunscreens, OTC and prescription medications, pet grooming aids

Open techniques can be used to test products that may cause irritation to the skin and can be helpful when suspected allergens are personal care products and cosmetics.[197] A "repeat open application test" (ROAT) involves placing the suspected allergen on the patient's antecubital fossa twice a day for 7 to 14 days and observing for the development of dermatitis. If positive, the patient is advised to avoid using the product. This test can be helpful in distinguishing an allergic from irritant response, as open testing is less likely to cause irritation than an occlusive PT.

TREATMENT

Identification and avoidance of the offending allergen are the most important aspects of ACD treatment. Since many agents are found in everyday products, avoidance can be difficult, even if the allergen has been identified. It is difficult to read through ingredient lists of products, especially as many of the common contact allergens bear long, similar-looking chemical names and many allergens cross-react with other allergens.[198] Thus, patients must be provided not only with a list of allergens they have to avoid but also a list of "safe products" that do not contain the allergens to which they are sensitized.[199]

If allergen/s cannot be avoided or patient continues to have chronic ACD, TCS can be used intermittently. Systemic corticosteroids should be avoided if possible, as the course of dermatitis may be very long and its use can result in rebound flares. Barrier creams and emollients can be helpful in reducing exposure, skin dryness, and subsequent pruritus of the affected areas.

Emollients should be fragrance-free to avoid risk of further sensitization. Calcineurin inhibitors (tacrolimus, pimecrolimus) have not been approved for use in ACD, but are a reasonable alternative in chronic cases and those that involve delicate areas (face, eyelid etc.). Phototherapy can be considered in the treatment of refractory cases.

If treatment with TCS does not improve or worsens the dermatitis, one should suspect ACD to the TCS, which has been described to affect 0.5% to 5.8% of patients.[200] If suspected, the patient should undergo patch testing to the suspected medication and ingredients that are known to be contact sensitizers.[201]

Antihistamines have not been shown to be helpful in treating the intense pruritus associated with ACD. Avoidance of wet work, excessive hand washing, hot water, soap, and sweating is advised. Personal protective equipment is particularly important in cases of occupation-related ACD.[202]

REFERRAL

Patch testing should be considered in patients with a localized or diffuse chronic, pruritic, eczematous, vesicular, or lichenified dermatitis in whom ACD is suspected. ACD can worsen the clinical course of AD patients, likely due to the impaired skin barrier increasing exposure and enhanced absorption of topically applied substances in personal products, ointments, and creams used for treating chronic AD. Therefore, patch testing is indicated to rule out concomitant ACD in any patient with AD that does not improve with the usual treatment, initially improves and then exacerbates, worsens with topical therapy, or has a change in their typical dermatitis pattern.

Although patch testing, especially the easy-to-use TRUE Test, is deceptively easy to apply, the interpretation of the PT results and the education and follow-up of patients with ACD is best done by providers with expertise on CD. Thus, a referral to an allergist or dermatologist with this expertise is indicated if ACD is suspected.

CONCLUSIONS REGARDING ACD

ACD is a common skin disorder seen in clinical practice. Diagnosis is based upon a thorough history, physical exam, and by the use of patch testing. Patch testing should be considered in patients with a localized or diffuse chronic, pruritic, eczematous, vesicular, or lichenified dermatitis in whom ACD is suspected and a referral to an allergist or dermatologist with the expertise to perform patch testing is indicated in such cases. Identification and avoidance of the offending allergen are the most important aspects of ACD treatment.

WHAT'S NEW IN ACD

- New work on allergic sensitization to common allergens (e.g., nickel, fragrance) has shown that different allergens have distinct molecular fingerprinting. For example, nickel shows strong Th17/Th1 polarization, while fragrance allergy involves Th2/Th22-skewing. These new data may influence therapeutic decisions for ACD patients based on the unique allergen polarity.
- ACD in the setting of concurrent AD shows a different and attenuated phenotype as compared to healthy individuals with ACD.[203]
- A large number of new, rare, and emerging allergens should be considered in the assessment of suspected ACD. Patch testing to these allergens has yet to be standardized; irritant and elicitation concentrations to patch testing need to be determined.
- Data about contact allergen sensitization in children with AD are limited but are continually expanding. Frequency and patterns of CD in children with AD and the results of patch testing have yet to be determined.
- Dupilumab, a human monoclonal antibody that inhibits the IL-4 receptor alpha subunit (IL-4Rα) and targets Th2 inflammation by inhibiting the signaling of IL-4 and IL-13, is approved for treatment of moderate-to-severe AD. Recent case reports and series show a variable modifying effect of dupilumab on PT results, with some patients showing loss of prior contact sensitization while on dupilumab.[204] These inconsistencies suggest that different contact allergens may elicit responses via diverse immune pathways.

REFERENCES

1. Davidson WF, Leung DYM, Beck LA, et al. Report from the National Institute of Allergy and Infectious Diseases workshop on "Atopic dermatitis and the atopic march: Mechanisms and interventions. J Allergy Clin Immunol. 2019;143:894–913.
2. Hill LW, Sulzberger MB. Evolution of atopic dermatitis. Arch Dermatol Syph. 1935;32:451–463.
3. Wallach D, Coste J, Tilles G, et al. The first images of atopic dermatitis: an attempt at retrospective diagnosis in dermatology. J Am Acad Dermatol. 2005;53:684–689.
4. Kapoor R, Menon C, Hoffstad O, et al. The prevalence of atopic triad in children with physician-confirmed atopic dermatitis. J Am Acad Dermatol. 2008;58:68–73.
5. Elias PM, Wakefield JS. Mechanisms of abnormal lamellar body secretion and the dysfunctional skin barrier in patients with atopic dermatitis. J Allergy Clin Immunol. 2014;134:781–791.
6. Schultz LF. Atopic dermatitis: a genetic-epidemiologic study in a population-based twin sample. J Am Acad Dermatol. 1993;28:719–723.
7. Schultz LF, Diepgen T, Svensson Å. The occurrence of atopic dermatitis in north Europe: an international questionnaire study. J Am Acad Dermatol. 1996;34:760–764.
8. Shaw TE, Currie GP, Koudelka CW, et al. Eczema prevalence in the United States: data from the 2003 National Survey of Children's Health. J Invest Dermatol. 2011;131:67–73.
9. Chiesa Fuxench ZC, Block JK, Boguniewicz M, et al. Atopic Dermatitis in America Study: a cross-sectional study examining the prevalence and disease burden of atopic dermatitis in the US adult population. J Invest Dermatol. 2019;139:583–590.
10. Sugiura H, Umemoto N, Deguchi H, et al. Prevalence of childhood and adolescent atopic dermatitis in a Japanese population: comparison with the disease frequency examined 20 years ago. Acta Derm Venereol. 1998;78:293–294.
11. Saeki H, Iizuka H, Mori Y, et al. Prevalence of atopic dermatitis in Japanese elementary schoolchildren. Br J Dermatol. 2005;152:110–114.
12. Williams HC. Is the prevalence of atopic dermatitis increasing? Clin Exp Dermatol. 1992;17:385–391.
13. Zeiger R, Heller S, Mellon M, et al. Genetic and environmental factors affecting the development of atopy through age 4 in children of atopic parents: a prospective randomized study of food allergen avoidance. Pediatr Allergy Immunol. 1992;3: 110–127.
14. Zeiger RS, Heller S. The development and prediction of atopy in high-risk children: follow-up at age seven years in a prospective randomized study of combined maternal and infant food allergen avoidance. J Allergy Clin Immunol. 1995;95:1179–1190.
15. Kay J, Gawkrodger DJ, Mortimer MJ, et al. The prevalence of childhood atopic eczema in a general population. J Am Acad Dermatol. 1994;30:35–39.
16. Williams HC, Strachan DP, Hay RJ. Childhood eczema: disease of the advantaged? Br Med J. 1994;308:1132–1135.
17. Hayashi T, Kawakami N, Kondo N, et al. Prevalence of and risk factors for allergic diseases: comparison of two cities in Japan. Ann Allergy Asthma Immunol. 1995;75:525–529.
18. International Study of Asthma and Allergies in Childhood (ISAAC) Steering Committee Worldwide variation in prevalence of symptoms of asthma, allergic rhinoconjunctivitis, and atopic eczema: ISAAC. Lancet. 1998;351:1225–1232.
19. Odhiambo JA, Williams HC, Clayton TO, et al. Global variations in prevalence of eczema symptoms in children from ISAAC Phase Three. J Allergy Clin Immunol. 2009;124:1251–1258.
20. Barnes KC. An update on the genetics of atopic dermatitis: scratching the surface in 2009. J Allergy Clin Immunol. 2010;125:16–29.
21. The EArly Genetics and Lifecourse Epidemiology (EAGLE) Eczema Consortium Multi-ancestry genome-wide association study of 21,000 cases and 95,000 controls identifies new risk loci for atopic dermatitis. Nat Genet. 2015;47(12):1449–1456.

22. Baurecht H, Hotze M, Brand S, et al. Genome-wide comparative analysis of atopic dermatitis and psoriasis gives insight into opposing genetic mechanisms. Am J Hum Genet. 2015;96(1):104–120.
23. Hirota T, Takahashi A, Kubo M, et al. Genome-wide association study identifies eight new susceptibility loci for atopic dermatitis in the Japanese population. Nat Genet. 2012;44(11):1222–1226.
24. Stevens ML, Zhang Z, Johansson E, et al. Disease-associated KIF3A variants alter gene methylation and expression impacting skin barrier and atopic dermatitis risk. Nat Commun. 2020;11:4092.
25. Irvine AD, McLean WH, Leung DY. Filaggrin mutations associated with skin and allergic diseases. N Engl J Med. 2011;365:1315–1327.
26. Brown SJ, Sandilands A, Zhao Y, et al. Prevalent and low-frequency null mutations in the filaggrin gene are associated with early-onset and persistent atopic eczema. J Invest Dermatol. 2008;128:1591–1594.
27. Henderson J, Northstone K, Lee SP, et al. The burden of disease associated with filaggrin mutations: a population-based, longitudinal birth cohort study. J Allergy Clin Immunol. 2008;121:872–877.
28. Bergmann RL, Edenharter G, Bergmann KE, et al. Atopic dermatitis in early infancy predicts allergic airway disease at 5 years. Clin Exp Allergy. 1998;28:965–970.
29. Vickers CF. The natural history of atopic eczema. Acta Derm Venerol. 1980;92:113–115.
30. Linna O, Kokkonen J, Lahtela P, et al. Ten-year prognosis for generalized infantile eczema. Acta Paediatr. 1992;81:1013–1016.
31. Kissling S, Wuthrich B. Sites, types of manifestations and micromanifestations of atopic dermatitis in young adults: a personal follow-up 20 years after diagnosis in childhood. Hautarzt. 1994;45:368–371.
32. Lammintausta K, Kalimo K, Raitala R, et al. Prognosis of atopic dermatitis: a prospective study in early adulthood. Int J Dermatol. 1991;30:563–568.
33. Gustafsson D, Sjoberg O, Foucard T, et al. Development of allergies and asthma in infants and young children with atopic dermatitis: a prospective follow-up to 7 years of age. Allergy. 2000;55:240–245.
34. Illi S, von Mutius E, Lau S, et al. The natural course of atopic dermatitis from birth to age 7 years and the association with asthma. J Allergy Clin Immunol. 2004;113:925–931.
35. Howell MD, Kim BE, Gao P, et al. Cytokine modulation of atopic dermatitis filaggrin skin expression. J Allergy Clin Immunol. 2007;120:150–155.
36. Nograles KE, Zaba LC, Shemer A, et al. IL-22-producing "T22" T cells account for upregulated IL-22 in atopic dermatitis despite reduced IL-17–producing TH17 T cells. J Allergy Clin Immunol. 2009;123:1244–1252.
37. Bisgaard H, Simpson A, Palmer CN, et al. Gene-environment interaction in the onset of eczema in infancy: filaggrin loss-of-function mutations enhanced by neonatal cat exposure. PLoS Med. 2008;5:e131.
38. Rodriguez E, Baurecht H, Herberich E, et al. Meta-analysis of filaggrin polymorphisms in eczema and asthma: robust risk factors for atopic disease. J Allergy Clin Immunol. 2009;123 1361–70, e7.
39. Van den Oord RA, Sheikh A. Filaggrin gene defects and risk of developing allergic sensitization and allergic disorders: systematic review and meta-analysis. BMJ. 2009;339:b2433.
40. De Benedetto A, Rafaels NM, McGirt LY, et al. Tight junction defects in patients with atopic dermatitis. J Allergy Clin Immunol. 2011;127:773–786, e1–7.
41. Broccardo CJ, Mahaffey S, Schwarz J, et al. Comparative proteomic profiling of patients with atopic dermatitis based on history of eczema herpeticum infection and Staphylococcus aureus colonization. J Allergy Clin Immunol. 2011;127:186–193, e1–11.
42. Hanifin JM, Rajka G. Diagnostic features of atopic dermatitis. Acta Derm Venereol (Stockh). 1980;92:44–47.
43. European Task Force on Atopic Dermatitis Severity scoring of atopic dermatitis: the SCORAD index. Dermatology. 1993;186:23–31.
44. Hanifin JM, Thurston M, Omoto M, et al. The eczema area and severity index (EASI): assessment of reliability in atopic dermatitis. EASI Evaluator Group. Exp Dermatol. 2001;10:11–18.
45. Brydensholt HL, Loland L, Buchvald FF, et al. Development of atopic dermatitis during the first 3 years of life. Arch Dermatol. 2006;142:561–566.
46. Bielory B, Bielory L. Atopic dermatitis and keratoconjunctivitis. Immunol Allergy Clin North Am. 2010;30:323–336.
47. Boguniewicz M, Leung DY. Recent insights into atopic dermatitis and implications for management of infectious complications. J Allergy Clin Immunol. 2010;125:4–13.
48. Howell MD, Wollenberg A, Gallo RL, et al. Cathelicidin deficiency predisposes to eczema herpeticum. J Allergy Clin Immunol. 2006;117:836–841.
49. Beck LA, Boguniewicz M, Hata T, et al. Phenotype of atopic dermatitis subjects with a history of eczema herpeticum. J Allergy Clin Immunol. 2009;124:260–269.
50. Leung DY, Gao PS, Grigoryev DN, et al. Human atopic dermatitis complicated by eczema herpeticum is associated with abnormalities in gamma interferon response. J Allergy Clin Immunol. 2011;127:965–973.
51. Gao PS, Leung DY, Rafaels NM, et al. Genetic variants in interferon regulatory factor 2 (IRF2) are associated with atopic dermatitis and eczema herpeticum. J Invest Dermatol. 2012;132:650–657.
52. Casagrande BF, Fluckiger S, Linder MT, et al. Sensitization to the yeast Malassezia sympodialis is specific for extrinsic and intrinsic atopic eczema. J Invest Dermatol. 2006;126:2414–2421.
53. Cho SH, Strickland I, Boguniewicz M, et al. Fibronectin and fibrinogen contributes to the enhanced binding of S. aureus to atopic skin. J Allergy Clin Immunol. 2001;108:269–274.
54. Leyden JE, Marples RR, Kligman AM. Staphylococcus aureus in the lesions of atopic dermatitis. Br J Dermatol. 1974;90:525–530.
55. Williams J, Vowels B, Honig P, et al. S. aureus isolation from the lesions, the hands, and the anterior nares of patients with atopic dermatitis. Pediatr Dermatol. 1998;15:194–198.
56. Leyden J, Kligman A. The case for steroid-antibiotic combinations. Br J Dermatol. 1977;96:179–187.
57. Schlievert PM, Strandberg KL, Lin YC, et al. Secreted virulence factor comparison between methicillin-resistant and methicillin-sensitive Staphylococcus aureus, and its relevance to atopic dermatitis. J Allergy Clin Immunol. 2010;125:39–49.
58. Torgerson TR, Ochs HD. Immune dysregulation, polyendocrinopathy, enteropathy, X-linked: Forkhead box protein 3 mutations and lack of regulatory T cells. J Allergy Clin Immunol. 2007;120:744–750.
59. Holland SM, DeLeo FR, Elloumi HZ, et al. STAT3 mutations in the hyper-IgE syndrome. N Engl J Med. 2007;357:1608–1619.
60. Zhang Q, Davis JC, Lamborn IT, et al. Combined immunodeficiency associated with DOCK8 mutations. N Engl J Med. 2009;361:2046–2055.

61. Kelsay K, Klinnert M, Bender B. Addressing psychosocial aspects of atopic dermatitis. Immunol Allergy Clin North Am. 2010;30:385–396.

62. Caubet JC, Eigenmann PA. Allergic triggers in atopic dermatitis. Immunol Allergy Clin North Am. 2010;30:289–307.

63. May CE. Objective clinical laboratory studies of immediate hypersensitivity reactions to foods in asthmatic children. J Allergy Clin Immunol. 1976;58:500–515.

64. Sampson HA, McCaskill CC. Food hypersensitivity and atopic dermatitis: evaluation of 113 patients. J Pediatr. 1985;107:669–675.

65. Sicherer SH, Sampson HA. Food hypersensitivity and atopic dermatitis: pathophysiology, epidemiology, diagnosis, and management. J Allergy Clin Immunol. 1999;104:S114–S122.

66. Van Reijsen FC, Felius A, Wauters EA, et al. T-cell reactivity for a peanut-derived epitope in the skin of a young infant with atopic dermatitis. J Allergy Clin Immunol. 1998;101:207–209.

67. Schade RP, Van Ieperen-van Dijk AG, Van Reijsen FC, et al. Differences in antigen-specific T-cell responses between infants with atopic dermatitis with and without cow's milk allergy: relevance of TH2 cytokines. J Allergy Clin Immunol. 2000;106:1155–1162.

68. Sampson HA, Broadbent K, Bernhisel-Broadbent J. Spontaneous basophil histamine release and histamine-releasing factor in patients with atopic dermatitis and food hypersensitivity. N Engl J Med. 1989;321:228–232.

69. Van der Heijden F, Wierenga EA, Bos JD, et al. High frequency of IL-4 producing CD4+ allergen-specific T lymphocytes in atopic dermatitis lesional skin. J Invest Dermatol. 1991;97:389–394.

70. Tuft L. Importance of inhalant allergens in atopic dermatitis. J Invest Dermatol. 1949;12:211–219.

71. Tupker RA, De Monchy JG, Coenraade PJ, et al. Induction of atopic dermatitis by inhalation of house-dust mite. J Allergy Clin Immunol. 1996;97:1064–1070.

72. Clark RA, Adinoff AD. The relationship between positive aeroallergen patch test reactions and aeroallergen exacerbations of atopic dermatitis. Clin Immunol Immunopathol. 1989;53:S132–S140.

73. Langeveld-Wildschut EG, Bruijnzeel PL, Mudde GC, et al. Clinical and immunologic variables in skin of patients with atopic eczema and either positive or negative atopy patch test reactions. J Allergy Clin Immunol. 2000;105:1008–1016.

74. Schafer T, Heinrich J, Wjst M, et al. Association between severity of atopic eczema and degree of sensitization to aeroallergens in schoolchildren. J Allergy Clin Immunol. 1999;104:1280–1284.

75. Tan BB, Weald D, Strickland I, et al. Double-blind controlled trial of effect of housedust-mite allergen avoidance on atopic dermatitis. Lancet. 1996;347:15–18.

76. Holm L, Ohman S, Bengtsson A, et al. Effectiveness of occlusive bedding in the treatment of atopic dermatitis: a placebo-controlled trial of 12 months' duration. Allergy. 2001;56:152–158.

77. Leung DY, Harbeck R, Bina P, et al. Presence of IgE antibodies to staphylococcal exotoxins on the skin of patients with atopic dermatitis: evidence for a new group of allergens. J Clin Invest. 1993;92:1374–1380.

78. Bunikowski R, Mielke M, Skarabis H, et al. Prevalence and role of serum IgE antibodies to the Staphylococcus aureus-derived superantigens SEA and SEB in children with atopic dermatitis. J Allergy Clin Immunol. 1999;103:119–124.

79. Nomura I, Tanaka K, Tomita H, et al. Evaluation of the staphylococcal exotoxins and their specific IgE in childhood atopic dermatitis. J Allergy Clin Immunol. 1999;104:441–446.

80. Strickland I, Hauk PJ, Trumble AE, et al. Evidence for superantigen involvement in skin homing of T cells in atopic dermatitis. J Invest Dermatol. 1999;112:249–253.

81. Bunikowski R, Mielke ME, Skarabis H, et al. Evidence for a disease-promoting effect of Staphylococcus aureus-derived exotoxins in atopic dermatitis. J Allergy Clin Immunol. 2000;105:814–819.

82. Herz U, Schnoy N, Borelli S, et al. A human-SCID mouse model for allergic immune response bacterial superantigen enhances skin inflammation and suppresses IgE production. J Invest Dermatol. 1998;110:224–231.

83. Hofer MF, Harbeck RJ, Schlievert PM, et al. Staphylococcal toxins augment specific IgE responses by atopic patients exposed to allergen. J Invest Dermatol. 1999;112:171–176.

84. Cardona ID, Goleva E, Ou L-S, et al. Staphylococcal enterotoxin B inhibits regulatory T cells by inducing glucocorticoid induced TNF receptor-related protein ligand on monocytes. J Allergy Clin Immunol. 2006;117:688–695.

85. Hauk PJ, Hamid QA, Chrousos GP, et al. Induction of corticosteroid insensitivity in human PBMCs by microbial superantigens. J Allergy Clin Immunol. 2000;105:782–787.

86. Strange P, Skov L, Lisby S, et al. Staphylococcal enterotoxin B applied on intact normal and intact atopic skin induces dermatitis. Arch Dermatol. 1996;132:27–33.

87. Skov L, Olsen JV, Giorno R, et al. Application of staphylococcal enterotoxin B on normal and atopic skin induces upregulation of T cells via a superantigen-mediated mechanism. J Allergy Clin Immunol. 2000;105:820–826.

88. Valenta R, Seiberler S, Natter S, et al. Autoallergy: a pathogenetic factor in atopic dermatitis? J Allergy Clin Immunol. 2000;105:432–437.

89. Valenta R, Natter S, Seiberler S, et al. Molecular characterization of an autoallergen, Hom s 1, identified by serum IgE from atopic dermatitis patients. J Invest Dermatol. 1998;111:1178–1183.

90. Schmid-Grendelmeier P, Fluckiger S, Disch R, et al. IgE-mediated and T cell-mediated autoimmunity against manganese superoxide dismutase in atopic dermatitis. J Allergy Clin Immunol. 2005;115:1068–1075.

91. Leung DYM, Boguniewicz M, Howell M, et al. New insights into atopic dermatitis. J Clin Invest. 2004;113:651–657.

92. Akdis CA, Akdis M, Simon D, et al. T cells and T cell-derived cytokines as pathogenic factors in the non-allergic form of atopic dermatitis. J Invest Dermatol. 1999;113:628–634.

93. Kimura M, Tsuruta S, Yoshida T. Unique profile of IL-4 and IFN-γ production by peripheral blood mononuclear cells in infants with atopic dermatitis. J Allergy Clin Immunol. 1998;102:238–244.

94. Kimura M, Tsuruta S, Yoshida T. Correlation of house dust mite-specific lymphocyte proliferation with IL-5 production, eosinophilia, and the severity of symptoms in infants with atopic dermatitis. J Allergy Clin Immunol. 1998;101:84–89.

95. Van Reijsen FC, Bruijnzeel-Koomen CA, Kalthoff FS, et al. Skin-derived aeroallergen-specific T-cell clones of Th2 phenotype in patients with atopic dermatitis. J Allergy Clin Immunol. 1992;90:184–193.

96. Teraki Y, Hotta T, Shiohara T. Increased circulating skin-homing cutaneous lymphocyte-associated antigen (CLA)+ type 2 cytokine-producing cells, and decreased CLA+ type 1 cytokine-producing cells in atopic dermatitis. Br J Dermatol. 2000;143:373–378.

97. Vercelli J, Jabara HH, Lauener RP, et al. IL-4 inhibits the synthesis of IFN-γ and induces the synthesis of IgE in human mixed lymphocyte cultures. J Immunol. 1990;144:570–573.

98. Beck LA, Thaci D, Hamilton JD, et al. Dupilumab treatment in adults with moderate-to-severe atopic dermatitis. New Engl J Med. 2014;371:130–139.

99. Boguniewicz M, Leung DY. Atopic dermatitis: a disease of altered skin barrier and immune dysregulation. Immunol Rev. 2011;242:233–246.

100. Vu AT, Baba T, Chen X, et al. *Staphylococcus aureus* membrane and diacylated lipopeptide induce thymic stromal lymphopoietin in keratinocytes through the Toll- like receptor 2-Toll-like receptor 6 pathway. J Allergy Clin Immunol. 2010;126:985–93, e1–3.

101. Ong PY, Ohtake T, Brandt C, et al. Endogenous antimicrobial peptides and skin infections in atopic dermatitis. N Engl J Med. 2002;347:1151–1160.

102. Schauber J, Gallo RL. Antimicrobial peptides and the skin immune defense system. J Allergy Clin Immunol. 2008;122:261–266.

103. Hata TR, Kotol P, Jackson M, et al. Administration of oral vitamin D induces cathelicidin production in atopic individuals. J Allergy Clin Immunol. 2008;122:829–831.

104. Camargo Jr. CA, Ganmaa D, Sidbury R, et al. Randomized trial of vitamin D supplementation for winter-related atopic dermatitis in children. J Allergy Clin Immunol. 2014;134:831–835.

105. Hamid Q, Boguniewicz M, Leung DY. Differential in situ cytokine gene expression in acute versus chronic atopic dermatitis. J Clin Invest. 1994;94:870–876.

106. Hamid Q, Naseer T, Minshall EM, et al. In vivo expression of IL-12 and IL-13 in atopic dermatitis. J Allergy Clin Immunol. 1996;98:225–231.

107. Thepen T, Langeveld-Wildschut EG, Bihari IC, et al. Biphasic response against aeroallergen in atopic dermatitis showing a switch from an initial TH2 response to a TH1 response in situ: an immunocytochemical study. J Allergy Clin Immunol. 1996;97:828–837.

108. Steinhoff M, Bienenstock J, Schmelz M, et al. Neurophysiological, neuroimmunological, and neuroendocrine basis of pruritus. J Invest Dermatol. 2006;126:1705–1718.

109. Bilsborough J, Leung DY, Maurer M, et al. IL-31 is associated with cutaneous lymphocyte antigen-positive skin homing T cells in patients with atopic dermatitis. J Allergy Clin Immunol. 2006;117:418–425.

110. Neis MM, Peters B, Dreuw A, et al. Enhanced expression levels of IL-31 correlate with IL-4 and IL-13 in atopic and allergic contact dermatitis. J Allergy Clin Immunol. 2006;118:930–937.

111. Sonkoly E, Muller A, Lauerma AI, et al. IL-31: a new link between T cells and pruritus in atopic skin inflammation. J Allergy Clin Immunol. 2006;117:411–417.

112. Kabashima K, Matsumura T, Komazaki H, et al. Trial of nemolizumab and topical agents for atopic dermatitis with pruritus. N Engl J Med. 2020;383:141–150.

113. Ziegler SF, Artis D. Sensing the outside world: TSLP regulates barrier immunity. Nat Immunol. 2010;11:289–293.

114. Gao PS, Rafaels NM, Mu D, et al. Genetic variants in thymic stromal lymphopoietin are associated with atopic dermatitis and eczema herpeticum. J Allergy Clin Immunol. 2010;125 1403–7, e4.

115. Muller KM, Jaunin F, Masouye I, et al. Th2 cells mediate IL-4-dependent local tissue inflammation. J Immunol. 1993;150:5576–5584.

116. Mudde GC, van Reijsen FC, Boland GJ, et al. Allergen presentation by epidermal Langerhans cells from patients with atopic dermatitis is mediated by IgE. Immunology. 1990;69:335–341.

117. Jürgens M, Wollenberg A, Hanau D, et al. Activation of human epidermal Langerhans cells by engagement of the high affinity receptor for IgE, FcεRI. J Immunol. 1995;155:5184–5189.

118. Abernathy-Carver KJ, Sampson HA, Picker LJ, et al. Milk-induced eczema is associated with the expansion of T cells expressing cutaneous lymphocyte antigen. J Clin Invest. 1995;95:913–918.

119. Santamaria Babi LF, Picker LJ, Soler MT, et al. Circulating allergen-reactive T cells from patients with atopic dermatitis and allergic contact dermatitis express the skin-selective receptor, the cutaneous lymphocyte-associated antigen. J Exp Med. 1995;181:1935–1940.

120. Schneider L, Tilles S, Lio P, et al. Atopic dermatitis: a practice parameter update 2012. J Allergy Clin Immunol. 2013;131: 295–9, e1–27.

121. Boguniewicz M, Fonacier L, Guttman-Yassky E, et al. Atopic dermatitis yardstick: practical recommendations for an evolving therapeutic landscape. Ann Allergy Asthma Immunol. 2018;120 10–22, e2.

122. Brar K, Nicol NH, Boguniewicz M. Strategies for successful management of severe atopic dermatitis. J Allergy Clin Immunol Pract. 2019;7:1–16.

123. Robison RG, Singh AM. Controversies in allergy: food testing and dietary avoidance in atopic dermatitis. J Allergy Clin Immunol Pract. 2019;7:35–39.

124. Nicol NH, Ersser SJ. The role of the nurse educator in managing atopic dermatitis. Immunol Allergy Clin North Am. 2010;30:369–383.

125. Zuberbier T, Orlow SJ, Paller AS, et al. Patient perspectives on the management of atopic dermatitis. J Allergy Clin Immunol. 2006;118:226–232.

126. Imokawa G, Abe A, Jin K, et al. Decreased level of ceramides in stratum corneum of atopic dermatitis: an etiologic factor in atopic dry skin? J Invest Dermatol. 1991;96:523–526.

127. Cardona ID, Kempe EE, Lary C, et al. Frequent versus infrequent bathing in pediatric atopic dermatitis: a randomized clinical trial. J Allergy Clin Immunol Pract. 2020;8:1014–1021.

128. Chopra R, Vakharia PP, Sacotte R, et al. Efficacy of bleach baths in reducing severity of atopic dermatitis: a systematic review and meta-analysis. Ann Allergy Asthma Immunol. 2017;119:435–440.

129. Lucky AW, Leach AD, Laskarzewski P, et al. Use of an emollient as a steroid- sparing agent in the treatment of mild to moderate atopic dermatitis in children. Pediatr Dermatol. 1997;14: 321–324.

130. Vilaplana J, Coll J, Trullas C, et al. Clinical and non-invasive evaluation of 12% ammonium lactate emulsion for the treatment of dry skin in atopic and non-atopic subjects. Acta Derm Venereol. 1992;72:28–33.

131. Lavker RM, Kaidbey K, Leyden J. Effects of topical ammonium lactate on cutaneous atrophy from a potent topical corticosteroid. J Am Acad Dermatol. 1992;26:535–544.

132. Hara J, Higuchi K, Okamoto R, et al. High expression of sphingomyelin deacylase is an important determinant of ceramide deficiency leading to barrier disruption in atopic dermatitis. J Invest Dermatol. 2000;115:406–413.

133. Chamlin SL, Kao J, Frieden IJ, et al. Ceramide-dominant barrier repair lipids alleviate childhood atopic dermatitis: changes in barrier function provide a sensitive indicator of disease activity. J Am Acad Dermatol. 2002;47:198–208.

134. Boguniewicz M, Zeichner JA, Eichenfield LF, et al. MAS063DP is effective monotherapy for mild to moderate atopic dermatitis in infants and children: a multicenter, randomized, vehicle-controlled study. J Pediatr. 2008;152:854–859.

135. Hajar T, Leshem YA, Hanifin JM, et al. A systematic review of topical corticosteroid withdrawal ("steroid addiction") in

patients with atopic dermatitis and other dermatoses. J Am Acad Dermatol. 2015;72:541–9, e2.

136. Matura M, Goossens A. Contact allergy to corticosteroids. Allergy. 2000;55:698–704.

137. Long CC, Mills CM, Finlay AY. A practical guide to topical therapy in children. Br J Dermatol. 1998;138:293–296.

138. Wolkerstorfer A, Strobos MA, Glazenburg EJ, et al. Fluticasone propionate 0.05% cream once daily versus clobetasone butyrate 0.05% cream twice daily in children with atopic dermatitis. J Am Acad Dermatol. 1998;39:226–231.

139. Lebwohl M. A comparison of once-daily application of mometasone furoate 0.1% cream compared with twice-daily hydrocortisone valerate 0.2% cream in pediatric atopic dermatitis patients who failed to respond to hydrocortisone. Mometasone Furoate Study Group. Int J Dermatol. 1999;38:604–606.

140. Suarez-Farinas M, Tintle SJ, Shemer A, et al. Nonlesional atopic dermatitis skin is characterized by broad terminal differentiation defects and variable immune abnormalities. J Allergy Clin Immunol. 2011;127 954–64, e1–4.

141. Schmitt J, von Kobyletzki L, Svensson A, et al. Efficacy and tolerability of proactive treatment with topical corticosteroids and calcineurin inhibitors for atopic eczema: systematic review and meta-analysis of randomized controlled trials. Br J Dermatol. 2011;164:415–428.

142. Stalder JF, Fleury M, Sourisse M. Local steroid therapy and bacterial skin flora in atopic dermatitis. Br J Dermatol. 1994;131:536–540.

143. Nimmagadda SR, Szefler SJ, Spahn JD, et al. Allergen exposure decreases glucocorticoid receptor binding affinity and steroid responsiveness in atopic asthmatics. Am J Respir Crit Care Med. 1997;155:87–93.

144. Herrscher RF, Kasper C, Sullivan TJ. Endogenous cortisol regulates immunoglobulin E-dependent late phase reaction. J Clin Invest. 1992;90:596–603.

145. Blotta MH, DeKruyff RH, Umetsu DT. Corticosteroids inhibit IL-12 production in human monocytes and enhance their capacity to induce IL-4 synthesis in CD4+ lymphocytes. J Immunol. 1997;158:5589–5595.

146. Charman CR, Morris AD, Williams HC. Topical corticosteroid phobia in patients with atopic eczema. Br J Dermatol. 2000;142:931–936.

147. Hanifin JM, Paller AS, Eichenfield L, et al. Efficacy and safety of tacrolimus ointment treatment for up to 4 years in patients with atopic dermatitis. J Am Acad Dermatol. 2005;53:S186–S194.

148. Papp KA, Werfel T, Folster-Holst R, et al. Long-term control of atopic dermatitis with pimecrolimus cream 1% in infants and young children: a two-year study. J Am Acad Dermatol. 2005;52:240–246.

149. Leung DY, Hanifin JM, Pariser DM, et al. Effects of pimecrolimus cream 1% in the treatment of patients with atopic dermatitis who demonstrate a clinical insensitivity to topical corticosteroids: a randomized, multicentre vehicle-controlled trial. Br J Dermatol. 2009;161:435–443.

150. Paul C, Cork M, Rossi AB, et al. Safety and tolerability of 1% pimecrolimus cream among infants: experience with 1133 patients treated for up to 2 years. Pediatrics. 2006; 117:e118.

151. Fonacier L, Spergel J, Charlesworth EN, et al. Report of the Topical Calcineurin Task Force of the American College of Allergy, Asthma and Immunology and the American Academy of Allergy, Asthma and Immunology. J Allergy Clin Immunol. 2005;115:1249–1253.

152. Arellano FM, Wentworth CE, Arana A, et al. Risk of lymphoma following exposure to calcineurin inhibitors and topical steroids in patients with atopic dermatitis. J Invest Dermatol. 2007;127:808–816.

153. Ho VC, Gupta A, Kaufmann R, et al. Safety and efficacy of nonsteroid pimecrolimus cream 1% in the treatment of atopic dermatitis in infants. J Pediatr. 2003;142:155–162.

154. Kapp A, Papp K, Bingham A, et al. Long-term management of atopic dermatitis in infants with topical pimecrolimus, a nonsteroid anti-inflammatory drug. J Allergy Clin Immunol. 2002;110:277–284.

155. Wahn U, Bos JD, Goodfield M, et al. Efficacy and safety of pimecrolimus cream in the long-term management of atopic dermatitis in children. Pediatrics. 2002;110:e2.

156. Guttman-Yassky E, Hanifin JM, Boguniewicz M, et al. The role of phosphodiesterase 4 in the pathophysiology of atopic dermatitis and the perspective for its inhibition. Exp Dermatol. 2019;28: 3–10.

157. Paller AS, Tom WL, Lebwohl MG, et al. Efficacy and safety of crisaborole ointment, a novel, nonsteroidal phosphodiesterase 4 (PDE4) inhibitor for the topical treatment of atopic dermatitis (AD) in children and adults. J Am Acad Dermatol. 2016;75: 494–503, e6.

158. Schlessinger J, Shepard JS, Gower R, et al. Safety, effectiveness, and pharmacokinetics of crisaborole in infants aged 3 to <24 months with mild-to-moderate atopic dermatitis: a phase IV open-label study (CrisADe CARE 1). Am J Clin Dermatol. 2020;21:275–284.

159. Langeveld-Wildschut EG, Riedl H, Thepen T, et al. Modulation of the atopy patch test reaction by topical corticosteroids and tar. J Allergy Clin Immunol. 2000;106:737–743.

160. Boguniewicz M, Sampson H, Harbeck R, et al. Effects of cefuroxime axetil on S. aureus colonization and superantigen production in atopic dermatitis. J Allergy Clin Immunol. 2001;108:651–652.

161. Rukwied R, Lischetzki G, McGlone F, et al. Mast cell mediators other than histamine induce pruritus in atopic dermatitis patients: a dermal microdialysis study. Br J Dermatol. 2000;142:1114–1120.

162. Metze D, Reimann S, Beissert S, et al. Efficacy and safety of naltrexone, an oral opiate receptor antagonist, in the treatment of pruritus in internal and dermatological diseases. J Am Acad Dermatol. 1999;41:533–539.

163. Berth-Jones J, Graham-Brown RA, Marks R, et al. Long-term efficacy and safety of cyclosporin in severe adult atopic dermatitis. Br J Dermatol. 1997;136:76–81.

164. Diepgen TL. Long-term treatment with cetirizine of infants with atopic dermatitis: a multi-country, double-blind, randomized, placebo-controlled trial (the ETAC trial) over 18 months. Early Treatment of the Atopic Child Study Group. Pediatr Allergy Immunol. 2002;13:278–286.

165. Drake LA, Fallon JD, Sober A, et al. Relief of pruritus in patients with atopic dermatitis after treatment with topical doxepin cream. J Am Acad Dermatol. 1994;31:613–616.

166. Shelley WB, Shelley ED, Talanin NY. Self-potentiating allergic contact dermatitis caused by doxepin hydrochloride cream. J Am Acad Dermatol. 1996;34:143–144.

167. Boguniewicz M. Biologic therapy for atopic dermatitis: moving beyond the practice parameter and guidelines. J Allergy Clin Immunol Pract. 2017;5:1477–1487.

168. Simpson EL, Paller AS, Siegfried EC, et al. Efficacy and safety of Dupilumab in adolescents with uncontrolled moderate to severe

atopic dermatitis: a phase 3 randomized clinical trial. JAMA Dermatol. 2019;156:44–56.

169. Paller A, Siegfried EC, Thaci D, et al. Efficacy and safety of dupilumab with concomitant topical corticosteroids in children 6 to 11 years old with severe atopic dermatitis: a randomized, double-blinded, placebo-controlled phase 3 trial. J Am Acad Dermatol. 2020;83:1282–1293.

170. Lee JH, Lee SJ, Kim D, et al. The effect of wet dressing on epidermal barrier in patients with atopic dermatitis. J Eur Acad Dermatol Venereol. 2007;21:1360–1368.

171. Wolkerstorfer A, Visser RL, de Waard-van der Spek FB, et al. Efficacy and safety of wet-wrap dressings in children with severe atopic dermatitis: influence of corticosteroid dilution. Br J Dermatol. 2000;143:999–1004.

172. Sidbury R, Davis DM, Cohen DE, et al. Guidelines of care for the management of atopic dermatitis: section 3. Management and treatment with phototherapy and systemic agents. J Am Acad Dermatol. 2014;71:327–349.

173. Glover MT, Atherton DJ. A double-blind controlled trial of hyposensitization to Dermatophagoides pteronyssinus in children with atopic eczema. Clin Exp Allergy. 1992;22:440–446.

174. Bussmann C, Bockenhoff A, Henke H, et al. Does allergen-specific immunotherapy represent a therapeutic option for patients with atopic dermatitis? J Allergy Clin Immunol. 2006;118:1292–1298.

175. Werfel T, Breuer K, Rueff F, et al. Usefulness of specific immunotherapy in patients with atopic dermatitis and allergic sensitization to house dust mites: a multi-centre, randomized, dose-response study. Allergy. 2006;61:202–205.

176. Bussmann C, Maintz L, Hart J, et al. Clinical improvement and immunological changes in atopic dermatitis patients undergoing subcutaneous immunotherapy with a house dust mite allergoid: a pilot study. Clin Exp Allergy. 2007;37:1277–1285.

177. Pajno GB, Caminiti L, Vita D, et al. Sublingual immunotherapy in mite-sensitized children with atopic dermatitis: a randomized, double-blind, placebo-controlled study. J Allergy Clin Immunol. 2007;120:164–170.

178. Cox L, Nelson H, Lockey R, et al. Allergen immunotherapy: a practice parameter, third update. J Allergy Clin Immunol. 2011;127 S1–55.

179. Tam H, Calderon MA, Manikam L, et al. Specific allergen immunotherapy for the treatment of atopic eczema. Cochrane Database Syst Rev. 2016;2:CD008774.

180. Wang HH, Li YC, Huang YC. Efficacy of omalizumab in patients with atopic dermatitis: a systematic review and meta-analysis. J Allergy Clin Immunol. 2016;138 1719–22, e1.

181. Chan S, Cornelius V, Cro S, et al. Treatment effect of Omalizumab on severe pediatric atopic dermatitis: the ADAPT randomized clinical trial. JAMA Pediatr. 2019;174:29–37.

182. Makrgeorgou A, Leonardi-Bee J, Bath-Hextall FJ, et al. Probiotics for treating eczema. Cochrane Database Syst Rev. 2018;11:CD006135.

183. Renert-Yuval Y, Guttman-Yassky E. New treatments for atopic dermatitis targeting beyond IL-4/IL-13 cytokines. Ann Allergy Asthma Immunol. 2020;124:28–35.

184. Alinaghi F, Bennike NH, Egeberg A, et al. Prevalence of contact allergy in the general population: a systematic review and meta-analysis. Contact Dermatitis. 2019;80:77–85.

185. Lim HW, Collins SAB, Resneck Jr. JS, et al. The burden of skin disease in the United States. J Am Acad Dermatol. 2017;76: 958–72, e2.

186. Schnuch A, Carlsen BA. Chapter 2: Genetics and individual predispositions in contact dermatitis. In: Johansen JD, Lepoittevin P, eds. Contact dermatitis. 5th ed. Berlin: Springer; 2011:14–28.

187. Zack B, Arrandale VH, Holness DK. Preventing occupational skin disease: a review of training programs. Dermatitis. 2017;28:169–182.

188. Boguniewicz M, Fonacier L, Leung DYM. Chapter 44: Atopic and contact dermatitis. In: Rich RF, Fleisher TA, Shearer WT, Shcroeder HE, Frew AJ, Weyand CM, eds. Clinical immunology: principles and practice. 5th ed. Amsterdam: Elsevier; 2019:620–621.

189. Bains SN, Nash P, Fonacier L. Irritant contact dermatitis. Clin Rev Allergy Immunol. 2019;56:99–109.

190. Nosbaum A, Nicolas JF, Lachapelle JM. Chapter 1: Pathophysiology of allergic and irritant contact dermatitis. In: Lachapelle JM, Maibach HI, eds. Patch testing and prick testing: A practical guide official publication of the ICDRG. 4th ed. Berlin: Springer; 2020:6–10.

191. DeKoven JG, Warshaw EM, Zug KA, et al. North American Contact Dermatitis Group patch test results: 2015–2016. Dermatitis. 2018;29:297–309.

192. Fonacier LS, Dreskin SC, Leung DYM. Allergic skin diseases. J Allergy Clin Immunol. 2010;125:S138–S149.

193. Warshaw EM, Ahmed RL, Belsito DV, et al. Contact dermatitis of the hands: cross-sectional analyses of North American Contact Dermatitis Group Data, 1994–2004. J Am Acad Dermatol. 2007;57:301–314.

194. Zirwas MJ. Contact dermatitis to cosmetics. Clin Rev Allergy Immunol. 2019;56:119–128.

195. Rietschel RL, Warshaw EM, Sasseville D, et al. Common contact allergens associated with eyelid dermatitis: data from the North American Contact Dermatitis Group 2003–2004 study period. Dermatitis. 2007;18:78–81.

196. Nassau S, Fonacier L. Allergic contact dermatitis. Med Clin North Am. 2020;104:61–76.

197. Schmidlin K, Sani S, Bernstein DI, et al. A hands-on approach to contact dermatitis and patch testing. J Allergy Clin Immunol Pract. 2020;8:1883–1893.

198. Zirwas MJ. Chapter 22: Treatment of contact dermatitis. In: Fowler JF, Zirwas MJ, eds. Fisher's Contact Dermatitis. 7th ed. Louisville: Contact Dermatitis Institute; 2019:689–694.

199. Fonacier L. A practical guide to patch testing. J Allergy Clin Immunol Pract. 2015;3:669–675.

200. Zmudzinska M, Czarnecka-Operacz M, Silny W. Contact allergy to glucocorticosteroids in patients with chronic venous leg ulcers, atopic dermatitis and contact allergy. Acta Dermatovenerol Croat. 2008;16:72–78.

201. Fonacier L, Bernstein DI, Pacheco K, et al. Contact dermatitis: a practice parameter-update 2015. J Allergy Clin Immunol Pract. 2015;3 S1–39.

202. NHS Plus, Royal College of Physicians, Faculty of Occupational Medicine Dermatitis: Occupational Aspects Of Management. A National Guideline. London: RCP; 2009.

203. Leonard A, Guttman-Yassky E. The unique molecular signatures of contact dermatitis and implications for treatment. Clin Rev Allergy Immunol. 2019;56:1–8.

204. Puza CJ, Atwater AR. Positive patch test reaction in a patient taking Dupilumab. Dermatitis. 2018;29:89.

12

Food Allergy and Gastrointestinal Syndromes

Anna Nowak-Węgrzyn, A. Wesley Burks, and Hugh A. Sampson

CHAPTER OUTLINE

SUMMARY OF IMPORTANT CONCEPTS

1. Food allergy affects 8% of US children and up to 10% of adults; the incidence of peanut allergy has quadrupled over the past decade in the US.
2. Sensitization to foods may occur in the gastrointestinal (GI) tract, through the inflamed skin in atopic dermatitis, or following sensitization to cross-reacting inhalant allergens (secondary or class 2 food allergy).
3. Food reactions may have immunoglobulin E (IgE)-mediated, non–IgE-mediated, or a combination of IgE- and non–IgE-mediated mechanisms. Foods are the most common triggers of anaphylaxis in children and major triggers in adults.
4. Increasing levels of food-specific serum IgE or skin-prick test wheals correlate with increasing probabilities of clinical reactivity, although the double-blind, placebo-controlled food challenge remains the gold standard for diagnosing food allergy.
5. Appropriate management of food-induced anaphylaxis requires education about recognizing symptoms and treating reactions promptly with epinephrine (adrenaline).

6. Cutaneous exposure to food protein through a disrupted skin barrier leads to allergic sensitization, whereas early ingestion generally induces tolerance. New immunotherapies for food allergy hold great promise for effective desensitization associated with successful immunomodulation.

INTRODUCTION

In the past decades, food allergy has emerged as an important public health problem affecting people of all ages in societies with a Western lifestyle, such as the US, Canada, the UK, Australia, and Western Europe.[1-4] The overall prevalence of food allergy in American children increased by 18% from 1997 to 2007.[5] Peanut allergy quadrupled during a similar period in the US, Canada, the UK, and Australia.[6,7] Food allergy is the most common cause of anaphylaxis in the outpatient setting for all ages, and it can lead to fatalities. The diagnosis of food allergy often requires labor-intensive, medically supervised oral food challenges (OFCs) that carry a risk for anaphylaxis and are not readily available to all patients. There is no cure for food allergy. Current management relies on food avoidance and timely treatment of acute reactions.[8] To facilitate diagnosis and management of food allergy, the first official US guidelines for food allergy were published in 2010, and European guidelines were published in 2014.[9,10] The growing recognition of the burden of food allergies and the challenges in diagnosis and management are driving multifaceted research approaches with the ultimate goal of finding a cure. Box 12.1 gives brief definitions of food allergies, food intolerances, and food aversions.

EPIDEMIOLOGY

Children

Food allergies are most common in the first few years of life. Cow's milk (CM), hen's egg, soybean, wheat, peanut, tree nuts, fish, and shellfish allergies cause more than 90% of food allergy in children.[2] These foods have relatively high protein contents and are introduced at early stages. Local dietary habits often result in the increased presence of various food allergens in the diet. Examples include sesame in Israel, buckwheat in Japan,

---

and mustard and lupine in France. Most allergies to CM, egg, soybean, and wheat are outgrown, whereas most allergies to peanut, nuts, seeds, and seafood persist into adulthood.[11]

Prospective studies from several countries indicate that about 2.5% of newborn infants experience hypersensitivity reactions to CM in the first year of life. Immunoglobulin E (IgE)–mediated reactions account for about 60% of these milk-allergic reactions. Hen's egg allergy is estimated to affect about 1.6% of young children in the US and UK. A rigorous, population-based study found an 8.9% prevalence of egg allergy diagnosed by OFC to raw egg in children younger than 12 months of age in Australia, suggesting that food allergies continue to increase in the youngest age groups.[6]

Most infants with non–IgE-mediated CM allergy outgrow their sensitivity by the third year of life, but about 10% to 25% of infants with IgE-mediated CM and egg allergies retain their sensitivity into the second decade of life, and about 50% develop allergic reactions to other foods.

Large, population-based studies have investigated the prevalence of peanut allergy and determined that peanut allergy affects more than 1% to 4% of children in Canada, the US, Australia, and the UK.[2] Adverse reactions to food additives affect 0.5% to 1% of children, especially those with atopic disorders, who have a higher prevalence of food allergy. About 35% of children with moderate-to-severe atopic dermatitis have IgE-mediated food allergies, many of whom exhibit skin symptoms provoked by ingestion of the food allergen.[12]

About 6% of children with asthma attending a general pulmonary clinic reportedly had food-induced wheezing. Among children with eosinophilic esophagitis (EoE), 50% have food-responsive disease (i.e., symptoms improve or resolve on elimination of the offending food).

Adults

Food allergy in adults was considered less common than in children. However, a large 2019 study ($n = 40,443$ adults, mean [SD] age, 46.6 [20.2] years) found a food allergy prevalence in adults of 10.8% compared to 8% in children in the US.[3] A survey from the UK identified 1.4% to 1.8% of adults reporting adverse food reactions, and a study in the Netherlands concluded that about 2% of the adult Dutch population was affected by adverse food reactions. The estimates of pollen-related food allergy are considerably higher. Among pollen-allergic individuals, 74% report symptoms (most had oral symptoms) to the pollen-associated foods (e.g., fruits, vegetables). Overall, 16.7% of young adults report pollen–food allergy symptoms.

Prevalence of Food Allergy

Studies of the prevalence of food allergy are hampered by the requirement of a physician-supervised OFC for the ultimate confirmation of food allergy. Food challenges are expensive, labor-intensive, and impractical in large-scale, population-based cohorts. For this reason, many studies use surrogate markers, such as evidence of specific IgE to food or self-reported food allergy to estimate prevalence figures. Several studies that applied similar methods over time showed a two- to three-fold increase in peanut allergy and peanut-IgE sensitization in

---

> ## BOX 12.1 Definitions
>
> - Food allergy is defined as an adverse health effect arising from a specific immune response that occurs reproducibly following exposure to a given food. Nonallergic adverse reactions to foods may be the result of food intolerances or adverse physiologic reactions.
> - Food intolerances are thought to comprise most adverse reactions to foods. They can be caused by factors inherent in the food ingested, such as toxic contaminants, toxins, pharmacologic properties of the food (e.g., caffeine in coffee), and host characteristics such as metabolic disorders (e.g., lactase deficiency) and idiosyncratic responses.
> - Food aversions may mimic adverse food reactions, but they typically cannot be reproduced when the patient ingests the food in a blinded fashion. Food allergy must be distinguished from a variety of adverse reactions to foods that do not have an immune basis, but whose clinical manifestations may resemble food allergy. Examples of adverse food reactions are presented in Table 12.1.

children in the US, the UK, Canada, and Australia over the past 10 to 20 years. Many studies reported rates of peanut allergy of 1% to 4% among young children.[2]

Food-induced anaphylaxis also appears to have increased. In the US, data from one geographic region in Minnesota from 1983 to 1987, and 1993 to 1997, show a 71% to 100% increase.[13,14] Studies focusing on pediatric food-related ambulatory and emergency department visits or food-induced anaphylaxis also suggest increases. In the UK, there was almost a doubling of anaphylaxis, from 5.6 to 10.2 cases per 100 000 hospital discharges over the 4 years from 1991 to 1995 ($p < 0.001$).[15]

The proportion of cases attributed to food-induced anaphylaxis also increased over the same period.[16]

The reasons for increased cases of food allergy are unknown. There appears to be a strong genetic contribution to peanut allergy. Monozygotic twins have 64% concordance for peanut allergy; dizygotic twins have 7% concordance. However, the rapid rate of increase suggests that environmental factors play a more important role, likely by affecting the expression of genetic susceptibility. Potential genetic and environmental risk factors contributing to the increase in prevalence of food allergy are discussed in Table 12.1.

TABLE 12.1 Potential Genetic and Risk Factors for Food Allergy Development

Potential Risk Factor for Food Allergy	Mechanism/Comments
Genetic	
Sex	Several studies report that gender could be related to food allergy, particularly peanut and tree nut allergies. Peanut allergy is significantly higher in male children; this ratio reverses during and after adolescence, possibly mediated through endocrine changes.
Ethnicity	The risk of possible and likely food allergy is increased in non-Hispanic Black people compared with White individuals. Black children were more likely to be sensitized to multiple foods than White children. As assessed by genetic ancestry informative markers, African ancestry is a notable risk factor for increased risk of peanut sensitization at levels associated with clinical reactivity.
Genetic polymorphism	Gene polymorphisms in interleukin-10 (IL-10) and interleukin-10 (IL-13) have been identified in association with food allergy, but these studies will need to be replicated in different populations. Variations in the two important single nucleotide polymorphisms (SNPs) of CD14 (rs2569190 and rs2569193) were associated with the presence of peanut allergy. More recent studies point to important gene–environment interactions in the development of food sensitization. In a prospective birth cohort study of 970 children, children who were ever breastfed (including exclusively breastfed children) were at 1.5 times higher risk of food sensitization than never-breastfed children. However, the association was altered by rs425648 in the IL-12 receptor β_1 gene (IL-12 rβ_1). Breastfeeding increased the risk of food sensitization in children carrying the GG genotype but significantly decreased the risk of food sensitization in breastfed infants carrying the GT/TT genotype. Similar interactions were observed for SNPs in the TSLP gene and the Toll-like receptor gene (TLR9).
Atopic dermatitis and filaggrin loss-of-function mutations	There is greater frequency of sensitization and allergy to foods with increasing severity of atopic dermatitis (AD); relative risk (RR) of 5.9 for IgE-mediated food allergy in an infant with severe eczema. The loss-of-function mutations within the filaggrin (*FLG*) gene are associated with development of AD. *FLG* was also studied as a candidate gene in the etiology of peanut allergy. The association of *FLG* mutation with peanut allergy is highly significant ($p = 0.0008$) even after controlling for coexistent AD. This indicates a role for epithelial barrier dysfunction in the pathogenesis of peanut allergy. It is possible that recent increases in food allergy might be related to the even more dramatic increases in the prevalence of AD worldwide, currently estimated to affect 20% of children and 10% adults in high-income countries.
Environmental	
Lack of microbial exposure	The *hygiene hypothesis* suggests that the lack of early life exposures to infectious agents (e.g., bacteria, parasites) may lead to a faulty programming of tolerogenic mechanisms, increasing the host's susceptibility to allergic diseases. Limited data for the hygiene hypothesis exist with respect to food allergy.
C-section	A metaanalysis of six studies showed a mild effect of cesarean delivery increasing the risk of food allergy (odds ratio [OR] = 1.32; 95% confidence interval [CI], 1.12–0.55). The proallergy skewing effect of cesarean section may be explained by the abnormal bacterial colonization of a newborn's gut in the absence of exposure to the protective bacterial flora in the birth canal. Alternatively, cesarean section is associated with higher maternal age, a higher number of first-born infants, and a higher number of male births, which all have been identified as independent risk factors for atopy.
Season of birth/vitamin D	Epidemiologic findings, such as the observations that season of birth is a risk factor, that food-induced pediatric anaphylaxis is more common in northern areas of the US (i.e., less sunlight exposure than in the southern states), and that maternal intake of vitamin D during pregnancy was associated with a decreased risk of food sensitization, support the hypothesis that relative deficiency of vitamin D may predispose offspring to development of atopy and food allergy. However, two independent studies showed that infants who received vitamin D supplementation were at increased risk of food allergy.
Obesity	The coinciding trend in increasing atopy with increasing childhood obesity has been well studied, especially in the context of asthma. Obesity induces an inflammatory state associated with an increased risk of atopy and could theoretically lead to an increased risk for food allergy. Atopy (defined by any positive specific IgE measurement) is increased in obese compared with normal-weight children. This association is driven primarily by allergic sensitization to foods (OR for food sensitization = 1.59; 95% CI, 1.28–1.98). Elevated C-reactive protein levels as a measure of inflammation were associated with total IgE levels, atopy, and food sensitization.

(Continued)

TABLE 12.1	Potential Genetic and Risk Factors for Food Allergy Development—cont'd
Potential Risk Factor for Food Allergy	Mechanism/Comments
n-3-Polyunsuturated fatty acids (n-3- PUFA)	The typical Western diet is characterized by the reduced consumption of n-3 PUFAs (found in oily fish) and increased consumption of proinflammatory omega-6 polyunsaturated fatty acids (found in margarine and vegetable oils) led to the increased production of prostaglandin E_2 (PGE_2). This presumably results in reduced production of interferon-γ (IFN-γ) by T cells and increased production of IgE by B cells, amplifying the risk of atopy and asthma.
Timing of food allergen introduction into the diet	Timing of exposure to food allergens may be critical for the development of oral tolerance. A review of 13 studies (only one was controlled) found a consistent association between the persistence of eczema and the introduction of solid foods before 4 months of age but not with an increased risk of asthma, food allergy, allergic rhinitis, or animal allergies. Several reports suggested that early introduction of peanut, cow's milk, egg, and wheat into the infant diet was associated with decreased risk of allergy to these foods. Countries in Asia, Africa, and the Middle East have low rates of peanut allergy, and peanut consumption is unrestricted during pregnancy and early childhood. A questionnaire-based study found that the prevalence of peanut allergy in the UK was 1.85% and the prevalence in Israel was 0.17% ($p < 0.001$). The adjusted risk ratio for peanut allergy between countries was 9.8 (95% CI, 3.1–30.5) in primary English school children. The only difference identified between the two populations was the timing of introduction of peanuts, which in Israel occurs during early weaning. Randomized clinical trials are underway to determine whether early introduction of peanuts and other solid foods protects against food allergy.

Natural History of Food Allergy

The prevalence of food hypersensitivity is greatest in the first few years of life. Most young children outgrow their food hypersensitivity (i.e., become tolerant) within a few years, except in most cases of peanut, tree nut, and seafood allergy.[11]

Most children outgrow CM allergy, and those with a milder phenotype of CM allergy become tolerant by school age. In a prospective, population-based study, most CM-allergic children lost their CM allergy by 3 years of age: 50% by 1 year, 70% by 2 years, and 85% by 3 years. All children with negative skin-prick test (SPT) results to CM at 1 year of age lost their sensitivity by their third birthday, whereas 25% of those with positive skin test results remained CM-allergic at 3 years of age. In contrast, among children with a more severe phenotype (i.e., multiple food allergies, asthma, and allergic rhinitis), 21% remained allergic to CM by 16 years of age. The highest serum concentration of CM-specific IgE for each patient (defined as the peak CM-IgE level) was highly predictive of outcome ($p < 0.001$), with few children whose peak CM-specific IgE concentration exceeded $50\,kU_A/L$ outgrowing milk allergy by their teenage years. Clinically, reactivity to baked milk is a useful marker of a more severe CM allergy. Children who were initially reactive to baked milk were 28 times less likely to become tolerant to unheated milk compared with children tolerant to baked milk over a median of 37 months (range, 8–75 months; $p < 0.001$).

Similar to milk allergy, 66% of egg-allergic children become egg tolerant by 5 years of age. However, among those with a more severe phenotype, 32% continued to avoid egg at the age of 16 years. A patient's highest recorded egg IgE level, presence of other atopic disease, and presence of other food allergies were significantly related to the persistence of egg allergy. In contrast to milk allergy, children reactive to baked egg have an excellent chance of outgrowing their egg allergy.

Approximately 20% of children with peanut allergy and 9% of children with tree nut allergy become tolerant to these foods with age. Unlike milk and egg allergies, peanut allergy occasionally recurs in children who appear to have outgrown their reactivity.

Risk of recurrence appears to be approximately 10% among children who refuse to eat peanuts on a regular basis, compared with rare recurrences in children eating peanuts regularly. The possibility of peanut allergy recurrence should be discussed before undertaking the OFC to peanut and before indicating that patients should ingest peanut frequently after a negative OFC result. Epinephrine should be carried for several months after a negative result until the patient has proven tolerance to multiple ingestions of regular servings of peanuts and peanut-containing foods. It appears that the natural history of allergy to seeds, fish, and shellfish is similar to that of tree nuts. Among 133 children with soy allergy evaluated in a food allergy referral center and followed for a median time of 5 years (range, 1–19 years), rates of resolution were 25% by 4 years, 45% by 6 years, and 69% by 10 years of age.

In a population of 103 children with IgE-mediated wheat allergy in a food allergy referral center, rates of resolution were 29% by 4 years, 56% by 8 years, and 65% by 12 years of age. Higher wheat-IgE levels were associated with poorer outcomes. The peak wheat IgE level recorded was a useful predictor of persistent allergy ($p < 0.001$), although many children, even those with the highest levels of wheat IgE, outgrew wheat allergy.[11]

Food Allergy in Adults

Although younger children are more likely to outgrow their food allergies, older children and adults also may lose their reactivity if the responsible food allergen is identified and eliminated from the diet. Approximately one-third of children and adults lose their clinical reactivity after 1 to 2 years of allergen avoidance. Skin-puncture test results typically remain positive and do not predict which patients will lose their clinical reactivity. Monitoring food allergen–specific IgE levels may be useful in predicting when patients outgrow their allergy. A significant drop in the specific IgE level to CM and egg by 50% over 1 to 2 years has been identified as a favorable prognostic factor in children.[17] The severity of the initial reaction does not appear to correlate with the ultimate likelihood of losing clinical reactivity, but the degree of compliance with the allergen avoidance diet and the food responsible for the reaction do affect the outcome.

Most non–IgE-mediated gastrointestinal (GI) food allergies occur in infants and are outgrown in the first 2 to 3 years of life. However, allergic EoE is frequently seen in adults, and the number of young children and adolescents affected appears to be increasing. Long-term studies have not been completed, and the prognosis of these disorders is unknown. Although most cases of dietary protein–induced enteropathy are outgrown, celiac disease is a lifelong sensitivity, and gluten-containing grains must be avoided for life. No formal studies on the natural history of non–IgE-mediated cutaneous or respiratory disorders have been undertaken, but these sensitivities are thought to be long-lasting.

Food Allergy as a Marker of Atopic Predisposition

In many children, food allergy coexists with other atopic conditions, such as atopic dermatitis, asthma, and allergic rhinitis. Sensitization to egg white in children with atopic dermatitis and a family history of atopy is associated with a 70% risk for respiratory allergic disease (i.e., asthma or allergic rhinitis) at 5 years of age. Individuals with past and current food allergy should be considered at high risk for asthma and environmental allergy.

Pathogenesis and Etiology

The GI tract processes ingested food into a form that can be absorbed and used for energy and cell growth. This requires the intestinal immune system to discriminate between harmful and harmless foreign proteins.[18] As shown in Table 12.2, a variety

TABLE 12.2 Gastrointestinal Barriers to Ingested Food Antigens

Barriers	Food Allergy Predisposition in Newborns and Infants
Immunologic Barriers	
Block penetration of ingested antigens	Newborn lacks IgA and IgM in exocrine secretions. Salivary sIgA is absent at birth, and levels remain low during early months of life
Antigen-specific sIgA in gut lumen	
Clear antigens penetrating GI barrier	Immaturity of the humoral immune system, low levels of circulating antibodies
Serum antigen-specific IgA and IgG Reticuloendothelial system	
Physiologic Barriers	
Breakdown of ingested antigens	Low basal acid output during first month of life
Gastric acid and pepsins Pancreatic enzymes Intestinal enzymes Intestinal epithelial cell lysozyme activity	Immaturity of the intestinal proteolytic activity until about 2 years of age
Block penetration of ingested antigens	Intestinal microvillus membranes are immature in infants, resulting in altered antigen binding and transport through mucosal epithelial cells
Intestinal mucous coat (i.e., glycocalyx) Intestinal microvillus membrane composition Intestinal peristalsis	

GI, Gastrointestinal; *IgM,* immunoglobulin M; *sIgA,* secretory immunoglobulin A.

of immunologic and nonimmunologic factors may destroy or block antigens from entering the body. However, developmental immaturity of these mechanisms in infants reduces the efficiency of their mucosal barriers and likely plays a major role in the increased prevalence of GI infections and food allergy seen in the first few years of life.

Normal Immune Response to the Ingested Food Antigens

Low concentrations of serum immunoglobulin G (IgG), immunoglobulin M (IgM), and immunoglobulin A (IgA) food-specific antibodies are commonly found in normal individuals. The younger an infant when a food antigen is introduced into the diet, the more pronounced the antibody response is likely to be. After introduction of CM, serum levels of CM protein-specific IgG antibodies rise over the first month, achieving peak antibody levels after several months, and then decline, even though CM proteins continue to be ingested.

Individuals with various inflammatory GI disorders (e.g., celiac disease, food allergy, inflammatory bowel disease) frequently have high levels of food-specific IgG and IgM antibodies. However, these antibodies do not indicate that the patient is allergic to these foods. The increased levels of food-specific antibodies (not IgE) appear to result from increased GI permeability to food antigens and reflect dietary intake.

Food Allergens

Among 399 described food allergens, only 71 of 14,831 (0.5%) protein families are represented, and the top 20 (0.13%) protein families account for 80% of all described food allergens, suggesting that food allergens share common characteristics that render them allergenic.[19] Functionally, based on the ability to induce allergic sensitization in the GI tract, food proteins can be classified as class I (traditional) food allergens or as class II food allergens that do not induce sensitivity through the GI tract but become allergenic as a consequence of sensitization to inhalant allergens.[20] The major food allergens that have been identified in class I allergy are water-soluble glycoproteins, which have molecular masses ranging from 10 to 70 kD and are more stable to treatment with heat, acid, and proteases. However, there are no obvious physicochemical properties common to the class II food allergens. The mostly plant-derived proteins are highly heat labile and difficult to extract intact, often making standardized extracts for diagnostic purposes unsatisfactory. Several class I and II food allergens have been identified, cloned, sequenced, and expressed as recombinant proteins. Many of the plant-related allergens are homologous to pathogenesis-related (PR) proteins, which are expressed by the plant in response to infections or other stress factors, or comprise seed-storage proteins, profilins, peroxidases, or protease inhibitors common to many plants.

Food additives and colorings derived from natural sources that contain proteins may induce allergic reactions. These include colors derived from turmeric, paprika, seeds (e.g., annatto), and insects (e.g., carmine, cochineal). Chemical additives are not likely to cause IgE-mediated food allergy, but some may have drug effects that cause adverse reactions, including allergy-like

BOX 12.2 Categories of Food Additives With Examples

Starches/Complex Carbohydrates	Cornstarch, Modified Starch
Preservatives (antimicrobials)	Potassium sorbate, sodium benzoate
Preservatives (antioxidants)	Butylated hydroxyanisole/hydroxytoluene (BHA/BHT)
Preservatives (antibrowning)	Potassium metabisulfite, sulfur dioxide
Nutrients	Vitamin A, ferrous sulfate
Flavors	Ethyl vanillin, cinnamic aldehyde
Anticaking agents	Sodium aluminosilicate
Emulsifying agents	Lecithin
Sequestrants	Citric acid
Stabilizers and gums	Tragacanth gum, xanthan gum
Acidulents	Phosphoric acid, hydrochloric acid
Flavor enhancers	Monosodium glutamate
Colors	Tartrazine, annatto
Enzymes	Papain
Leavening agents	Sodium bicarbonate

symptoms, or they may invoke immune responses.[21] Tartrazine (yellow #5) is a synthetic color that has been extensively investigated because of concerns that it may trigger urticaria, allergic reactions, and asthma. However, well-conducted studies have not validated these concerns. Sulfites are added to foods as a preservative, an antibrowning agent, or for its bleaching effect. In sensitive persons, sulfites may induce asthma (Box 12.2).

Cross-Reactivity

Structural homology among allergens underlies immunologic and clinical cross-reactivity. More than 70% identity in the primary sequence is considered necessary for clinical cross-reactivity. However, the expression of clinical cross-reactivity is modulated by additional factors, including protein solubility and digestibility, concentration and affinity of the specific IgE antibodies, and the dose and route of allergen exposure. High

rates of clinical cross-reactivity are observed among milks from cows, goats, and sheep (>90%); melons (90%); crustacean shellfish (75%); fruits from the Rosaceae family, such as apple, pear, and peach (55%); and bony fish (50%). Lower rates are observed among tree nuts (37%), grains (20%), CM and beef (10%), and peanuts and other legumes (5%). The rates of pollen-fruit cross-reactivity are about 50% for birch pollen and Rosaceae (e.g., apple, peach, pear, cherry) fruits. The rate of reactions to kiwi, banana, or avocado among latex-allergic individuals is about 11%. The risk of latex allergy among kiwi-, banana-, or avocado-allergic individuals is about 35%.[21]

Pathophysiologic Mechanisms of Food Allergy

In the susceptible host, a failure to develop or a breakdown in oral tolerance, commonly as a result of heavy occupational exposure or sensitization to cross-reactive allergens, may result in allergic responses to ingested food antigens. The extended Gell[1] and Coombs classification provides a framework for discussing hypersensitivity reactions, but food-allergic disorders usually involve more than one of the classic mechanisms (Table 12.3).

IgE-Mediated Food Allergy

The best characterized food-allergic reactions involve IgE antibodies that bind to high-affinity receptors on mast cells and basophils as well as low-affinity receptors on macrophages, monocytes, lymphocytes, and platelets. When food allergens penetrate mucosal barriers and reach IgE, antibodies bind to mast cells or basophils, mediators are released that induce vasodilatation, smooth muscle contraction, and mucus secretion, producing the symptoms of immediate hypersensitivity. IgE-mediated allergic reactions are associated with a variety of symptoms: generalized (e.g., hypotension, shock); cutaneous (e.g., urticaria, angioedema, pruritic morbilliform rash); oral and GI (e.g., lip, tongue, palatal pruritus and swelling, laryngeal edema, vomiting, and diarrhea); and upper and lower respiratory systems (e.g., ocular pruritus and tearing, nasal congestion, pharyngeal edema, and wheezing). A rise in plasma histamine has been associated with the development of these symptoms after blinded food challenges. In contrast, serum β-tryptase levels are usually not elevated.

In one study, increased levels of serum platelet-activating factor (PAF) were reported for subjects with peanut-induced

TABLE 12.3 Classification of Food-Allergic Disorders Based on Pathophysiology

Disorder	IgE-Mediated Response	IgE- and Cell-Mediated Response	Non–IgE-Mediated Response
Generalized	Food-dependent, exercise-induced anaphylaxis		
Cutaneous	Urticaria, angioedema, flushing, acute morbilliform rash, acute contact urticaria	Atopic dermatitis, contact dermatitis	Contact dermatitis, dermatitis herpetiformis
Gastrointestinal	Oral allergy syndrome, gastrointestinal anaphylaxis	Allergic eosinophilic esophagitis, allergic eosinophilic gastroenteritis	Allergic proctocolitis, food protein–induced enterocolitis syndrome, celiac disease, infantile colic
Respiratory	Acute rhinoconjunctivitis, acute bronchospasm	Asthma	Pulmonary hemosiderosis (Heiner syndrome)

Modified from Nowak-Węgrzyn A, Sampson HA. Adverse reactions to foods. Med Clin North Am 2006;90:97–127.

anaphylaxis who presented to the emergency department.[22] Serum PAF acetylhydrolase activity was significantly lower in patients with fatal peanut anaphylaxis than in control patients, which suggested that impaired ability to break down PAF might contribute to severe anaphylaxis. However, these findings require replication.

Augmentation Factors

Several factors have been associated with increased risk of developing food allergy and with increased severity of food-allergic reactions. Drugs lowering the gastric acidity predisposed to de novo sensitization to food allergen (i.e., hazelnut and codfish) in a mouse model and in treated humans.[23,24] In allergic individuals, antacids increased the severity of codfish-induced anaphylaxis.[25,26] Exercise, sleep deprivation, ingestion of alcohol and nonsteroidal antiinflammatory drugs (NSAIDs) are also associated with increased severity of food-induced anaphylaxis.

CLINICAL FEATURES

Classification of food hypersensitivity disorders into those primarily involving IgE-mediated reactions, those not involving IgE-mediated mechanisms, and those that may involve both IgE- and non–IgE-mediated mechanisms is most useful for clinical and diagnostic purposes.

Gastrointestinal Food Allergy
Gastrointestinal IgE-Mediated Food Allergy

Pollen-food allergy syndrome (*oral allergy syndrome*) is elicited by a variety of plant proteins, especially PR proteins cross-reacting with airborne allergens (Table 12.4). Sensitization to inhaled pollen is the primary event, with secondary reactions occurring following ingestion of the cross-reactive plant foods. It is estimated that pollen-food allergy syndrome affects 50% to 70% of adults suffering from pollen allergy, especially to birch, ragweed, and mugwort pollens. Symptoms are provoked almost exclusively in the oropharynx and rarely involve other target organs. Little is known regarding its prevalence among children. Local contact induces IgE-mediated mast cell activation and provokes the rapid onset of pruritus, tingling, and angioedema of the lips, tongue, palate, and throat, and it occasionally elicits a sensation of pruritus in the ears or tightness in the throat. Symptoms are usually induced by raw fruits and vegetables and are short-lived due to exquisite susceptibility of the allergens to digestion. The cooked forms of these foods typically do not induce symptoms.

Ragweed-allergic patients may experience pollen-food allergy syndrome after contact with raw melons (e.g., watermelon, cantaloupe, honeydew) and bananas. Symptoms may vary throughout the year, as shown for birch pollen–related food allergies. Symptoms are more prominent during the birch pollen season, corresponding to the seasonal rise in birch-specific IgE levels. Birch pollen–allergic patients may develop symptoms after the ingestion of raw carrots, celery, apples, pears, hazelnuts, and kiwi. Cross-reactivity between birch pollen and various fruits and vegetables is due to homology among various PR proteins. For example, Mal d 1, the major apple allergen, is 63% homologous with the major birch pollen allergen, Bet v 1 (Table 12.4).

Immediate GI food allergy (i.e., *GI anaphylaxis*) is a form of IgE-mediated GI hypersensitivity that often accompanies allergic manifestations in other target organs and results in a variety of symptoms. Symptoms usually develop within minutes to 2 hours of consuming the responsible food and consist of nausea, abdominal pain, cramps, vomiting, and diarrhea. In food-allergic children with atopic dermatitis, frequent ingestion of a food allergen appears to induce partial desensitization of GI mast cells, resulting in less pronounced symptoms, such as occasional minor complaints of poor appetite and periodic abdominal pain. A similar diminution of symptoms is seen in young infants with frequent vomiting, leading to a loss of consistent vomiting immediately after feeding.

Diagnosis is established by clinical history, determination of food-specific IgE antibodies (i.e., SPTs or in vitro IgE measurement), complete elimination of the suspected food allergen for up to two weeks with resolution of symptoms, and OFC. OFCs usually provoke typical symptoms if the allergen has been strictly eliminated from the patient's diet for 10 to 14 days.

Non–IgE-Mediated Gastrointestinal Food Allergy

Several GI disorders are thought to result from cell-mediated hypersensitivities (Table 12.4). Allergic EoE, gastritis, and gastroenteritis are characterized by infiltration of the esophagus, stomach, and intestinal walls with eosinophils, basal zone hyperplasia, papillary elongation, absence of vasculitis, and peripheral eosinophilia in about 50% of patients. These eosinophilic gastroenteropathies were previously classified as mixed pathophysiology, but the underlying pathophysiology involves an antigen-mediated Th2 immune response that draws eosinophils to the esophagus, causing mucosal inflammation, esophageal remodeling, and fibrosis, without a contribution by allergen-specific IgE antibodies. EoE is increasingly seen during infancy through adolescence, although the diagnosis appears to be occurring more frequently in adults.[27] EoE typically manifests with symptoms of chronic gastroesophageal reflux disease, intermittent emesis, food refusal, abdominal pain, dysphagia, irritability, sleep disturbance, and failure to respond to conventional reflux medications.[28] In adults, abdominal discomfort, dysphagia, and food impaction are more common. Diagnosis depends on the GI biopsy demonstrating a characteristic eosinophilic infiltration, typically more than 15 eosinophils per high-power field (×40).[29]

Elimination of the responsible food allergens from the diet for up to 8 weeks may be necessary to bring about resolution of symptoms and for up to 12 weeks to bring about normalization of intestinal histology. This diet often requires the use of an amino acid–derived formula or an oligoantigenic diet.[30] To identify the responsible foods, challenges are required that consist of reintroducing the suspect food allergen and demonstrating recurrence of symptoms and a significant eosinophilic infiltrate on biopsy.[31]

Dietary intervention is effective, and about 50% of children respond favorably to dietary modifications. However, an elemental diet (e.g., amino acid–based formulas) may be necessary to identify the food allergens that provoke symptoms. A six-food empiric elimination diet was effective in resolving symptoms and

TABLE 12.4   Gastrointestinal Food-Allergic Disorders

Disorder	Age Group	Characteristics	Diagnosis	Prognosis and Course
IgE-Mediated Disorders				
Acute gastrointestinal hypersensitivity	Any	Onset: minutes to 2 h; nausea, abdominal pain, emesis, diarrhea; typically in conjunction with cutaneous and/or respiratory symptoms	History, positive SPT, and/or serum food-IgE level; confirmatory OFC	Varies, food-dependent; milk, soy, egg, and wheat typically outgrown; peanut, tree nuts, seeds, and shellfish typically persistent
Pollen-food allergy syndrome (oral allergy syndrome)	Any; most common in young adults (50% of birch pollen–allergic adults)	Immediate symptoms on contact of raw fruit with oral mucosa: pruritus, tingling, erythema, or angioedema of the lips, tongue, oropharynx; throat pruritus/tightness	History, positive SPT with raw fruits or vegetables; OFC positive with raw fruit, negative with cooked	Severity of symptoms varies with pollen season; may improve in a subset of patients with pollen immunotherapy
Non–IgE-mediated Disorders				
Eosinophilic esophagitis	Any, but especially infants, children, and adolescents	*Children*: chronic or intermittent symptoms of gastroesophageal reflux, emesis, dysphagia, abdominal pain, and irritability *Adults*: abdominal pain, dysphagia, and food impaction	History, positive SPT, and/or food-IgE level in 50% but poor correlation with clinical symptoms; patch testing may be of value; elimination diet and OFC; endoscopy or biopsy provides conclusive diagnosis and information about treatment response	Varies, not well established; improvement with elimination diet within 6–8 weeks; elemental diet may be required; often responds to swallowed topical steroids
Food protein–induced allergic proctocolitis	Young infants (<6 months), frequently breastfed	Blood-streaked or heme-positive stools; otherwise healthy appearing	History, prompt response (resolution of gross blood in 48 h) to allergen elimination; biopsy conclusive but not necessary for most	Most able to tolerate milk or soy by 1–2 years
Food protein–induced enterocolitis syndrome	Young infants	*Chronic*: emesis, diarrhea, failure to thrive on chronic exposure *Subacute*: repetitive emesis, dehydration (15% shock), diarrhea on repeat exposure after elimination period; breastfeeding protective	History, response to dietary restriction; OFC	Most have resolution in 1–3 years; rarely persists into late teenage years
Food protein–induced enteropathy	Young infants; incidence has decreased	Protracted diarrhea, (steatorrhea), emesis, failure to thrive, anemia in 40%	History, endoscopy and biopsy; response to dietary restriction	Most have resolution in 1–2 years
Celiac disease (gluten-sensitive enteropathy)	Any	Chronic diarrhea, malabsorption, abdominal distention, flatulence, failure to thrive or weight loss; may be associated with oral ulcers and/or dermatitis herpetiformis (DH)	Biopsy diagnostic, shows villous atrophy; screening with serum IgA anti-tissue transglutaminase and anti-gliadin; resolution of symptoms with gluten elimination and relapse on oral challenge	Lifelong

IgE, Immunoglobulin E; *OFC*, oral food challenge; *SPT*, skin-prick test.
Modified from Nowak-Węgrzyn A, Sampson HA. Adverse reactions to foods. Med Clin North Am 2006; 90:97–127.

esophageal pathology in more than 70% of patients treated.[30] An alternative approach is to use swallowed inhaled or oral corticosteroids, which usually bring about rapid symptomatic relief.[32]

Infantile colic is an ill-defined syndrome of paroxysmal fussiness characterized by inconsolable agonized crying, drawing up of the legs, abdominal distention, and excessive gas. It usually develops in the first 2 to 4 weeks of life and persists through the third or fourth month. Although a variety of psychosocial and dietary factors have been implicated, it is difficult to establish the cause of infantile colic. Double-blind, crossover trials of bottle-fed and breast-fed infants suggest that IgE-mediated hypersensitivity may be a pathogenic factor in some infants.

Allergic mechanisms may account for only 10% to 15% of colicky infants. Diagnosis of food-induced colic can be established by implementation of several brief trials of hypoallergenic formula. Symptoms should resolve when the child is placed on the hypoallergenic formula and recur when the regular formula or breastfeeding resumes.

Food protein–induced enterocolitis syndrome (FPIES) is a disorder most commonly seen in infants within the first 6 months of life who present with protracted vomiting and diarrhea, which may result in dehydration.[33] A study from Israel reported a prevalence for milk-induced FPIES of 0.34% in a large (>14,000 infants), population-based birth cohort.[34] A recent population-based survey reported that 0.51% of American children less than 18 years old suffer from FPIES.[35] Vomiting usually occurs 1 to 4 hours after feeding, and continued exposure may result in watery or bloody diarrhea, anemia, abdominal distention, and failure to thrive. Symptoms are most commonly provoked by CM or soy protein–based formulas.

FPIES has been reported in older infants and children caused by rice, oatmeal, egg, wheat, oat, peanut, nuts, chicken, turkey, and fish. Hypotension occurs in about 15% of cases after allergen ingestion, and 10% to 15% of patients present with methemoglobinemia. In adults, shellfish sensitivity may provoke a similar syndrome, with symptoms of severe nausea, abdominal cramps, and protracted vomiting. After an acute reaction, there is a prominent increase in the number of peripheral blood neutrophils, peaking at 4 to 6 hours from the onset of symptoms. Stools often contain occult blood, neutrophils, eosinophils, and Charcot–Leyden crystals. SPT results for the suspected foods are negative. Jejunal biopsies reveal flattened villi, edema, and increased numbers of lymphocytes, eosinophils, and mast cells.

Diagnosis can be established when elimination of the responsible allergen leads to resolution of symptoms within 72 hours and oral challenge provokes symptoms. However, secondary disaccharidase deficiency may uncommonly persist longer and may result in ongoing diarrhea for up to 2 weeks. OFCs consist of administering 0.3 to 0.6 g/kg of body weight of the suspected food protein.[36] Vomiting usually develops within 1 to 4 hours of administering the challenge food, often accompanied by pallor and lethargy. Diarrhea or loose stools may develop after 4 to 8 hours. In conjunction with a positive food challenge result, the peripheral blood absolute neutrophil count increases to at least 1500 cells/mm[5] within 4 to 6 hours of developing symptoms, and neutrophils and eosinophils may be found in the stools. Because about 15% of OFC lead to profuse vomiting, dehydration, and hypotension, they must be performed under medical supervision.

Food protein–induced allergic proctocolitis usually manifests in the first few months of life. Although such reactions are often caused by CM or soy protein hypersensitivity, most occur in breastfeeding infants.[37] Infants typically appear well, often have normally formed stools, and usually are discovered because of the presence of blood (gross or occult) in their stools. Blood loss is usually minor but occasionally can produce anemia. The diagnosis can be established when elimination of the responsible allergen leads to resolution of gross blood passage (hematochezia), usually with dramatic improvement within 72 hours of appropriate food allergen elimination, but complete clearance and resolution of mucosal lesions may take up to 1 month. Reintroduction of the allergen leads to recurrence of symptoms within several hours to days. Lesions are confined to the distal large bowel. Sigmoidoscopy findings vary, ranging from areas of patchy mucosal injection to severe friability with small, aphthoid ulcerations and bleeding. Colonic biopsy reveals a prominent eosinophilic infiltrate in the surface and crypt epithelia and the lamina propria. In severe lesions with crypt destruction, neutrophils are prominent.

CM and soy protein–induced allergic proctocolitis usually resolve within 6 months to 2 years of allergen avoidance, but occasional refractory cases are seen.[38]

Food protein–induced enteropathy (excluding celiac disease) usually manifests in the first several months of life with diarrhea (mild-to-moderate steatorrhea in about 80%) and poor weight gain. Symptoms include protracted diarrhea, vomiting in up to two-thirds of patients, failure to thrive, and malabsorption, which is demonstrated by the presence of reducing substances in the stools, increased fecal fat, and abnormal D-xylose absorption. CM hypersensitivity is the most frequent cause of this syndrome, but it also has been associated with sensitivity to soy, egg, wheat, rice, chicken, and fish.[39]

Diagnosis requires the identification and exclusion of the responsible allergen from the diet, which brings about a resolution of symptoms within several days to weeks. On endoscopy, a patchy villous atrophy is evident, and biopsy reveals a prominent mononuclear round cell infiltrate and a small number of eosinophils, which is not unlike celiac disease but usually is much less extensive. Colitis-like features are usually absent, but anemia occurs in about 40% of affected infants, and protein loss occurs in most. Complete resolution of the intestinal lesions may require 6 to 18 months of allergen avoidance. Unlike celiac disease, loss of clinical reactivity frequently occurs, but the natural history of this disorder has not been well studied.

Celiac disease is an extensive enteropathy that leads to malabsorption.[40] The disease occurs in adults and children at rates approaching 1% of the population. Total villous atrophy and extensive cellular infiltrates are associated with sensitivity to gliadin, the alcohol-soluble portion of gluten found in wheat, rye, and barley. Celiac disease represents an interplay between the environment and genetics, with a strong association with human leukocyte antigen (HLA)-DQ2 ($\alpha1*0501$, $\beta1*0201$), which is present in more than 90% of patients. Introduction of gluten into infant diets before 4 months of age has been identified as a risk factor for celiac disease by some studies, whereas introduction after 6 months has been identified as a risk factor for wheat allergy. The intestinal inflammation in celiac disease is precipitated by exposure to gliadin. Gluten-specific T cells are found in the biopsies of these patients, and without exception, they respond to gluten-derived peptides bound to the disease-associated HLA-DQ2 or HLA-DQ8 molecules. Most patients develop IgA antibodies against gliadin and tissue transglutaminase (tTGase). Virtually all celiac disease patients possess autoantibodies to distinct epitopes on the tTGase molecule, but the antibodies do not appear to be responsible for the pathology.[41]

Initial symptoms often include diarrhea or frank steatorrhea, abdominal distention and flatulence, weight loss, and occasionally nausea and vomiting. Oral ulcers and other extra-intestinal symptoms caused by malabsorption are not uncommon. Villous atrophy of the small bowel is a characteristic feature of celiac patients who ingest gluten. IgA antibodies to gluten are present in more than 80% of adults and children with untreated celiac disease. Patients usually have increased levels of IgG antibodies to a variety of foods, which is presumably the result of increased food antigen absorption. Diagnosis depends on demonstrating biopsy evidence of villous atrophy and inflammatory infiltrate, resolution of biopsy findings after 6 to 12 weeks of gluten elimination, and recurrence of biopsy changes after a gluten challenge. Revised diagnostic criteria have eliminated the requirement for a gluten challenge and instead place a greater focus on serologic studies.

Quantification of IgA anti-gliadin and IgA anti-endomysial antibodies may be used for screening with IgA anti-tTGase antibodies in patients older than 2 years of age. After the diagnosis of celiac disease is established, lifelong elimination of gluten-containing foods is necessary to control symptoms and to avoid the increased risk of malignancy.

Cutaneous Food Allergy

The skin is a frequent target organ in IgE- and non–IgE-mediated food hypersensitivity reactions (Table 12.5). Ingestion of food allergens may lead to the rapid onset of cutaneous symptoms or aggravate chronic conditions.[1,2]

Cutaneous IgE-Mediated Food Allergy

Urticaria and angioedema are the most common acute symptoms of food-allergic reactions, although the prevalence of these reactions is unknown. Because the onset of symptoms follows within minutes of ingesting the responsible allergen, the cause-and-effect nature of the reaction is often obvious. Most individuals with these reactions do not seek medical assistance or necessarily report these to their physicians. The foods most commonly incriminated in adults are fish, shellfish, tree nuts, and peanut, and in children, they include egg, milk, peanut, and nuts.

Acute contact urticaria has been reported with raw meats, fish, shellfish, milk, raw egg, vegetables, and fruits. Most studies of patients with chronic urticaria and angioedema (i.e., symptoms lasting >6 weeks) indicate that allergy to foods or food additives are rarely (2%–4%) implicated. Diagnosis is based on the demonstration of food-specific IgE antibodies (i.e., skin test or in vitro IgE), resolution of skin symptoms with complete elimination of the putative food from the diet, and development of symptoms after challenge.

Mixed IgE- and Non–IgE-Mediated Cutaneous Food Allergy

Atopic dermatitis usually begins in early infancy (90% younger than 1 year of age). It is characterized by a typical distribution, extreme pruritus, chronically relapsing course, and association with asthma and allergic rhinitis.[42]

In one study, 35% to 40% of children with moderate-to-severe atopic dermatitis presenting to a university-based dermatologist were found to be food allergic after allergy evaluations and double-blind, placebo-controlled food challenges (DBPCFCs).[12,43] An earlier study demonstrated a direct correlation between disease severity and the likelihood of food allergy. In a follow-up study of 34 children with atopic dermatitis, 17 children with food allergy placed on an appropriate allergen elimination diet experienced marked, significant improvement in their eczematous rash over the 4-year follow-up period compared

TABLE 12.5 Cutaneous Food-Allergic Disorders

Disorder	Age Group	Characteristics	Diagnosis	Prognosis and Course
IgE-Mediated Disorders				
Acute urticaria and angioedema	Any	Pruritic, evanescent skin rash (hives) and swelling within minutes to 2 h after food ingestion; food identified as a culprit in 20%	History, positive SPT, and/or serum food-IgE level; confirmed by OFC if necessary	Varies, food-dependent; milk, soy, egg, and wheat typically outgrown; peanut, tree nuts, seeds, and shellfish typically persistent
Chronic urticaria and angioedema (rare)	Any	Hives and swelling for >6 weeks; approximately 2% caused by food	History, positive SPT, and/or serum food-IgE level; confirmed by OFC if necessary	Varies
IgE- and Non–IgE-Mediated Disorders				
Atopic dermatitis	Infant and child; 90% start <5 years	Relapsing pruritic vesiculopapular rash; generalized in infants, localized to flexor areas in older children; food allergy in about 35% of children with moderate-to-severe atopic dermatitis	History, SPT, and/or serum food-IgE level; elimination diet and OFC	60–80% improve significantly or allergy resolves by adolescence
Non–IgE-mediated Disorders				
Contact dermatitis	Any; more common in adults	Relapsing pruritic eczematous rash, often on hands or face; often occurs in occupational contact with food stuff	History, patch testing	Varies
Dermatitis herpetiformis	Any	Intensely pruritic vesicular rash on extensor surfaces and buttocks	Biopsy diagnostic, shows IgA granule deposits at the dermal-epidermal junction; resolves with dietary gluten avoidance	Lifelong

Ig, Immunoglobulin; *OFC*, oral food challenge; *SPT*, skin-prick test.
Modified from Nowak-Węgrzyn A, Sampson HA. Adverse reactions to foods. Med Clin North Am 2006;90:97–127.

with non–food-allergic children and food-allergic children not adhering to an allergen-elimination diet. In a series of almost 500 children with atopic dermatitis and food allergy, approximately one-third of symptomatic food hypersensitivities were outgrown in 2 to 3 years. The probability of developing tolerance appeared to depend on the food antigen responsible; development of tolerance to soy was common, whereas development of tolerance to peanut was rare. Results of SPTs often became negative or remained unchanged, but concentrations of allergen-specific IgE dropped significantly. The pathogenic role of food allergy in adults with atopic dermatitis requires further investigation.

Diagnosis is based on demonstration of food-specific IgE antibodies, elimination diets, and OFCs. At the time of first evaluation, skin symptoms provoked by a DBPCFC usually consist of a markedly pruritic, erythematous, morbilliform rash that develops in sites for which atopic dermatitis has a predilection. Urticarial lesions are rarely seen. However, urticaria is frequently seen in follow-up challenges conducted 1 to 2 years later in patients who had adhered to an appropriate allergen elimination diet and had experienced clearing of their eczema but who remained food sensitive. Attempts at reintroducing food should be under a physician's supervision.[12] Although the history may not suggest other food-induced complaints, food challenges can provoke intestinal symptoms (e.g., nausea, abdominal cramping, vomiting, diarrhea) in almost half of patients; upper respiratory symptoms (e.g., laryngeal edema, sensation of itching and tightness in the throat; persistent throat clearing with a dry, hacking cough; hoarseness) in about one-third; and wheezing in about 10% of positive challenges. When absorption studies are performed (e.g., lactulose-rhamnose, lactulose-mannitol), most patients are found to have malabsorption, even though GI complaints are minimal.

Non–IgE-Mediated Cutaneous Food Allergy

Food-induced contact dermatitis is seen frequently among food handlers, especially among those who handle raw fish, shellfish (e.g., snow crabs), meats, and eggs. Patch tests can be used if necessary to confirm the diagnosis.

Dermatitis herpetiformis (*DH*) is a chronic, blistering skin disorder associated with a gluten-sensitive enteropathy.[44] It is characterized by a chronic, intensely pruritic papulovesicular rash symmetrically distributed over the extensor surfaces and buttocks. The histology of the intestinal lesion is virtually identical to that seen in celiac disease, but villous atrophy and inflammatory infiltrates are usually milder. As in patients with celiac disease, virtually all DH patients have circulating IgA antibodies against tTGase, the quantity of which appears to correlate with the extent of the jejunal mucosal lesions.

Diagnosis of DH depends on the presence of the characteristic skin lesions and demonstration of IgA deposition at the dermal-epidermal junction of the skin. Although many patients have minimal or no GI complaints, biopsy of the small bowel usually reveals intestinal involvement. Elimination of gluten from the diet usually leads to resolution of skin symptoms and normalization of intestinal findings over several months. Administration of sulfones, the mainstay of therapy, leads to rapid resolution of skin symptoms but has virtually no effect on intestinal symptoms.[45]

Respiratory Food Allergy

Acute respiratory symptoms caused by food allergy represent pure IgE-mediated reactions, whereas chronic respiratory symptoms represent a mix of IgE-mediated and non–IgE-mediated symptoms (Table 12.6). Upper and lower respiratory reactions

TABLE 12.6 Respiratory Food-Allergic Disorders

Disorder	Age Group	Characteristics	Diagnosis	Prognosis and Course
IgE-Mediated Disorders				
Allergic rhinoconjunctivitis	Any	Ocular pruritus, conjunctival injection and watery discharge, nasal pruritus, congestion, rhinorrhea, sneezing within minutes to 2 h after food ingestion or inhalation; cutaneous and gastrointestinal manifestations typical	History, SPT, and/or serum food-IgE level; OFC	Varies
Acute bronchospasm	Any	Cough, wheezing, dyspnea on food ingestion or inhalation; possible risk factor for severe anaphylaxis; cutaneous and gastrointestinal manifestations typical	History, SPT, and/or serum food-IgE level; OFC	Varies
IgE- and Non–IgE-mediated Disorders				
Asthma	Any	Chronic cough, wheezing, dyspnea; food allergy is risk factor for intubation in children who have asthma	History, SPT, and/or serum food-IgE level; OFC	Varies
Non–IgE-mediated Disorders[a]				
Pulmonary hemosiderosis (Heiner syndrome)	Infants, children (rare)	Chronic cough, hemoptysis, lung infiltrates, wheezing, anemia; described in cow's milk– and buckwheat-allergic infants	History, SPT, and serum food-IgE negative, but milk and buckwheat IgG precipitins positive; lung biopsy with deposits of IgG and IgA	Unknown

Ig, Immunoglobulin; *OFC*, oral food challenge; *SPT*, skin-prick test.
[a]Presumed.
Modified from Nowak-Węgrzyn A, Sampson HA. Adverse reactions to foods. Med Clin North Am 2006;90:97–127.

have been provoked in some children by DBPCFCs, with spirometry demonstrating significant reductions in forced vital capacity, forced expiratory volume in 1 second, and maximum end-expiratory flow values during positive food challenges.[46,47]

Rhinoconjunctivitis alone is infrequently a manifestation of food allergy, and when present, it is typically accompanied by other allergic symptoms. Within minutes to 2 hours of ingestion, food allergens may induce typical signs and symptoms of rhinoconjunctivitis, including periocular erythema, ocular pruritus, and tearing; nasal congestion, pruritus, sneezing, and rhinorrhea.

Approximately 25% of 112 patients with histories of adverse food reactions occurring after 10 years of age developed respiratory symptoms after an OFC, and most were nasal symptoms caused by fruit or vegetables.[48] Despite the notion that milk ingestion frequently leads to nasal congestion in young infants, the objective evidence from oral milk challenges shows that only 0.08% to 0.2% of infants develop nasal symptoms after a milk challenge.

In children with atopic dermatitis, nasal symptoms typically develop within 15 to 90 minutes of initiating the DBPCFC and last about 0.5 to 2 hours. Nasal and periocular pruritus are commonly followed by prolonged bursts of sneezing and copious rhinorrhea.

Asthma or isolated wheezing alone is an infrequent manifestation of food allergy. Although ingestion of food allergens is rarely the main aggravating factor in chronic asthma, some evidence suggests that food antigens can provoke bronchial hyperreactivity. In surveys of children with asthma attending pulmonary clinics, food-induced respiratory reactions were demonstrated in about 6% to 8.5% of children.[49] About 25% of 279 children referred for evaluation with histories of food-induced wheezing or asthma experienced wheezing as one of the symptoms during a DBPCFC. Asthmatic reactions to airborne food allergens have been reported when susceptible individuals are exposed to vapors or steam emitted from cooking food (e.g., milk, fish, mollusks, crustaceans, eggs, garbanzo beans).[21] One study suggested that children with asthma sensitized to food allergens are at greater risk for severe asthma, as judged by hospitalizations, emergency visits, days missed from school, and rescue medication use.

Diagnosis of food-induced respiratory disease is based on a patient's history, evidence of food-specific IgE (e.g., positive skin test results, serology), and OFCs. DBPCFCs after strict elimination of suspected food allergens are usually the only way to confirm the diagnosis of food-induced wheezing. Because many factors can exacerbate wheezing, elimination diets alone typically are not useful.

Non–IgE-Mediated Respiratory Food Allergy

Food-induced pulmonary hemosiderosis (Heiner syndrome) is a rare syndrome of recurrent episodes of pneumonia associated with pulmonary infiltrates and hemorrhage, hemosiderosis, GI blood loss, iron-deficiency anemia, and failure to thrive. Hemosiderin-laden macrophages may be found in morning aspirates of the stomach or seen in biopsy specimens of the lung.[1] Heiner syndrome is most often associated with a

non–IgE-mediated hypersensitivity to CM, but reactivity to egg, pork, and buckwheat have also been reported. Although peripheral blood eosinophilia and multiple serum precipitins to CM are a relatively constant feature, the immunologic mechanisms responsible for this disorder are unknown. Diagnosis is based on the elimination of the precipitating allergen and subsequent resolution of symptoms. Characteristic laboratory data, including precipitating IgG antibodies to CM (or the responsible antigen), are also necessary for diagnosis.

Food-Induced Generalized Anaphylaxis

Food allergies are the single leading cause of generalized anaphylaxis seen in hospital emergency departments in the US and account for at least one-third of cases.[50,51] In addition to the cutaneous, respiratory, and GI symptoms described earlier, patients may develop cardiovascular symptoms, including hypotension, vascular collapse, and cardiac dysrhythmias, presumably due to massive mediator release by mast cells. However, most food-induced anaphylactic reactions are not associated with major increases in serum levels of β-tryptase. In a series of 12 fatal or near-fatal food-induced anaphylactic reactions, all patients experienced severe respiratory compromise, 10 of 12 had nausea and vomiting, and only 7 of 12 patients (or one of six fatal reactions) had cutaneous symptoms.[52] About one-third of patients developed a biphasic reaction and one-quarter experienced prolonged symptoms, typically lasting 2 to 3 days.

Factors that appear to be associated with severe reactions include the presence of asthma; a history of severe reactions; denial of symptoms; and failure to initiate therapy expeditiously.[53] Surveys of food-induced anaphylactic deaths found that anaphylactic reactions to foods affected both sexes equally, most victims were adolescents or young adults, and almost all individuals with a food allergy had a history of some type of reaction to the food culprit that caused the fatal reaction. Among the subjects for whom data were available, virtually all were known to have asthma, very few had epinephrine available for use at the time of their reaction, and about 10% of those who received epinephrine in a timely fashion did not survive. Peanuts or tree nuts were responsible for more than 85% of the fatalities in the US.

Food-Dependent, Exercise-Induced Anaphylaxis

Food-dependent, exercise-induced anaphylaxis (FDEIA) occurs only when the patient exercises within 2 to 4 hours of ingesting a food, but in the absence of exercise, the patient can ingest the food without any apparent reaction.[2,54] Amongst patients with exercise-induced anaphylaxis, approximately 30% to 50% report associated food triggers. Patients usually have asthma and other atopic disorders, positive SPT results for the food that provokes their symptoms, and occasionally a history of reacting to the food when they were younger. This disorder appears to be more common in females than males and most prevalent in the late teens to the mid-30s. The exact mechanism of this disorder is unknown, but several foods have been implicated, including wheat (i.e., omega-5 gliadin portion), shellfish, fruit, milk, celery, and fish. Diagnosis is based on an unequivocal history of food ingestion followed by exercise, the rapid onset (within 1–2 h) of classic IgE-mediated symptoms, and the demonstration of food-specific IgE antibodies by skin-prick testing or in vitro serologic tests. Lacking this evidence, a physician-supervised food challenge is usually warranted to ensure that the suspected food is truly responsible for the anaphylactic reaction. Challenges should be done in a hospital setting by a physician experienced in the treatment of anaphylactic reactions.[24]

Delayed Anaphylaxis Caused by Mammalian Meat

Galactose-α-1,3-galactose (α-gal) has been identified as a cause of serious, even fatal, anaphylaxis.[55] In contrast to previously described cross-reactive carbohydrate determinants expressed in plants and insects, the oligosaccharide α-gal is abundantly expressed on cells and tissues of nonprimate mammals. This expression pattern makes α-gal potentially clinically relevant as a food allergen (e.g., beef, pork, lamb) or as an inhaled allergen (e.g., cat, dog). IgE antibodies to α-gal are associated with an unusual form of delayed anaphylaxis, which occurs 3 to 6 hours after ingestion of mammalian meat that carries α-gal. Patients with IgE to α-gal describe generalized urticaria or frank anaphylaxis starting 3 to 6 hours after eating beef, pork, or lamb and have a consistent pattern of skin testing (likelihood of positive results is increased by testing with freshly ground meat or with intradermal testing) and serum IgE antibody results.

Most patients developed anaphylaxis to red meat in adulthood; some reported receiving multiple tick bites, suggesting that tick bites, especially the lone star tick (*Amblyomma americanum*) in the US, may predispose to sensitization to α-gal.[56]

Other Food-Induced Hypersensitivity Reactions

Ingestion of pasteurized, whole CM by infants, especially those younger than 6 months of age, frequently leads to occult GI blood loss and occasionally to *iron-deficiency anemia*. Substitution of infant formula (including CM-derived formulas that have been subjected to extensive heating) for whole CM usually normalizes fecal blood loss within 3 days.

PATIENT EVALUATION, DIAGNOSIS, AND DIFFERENTIAL DIAGNOSIS

Food Allergy Guidelines are available online (http://www.niaid.nih.gov/topics/foodallergy, accessed on 9/10/200)[9,57] in a full format, with an executive summary, and a lay-language summary for patients, families, and caregivers. The European Academy of Allergy and Clinical Immunology (EAACI) has also published guidelines for anaphylaxis and food allergy.[10]

The diagnostic approach to food allergy begins with the medical history and physical examination. These assessments guide the selection of the laboratory tests (Fig. 12.1).

The value of the medical history largely depends on the patient's recollection of symptoms and the examiner's ability to differentiate between disorders provoked by food hypersensitivity and other causes (Table 12.7). In some cases, it may be useful in diagnosing food allergy (e.g., acute events such as systemic anaphylaxis after isolated ingestion of shrimp), but history alone should never be used to make a diagnosis.

In several series, <50% of reported food-allergic reactions could be verified by DBPCFCs. Information required to establish that a food-allergic reaction occurred and to construct an appropriate blinded challenge at a later date include the following: the food presumed to have provoked the reaction; the quantity of the suspected food ingested; the length of time between ingestion and development of symptoms; whether similar symptoms developed on other occasions when the food was eaten; whether other factors (e.g., exercise, alcohol, drugs) are necessary; and how long since the last reaction to the food occurred. In chronic disorders (e.g., atopic dermatitis, asthma, chronic urticaria), the history is often an unreliable indicator of the offending allergen.

Diet diaries are frequently discussed as an adjunct to history. Patients are instructed to keep a chronologic record of all foods ingested over a specified period, including items placed in the mouth but not swallowed, such as chewing gum. Any symptoms experienced by the patient are also recorded. The diary is then reviewed to determine whether there are any relationships between foods ingested and symptoms experienced. Occasionally, this method detects an unrecognized association between a food and a patient's symptoms. Unlike the medical history, it collects information on a prospective basis and does not depend on a patient's memory. This approach should be used selectively because it often causes patients and families to focus obsessively on foods instead of other potential triggers of their reactions.

Elimination diets are frequently used in the diagnosis and management of food allergy. Suspected foods are completely omitted from the diet. The success of these diets depends on the identification of the correct allergens, the ability of the patient to maintain a diet free of all forms of the offending allergens, and the assumption that other factors do not provoke similar symptoms during the period of study. Unfortunately, these conditions are rarely met. In a young infant reacting to CM-formula, resolution of symptoms after substitution with a soy formula or casein hydrolysate or with an elemental amino acid–based formula is highly suggestive of CM or other food allergies, respectively, but it also could be caused by lactose intolerance. Although avoidance of suspected food allergens is recommended before blinded challenges, elimination diets alone are rarely diagnostic of food allergy, especially in chronic disorders such as atopic dermatitis or asthma. A trial of a diagnostic elimination diet should be followed by a reintroduction of the food either under physician supervision (with positive food-specific IgE tests or suspected FPIES) or at home, in the case of other GI food-allergic disorders.

SPTs are reproducible and frequently used to screen patients with suspected IgE-mediated food allergies. Glycerinated food extracts (1:10 or 1:20) and appropriate positive (e.g., histamine) and negative (e.g., saline) controls are applied by the prick or puncture technique.

Any food allergens eliciting a wheal with a diameter at least 3 mm greater than the negative control are considered to be positive; all other results are considered to be negative. A positive SPT should be interpreted as indicating the *possibility* that the patient has symptomatic reactivity to the specific food, whereas

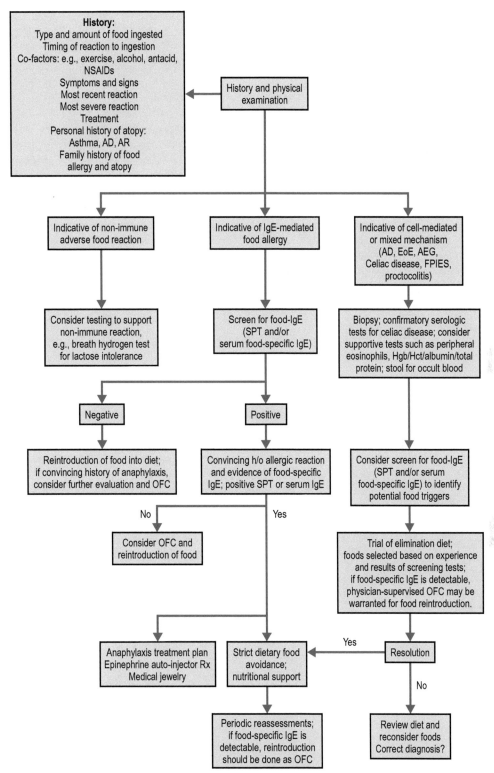

Fig. 12.1 Current approach to the diagnosis and management of food allergy. *AD*, Atopic dermatitis; *AEG*, allergic eosinophilic gastroenteritis; *AR*, allergic rhinitis; *EoE*, eosinophilic esophagitis; *FPIES*, food protein–induced enterocolitis syndrome; *Hct*, hematocrit; *Hgb*, hemoglobin; *IgE*, immunoglobulin E; *NSAIDs*, nonsteroidal antiinflammatory drugs; *OFC*, oral food challenge; *Rx*, treatment; *SPT*, skin-prick test. (Modified from Nowak-Węgrzyn A, Sampson HA. Adverse reactions to foods. Med Clin North Am 2006;90:97–127.)

negative skin test results confirm the absence of IgE-mediated reactions (negative predictive accuracy is >95%) if good-quality food extracts are used. The SPT may be considered an excellent means of excluding IgE-mediated food allergies, but it can only

suggest the presence of clinical food allergies. There are some exceptions to this general statement. First, IgE-mediated allergy to several fruits and vegetables (e.g., apples, oranges, bananas, pears, melons, potatoes, carrots, celery) is frequently not

TABLE 12.7 Nonallergic Adverse Reactions to Consider in the Differential Diagnosis of Food Allergy

Condition	Symptoms	Mechanism and comments
Enzyme Deficiencies		
Lactose intolerance	Bloating, abdominal pain, diarrhea (dose-dependent)	Lactase deficiency
Fructose intolerance	Emesis, poor feeding, jaundice, hypoglycemia, seizures	Hereditary fructose aldolase B deficiency; rare
Fructose malabsorption	Bloating, abdominal pain, diarrhea (dose-dependent)	Deficiency of fructose carrier GLUT5 in the enterocytes in small intestines; 10% prevalence in Asia, up to 30% in Western Europe and Africa
Pancreatic insufficiency	Malabsorption	Deficiency of pancreatic enzymes, acquired or congenital (e.g., cystic fibrosis, Shwachman–Diamond syndrome)
Alcohol	Nasal congestion, flushing, vomiting	Polymorphism of the aldehyde dehydrogenase gene (*ALDH*), resulting in deficiency of ALDH, which metabolizes alcohol in the liver; common in Asians
Gallbladder or liver disease	Malabsorption	Deficiency of liver enzymes
Gastrointestinal Disorders		
Gastroesophageal reflux disease	Nausea, emesis, abdominal pain, heartburn, dysphagia	Chronic symptom of mucosal damage caused by stomach acid refluxing into the esophagus
Peptic ulcer disease	Abdominal pain, bloating, loss of appetite, weight loss, melena	Ulcer of the gastrointestinal tract (commonly duodenum); 70–90% are associated with *Helicobacter pylori* infection
Anatomic Defects		
Hiatal hernia	Abdominal pain, shortness of breath, nausea, emesis	Protrusion (or herniation) of the upper part of the stomach into the thorax through a tear or weakness in the diaphragm
Pyloric stenosis	Severe, nonbilious, projectile vomiting in the first few months of life	Stenosis due to hypertrophy of muscle around pylorus, which spasms when stomach empties; rare case reports of eosinophilic infiltrates in pylorus and reported resolution of muscle hypertrophy with hypoallergenic formula or steroids
Hirschsprung disease	Delayed passage of meconium, constipation, ileus, emesis	Failure of neural crest cells to migrate completely during fetal development of the intestine, causing agangliosis; usually affects short segment of the distal colon
Tracheoesophageal fistula	Copious salivation associated with choking, coughing, vomiting, and cyanosis coincident with the onset of feeding in newborns and young infants	*Congenital*: failed fusion of tracheoesophageal ridges during third week of embryologic development *Acquired*: usually sequela of surgical procedures (e.g., laryngectomy)
Physiologic Effects of Active Substances		
Caffeine	Tremors, cramps, diarrhea	Xanthine alkaloid acts as stimulant drug; found in seeds, leaves, and fruit of some plants, where it acts as a natural pesticide; consumed in coffee, tea, and drinks containing kola nut, yerba mate, guarana berry, or guayusa derivatives
Theobromine	Sleeplessness, tremors, restlessness, anxiety, increased urination, loss of appetite, nausea, vomiting	Bitter alkaloid in cocoa bean and tea leaves; elderly more susceptible
Tyramine	Migraine	Naturally occurring monoamine compound derived from tyrosine; acts as a catecholamine-releasing agent; pharmacologic effects in susceptible individuals; found in pickled, aged, smoked, fermented, or marinated foods (e.g., hard cheeses, tofu, sauerkraut, fava beans)
Histamine	Flushing, headache, nausea	Naturally occurring in fermented foods and beverages (e.g., fish, sauerkraut) due to a conversion from histidine to histamine performed by fermenting bacteria or yeasts; sake contains histamine in the 20–40 mg/L range and wines in the 2–10 mg/L range
Serotonin	Flushing, diarrhea, palpitations	Monoamine neurotransmitter derived from tryptophan; found in nuts, mushrooms, fruits, and vegetables; highest values (25–400 mg/kg) in nuts of walnut and hickory genera; concentrations of 3–30 mg/kg found in plantain, pineapple, banana, kiwi, plums, and tomatoes

(Continued)

TABLE 12.7 Nonallergic Adverse Reactions to Consider in the Differential Diagnosis of Food Allergy—cont'd

Condition	Symptoms	Mechanism and comments
Food Additives and Contaminants		
Sodium metabisulfite	Rare reports of bronchospasm in sensitive individuals	Antioxidant and preservative in food, also known as E223
Monosodium glutamate (MSG)	Chinese restaurant syndrome begins 15–20 min after the meal and lasts for about 2 h; symptoms include numbness at the back of the neck and gradually radiating to the arms and back, general weakness, and palpitations	Naturally occurring nonessential amino acid; flavor enhancer; in a DBPCFC study, objective reactions to MSG were observed in only 2 of 130 self-selected MSG-reactive adult volunteers[2]
Accidental contaminants	Abdominal pain, diarrhea, nausea	Include heavy metals (e.g., mercury, copper), pesticides, antibiotics (e.g., penicillin), dust or storage mites
Infectious agents	Pain, fever, nausea, emesis, diarrhea	Include bacteria (e.g., *Salmonella*, *Shigella*, *Escherichia coli*, *Yersinia*, *Campylobacter*); parasites (e.g., *Giardia*, *Trichinella*); viruses (e.g., hepatitis, rotavirus, enterovirus)
Neurologic Disorders		
Auriculotemporal syndrome (Frey syndrome)	Facial flush in trigeminal nerve distribution associated with spicy foods	Neurogenic reflex, frequently associated with birth trauma to trigeminal nerve (forceps delivery)
Gustatory rhinitis	Profuse watery rhinorrhea associated with spicy foods	Neurogenic reflex
Conditions Confused with Food Reactions		
Panic disorder	Subjective reactions, fainting on smelling or seeing the food; tachycardia, perspiration, dyspnea, shivers, uncontrollable fear (fear of dying)	Psychological; anxiety disorder affects children and adults; usually leads to extensive medical testing; controlled with medications and behavioral therapy

DBPCFC, Double-blind, placebo-controlled food challenge.
Modified from Nowak-Węgrzyn A, Sampson HA. Adverse reactions to foods. Med Clin North Am 2006; 90:97–127.

detected with commercially prepared reagents, presumably due to the lability of the responsible allergen. Second, commercial extracts sometimes lack the appropriate allergen to which an individual is reactive, as demonstrated by the use of fresh foods for skin test reagents. Third, children younger than 1 year of age may have IgE-mediated food allergy in the absence of positive skin test results, and infants younger than 2 years of age may have smaller wheals, presumably due to a lack of skin reactivity. Fourth, a positive skin test result for a food, that when ingested in the absence of other foods provokes a serious systemic anaphylactic reaction, may be considered diagnostic. In general, the larger the SPT wheal diameter, the higher the likelihood of a reaction upon ingestion of the food. For some foods, the diagnostic decision points have been established, above which there is more than a 95% likelihood that the patient is allergic. The examples are cow milk wheal size ≥10 mm and peanut wheal size ≥8 mm in children.[58]

Intradermal skin testing is more sensitive than the SPT but is much less specific than a DBPCFC. Intradermal skin testing increases the risk of inducing a systemic reaction compared with skin-prick testing and is therefore not recommended.

In the past, the atopy patch test was explored for the diagnosis of non–IgE-mediated food allergy in several disorders. The lack of standardized reagents and method limits the utility of this approach. In one large study of children with atopic dermatitis,

the investigators concluded that the patch test added little diagnostic benefit compared with standard diagnostic tests.[21]

In vitro allergen-specific IgE tests are used for measuring serum for IgE-mediated food allergies. In the past 10 years, the quantitative measurement of food-specific IgE antibodies (i.e., CAP System FEIA or UniCAP) has been shown to be more predictive of symptomatic IgE-mediated food allergy than other methods. Food-specific IgE levels exceeding the diagnostic values (Table 12.8) indicate that patients are >95% likely to experience an allergic reaction if they ingest the specific food.[36,59] The IgE levels can be monitored, and if they fall to <2 kU_A/L for egg, milk, or peanut, the patient without recent severe reactions should be challenged again to determine whether he or she has outgrown the food allergy.

Periodic evaluations should be offered to children with peanut allergy, and an OFC for peanut should be considered in patients who have not had reactions in the past 1 to 2 years and who have a serum peanut-IgE level of <2.0 kU_A/L.

Component-resolved diagnosis (CRD) is based on individual natural or recombinant allergenic proteins that are purified. Specified amounts of allergens can be spotted on an activated biochip surface, and minute quantities of serum are needed to detect IgE antibody to almost any number of specific allergens in a single-step process. CRD potentially offers superior specificity due to the purity of the components compared with wholefood

TABLE 12.8 Food-specific IgE Serum Concentrations Highly Predictive of Clinical Reactivity

Allergen	Diagnostic Decision Level (kU$_A$/L)[a]	Sensitivity (%)	Specificity (%)	Positive Predictive Value (%)	Negative Predictive Value (%)
Egg white	7	61	95	98	38
Infants ≤2 years	0.35	91	77	95	68
Ovomucoid for baked egg	10.8	55	96	88	80
Milk	15	57	94	95	53
Infants ≤1 year	5	30	99	95	64
Peanut	14	57	99	99	36
Fish	20	25	100	99	89
Soybean	30	44	94	73	82
Wheat	26	61	92	74	87
Tree nuts	15	Other values were not calculated and are not available		95	

[a]kU$_A$/L = allergen-specific kilo units per liter.

extracts. OFCs were used in several studies to evaluate the clinical applications of CRD in cases of food allergy. Patients with IgE antibodies directed exclusively against birch Bet v 1 cross-reactive components in peanut Ara h 8 and hazelnut Cor a 1 are at low risk for systemic reaction to peanut and hazelnut; many may ingest these nuts without any allergic symptoms and therefore such patients are excellent candidates for supervised OFCs.[60] In contrast, patients with IgE directed against Ara h 2 or Cor a 9 and/or 14 are at higher risk for systemic reactions.[61] High levels of IgE against heat stable casein in CM and ovomucoid in egg white are associated with higher risk of reactions to baked milk and egg products.[62] A new generation of specific antibody testing is focused on identifying antibodies directed at particular epitopes (binding sites) on the allergenic molecules. Specific recognition patterns and higher numbers of the bound epitopes have been detected in patients with more severe and more persistent phenotypes of peanut and CM allergy and could predict response to food oral 5immunotherapy and "high-risk" infants who would go on to develop peanut allergy.[63,64] The basophil activation test (BAT) is a functional assay that uses live basophils in whole blood to detect IgE-mediated activation of basophils after stimulation with allergen.[65] The basophils of allergic patients typically show a dose-dependent expression of activation markers, such as CD63 or CD203c (detected by flow cytometry), whereas the basophils of sensitized but tolerant patients fail to express or have a much lower expression of activation markers after stimulation with allergen. The difference in upregulation of basophil activation markers in response to allergen between allergic and nonallergic patients forms the basis of the use of the BAT to diagnose FA. Currently, epitope-based assays and BAT are restricted to research studies, but the efforts to incorporate them into clinical diagnostics are ongoing.[66]

OFCs are an important element in the management of food allergies in patients, and they remain the most accurate tests for the diagnosis of food allergy.[36] Food challenges may be conducted at home without medical supervision only if the physician determines that there is no risk of a severe reaction. This approach may be appropriate for patients who present with complaints that are usually not associated with food allergy and when skin or in vitro testing results have been negative. It may also be appropriate to do a home reintroduction of a food that has been temporarily discontinued as part of an elimination diet but had been present in the diet previously. However, if there has been prolonged avoidance lasting weeks to a few months, the pattern of reactivity might have changed, and a home introduction may no longer be safe. In the majority of the cases, OFCs are performed under physician supervision.

The DBPCFC has been labeled the gold standard for the diagnosis of food allergies. Many investigators have used DBPCFCs successfully in children and adults to examine a variety of food-related complaints. In clinical practice, open (unblinded) and single-blinded OFCs are frequently used. The selection of foods to be tested in an OFC is usually based on history and skin test or in vitro IgE test results. The basic methodology underlying all OFCs is administration of the suspect food in gradually increasing doses under close observation in a medical setting. Challenges should be terminated and treatment administered at the first sign that a reaction is occurring. OFCs carry the potential for significant risk, but these risks can be minimized by appropriate dosing and by performing challenges in a controlled setting with experienced personnel (Box 12.3). Oral challenge testing should be considered for clinical and research purposes. As shown in the algorithm in Fig. 12.2, in the clinical setting, challenges are typically done for three major reasons. First, OFCs are used to establish an accurate diagnosis when the diagnosis remains unclear after other standard diagnostic methods have been tried, including obtaining the patient's history, skin testing, measurement of specific IgE levels, and elimination diets. Second, to determine the role food allergy plays in chronic conditions, such as atopic dermatitis or EoE. Third, OFCs are frequently used to determine whether a patient with a known food allergy has developed tolerance to that food.

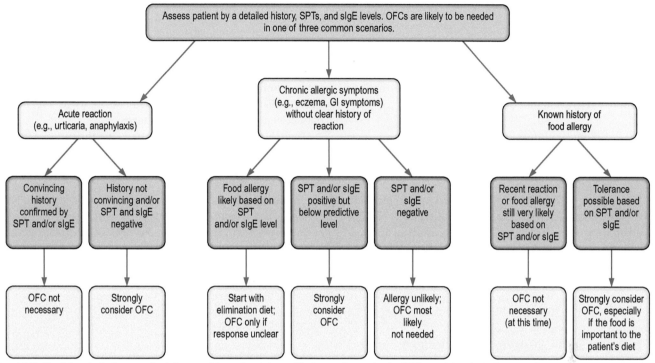

Fig. 12.2 Oral food challenge decision-making algorithm. *GI,* Gastrointestinal; *OFC,* oral food challenge; *SPT,* skin-prick test; *sIgE,* specific IgE.

BOX 12.3   Steps to Minimize Challenge Risks

- Adjust the starting dose and challenge protocol for individual patients who may be at higher risk for severe reactions.
- Use experienced observers who have been trained to do food challenges and are present throughout the challenge, continually interacting with and reexamining the patient at regular intervals.
- Stop the challenge as soon as the observer is convinced that a reaction is occurring. Prepare all medications that may be needed before the challenge so that they can be administered without delay.
- Perform challenges only in settings where all measures that might be needed to treat a severe reaction are readily available.

Unproven Tests for Food Allergy

There are no controlled trials supporting the diagnostic value of food-specific IgG or IgG_4 antibody levels, food antigen–antibody complexes, evidence of lymphocyte activation (e.g., ^{3}H-uptake, IL-2 production, leukocyte inhibitory factor production), or sublingual or intracutaneous provocation.[1]

FOOD ALLERGY TREATMENT

Practical Management

Management of food allergies requires avoidance of the offending allergens and prompt treatment of allergic reactions.[21,58] Food allergen avoidance is challenging because food is necessary for sustenance and allergens are ubiquitous. Patients and caregivers must understand food-labeling laws, prevention of cross-contact of safe foods with allergens, and means of acquiring safe meals in settings such as restaurants and schools. Adding to the complexity of avoidance is the possibility of exposure to food allergens in occupational settings, in nonfood items such as cosmetics and medications, and through non-ingestion exposures by skin contact or inhalation. Nutritional concerns arise when multiple foods are removed from the diet. Successful emergency management requires prompt recognition and treatment of an allergic reaction or anaphylaxis.

The daily burden of managing food allergies seriously impacts quality of life.[67] Successful management requires detailed education of patients and caregivers about avoidance and treatment.

Food Allergen Avoidance Strategies
General Approach to Avoidance

Allergen avoidance should be prescribed based on a confirmed diagnosis. Avoidance education must include all persons responsible for obtaining or preparing foods. Educational materials are available through a variety of resources, including Food Allergy Research & Education (www.foodallergy.org).

Strict avoidance is typically prescribed to avoid any risk of allergic reaction, although it may not always be necessary. Examples where ingestion of the allergenic protein may be acceptable include raw fruits and vegetables in persons with mild symptoms of pollen-food–related syndrome; extensively heated forms of milk or egg (e.g., bakery goods) in persons who tolerate them, despite reacting to whole forms; and maternal ingestion of allergens when breastfeeding allergic infants who show no evidence of reactions. Patients who tolerate these forms of exposure are identified through their medical history or by medically supervised OFC. Caution is needed because anaphylaxis can occur in some persons. The risk or benefit of allowing exposure to tolerated forms of the allergen should be individualized. There is no evidence that strict food avoidance (compared with less strict avoidance) has an effect on the rate of natural remission. Avoidance of foods that are related and may have cross-reactive proteins can be individualized according to risk of clinical cross-reactivity. Table 12.9 summarizes options for the approach to avoidance of dietary allergens.

Labeling of Manufactured Products

In the US, the Food Allergen Labeling and Consumer Protection Act (FALCPA) of 2004 requires that milk, egg, peanut, tree nuts, fish, crustacean shellfish, wheat, and soy, be declared on ingredient labels using plain English words. These foods and food categories are often referred to as "major allergens." The law does not apply to any other foods or to noncrustacean seafood. The common names used to identify the foods may be listed within the ingredient list or in a separate statement (e.g., "contains peanut"). Although not required, if a "contains statement" is used, all the major allergens must be included. The law also requires that the specific type of allergen within a category be named, such as "walnut" or "shrimp."

FALCPA applies to foods manufactured in or imported into the US; it does not apply to agricultural products (e.g., fresh meat, eggs, poultry, fruits, vegetables) or alcoholic beverages, which may use food proteins as ingredients or processing agents. The law is subject to revisions, as described at http://www.fda.gov/Food/FoodSafety/FoodAllergens.

Labeling laws vary among countries, and some have none. Many countries have laws that include more than just the eight food allergen groups currently covered by US laws. For example, the European Union enacted legislation in 2005 requiring that six allergens not covered in US laws be listed: rye, barley, oats, celery, mustard, and sesame seeds.

The FALCPA of 2004 does not regulate the use of advisory labeling, including statements describing the potential presence of unintentional ingredients in food products; such declarations are done voluntarily in the US, and approaches are evolving internationally.[68] Although many terms are used (e.g., "may contain," "manufactured on equipment with") to describe possible cross-contact, these do not convey risk. Therefore, general advice is to avoid products with these advisories. Nonetheless, there may be lower thresholds that would pose virtually no risk, and improved labeling based on studies of thresholds and adequate testing of final products may be possible. Consumers should be aware that food proteins might be a component of nonfood items (Table 12.10).

Cross-Contact

Cross-contact (cross-contamination) of an otherwise safe food with an allergen is a concern for food preparation in commercial

TABLE 12.9 Options for Allergen Avoidance in Select Circumstances

Circumstance	Options	Risk or Benefit[a]
Raw fruits and vegetables causing oral symptoms (pollen-related)	Allow ingestion on case-by-case basis based on preference and severity	Small risk of systemic reaction or anaphylaxis
Products with extensively heated (baked-in) egg or milk in persons with allergy to whole forms	Allow ingestion if tolerated by history or challenge (caution for possible anaphylaxis)	Unclear whether this approach speeds, hinders, or has no influence on recovery. Risk of reaction despite initial apparent tolerance. Possible risk of chronic inflammation from exposure
Maternal ingestion of an allergen while breastfeeding, when same allergen caused a reaction when ingested by infant	Allow mother to continue previously ingested amounts if infant showed no sign of acute or chronic reaction	May risk reaction. No data on influence on natural course. Variations in dose ingested may alter the risk
Allergy to peanut, not tree nuts	Allow ingestion of tolerated tree nuts	Cross-contact or misidentification may lead to reactions. New onset of allergy to allowed food is possible, although degree of risk uncertain
Allergy to some but not all tree nuts	Allow peanut in forms that are free from tree nuts. Allow ingestion of tolerated tree nuts	As above, with less risk for commercial peanut butter and various commercial products with isolated nut ingredients (e.g., almond in almond milk)
Allergy to some but not all fish	Allow tolerated fish. Allow canned fish that are tolerated	Risk of cross-contact, misidentification, or new onset of allergy. Less risk for processed (canned) fish
Allergy to some but not all shellfish	Allow tolerated shellfish	Risk of cross-contact, misidentification, or new onset of allergy
Allergy to some but not all botanically related foods (e.g., fruits, legumes, vegetables, grains)	Allow tolerated types	Many options to ingest 'related' foods if proved tolerated with lower risk of cross-contact, misidentification, or new onset of allergy

[a]Individual quality of life or nutritional benefits are assumed. Decisions are individualized based on patient preferences, physician judgment, risk assessment, and past history.

TABLE 12.10	Examples of Food Allergens in Unexpected and Nonfood Items	
Product type	**Examples**	**Relevance**
Cosmetics	Almond or milk in shampoos or ointments	Contact urticaria or dermatitis is possible. Some derivatives (e.g., shea nut butter) may have negligible protein
Pet food	Milk, egg, fish, soy, etc.	Animal lick may cause contact urticaria. Fish food on fingers may transfer to eyes or mouth causing symptoms
School supplies	Wheat in play-doh, milk casein contained in fingerpaints or dustless chalk, etc.	Contact urticaria or dermatitis is possible. Food residue on fingers may transfer to eyes or mouth causing symptoms
Medications	Lactose in dry powder inhaler (DPI) or tablets may have trace milk. Soy lecithin, egg lecithin	Case reports of reactions to casein identified in DPI, relevance in pills/pharmaceutical grade lactose unclear. Relevance of potential trace protein in lecithin (fatty derivative) unclear, likely low risk
Vaccines	Egg (yellow fever), gelatin (MMR), possibly milk (DTAP)	Relevant for those with severe phenotype
Nutrition supplements	Glucosamine-chondroitin supplements (shark cartilage or shrimp shell), chitosan or chitin products (derived from crustacean shell)	Relevance uncertain, likely low risk
Saliva (kissing)	Residual protein from meals	Relevant for intimate contact
Transfusion	Packed red blood cells, plasma (containing allergens from donor ingestion)	Risk presumably low, theoretically higher for products that include serum proteins rather than washed blood products

facilities, in restaurants and food establishments, and at home. Examples of cross-contact include a knife used to spread peanut butter then contaminating jelly; shared grills, pans, food processors, and other equipment used without thorough cleaning between preparation of different foods; dipping ice cream scoops from one flavor to the next; using a fryer for both shrimp and potatoes; and preparing foods in a workspace not cleaned between preparations. Patients and caregivers must be educated about these concerns and address them when obtaining or preparing meals.

Manner of Exposure

The three primary manners of exposure are skin contact, inhalation, and ingestion. The primary concern regarding avoidance of an allergen relates to *ingestion*. Although exposures through skin contact or inhalation are unlikely to cause anaphylaxis, skin rashes and respiratory symptoms may occur. For young children, there is a concern that skin contact could lead to ingestion (e.g., sucking fingers). Food odors may be caused by volatile organic compounds that lack appreciable proteins and present minimal allergic risk (e.g., odor of peanut butter would not trigger anaphylaxis) or may include proteins when the food is aerosolized (e.g., during cooking, dust from powdery forms). In the latter case (e.g., in proximity to boiling milk, frying fish, or powdered milk), respiratory or skin symptoms could occur. Non-ingestion reactions occur in occupational settings as well (e.g., food handlers, see Chapter 14). Baker's asthma describes airborne sensitivity to wheat flour. Individuals with baker's asthma can typically tolerate wheat ingestion. Persons with occupational allergy caused by foods may need to wear gloves and masks or find alternative employment. Aside from occupational exposures, individuals with food allergies may need to avoid situations where the food allergen is aerosolized nearby. Young children may need to be supervised around food allergens to avoid hand-to-mouth contact. Standard cleaning procedures (soap and water and wiping with friction) should suffice to remove allergens from surfaces. Antibacterial foams and gels do not remove allergens from hands. Minor allergic reactions from kissing are common because allergen can be transferred in saliva or residual protein on the lips. Skin contact with the saliva is unlikely to cause a severe reaction, but intimate kissing is similar in risk to ingestion, and a partner may need to avoid the allergen.

Restaurants, Food Establishments, Travel

Restaurants and other food establishments, such as bakeries or ice cream stores, present challenges for food-allergic individuals. Consumers should identify themselves as allergic so that instructions about avoidance are not misperceived as being taste preferences. Clear communication is crucial because those preparing the foods may have limited understanding of the needs of an allergic consumer. It may be prudent for consumers to review concerns such as cross-contact and hidden ingredients with the relevant personnel. All persons handling the food should be involved in discussions about meal preparation. This could prevent errors, such as a "prep" worker adding butter to a food that appears dry. Consumers may present written materials that describe the allergies ("chef cards"), and food establishments may follow guidelines; both are available from several sources, including Food Allergy Research & Education (www.foodallergy.org). Buffets or specialty or ethnic restaurants (e.g., seafood, Asian) may pose high risks and should be avoided depending on the consumer's specific allergies. Traveling with food allergies requires considerations beyond obtaining meals safely in restaurants. Allergic reactions to peanut and tree nuts have been reported on commercial airliners, but the studies rely heavily on self-report.[69] Overall, exposure to the cabin air seems unlikely to trigger severe reactions for most persons with food allergies. Travelers with food allergies should avoid eating potentially unsafe airline foods and carry safe alternatives.

Adults traveling with young children with food allergies might inspect crevices around their seats and wipe surfaces to avoid ingestion of residual allergens by toddlers. Some airlines may provide additional accommodations when requested in advance (e.g., flight with no peanuts served). Vacation choices, including all-inclusive resorts, cruises, and international travel, are circumstances in which advance planning is required because meals are prepared by others.

Potentially less risky alternatives include accommodations with a kitchenette so that some meals can be self-prepared.

Avoidance for Schools and Camp

School-based strategies must be practical and must focus on policies to avoid ingestion of the allergen and promptly recognize and treat anaphylaxis.[2,70] Allergen avoidance may vary depending on the age of the children, with more supervision, cleaning, and containment of allergen needed for younger children. Risk-taking behaviors among adolescents with food allergy, such as eating unsafe foods and delaying treatment of a reaction, are likely contributing factors to the observation that this age group is at increased risk for fatal allergic reactions.

Therefore, peer and patient education is suggested to improve safety for adolescents. Physicians can encourage parents to request to meet with key school staff members who have responsibility for the care of their child and to work cooperatively with schools to ensure their child's safety. Key staff members may include the school nurse, principal, and directors of transportation and food service, and classroom teachers. Avoidance strategies and emergency management must also be communicated to personnel who may not have primary responsibilities for the student, such as coaches, specialty teachers (art, music), substitute teachers, and field trip personnel. These individuals should also be familiar with emergency plans, should be trained to use epinephrine autoinjectors, and should recognize indicators for activating the emergency medical response system.

It may be helpful to counsel parents about the degree and manner of exposure that might be dangerous for a specific child, such as ingestion versus inhalation or touching food residues, so that parents are appropriately vigilant without becoming needlessly hypervigilant or anxious about avoidance strategies. Care must be taken not to ostracize or physically separate the child with food allergies. For example, an "allergen-aware" table should include the child's friends who are eating safe meals. Experts have not espoused blanket "bans" on foods, particularly because peanut butter, milk, egg, and other common allergens may be a protein staple of another child's diet. In specific cases, individual schools or classrooms might pursue these options. For example, removal of highly allergenic foods from the vicinity of very young children or children with significant developmental disabilities might be warranted when transfer of the allergen among the children is likely. Schools may choose to ban children from bringing food from home to share with classmates for celebratory functions and may offer acceptable alternative options. Table 12.11 provides suggestions to reduce accidental ingestion of allergens. Management of food allergy is similar for schools and camps. However, the persons providing supervision in camps may be young and inexperienced, necessitating

TABLE 12.11	Preventive Measures to Reduce Risk of Allergen Ingestion in School Settings	
Setting	**Measures**
School-wide	Institute policy on no food sharing or trading.
	Educate teachers, including substitutes, coaches, special program teachers, and cafeteria staff.
	Consider allergen-safe cafeteria tables or schools, depending on student ages and needs (supervision, selective allergen exclusion).
	Enforce strict no-bullying policies.
Selected classroom	Allow no food in craft projects.
	Reduce food rewards, and provide a substitute.
	Maintain safe, nonperishable snacks as substitute, if needed.
	Consider 'bans,' depending on food (peanut) and age.
	Encourage handwashing.
School bus	Permit no eating or food parties.
	Have communication device for emergency calls.
	Allow younger child to sit at front.

additional safeguards, such as additional supervision at mealtimes or having more experienced supervisors available when away from first-aid and nursing services.

Nutritional Issues

Allergen avoidance diets can result in failure to thrive and deficiencies in specific macronutrients and micronutrients. These concerns, in addition to the daily lifestyle impact of following avoidance diets, underscore the importance of having an accurate diagnosis to allow the broadest diet possible.[71] Additionally, food aversion and anxiety may result in insufficient nutrient intake. Food allergy–related disorders such as EoE may be associated with poor appetite and early satiety, and children with untreated food allergy–related atopic dermatitis may experience malabsorption and increased energy needs from skin damage. Therefore, addressing nutritional concerns may require a multifaceted approach, including consultation with a registered dietitian. Nutritional counseling and regular growth monitoring are recommended for children with food allergies.

Nutritional deficits caused by allergen-restricted diets include poor caloric intake (proteins, carbohydrates, fats) and insufficient vitamins, minerals, and trace elements. Many sources of protein, including milk, egg, soy, fish, shellfish, peanut, and tree nuts, are also common allergens. The *acceptable macronutrient distribution range* (AMDR) for protein is 5% to 20% for children 1 to 3 years of age, 10% to 30% for children 4 to 18 years of age, and 10% to 35% for adults. Quality proteins that include essential amino acids are typically obtained from meats. Complementary foods (e.g., rice, beans) may be needed for those who are vegetarian or meat allergic. The AMDR for fat is 25% to 35% of total energy intake for older children and adults (30%–40% for children 1 to 3 years of age). Essential fatty acids (linoleic and linolenic) are found in fish. However, essential fatty acids are also available in vegetable oils such as canola, corn, soy, and olive. The diet should consist of a blend of saturated fats,

TABLE 12.12 Nutritional Concerns and Substitutions for Diets Devoid of Select Allergens[a]

Allergen	Key Nutrients	Substitutions
Milk	Protein, fat, calcium, vitamin A, vitamin D, vitamin B_{12}	Meats, fish, or poultry (protein, fat, vitamin B_{12}); fortified soy drinks (calcium, protein, vitamins D and B_{12}), legumes (protein), avocado (fat), enriched milks from rice, almond, oat or fortified juices (calcium; vitamins D, A, and B_{12}), dark-green leafy vegetables (vitamin A)[b]
Soy	Protein, thiamine, folate, magnesium, phosphorus, zinc, riboflavin, iron	Meat (protein, thiamine, phosphorus, iron); other legumes (protein, thiamine, folate, iron); fish (protein, phosphorus, iron); dark-green leafy vegetables (riboflavin, folate); whole grains (thiamine, riboflavin, folate, magnesium, iron); alternative fortified "milks" (see previous entry)
Wheat	Carbohydrates, fiber, niacin, riboflavin, iron, folate	Enriched flours, including rice, oat, corn, and potato (carbohydrates, niacin, thiamine, riboflavin, iron, folate); fruits and vegetables (fiber, carbohydrates); meat (niacin, iron, thiamine); leafy green vegetables (riboflavin, folate)
Egg	Protein, vitamin B_{12}, selenium, biotin	Meat/fish (protein, vitamin B_{12}, selenium), soy (protein, biotin)

[a]This table cannot be used in isolation to construct adequate nutritional plans.
[b]Adults can obtain calcium and vitamin D from nondairy sources (fortified juices, alternative "milks" and supplements). However, infants and children require a replacement source of fat and protein and fortified juices or rice milk are otherwise insufficient; complete fortified nutritional formulas (soy, casein hydrolysates, amino acid–based, etc.) may suffice, but children avoiding milk/soy may benefit from more complete dietary assessments. A diet devoid of egg, peanut, fish, or shellfish is typically easily substituted with other protein sources.

which are usually obtained from animal origin, but also monosaturated and polyunsaturated fats, which are components of vegetable oils. The AMDR for carbohydrate is 45% to 65% of total caloric intake. Carbohydrates, particularly grains, contribute to dietary fiber, iron, thiamine, niacin, riboflavin, and folic acid. Micronutrients include vitamins, minerals, and trace elements. The Department of Agriculture maintains documents regarding dietary recommendations via www.usda.gov or www.choosemyplate.gov. Table 12.12 describes nutritional concerns and possible solutions for diets devoid of some of the key common allergens.

EMERGENCY MANAGEMENT

The emergency management of food-induced anaphylaxis is similar to the treatment of anaphylaxis from any cause (see Chapter 13). Any food can potentially trigger anaphylaxis, but peanut, tree nuts, milk, fish, and shellfish appear to account for most of the episodes leading to fatalities.[53,72] Prompt recognition of anaphylaxis and treatment with epinephrine are crucial for a good outcome. In a study of 45 episodes of anaphylaxis in children, those who received epinephrine early were less likely to require hospital admission (14% versus 47%, respectively; $p < 0.05$).[73] Box 12.4 lists risk factors for fatal food-induced anaphylaxis and comorbid conditions that increase risk. The treatment of severe reactions caused by FPIES is different and involves intravenous hydration and corticosteroids, although proof for the efficacy of the latter is lacking.

Recognition of Reactions

Patients diagnosed with potentially severe food allergies, and their caretakers, must be educated regarding recognition of reactions. Signs, symptoms, and time course should be reviewed, as well as when and how to inject epinephrine and alert emergency services. Anaphylaxis caused by food allergy may occur without urticaria or skin symptoms in up to 20% of patients, which

BOX 12.4 Risks for Fatal Food Anaphylaxis and Comorbid Conditions

Risks Associated with Fatal Food Anaphylaxis
- Delayed treatment with epinephrine
- Allergy to peanut, tree nuts, fish, or shellfish
- Adolescent or young adult
- Asthma
- Cardiovascular disease in middle-aged or older patient
- Lack of skin symptoms

Comorbid Conditions Associated With Increased Food Anaphylaxis Risk or That Affect Severity or Treatment
- Asthma
- Exercise
- Alcohol
- Mastocytosis
- Chronic lung disease
- Medications:
  - pH lowering drugs
  - Nonsteroidal antiinflammatory drugs
  - β-Adrenergic antagonists
  - Angiotensin-converting enzyme (ACE) inhibitors
  - α-Adrenergic blockers

may account for delays in treatment leading to poor outcomes. Additionally, biphasic reactions, with recurrence of symptoms several hours after resolution of initial reactions, are described in 1% to 20% of patients. Given the possibility of biphasic reactions, victims of food-induced anaphylaxis should remain under medical observation for 4 to 6 hours or longer after anaphylaxis to ensure that symptoms have subsided.

Treatment With Epinephrine and Antihistamines

Although antihistamines are indicated to treat symptoms such as urticaria or oral pruritus, dependence on antihistamines is a common reason for delaying anaphylaxis treatment with epinephrine, which may result in an increased risk of a progressively severe reaction. Patients and caregivers should be counseled on the appropriate use of self-injectable epinephrine and not to depend on antihistamines or bronchodilators for treatment of anaphylaxis. Repeated doses of epinephrine may be needed in 10% to 20% of episodes of food-induced anaphylaxis.[51] Prompt transfer to a facility capable of managing anaphylaxis should be sought. Patients and families should understand that although subsequent reactions are not necessarily more severe than initial reactions, they can be. For example, initial mild reactions to peanut may be followed by more severe reactions on subsequent exposures. Similarly, specific IgE levels do not predict the severity of a reaction. Epinephrine autoinjectors may be prescribed for anyone diagnosed with a food allergy but definitely *should* be prescribed for patients with a prior history of anaphylaxis, those with food allergy and asthma, and those with a known food allergy to potent allergens such as peanut, tree nuts, fish, and shellfish.

Emergency Plans and Special Considerations for School

Patients with potentially severe food allergies should be given a written emergency plan that describes when to inject epinephrine and instructions on how to self-inject. (The prescriptions of epinephrine, plans for monitoring expiration dates of autoinjectors, avoidance measures, and follow-up instructions are detailed in Chapter 13.) Autoinjector dosing is limited, in general two doses are available: the 0.15 mg dose is recommended for children weighing 10 to 25 kg (22–55 lb) and the 0.3 mg dose for those over 25 kg. In the US, 0.1 mg autoinjector is available for infants weighing less than 10 kg, and in Europe, a 0.5 mg autoinjector is available for those weighing more than 45 kg.

There are special considerations for treating children in schools or camps. The family must notify the school about the child's potentially life-threatening food allergy and provide written treatment plans, including the child's name, identifying information (child's photograph, if possible), specifics about the food allergies, symptoms and treatments, instructions to activate emergency services, and medical and family contact information. In some circumstances, a child may be allowed to carry autoinjectors and to self-inject, but a supervising adult should have the primary responsibility to recognize and treat anaphylaxis. In the school setting, this is ideally a health professional, but a delegate might be needed. Epinephrine autoinjectors should be available promptly in the event of anaphylaxis. Children should be encouraged to wear medical identification jewelry. Because 25% of anaphylaxis episodes in schools occur without a previous diagnosis, a prescription for unassigned epinephrine for general use, consistent with district regulations and state laws, should be considered. When to inject epinephrine can be confusing for lay personnel. The safety of the drug should be emphasized such that injections should be given if there is suspicion of anaphylaxis. It may be advisable to inject epinephrine at the time of first symptoms if an allergen was ingested that previously caused anaphylaxis, or before symptoms if an allergen was ingested that previously caused severe anaphylaxis with cardiovascular collapse.[74]

TABLE 12.13	Changes in Notions About Allergy Prevention Through Diet
Prior Notion/ Recommendation (For Those at Risk for Atopy)	Recent Notions/ Recommendations
Avoid peanut during pregnancy	No proof of effectiveness
Avoid food allergens during lactation	Possible reduction in atopic dermatitis, no evidence regarding food allergy
Breastfeeding exclusively for 3–4 months	May protect for atopy, but evidence is modest; lack of evidence for food allergy prevention
Alternative hypoallergenic formulas	May protect for atopy, but evidence is modest; lack of evidence for food allergy prevention
Delay complementary foods until 4–6 months	Lack of evidence to prevent atopic disease
Avoid allergens: milk to age 1 year; egg to 2 years; and peanut, nuts, and fish to 3 years	Early introduction of allergenic foods at 4–6 months protect against development of peanut and egg allergy

Prevention of Food Allergy

Considering the global burden of food allergy, there is a significant interest in strategies to prevent its development. Given the known benefits of breastfeeding, it is globally recommended as the preferred infant nutrition in the first 4 to 6 months of life in the absence of other contraindications. The current WHO guideline on breastfeeding was implemented in 2001 and recommends exclusive breastfeeding until 6 months of life and continuation of breastfeeding until 2 years of age and beyond (https://www.who.int/nutrition/topics/en/, accessed online on August 30, 2020). However, the available evidence does not support the notion that breastfeeding is protective against food allergy (Table 12.13).[75–77]

Trials based on the hypothesis that early introduction of peanut takes advantage of the oral tolerance pathways activated by ingestion that precedes the potential sensitization to peanut via the disrupted skin barrier changed the previous prevention paradigm (Fig. 12.3).[78–80] The 2015 landmark Learning Early About Peanut Allergy (LEAP) study established that early introduction to peanut and continued consumption in an infant population at high risk of allergy (severe eczema and or egg allergy) was associated with an 81% relative risk reduction of peanut allergy at 60 months of age (p < 0.0005). In addition, the Enquiring About Tolerance (EAT) study randomized breastfed infants not selected for high risk of allergy to early introduction of six allergens, including milk, egg, peanut, sesame, fish and wheat with a goal ingestion of 4 grams/week of each food.[81] Only 43% of the participants randomized to the early introduction group adhered to the protocol, but the per-protocol analysis showed a comparative reduction of allergy to peanut (standard 2.5% versus early introduction 0%, p = 0.003) and egg (standard 5.5% versus early introduction 1.4%, p = 0.009) Box 12.5.[82] A 2016 metaanalysis concluded with a moderate degree of certainty

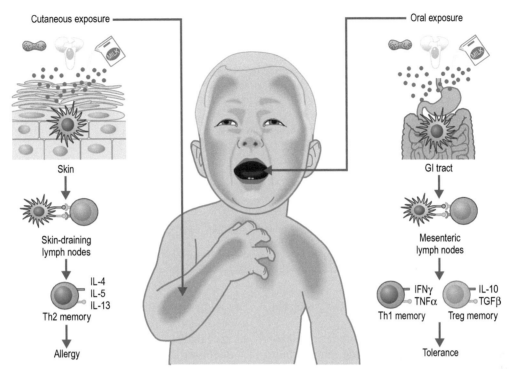

Fig. 12.3 Dual-allergen-exposure hypothesis for pathogenesis of food allergy. Tolerance occurs as a result of oral exposure to food, and allergic sensitization results from cutaneous exposure. *GI*, Gastrointestinal; *IFN-γ*, interferon-γ; *TGF-β*, transforming growth factor beta; *Th2*, T helper type 2 lymphocyte; *TNF-α*, tumor necrosis factor alpha; *Treg*, T regulatory lymphocyte. (Modified from Lack G. Epidemiologic risks of food allergy. J Allergy Clin Immunol 2008;121:1331–1336.)

BOX 12.5 Allergy Prevention Studies

LEAP Study (Learning Early About Peanut Allergy: www.leapstudy.co.uk[79,80])

- In total, 640 high-risk children were enrolled at age 4 to 11 months.
- Each child was randomized to an avoidance group (complete avoidance of peanut-containing foods) or a consumption group (consume a peanut snack three times a week; 6 g of peanut protein/week) for 60 months.
- Among 530 infants in the intention-to-treat population who initially had negative results on the skin-prick test, the prevalence of peanut allergy at 60 months of age was 13.7% in the avoidance group and 1.9% in the consumption group ($p < 0.001$).
- Among 98 participants in the intention-to-treat population who initially had positive test results, the prevalence of peanut allergy was 35.3% in the avoidance group and 10.6% in the consumption group ($p = 0.004$).

LEAP-On[80]

At the end of LEAP trial, all the participants were instructed to avoid peanuts for 12 months.

556 of 628 eligible participants (88.5%) from LEAP enrolled into LEAP-On.

Adherence to avoidance was high: 90.4% in the peanut-avoidance group and 69.3% in the peanut-consumption group.

Peanut allergy at 72 months was significantly more prevalent in the peanut-avoidance than in the peanut-consumption group (18.6% [52 of 280 participants] versus 4.8% [13 of 270], $P < 0.001$).

Three new cases of allergy developed in each group, but after 12 months of avoidance there was no significant increase in the prevalence of allergy in the consumption group (3.6% [10 of 274 participants] at 60 months and 4.8% [13 of 270] at 72 months, $p = 0.25$).

Fewer participants in the peanut-consumption group than in the peanut-avoidance group had high levels of Ara h2 (a component of peanut protein)–specific IgE and peanut-specific IgE; in addition, participants in the peanut-consumption group continued to have a higher level of peanut-specific IgG$_4$ and a higher peanut-specific IgG$_4$:IgE ratio.

EAT Study (Enquiring About Tolerance: www.eatstudy.co.uk[81])

- Infants ($n = 1302$) were randomized to one of two groups.
- In one group ($n = 651$), six allergenic foods (peanut, cooked egg, cow's milk, sesame, whitefish, and wheat) were introduced from 3 months of age, while the infant continued to breastfeed (early introduction group).
- The other group ($n = 651$) followed current UK government weaning advice: aim for exclusive breastfeeding for 6 months (standard weaning group).
- The children were monitored until 3 years of age to see whether early diet has an effect in reducing the prevalence of food allergy, as determined by double-blind, placebo-controlled food challenges.

(Continued)

BOX 12.5   Allergy Prevention Studies—cont'd

Results

Intention-to-treat analysis: food allergy to one or more of the six intervention foods developed in 7.1% of the participants in the standard-introduction (42 of 595 participants) and in 5.6% of those in the early introduction group (32 of 567) ($p = 0.32$).

  Per-protocol analysis: the prevalence of any food allergy was significantly lower in the early introduction than in the standard-introduction group (2.4% versus 7.3%, $p = 0.01$), as was the prevalence of peanut allergy (0% versus 2.5%, $p = 0.003$) and egg allergy (1.4% versus 5.5%, $p = 0.009$); there were no significant effects with respect to milk, sesame, fish, or wheat.

  The consumption of 2 g per week of peanut or egg-white protein was associated with a significantly lower prevalence of these respective allergies than was less consumption.

Issues with adherence[99]

Adherence was 92.9% in the standard-introduction versus 42.8% in the early introduction group.

  Four factors accounted for 78% of the nonadherence:

- non-White race (odds ratio [OR], 2.21; 95% CI, 1.18 to 4.14)
- parentally perceived symptoms in the child related to any of the early introduction foods (OR, 1.70; 95% CI, 1.02 to 2.86)
- reduced maternal quality of life (psychological domain) (OR, 0.69; 95% CI, 0.47 to 1.00)
- the presence of eczema in the child at enrollment (OR, 1.38; 95% CI, 0.87 to 2.19).

that introduction of egg between 4 and 6 months was associated with reduced egg allergy.[83]

The findings of these studies prompted the updated guidelines throughout the world, recommending early introduction of peanut in most countries, including the US, and early introduction of egg in other countries, including Australia and the UK. The Task Force of the EAACI suggests introducing well-cooked egg into the infant diet as part of complementary feeding and introducing peanut in age-appropriate forms in populations with a high prevalence of peanut allergy. They further state that the best age to introduce egg and peanut is from 4 to 6 months of life.[84] In the US, the most recent American Academy of Pediatrics guidance states there is no evidence that delaying the introduction of allergenic foods beyond 4 to 6 months of age prevents atopic disease and that early introduction of peanut may prevent peanut allergy.[75] The National Institutes of Allergy and Infectious Diseases Addendum Guidelines published in January of 2017 recommend introducing peanut between 4 and 6 months of age in those with severe eczema or egg allergy after other solids have been introduced and after physician evaluation, around 6 months of age for those with moderate eczema, and according to family and cultural practices for those without additional risk of peanut allergy.

Another direction in food allergy prevention focuses on meticulous skin care and restoration of the skin barrier to minimize transcutaneous exposure to allergens in the environment, but the results from two large randomized clinical trials (BEEP and PreventADALL) do not support this hypothesis.[85,86]

Future Therapeutic Strategies

The apparent rising prevalence of food allergies, lack of effective prevention strategies, and inadequate treatment that relies on allergen avoidance and injection of epinephrine for anaphylaxis have considerably increased the urgency to develop effective treatments. There are no therapies proven to accelerate the development of oral tolerance or provide effective protection from accidental exposures. However, novel allergen-specific and allergen-nonspecific approaches to food allergy therapy are being developed and studied. Both allergen-specific therapies

and more generalized immunomodulatory approaches are under investigation in animal and human models of food allergy (Table 12.14).

Because it is important to delineate the responses to therapeutic interventions, the terms *desensitization* and *tolerance* are often used to better define the clinical and immunologic state during therapy (Box 12.6). Desensitization is defined as temporary state of increased threshold for allergic reactions while immunotherapy is ongoing. The ultimate goal of effective immunotherapy is long-term tolerance induction through active immunomodulation to promote regulatory T cell development and immunologic skewing away from the classic Th2 response seen with many of the emerging therapies (Fig. 12.4).[87]

Oral immunotherapy (OIT) has been studied for several years in clinical trials and has accumulated the most convincing evidence for effectiveness among emerging therapies for food allergy. OIT is associated with a robust response to therapy, but with limitations related to its side effects profile. Early open-label trials have shown a beneficial response to OIT with a variety of allergens, including milk, egg, and fish, with evidence of clinical desensitization in up to 80% of patients treated.

The concepts of clinical desensitization and tolerance have been more fully explored in recent studies. Current OIT protocols are typically conducted using an allergen powder ingested in a food vehicle and consist of the following three phases:

1. Modified rush desensitization, with six to eight doses of allergen given under observation in rapid succession during day 1 to obtain a relative "desensitized state."
2. Dosing buildup, with a daily dose of the food protein at home with scheduled dose escalations under observation every 1 to 2 weeks until a target dose is reached.
3. Home maintenance therapy, with daily ingestion of a target dose (typically for years).

These phases are sometimes followed by OFC to assess clinical desensitization (while receiving therapy) and functional tolerance/sustained unresponsiveness (SU) (while off therapy on diet restriction). Clinical desensitization has been well documented in open-label studies for peanut, milk, and egg, with success rates ranging from 75% to 100% after 1 to 2 years of therapy.

TABLE 12.14　Emerging Therapies for Food Allergy[a]

Therapy	Use	Stage of Study	Allergen Studied
Allergen-Nonspecific Therapy			
Anti-IgE therapy (omalizumab)	Treatment	Human phase I–III	Peanut, milk, multi-food; monotherapy or combined with OIT
Anti-IL-4/IL-13 receptor monoclonal antibody (dupilumab)	Treatment	Human phase II–III	Peanut; monotherapy or combined with OIT
Anti-IL-33	Treatment	Human phase II	Peanut
Bruton's tyrosine kinase inhibitor (ibrutinib)	Treatment	Human phase II	Peanut
Probiotic mix (VE416); clonal human commensal bacterial strains selected for their ability to suppress allergic responses and manufactured under cGMP conditions	Treatment	Human phase I–II	Peanut; monotherapy or combined with OIT
Lactobacillus rhamnosus CGMCC 1.3724 (NCC4007)	Treatment	Human phase II–III	Peanut; combined with OIT
Traditional Chinese Medicine	Treatment	Human phase I–II	Peanut, tree nut, fish, shellfish, sesame
Probiotics	Prevention	Longitudinal study	Nonspecific
Prebiotics	Prevention	Longitudinal study	Nonspecific
Allergen-specific Therapy			
Subcutaneous IT	Treatment	Human phase I (aborted due to safety)	Peanut
Oral IT	Treatment	Human phase I–III	Peanut, milk, egg, wheat, fish, fruits
Heated antigen	Treatment	Human phase I–II	Egg, milk
Sublingual IT	Treatment	Human phase I–II	Peanut, milk, hazelnut, kiwi, peach
Epicutaneous IT	Treatment	Human phase I–III	Peanut, milk
Recombinant protein IT with adjuvants	Treatment	Human phase I–II	Peanut
Engineered allergen IT	Treatment	Phase I–II	Peanut

cGMP, Current Good Manufacturing Practice; *IL*, Interleukin; *IT*, immunotherapy.
[a]For detailed information on clinical trials, see clinicaltrials.gov.

BOX 12.6　The Clinical Outcomes of Food Immunotherapy

Desensitization
- A change in threshold dose of ingested allergen required to induce allergic symptoms after food exposure occurring while on therapy.
- This is a reversible state typically induced by allergen exposure, in which effector cells are rendered less reactive or nonreactive by daily uninterrupted administration of allergen.
- Discontinuation of therapy leads to gradual loss of desensitization.
- It can be achieved by the majority of the treated patients.
- Desensitization can be vulnerable to augmentation factors (e.g., acute febrile illness, dosing on empty stomach, exercise, menstruation, etc.).

Tolerance
- The long-lasting effects of treatment, presumably due to effects on T cell responsiveness that persist after the treatment is stopped.
- The immunomodulatory effects of desensitization can be seen early in the course of immunotherapy; however, evidence suggests that the length of time to reach tolerance varies with the type and amount of specific food allergen, the duration of therapy, and the individual patient.

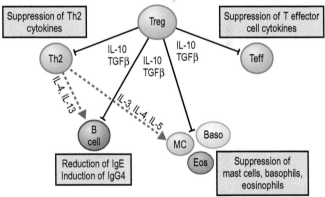

Fig. 12.4 Food allergy treatments modulate the food-allergic response through activation of regulatory T cells and suppression of a variety of effector cell types. *Baso*, Basophil; *Eos*, eosinophil; *IL*, interleukin; *MC*, mast cell; *Teff*, T effector lymphocyte; *TGF-β*, transforming growth factor beta; *Th2*, T helper type 2 lymphocyte; *Treg*, T regulatory lymphocyte.

While early desensitization is associated with decreased reactivity of effector cells, for example, mast cells and basophils, due to systemic exposure to minute quantities of allergen, longer-term desensitization has been associated with immunomodulation with reduced markers of mast cell (skin tests) and basophil activation, changes in IgE and IgG profiles, reduced Th2 cytokine profile, and activation of Tregs (Table 12.15).[87]

The prevailing question is whether OIT induces *tolerance*, not just desensitization. The longest study of peanut-OIT treated 50 subjects with daily maintenance dose of 4 mg of

TABLE 12.15 Immunologic Changes in IgE-Mediated Food Allergy Compared With Effective Immunotherapy

Immune parameters	Food Allergy	Effective Immunotherapy
Serum IgE	↑	↓
Serum IgG$_4$	↔	↑
Mast cell reactivity	↑	↓
Basophil activation	↑	↓
Helper T cell (Th2) cytokines	↑	↓
Regulatory T cell activation	↓	↑

BOX 12.7 Side Effects Reported in the Trials of Food Oral Immunotherapy

- *Common*: Mild to moderate, predominantly oropharyngeal pruritus and gastrointestinal (discomfort, pain, nausea, diarrhea, vomiting) side effects are most common, and easily treated.
- *Rare*: More severe reactions have been rarely reported, including generalized urticaria/angioedema, wheezing/respiratory distress, laryngeal edema, and repetitive emesis.
- *Discontinuation of therapy*: Of participants treated with OIT, about 20% experienced dose-limiting GI side effects, preventing continuation of therapy.
- *Augmentation factors*: Viral infections, menses, dosing on empty stomach, hot showers, and exercise have been associated with lowering the reaction threshold for subjects receiving stable OIT dosing. These often require temporary interruption of dosing and dose adjustments to compensate for illness.

peanut protein for an average 3 years.[88] At the end of the treatment period, 50% of the subjects were able to safely ingest a full serving of peanut (5 g of peanut protein) after 1 month of stopping the daily dosing. In a single center, phase II clinical trial of peanut OIT with high daily maintenance dose 4000 mg of peanut protein for 2 years, 35% of participants (median age 11 years) maintained the ability to ingest 4000 mg of peanut protein without allergic symptoms following 3 months of discontinuation of OIT and strict peanut avoidance.[89] Following the successful phase III clinical trial, in early 2020, the US FDA approved the first commercial biologic drug for peanut OIT, for children 4 to 17 years old at the time of the initiation and with the indication of "the mitigation of allergic reactions, including anaphylaxis that may occur with accidental exposure to peanut" (https://www.fda.gov/vaccines-blood-biologics/allergenics/palforzia; accessed 9/1/2020).[90] In combination, the results from several studies suggest SU is possible in at least a portion of patients; however, further study is needed to determine the duration of unresponsiveness and the persistence of immunomodulation.

Clinical trials using OIT have focused primarily on single-allergen delivery to impact single-food allergy. In a small phase II clinical trial, 48 participants, aged 4 to 15 years, with multi-food allergies validated by DBPCFCs were treated with multi-food OIT to two to five foods, together with omalizumab ($n = 36$) or with placebo ($n = 12$). Omalizumab or placebo was administered subcutaneously for 16 weeks with OIT starting at week 8; omalizumab or placebo was stopped 20 weeks before exit DBPCFCs (week 36) to determine the primary endpoint: the proportion of participants who passed DBPCFCs to at least 2 of their offending foods. At week 36, a significantly greater proportion of the omalizumab (30/36, 83%) versus placebo (4/12, 33%) participants passed DBPCFCs to 2 g protein for ≥2 of their offending foods (odds ratio [OR]: 10, 95% confidence interval CI]: 1.8, 58.3, $p = 0.004$), suggesting that omalizumab improves the efficacy of multi-food OIT and enables safe and rapid desensitization.[91] Large multicenter studies evaluating multi-food OIT are ongoing.

Although OIT has demonstrated significant clinical successes, safety remains a concern for wide-scale implementation (Box 12.7).[92]

Extensively Heated Milk and Egg Protein

A possible alternative or treatment adjunct to OIT is the use of crude, heat-denatured allergen. Because high-temperature cooking of egg and milk proteins results in conformational changes of native protein structure and reduced IgE binding, some children with milk or egg allergy may tolerate baked products.

Two clinical trials have been conducted in milk-allergic and egg-allergic children. The results suggest that up to 80% of milk-allergic or egg-allergic children can safely ingest extensively heated milk products in a muffin or egg products in a waffle.[93] OFC was done to confirm the allergy and ability to tolerate the baked product. Side effects were negligible, and no subjects who tolerated the baked product required epinephrine during OFC, although 35% of baked milk-reactive subjects and 19% of baked egg-reactive subjects did. Clinical successes were associated with reduced allergen-specific IgE and SPT, increased allergen-specific IgG$_4$, and activated Tregs. Similar findings were noted in ovalbumin (OVA)-sensitized mice treated with heated OVA or ovomucoid. Heat treatment reduced allergenicity of the egg antigens through enhanced GI digestibility and reduced absorption in a form capable of triggering basophils.

These findings suggest that ingestion of extensively heated egg or milk products may serve as a safe and effective treatment modality, although less efficacious than OIT.[94] In a head-to-head comparison between a baked egg diet versus egg OIT, baked egg tolerant, nonbaked egg-reactive children, ages 3 to 16 years were randomized to 2 years of treatment with either baked egg diet or egg OIT.[95] Double-blind, placebo-controlled food challenges were conducted after 1 and 2 years of treatment to assess for desensitization, and after 2 years of treatment followed by 8 to 10 weeks off of treatment to assess for SU (a surrogate for permanent tolerance). SU was achieved in 3 of 27 participants assigned to baked egg diet (11.1%) versus 10 of 23 participants assigned to egg OIT (43.5%) ($p = 0.009$).

Questions remain about the dose required for efficacy, degree of heating needed, role of the food matrix in the observed response, ability of extensively heated proteins to induce lasting tolerance, and the role of heated allergens as treatment adjuncts to other forms of immunotherapy.

TABLE 12.16 Comparison of OIT, SLIT, and EPIT

	OIT	SLIT	EPIT
Typical daily dose	300–4000 mg	2–7 mg	250 mcg
Predominant side effects	Oral, gastrointestinal (systemic increases with infection, exercise, menses)	Oropharyngeal	Local cutaneous: pruritus, eczematous rash
Desensitization	Large effect	Lesser effect	Lesser effect
Functional tolerance	Effective in subset of patients	Unknown to date	Unknown to date
Immunomodulation	Significant	Modest	Modest

EPIT, Epicutaneous immunotherapy; *OIT*, oral immunotherapy; *SLIT*, sublingual immunotherapy.

Sublingual Immunotherapy

Sublingual immunotherapy (SLIT) has shown efficacy for treatment of inhalant allergies and asthma. In the treatment of aeroallergens, SLIT has clinical advantages similar to subcutaneous immunotherapy (SCIT), but lower risks for severe, fatal reactions. SLIT employs a liquid concentrate administered sublingually in small, increasing doses in a controlled setting coupled with home dosing to reach a target maintenance dose. SLIT-tablet preparations are in frequent use for inhalant allergies in Europe and Australia. Although the mechanism of action is not fully elucidated, data suggest that it is similar to that in other forms of immunotherapy. In a single center clinical trial, children with peanut allergy aged 1 to 11 years underwent extended maintenance SLIT with 2 mg/d peanut protein for up to 5 years.[96] Thirty-seven of 48 subjects completed 3 to 5 years of peanut SLIT, with 67% (32/48) successfully consuming 750 mg or more peanut protein during DBPCFCs. Furthermore, 25% (12/48) passed the 5000-mg DBPCFC (equivalent to a full serving of peanut) without clinical symptoms, with 10 of these 12 demonstrating SU after 2 to 4 weeks. Side effects were reported with 4.8% of doses (mild, oral), only 0.21% were treated with antihistamines, and no epinephrine was administered. Extended-therapy peanut SLIT provided clinically meaningful desensitization in the majority of children with peanut allergy that was accompanied by ease of administration and generally a favorable safety profile.

Epicutaneous Immunotherapy

Epicutaneous immunotherapy (EPIT) acts by delivering a very small dose of allergenic protein directly to the epidermal layer of the skin. In a phase III pivotal clinical trial (PEPITES), children 4 to 11 years with peanut allergy applied peanut patch containing either 250 µg of peanut protein (n = 238) or placebo (n = 118) daily for 12 months.[97] The primary outcome was the percentage difference in responders between the peanut patch and placebo patch based on eliciting dose (highest dose at which objective signs/symptoms of an immediate hypersensitivity reaction developed) determined by food challenges at baseline and month 12. Among 356 participants (median age, 7 years; 61.2% male), 89.9% completed the trial; with the mean treatment adherence 98.5%. The response rate was 35.3% with peanut-patch treatment and 13.6% with placebo (difference, 21.7% [95% CI, 12.4%–29.8%; p < 0.001]). However, the prespecified lower bound of the 95% CI threshold was not met. Subjects who completed PEPITES were offered enrollment in an open-label

extension study. Following an additional 2 years of daily peanut patch 250 µg, subjects underwent month-36 DBPCFC. Of 213 eligible subjects who had received peanut patch in PEPITES, 198 (93%) entered the extension study and 141 (71%) had completed DBPCFC at month 36.[98] At month 36, 51.8% of subjects (73 of 141) reached an eliciting dose of ≥1000 mg, compared with 40.4% (57 of 141) at month 12; 75.9% (107 of 141) demonstrated increased eliciting dose compared with baseline; and 13.5% (19 of 141) tolerated the full DBPCFC of 5444 mg. Median cumulative reactive dose increased from 144 (equivalent to 1/2 peanut) to 944 mg (equivalent to approximately three peanuts). Local patch-site skin reactions were common and decreased over time. There was no treatment-related epinephrine use in years 2 or 3. Treatment adherence was high (96.9%), and withdrawals due to treatment-related adverse events were low (1%). The peanut patch is undergoing review by the US FDA at this time.

Although OIT, SLIT, and EPIT can confer benefits to patients, these therapies differ in dosing limitations, effectiveness, side effects, and extent of immunomodulation (Table 12.16).[92] Even when effective, these forms of therapy will not likely be applicable and/or acceptable across all ages and risk categories of food allergies, and thus specific paradigms and alternate treatments are needed. Various allergen-nonspecific therapies, for example, monoclonal antibodies directed against IgE (omalizumab), IL-4/IL-13 receptor (dupilumab), IL-33, Bruton's tyrosine kinase (ibrutinib), as well as probiotics are under active investigation, either as monotherapy or in combination with OIT.

CONCLUSIONS

Ingested foods represent the greatest foreign antigenic load confronting the human immune system. In the vast majority of individuals, tolerance develops to food antigens, which are constantly gaining access to the body proper. However, when tolerance fails to develop, the immune system responds with an allergic reaction. Allergic reactions to milk were first described by Hippocrates more than 2000 years ago; however, it is only in the past few decades that food allergy has emerged as an important public health problem affecting people of all ages in societies with a Western lifestyle, such as the US, Canada, the UK, Australia, and Western Europe. Allergies to food affect up to 8% of children under 5 years of age and approximately 3.5% of the general population. Inadvertent ingestion of food allergens may provoke various GI, cutaneous, respiratory symptoms, and/or systemic anaphylaxis with shock.

Food allergy guidelines have been developed to help facilitate uniform approaches to diagnosis and management. While OFCs remain the standard for food allergy diagnosis, skin-prick testing and detection of specific IgE directed against complete foods and specific allergenic components are useful noninvasive tools.

Current therapy for food allergy requires education about avoidance in a variety of settings and instructions on when and how to treat inevitable allergic reactions. These approaches require constant vigilance and affect quality of life. Increasing attention has therefore focused on primary prevention and improved therapies, with a shift in our approach to the prevention of food allergy. Previous guidelines on food allergen avoidance during pregnancy, breastfeeding, and infancy have been questioned. The relationship between allergen exposure and development of food allergy is complex. Allergen exposure through a disrupted skin barrier may be involved in establishing allergy, whereas allergen exposure through the GI mucosa may be involved in establishing tolerance. Immune responses to such allergen exposures are likely to be modulated by nonspecific factors, such as GI microflora, infectious exposure, other dietary factors, and possibly sunlight exposure.

Interventional trials are in progress and in the next few years should help to determine the relative contribution of these different factors and allow us to reduce the burden caused by food allergy. Advances in our understanding of the immunologic mechanisms underlying food allergy and the complexities of the mucosal immune response have resulted in substantial progress toward definitive therapeutic options for food-allergic individuals. Current therapeutic strategies are focused on harnessing oral tolerance to modulate the allergic response using antigen-specific and antigen-nonspecific approaches. Although significant gains and positive clinical and immunomodulatory insights have been appreciated, these approaches are often associated with significant risk and unanswered long-term safety and efficacy questions. Ongoing studies will fill our current therapeutic knowledge gaps and carefully move toward broader clinical application in the future.

REFERENCES

1. *Renz H, Allen KJ, Sicherer SH, et al. Food allergy. Nat Rev Dis Prim. 2018;4:17098.
2. *Sicherer SH, Warren CM, Dant C, Gupta RS, Nadeau KC. Food allergy from infancy through adulthood. J Allergy Climmunol Pract. 2020;8:1854–1864.
3. Gupta RS, Warren CM, Smith BM, et al. Prevalence and severity of food allergies among US adults. JAMA Netw Open. 2019;2:e185630.
4. Gupta RS, Warren CM, Smith BM, et al. The public health impact of parent-reported childhood food allergies in the United States. Pediatrics. 2018;142:e20181235.
5. Branum AM, Lukacs SL. Food allergy among children in the United States. Pediatrics. 2009;124:1549–1555.
6. Osborne NJ, Koplin JJ, Martin PE, et al. Prevalence of challenge-proven IgE-mediated food allergy using population-based sampling and predetermined challenge criteria in infants. J Allergy Clin Immunol. 2011;127:668–676. e1-e2.
7. Bunyavanich S, Rifas-Shiman SL, Platts-Mills TA, et al. Peanut allergy prevalence among school-age children in a US cohort not selected for any disease. J Allergy Clin Immunol. 2014;134:753–755.
8. Jones SM, Burks AW. Food allergy. N Engl J Med. 2017;377:2294–2295.
9. *Boyce JA, Assa'ad A, Burks AW, et al. Guidelines for the diagnosis and management of food allergy in the United States: report of the NIAID-sponsored expert panel. J Allergy Clin Immunol. 2010;126:S1–S58.
10. Muraro A, Werfel T, Hoffmann-Sommergruber K, et al. EAACI food allergy and anaphylaxis guidelines: diagnosis and management of food allergy. Allergy. 2014;69:1008–1025.
11. Savage J, Sicherer S, Wood R. The natural history of food allergy. J Allergy Climmunol Pract. 2016;4:196–203.
12. Eigenmann PA, Beyer K, Lack G, et al. Are avoidance diets still warranted in children with atopic dermatitis? Pediatric Allergy Immunol: Off Publ Eur Soc Pediatric Allergy Immunol. 2020;31:19–26.
13. Yocum MW, Butterfield JH, Klein JS, Volcheck GW, Schroeder DR, Silverstein MD. Epidemiology of anaphylaxis in Olmsted County: a population-based study. J Allergy Clin Immunol. 1999;104:452–456.
14. Decker WW, Campbell RL, Manivannan V, et al. The etiology and incidence of anaphylaxis in Rochester, Minnesota: a report from the Rochester Epidemiology Project. J Allergy Clin Immunology. 2008;122:1161–1165.
15. Sheikh A, Alves B. Hospital admissions for acute anaphylaxis: time trend study. BMJ (Clin Res ed). 2000;320:1441.
16. Sheikh A, Alves B. Age, sex, geographical and socio-economic variations in admissions for anaphylaxis: analysis of four years of English hospital data. Clin Exp Allergy: J Br Soc Allergy Clin Immunol. 2001;31:1571–1576.
17. Shek LP, Soderstrom L, Ahlstedt S, Beyer K, Sampson HA. Determination of food specific IgE levels over time can predict the development of tolerance in cow's milk and hen's egg allergy. J Allergy Clin immunol. 2004;114:387–391.
18. Iweala OI, Burks AW. Food allergy: our evolving understanding of its pathogenesis, prevention, and treatment. Curr Allergy Asthma Rep. 2016;16:37.
19. Radauer C, Bublin M, Wagner S, Mari A, Breiteneder H. Allergens are distributed into few protein families and possess a restricted number of biochemical functions. J Allergy Clin Immunol. 2008;121:847–852. e7.
20. Sampson HA, O'Mahony L, Burks AW, Plaut M, Lack G, Akdis CA. Mechanisms of food allergy. J Allergy Clin Immunol. 2018;141:11–19.
21. Sampson HA, Aceves S, Bock SA, et al. Food allergy: a practice parameter update-2014. J Allergy Clin Immunol. 2014;134:1016–1025. e43.
22. Vadas P, Gold M, Perelman B, et al. Platelet-activating factor, PAF acetylhydrolase, and severe anaphylaxis. N Engl J Med. 2008;358:28–35.
23. Simons FE, Ardusso LR, Bilò MB, et al. International consensus on (ICON) anaphylaxis. World Allergy Organ J. 2014;7:9.
24. Roberts G, Allen K, Ballmer-Weber B, et al. Identifying and managing patients at risk of severe allergic reactions to food: report from two iFAAM workshops. Clin Exp Allergy: J Br Soc Allergy Clin Immunol. 2019;49:1558–1566.
25. Bartra J, Araujo G, Muñoz-Cano R. Interaction between foods and nonsteroidal anti-inflammatory drugs and exercise in

the induction of anaphylaxis. Curr Opallergy Climmunol. 2018;18:310–316.

26. Muñoz-Cano R, Pascal M, Araujo G, et al. Mechanisms, cofactors, and augmenting factors involved in anaphylaxis. Front Immunol. 2017;8:1193.

27. Arias Á, Lucendo AJ. Epidemiology and risk factors for eosinophilic esophagitis: lessons for clinicians. Expert Rev Gastroenterol & Hepatol. 2020;14:1–14.

28. Lucendo AJ, Molina-Infante J, Arias Á, et al. Guidelines on eosinophilic esophagitis: evidence-based statements and recommendations for diagnosis and management in children and adults. U Eur Gastroenterol J. 2017;5:335–358.

29. *Chehade M, Jones SM, Pesek RD, et al. Phenotypic characterization of Eosinophilic esophagitis in a large multicenter patient population from the consortium for food allergy research. J Allergy Climmunol Pract. 2018;6:1534–1544. e5.

30. *Groetch M, Venter C, Skypala I, et al. Dietary therapy and nutrition management of Eosinophilic esophagitis: a work group report of the American Academy of Allergy, Asthma, and Immunology. J Allergy Climmunol Pract. 2017;5:312–324. e29.

31. Chehade M, Brown S. Elimination diets for eosinophilic esophagitis: making the best choice. Expert Rev Clin Immunol. 2020;16:1–9.

32. Greuter T, Godat A, Ringel A, et al. Effectiveness and safety of high versus low dose swallowed topical steroids for maintenance treatment of Eosinophilic esophagitis: a multi-center observational study. Clin Gastroenterol Hepatol: Off Clin Pract J Am Gastroenterological Assoc. 2020 Aug 13;S1542–3565(20)31136–8. https://doi.org/10.1016/j.cgh.2020.08.027.

33. *Nowak-Węgrzyn A, Chehade M, Groetch ME, et al. International consensus guidelines for the diagnosis and management of food protein-induced enterocolitis syndrome: Executive summary-Workgroup Report of the Adverse Reactions to Foods Committee, American Academy of Allergy, Asthma & Immunology. J Allergy Clin Immunol. 2017;139:1111–1126. e4.

34. Katz Y, Goldberg MR, Rajuan N, Cohen A, Leshno M. The prevalence and natural course of food protein-induced enterocolitis syndrome to cow's milk: a large-scale, prospective population-based study. J Allergy Clin Immunol. 2011;127:647–653. e1–3.

35. Nowak-Wegrzyn A, Warren CM, Brown-Whitehorn T, Cianferoni A, Schultz-Matney F, Gupta RS. Food protein-induced enterocolitis syndrome in the US population-based study. J Allergy Clin Immunol. 2019;144:1128–1130.

36. Bird JA, Leonard S, Groetch M, et al. Conducting an oral food challenge: an update to the 2009 Adverse Reactions to Foods Committee Work Group Report. J Allergy Climmunol Pract. 2020;8:75–90. e17.

37. Lake AM. Food-induced eosinophilic proctocolitis. J Pediatric Gastroenterol Nutr. 2000;30(Suppl):S58–S60.

38. Martin VM, Virkud YV, Seay H, et al. Prospective assessment of pediatrician-diagnosed food protein-induced allergic proctocolitis by gross or occult blood. J Allergy Climmunol Pract. 2020;8:1692–1699. e1.

39. Nowak-Węgrzyn A, Katz Y, Mehr SS, Koletzko S. Non-IgE-mediated gastrointestinal food allergy. J Allergy Clin Immunol. 2015;135:1114–1124.

40. Lebwohl B, Sanders DS, Green PHR. Coeliac disease. Lancet (London, Engl). 2018;391:70–81.

41. Lebwohl B, Green PHR. New developments in celiac disease. Gastroenterol Clin North Am. 2019;48:xv–xvi.

42. Davidson WF, Leung DYM, Beck LA, et al. Report from the National Institute of Allergy and Infectious Diseases workshop on "Atopic dermatitis and the atopic march: mechanisms and interventions". J Allergy Clin Immunol. 2019;143:894–913.

43. Eigenmann PA, Sicherer SH, Borkowski TA, Cohen BA, Sampson HA. Prevalence of IgE-mediated food allergy among children with atopic dermatitis. Pediatrics. 1998;101:E8.

44. Gudjonsson JE, Kabashima K, Eyerich K. Mechanisms of skin autoimmunity: cellular and soluble immune components of the skin. J Allergy Clin Immunol. 2020;146:8–16.

45. Taraghikhah N, Ashtari S, Asri N, et al. An updated overview of spectrum of gluten-related disorders: clinical and diagnostic aspects. BMC Gastroenterol. 2020;20:258.

46. James JM, Bernhisel-Broadbent J, Sampson HA. Respiratory reactions provoked by double-blind food challenges in children. Am J Respiratory Crit Care Med. 1994;149:59–64.

47. James JM, Eigenmann PA, Eggleston PA, Sampson HA. Airway reactivity changes in asthmatic patients undergoing blinded food challenges. Am J Respiratory Crit Care Med. 1996;153:597–603.

48. Kivity S, Dunner K, Marian Y. The pattern of food hypersensitivity in patients with onset after 10 years of age. Clin Exp Allergy: J Br Soc Allergy Clin Immunol. 1994;24:19–22.

49. Novembre E, de Martino M, Vierucci A. Foods and respiratory allergy. J Allergy Clin Immunol. 1988;81:1059–1065.

50. Michelson KA, Dribin TE, Vyles D, Neuman MI. Trends in emergency care for anaphylaxis. J Allergy Climmunol Pract. 2020;8:767–768. e2.

51. Shaker MS, Wallace DV, Golden DBK, et al. Anaphylaxis-a 2020 practice parameter update, systematic review, and grading of recommendations, assessment, development and evaluation (GRADE) analysis. J Allergy Clin Immunol. 2020;145:1082–1123.

52. Sampson HA, Mendelson L, Rosen JP. Fatal and near-fatal anaphylactic reactions to food in children and adolescents. N Engl J Med. 1992;327:380–384.

53. Shaker MS, Oppenheimer J, Wallace DV, et al. Making the GRADE in anaphylaxis management: toward recommendations integrating values, preferences, context, and shared decision making. Ann Allergy, Asthma & Immunol: Off Publ Am Coll Allergy, Asthma, & Immunol. 2020;124:526–535. e2.

54. *Christensen MJ, Eller E, Kjaer HF, Broesby-Olsen S, Mortz CG, Bindslev-Jensen C. Exercise-induced anaphylaxis: causes, consequences, and management recommendations. Expert Rev Clin Immunol. 2019;15:265–273.

55. *Platts-Mills TAE, Commins SP, Biedermann T, et al. On the cause and consequences of IgE to galactose-α-1,3-galactose: a report from the National Institute of Allergy and Infectious Diseases Workshop on Understanding IgE-Mediated Mammalian Meat Allergy. J Allergy Clin Immunol. 2020;145:1061–1071.

56. Commins SP. Diagnosis and management of alpha-gal syndrome: lessons from 2,500 patients. Expert Rev Clin Immunol. 2020;16:1–11.

57. *Togias A, Cooper SF, Acebal ML, et al. Addendum guidelines for the prevention of peanut allergy in the United States: Report of the National Institute of Allergy and Infectious Diseases-sponsored expert panel. J Allergy Clin Immunol. 2017;139:29–44.

58. Sicherer SH, Sampson HA. Food allergy: a review and update on epidemiology, pathogenesis, diagnosis, prevention, and management. J Allergy Clin Immunol. 2018;141:41–58.

59. *Bird JA, Groetch M, Allen KJ, et al. Conducting an oral food challenge to peanut in an infant. J Allergy Climmunol Pract. 2017;5:301–311. e1.

60. Greenhawt M, Shaker M, Wang J, et al. Peanut allergy diagnosis-a 2020 practice parameter update, systematic review, and GRADE analysis. J Allergy Clin Immunol. 2020;146:1302.

61. Masthoff LJ, Mattsson L, Zuidmeer-Jongejan L, et al. Sensitization to Cor a 9 and Cor a 14 is highly specific for a hazelnut allergy

with objective symptoms in Dutch children and adults. J Allergy Clin Immunology. 2013;132:393–399.

62. Bartuzi Z, Cocco RR, Muraro A, Nowak-Węgrzyn A. Contribution of molecular allergen analysis in diagnosis of milk allergy. Curr Allergy Asthma Rep. 2017;17:46.

63. *Suprun M, Sicherer SH, Wood RA, et al. Early epitope-specific IgE antibodies are predictive of childhood peanut allergy. J Allergy Clin Immunol. 2020;146:1080–1088.

64. Wang J, Lin J, Bardina L, et al. Correlation of IgE/IgG₄ milk epitopes and affinity of milk-specific IgE antibodies with different phenotypes of clinical milk allergy. J Allergy Clin Immunol. 2010;125:695–702. e1–e6.

65. Santos AF, Couto-Francisco N, Bécares N, Kwok M, Bahnson HT, Lack G. A novel human mast cell activation test for peanut allergy. J Allergy Clin Immunol. 2018;142:689–691. e9.

66. *Santos AF, Brough HA. Making the most of in vitro tests to diagnose food allergy. J Allergy Climmunol Pract. 2017;5:237–248.

67. Warren CM, Jiang J, Gupta RS. Epidemiology and burden of food allergy. Curr Allergy Asthma Rep. 2020;20:6.

68. DunnGalvin A, Chan CH, Crevel R, et al. Precautionary allergen labelling: perspectives from key stakeholder groups. Allergy. 2015;70:1039–1051.

69. Sánchez-Borges M, Cardona V, Worm M, et al. In-flight allergic emergencies. World Allergy Organ J. 2017;10:15.

70. Greenhawt M, Shaker M, Stukus DR, et al. Managing food allergy in schools during the COVID-19 pandemic. J allergy Climmunology Pract. 2020;8:2845–2850.

71. Nowak-Węgrzyn A, Groetch M. Nutritional aspects and diets in food allergy. Chem Immunol Allergy. 2015;101:209–220.

72. *Turner PJ, Campbell DE, Motosue MS, Campbell RL. Global trends in anaphylaxis epidemiology and clinical implications. J Allergy Climmunol Pract. 2020;8:1169–1176.

73. Gold MS, Sainsbury R. First aid anaphylaxis management in children who were prescribed an epinephrine autoinjector device (EpiPen). J Allergy Clin Immunol. 2000;106:171–176.

74. Turner PJ, Regent L, Jones C, Fox AT. Keeping food-allergic children safe in our schools-Time for urgent action. Clin Exp allergy: J Br Soc Allergy Clin Immunol. 2020;50:133–134.

75. *Greer FR, Sicherer SH, Burks AW. The effects of early nutritional interventions on the development of atopic disease in infants and children: the role of maternal dietary restriction, breastfeeding, hydrolyzed formulas, and timing of introduction of allergenic complementary foods. Pediatrics. 2019;121:143.

76. *Baker MG, Nowak-Wegrzyn A. Food allergy prevention: current evidence. Curr Op Cl Nutr Metab Care. 2020;23:196–202.

77. Bird JA, Parrish C, Patel K, Shih JA, Vickery BP. Prevention of food allergy: beyond peanut. J Allergy Clin Immunol. 2019;143:545–547.

78. Fox AT, Kaymakcalan H, Perkin M, du Toit G, Lack G. Changes in peanut allergy prevalence in different ethnic groups in 2 time periods. J Allergy Clin Immunol. 2015;135:580–582.

79. *Du Toit G, Roberts G, Sayre PH, et al. Randomized trial of peanut consumption in infants at risk for peanut allergy. N Engl J Med. 2015;372:803–813.

80. *Du Toit G, Sayre PH, Roberts G, et al. Effect of avoidance on peanut allergy after early peanut consumption. N Engl J Med. 2016;374:1435–1443.

81. Perkin MR, Logan K, Tseng A, et al. Randomized trial of introduction of allergenic foods in breast-fed infants. N Engl J Med. 2016;374:1733–1743.

82. Perkin MR, Bahnson HT, Logan K, et al. Factors influencing adherence in a trial of early introduction of allergenic food. J Allergy Clin Immunol. 2019;144:1595–1605.

83. Ierodiakonou D, Garcia-Larsen V, Logan A, et al. Timing of allergenic food introduction to the infant diet and risk of allergic or autoimmune disease: a systematic review and meta-analysis. Jama. 2016;316:1181–1192.

84. de Silva D, Halken S, Singh C, et al. Preventing food allergy in infancy and childhood: systematic review of randomised controlled trials. Pediatric Allergy Immunol: Off Publ Eur Soc Pediatric Allergy Immunol. 2020;31:813–826.

85. Chalmers JR, Haines RH, Bradshaw LE, et al. Daily emollient during infancy for prevention of eczema: the BEEP randomised controlled trial. Lancet (London, Engl). 2020;395:962–972.

86. Skjerven HO, Rehbinder EM, Vettukattil R, et al. Skin emollient and early complementary feeding to prevent infant atopic dermatitis (PreventADALL): a factorial, multicentre, cluster-randomised trial. Lancet (London, Engl). 2020;395:951–961.

87. Kulis MD, Patil SU, Wambre E, Vickery BP. Immune mechanisms of oral immunotherapy. J Allergy Clin Immunol. 2018;141:491–498.

88. *Vickery BP, Scurlock AM, Kulis M, et al. Sustained unresponsiveness to peanut in subjects who have completed peanut oral immunotherapy. J Allergy Clin Immunol. 2014;133:468–475.

89. *Chinthrajah RS, Purington N, Andorf S, et al. Sustained outcomes in oral immunotherapy for peanut allergy (POISED study): a large, randomised, double-blind, placebo-controlled, phase 2 study. Lancet (London, Engl). 2019;394:1437–1449.

90. Vickery BP, Vereda A, Casale TB, et al. AR101 oral immunotherapy for peanut allergy. N Engl J Med. 2018;379:1991–2001.

91. Andorf S, Purington N, Kumar D, et al. A phase 2 randomized controlled multisite study using omalizumab-facilitated rapid desensitization to test continued vs discontinued dosing in multifood allergic individuals. EClinicalMedicine. 2019;7:27–38.

92. *Kim EH, Patel C, Burks AW. Immunotherapy approaches for peanut allergy. Expert Rev Clin Immunol. 2020;16:167–174.

93. Upton J, Nowak-Wegrzyn A. The impact of baked egg and baked milk diets on IgE- and non-IgE-mediated allergy. ClRev Allergy & Immunol. 2018;55:118–138.

94. *Nowak-Węgrzyn A, Lawson K, Masilamani M, Kattan J, Bahnson HT, Sampson HA. Increased tolerance to less extensively heat-denatured (baked) milk products in milk-allergic children. J Allergy Climmunol Pract. 2018;6:486–495. e5.

95. *Kim EH, Perry TT, Wood RA, et al. Induction of sustained unresponsiveness after egg oral immunotherapy compared to baked egg therapy in children with egg allergy. J Allergy Clin Immunol. 2020;146:851–862.

96. Kim EH, Yang L, Ye P, et al. Long-term sublingual immunotherapy for peanut allergy in children: clinical and immunologic evidence of desensitization. J Allergy Clin Immunol. 2019;144:1320–1326. e1.

97. *Fleischer DM, Greenhawt M, Sussman G, et al. Effect of epicutaneous immunotherapy vs placebo on reaction to peanut protein ingestion among children with peanut allergy: the PEPITES randomized clinical trial. Jama. 2019;321:946–955.

98. Fleischer DM, Shreffler WG, Campbell DE, et al. Long-term, open-label extension study of the efficacy and safety of epicutaneous immunotherapy for peanut allergy in children: PEOPLE 3-year results. J Allergy Clin Immunol. 2020;146:863.

99. Voorheis P, Bell S, Cornelsen L, et al. Challenges experienced with early introduction and sustained consumption of allergenic foods in the enquiring about tolerance (EAT) study: a qualitative analysis. J Allergy Clin Immunol. 2019;144:1615–1623.

Key references are preceded by an asterisk.

Anaphylaxis

Paul J. Turner and Simon G.A. Brown

SUMMARY OF IMPORTANT CONCEPTS

- Anaphylaxis lies along a spectrum of symptom severity, ranging from mild-moderate respiratory symptoms to circulatory "shock" and/or collapse ("anaphylactic shock").
- Medication, foods, and insect stings are the most common triggers of anaphylaxis.
- Activation of multiple inflammatory pathways causes fluid extravasation (tissue edema, hypovolemia), vascular dilation (erythema, reduced venous return to the heart), bronchospasm, and smooth muscle contraction (bronchospasm, abdominal, and pelvic cramps).
- The cornerstones of emergency management are support of the airway and/or ventilation, supine positioning of the patient, epinephrine (adrenaline) that is usually intramuscular but occasionally intravenous (IV), and volume expansion with IV isotonic crystalloid.
- Mortality from anaphylaxis may be increased in patients with a history of severe reactions, those with asthma (risk of severe bronchospasm), teenagers and young adults (possible risk-taking behaviors), and older people with comorbidities (limited cardiorespiratory reserve).
- Following an episode of anaphylaxis, prevention of further episodes and reducing risks should these occur requires identification of likely triggers and cofactors, optimizing the management of comorbidities, allergen avoidance strategies, provision of rescue medication (epinephrine autoinjector device and anaphylaxis action plan), patient education, and consideration for immunotherapy, if available.

INTRODUCTION

Anaphylaxis is a serious, immediate-type systemic hypersensitivity reaction affecting multiple organ systems and characterized at its most severe by bronchospasm, upper airway angioedema, hypotension, and collapse.[1] Immediate recognition and relatively simple emergency management will prevent death on most occasions, but avoidable deaths occur due to lack of familiarity with the condition, poor recognition of atypical presentations, and/or inappropriate management. Once the acute episode has resolved, patients will also benefit from a careful assessment of likely causes and potential cross-reactivities, avoidance strategies, attention to relevant comorbidities, immunotherapy if available, and action management plans for future reactions including an assessment for provision of rescue medication—in particular, epinephrine (adrenaline) autoinjector(s).

HISTORICAL PERSPECTIVE

The term *anaphylaxis* (from the Greek words *ana*, "contrary to," and *phylaxis*, "protection") was coined by Portier and Richet in 1902, after they observed the sudden cardiorespiratory collapse that occurred in dogs after repeated exposure to small amounts of jellyfish venom. This response was eventually attributed to an immunoglobulin E (IgE) to the venom, and so the term ana*phylaxis* was initially applied to systemic, immediate hypersensitivity reactions caused by IgE-mediated immunologic release of mediators from mast cells and basophils, and

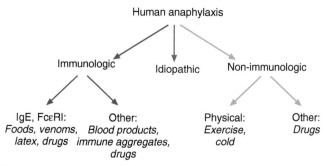

Fig. 13.1 Visual schema of change in anaphylaxis terminology. (From Simons FE. Anaphylaxis, killer allergy: long-term management in the community. J Allergy Clin Immunol 2006;117:367–77.)

BOX 13.1 WAO Clinical Criteria for Diagnosing Anaphylaxis (Updated 2020)

Anaphylaxis is highly likely when any one of the following two criteria are fulfilled:

1. Acute onset of an illness (minutes to several hours) with simultaneous involvement of the skin, mucosal tissue, or both (e.g., generalized hives, pruritus or flushing, swollen lips-tongue-uvula)

   AND AT LEAST ONE OF THE FOLLOWING:

   a. Respiratory compromise (e.g., dyspnea, wheeze-bronchospasm, stridor, reduced PEF, hypoxemia)

   b. Reduced BP or associated symptoms of end-organ dysfunction (e.g., hypotonia [collapse], syncope, incontinence)

   c. Severe gastrointestinal symptoms (e.g., severe crampy abdominal pain, repetitive vomiting), especially after exposure to nonfood allergens

2. Acute onset of hypotension[a] or bronchospasm[b] or laryngeal involvement[c] after exposure to a known or highly probable allergen for that patient (minutes to several hours), even in the absence of typical skin involvement.

BP, Blood pressure; *PEF*, peak expiratory flow.
[a]Hypotension defined as a decrease in systolic BP greater than 30% from that person's baseline, OR
(i) Infants and children under 10 years: systolic BP less than (70 mmHg + [2 × age in years]).
(ii) Adults and children over 10 years: systolic BP less than <90 mmHg.
[b]Excluding lower respiratory symptoms triggered by common inhalant allergens or food allergens perceived to cause "inhalational" reactions in the absence of ingestion.
[c]Laryngeal symptoms include: stridor, vocal changes, odynophagia.

the term *anaphylactoid reaction* was later introduced to refer to a clinically similar event not mediated by IgE.

Anaphylaxis may be triggered by both immune and nonimmune mechanisms. The classical (and most common) pathway for anaphylaxis involves IgE-mediated allergen recognition, which results in the release of preformed mediators from effector cells such as mast cells and basophils. Other non–IgE-mediated mechanisms (immunoglobulin G [IgG], immune complex, complement related) have been reported but are thought to be rare in humans. Direct mast cell activation (also called non-immunologic anaphylaxis) has been described for some drugs (e.g., opioids) as well as for ethanol and physical exertion. To avoid confusion, and to emphasize that for emergency management the mechanism by which anaphylaxis has been triggered is irrelevant, the term *anaphylactoid* is no longer used (Fig. 13.1).

A consensus for the clinical criteria used to diagnose anaphylaxis was published following a symposia jointly sponsored by the US National Institutes of Health (Allergy and Infectious Disease) and the Food Allergy and Anaphylaxis Network (NIAID/FAAN) in 2005,[2] and was subsequently adopted by the World Allergy Organization (WAO).[3] More recently, it has become clear that some refinement to these criteria might be helpful: the concept that anaphylaxis is a systemic or multiorgan reaction is potentially problematic, as it often involves isolated respiratory or cardiovascular symptoms, and such presentations are not uncommon in fatal anaphylaxis.[4] Isolated respiratory symptoms following allergen exposure, particularly to food, are not considered to be anaphylaxis under the previous NIAID/FAAN criteria nor can they be described as a generalized reaction. Consequently, new revised clinical criteria for the diagnosis of anaphylaxis were proposed by WAO in 2020 (Box 13.1).[1]

EPIDEMIOLOGY

Although the exact incidence of anaphylaxis is unknown, estimates range from 50 to 2000 episodes per 100,000 person-years, with a "lifetime" prevalence of 0.05% to 2%. The incidence of anaphylaxis appears to be increasing, at least in industrialized populations, although the uncertainties introduced by retrospective methodologies and changes in clinical practice (decision to admit) and coding can be hard to dissect. Despite this, the available data from the US, the UK, and Australia indicate that fatal anaphylaxis is rare, with an annual incidence

of around 0.05 cases per 100,000 population.[5] Furthermore, despite significant increases in hospital admissions for anaphylaxis globally, in most countries where data are available, there has been no observed increase in the rate of fatal anaphylaxis (of any cause) over the same time periods. Furthermore, even in Australia, where anaphylaxis fatalities have increased, the case fatality rate (proportion of case fatalities as a total of anaphylaxis hospitalizations) has decreased to less than 1% (Fig. 13.2). In the UK, iatrogenic causes (medication, blood products, contrast media) are the most common triggers for fatal anaphylaxis in 55% of cases, followed by food (26%) and insect stings (19%) (Fig. 13.3).[6] Admission and fatality rates for drug-induced and insect sting–induced anaphylaxis increase with age. In contrast, younger adults appear to be most at risk of fatal food-triggered anaphylaxis, with a marked peak in the incidence of fatal reactions during the second and third decades of life.[6] These data are similar to those found in a smaller cohort of fatal anaphylaxis over nine years in Australia, although in the latter study, an increase in drug-related fatal anaphylaxis but not food-induced anaphylaxis was observed.[7]

In the US and Australia, epinephrine autoinjector prescriptions and anaphylaxis admissions are fewer in states with warmer climates and more year-round sunlight, suggesting that lower vitamin D levels might predispose to anaphylactic events.[8] Anaphylaxis is more frequent in adults than children for some agents (radiocontrast media, plasma expanders, anesthetics, antibiotics, insect stings), which may be a function of exposure frequency. Anaphylaxis is also more common in females overall, although for food anaphylaxis, males are affected more frequently prior to puberty.[6] Atopy has been identified as a risk

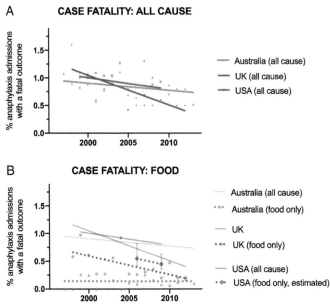

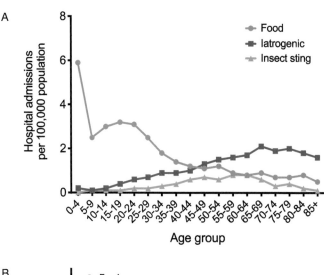

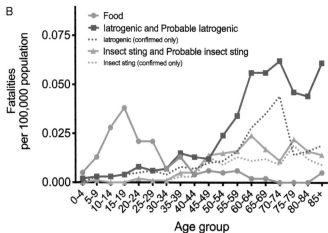

Fig. 13.2 Incidence of fatal anaphylaxis expressed as a proportion of hospital admissions, for all cause (A) and due to food (B). (From Turner PJ, Campbell DE, Motosue MS, Campbell RL. Global trends in anaphylaxis epidemiology and clinical implications. J Allergy Clin Immunol Pract 2020;8(4):1169–1176. Fig. 4.)

Fig. 13.3 Age distribution for anaphylaxis admissions *(top panel)* and fatalities *(lower panel)* by triggering agent (food, iatrogenic causes, and insect stings) from 1992 to 2012 in the UK. (From Turner PJ, Gowland MH, Sharma V, et al. Increase in anaphylaxis-related hospitalizations but no increase in fatalities: an analysis of United Kingdom national anaphylaxis data, 1992–2012. J Allergy Clin Immunol 2015;135(4):956–963. Fig. 2.)

factor for anaphylaxis caused by food, exercise, radiocontrast media, and latex and for idiopathic anaphylaxis, but it does not appear to be a risk factor for reactions triggered by insulin, penicillin, and Hymenoptera sting reactions. Several studies have shown that asthma is a risk factor for anaphylaxis, but the link between asthma control and anaphylaxis severity is unclear.[9]

PATHOPHYSIOLOGY

Triggering

Anaphylaxis can result from several triggers (Table 13.1). The classic *IgE-dependent* immunologic mechanism is best understood and characterized by allergen cross-linking of FcεRI receptors (high-affinity IgE receptors) on mast cells and basophils. Other immunologic mechanisms involving other types of antibody and various inflammatory pathways are referred to as *IgE-independent*. These are not as well understood and are possibly overlapping. For example, aspirin and other nonsteroidal antiinflammatory drugs (NSAIDs) can cause agent-specific reactivity or class reactivity. This suggests an immune-mediated mechanism for the former and a metabolic mechanism (e.g., arachidonic acid metabolism) for the latter. Reactions to NSAIDs also tend to have delayed onset and protracted course, which suggests antibody-dependent reactivity to a metabolite. In animal models in mice, anaphylaxis can be triggered by the IgG FcγRIII receptor, requiring proportionately more antigen and antibody than the IgE-dependent pathway.[10] IgG-dependent anaphylaxis has not been demonstrated in humans.[10] However, human IgG receptors are capable of activating macrophages to release platelet-activating factor (PAF), which can activate mast cells in vitro. There are also emerging data from both human

and animal studies that allergen-specific IgG can interfere with IgE-dependent anaphylaxis, modulating the response. Some agents can initiate degranulation of mast cells and basophils without help from immune pathways, and this is termed *non-immunologic* anaphylaxis. Examples include physical factors, such as heat or cold, and opioids and vancomycin, which directly activate mast cells, for example via the Mas-related G-protein Coupled Receptor X2 (MRGPRX2). Importantly, anaphylaxis can also be *summative*, in which a combination of physical stimulus (usually exercise) in close proximity to allergen ingestion (to which the patient has allergen-specific IgE [sIgE]) results in a reaction.

Biochemical Mediators and Effects

Many of the pathophysiologic events that occur during anaphylaxis are easily explained by the actions of mediators, summarized in Table 13.2, all of which have overlapping actions of similar clinical importance. This results in the triad of smooth muscle contraction, vasodilation, and increased vascular permeability

TABLE 13.1   Summary of Incidence for Common Triggers of Anaphylaxis

Agent	Comment/Findings
Antibiotics[11]	Arguably most common cause of drug-induced anaphylaxis, most frequently β-lactams, accounting for as many as 22% of all drug-related episodes. Nonfatal drug-induced anaphylaxis to penicillin may affect 1.9–27.2 million Americans.
Latex[12]	Populations at risk experience multiple mucosal exposures to latex, for example, healthcare workers, patients with multiple catheterizations/surgeries. Overall incidence of latex allergy in the US is 2.7–16 million. Although incidence of latex allergy has risen greatly over last 15 years, with reduced use of powdered gloves and substitution of nonlatex gloves in hospitals, incidence appears to have stabilized.
Perioperative anaphylaxis[13,14]	Depending on the country, perioperative anaphylactic reactions represent 9%–19% of complications of anesthesia. Fatality rate approximates 5%–7%. Muscle relaxants account for 62% and latex 16%; the remainder of reactions result from hypnotics, antibiotics, plasma substitutes, and opioids. Serial data collected in France showed increased incidence of perioperative anaphylactic events. Muscle relaxants still remain the most common cause.
Radiocontrast media[15]	Adverse reactions to ionic contrast media (hyperosmolar agents) occur with a frequency of 4%–12% and to nonionic (lower osmolar agents) of 1%–3%. Severe adverse reactions occur in 0.16% of ionic media administration and 0.03% with nonionic media. Paradoxically, mortality rate (1–3 per 100,000 contrast administrations) appears similar for both ionic and nonionic media.
Hymenoptera stings[16]	Potentially life-threatening systemic reactions to insect stings occur in an estimated 0.4%–0.8% of children and 3% of adults.
Food[17,18]	As many as 6% of children and 3%–4% of adults have food allergy. Based on incidence in Colorado, approximately 0.0004% of the US population, or 1080 Americans, have anaphylaxis to food each year. Shellfish is probably the most common source in adults and peanuts in children. Also, 1.1% of the US population may be allergic to tree nuts or peanuts.
Nonsteroidal antiinflammatory drugs[19]	Incidence varies depending on whether or not asthmatic patients are included. NSAIDs are probably the second most common medication offender after antibiotics.
Antisera	Once the most important cause of anaphylaxis, antisera have greatly diminished in importance with their decreased use as therapeutic agents, but antiserum is still used for snakebites and immunosuppression. Incidence in patients receiving antilymphocyte globulin may be as high as 2%, and incidence to antivenom 4.6%–10%. Incidence may decline further with recent release of Crotalidae Polyvalent ImmunFab, a purified preparation of Fab fragment obtained from sheep immunized with venom. Although urticaria has been reported, no anaphylactic episodes have occurred with this agent.
Reactions associated with hemodialysis[20]	Incidence appears to be increasing. Drug administration data show 3.5 severe hypersensitivity reactions per 100,000 hollow-fiber dialyzers sold. In 260,000 dialysis treatments, 21 severe reactions occurred, including one fatality.
Idiopathic anaphylaxis[21]	Cause remains unidentified in as many as two-thirds of adults presenting to allergist/immunologist for evaluation of anaphylaxis. Survey of 75 US allergists found 633 cases encountered. The authors extrapolated data to the US population and estimated as many as 20,592–47,024 cases.
Biologic agents[22]	With increased use of biologic agents, anaphylactic reactions to these products have also increased, including omalizumab, tumor necrosis factor antagonists, cetuximab, tocilizumab, and natalizumab.

TABLE 13.2   Mast Cell and Basophil Mediators and Roles in Producing Anaphylactic Events

Mediators	Pathophysiologic Activity	Clinical Correlates
Histamine and products of arachidonic acid metabolism (leukotrienes, thromboxane, prostaglandins, platelet-activating factor)	Smooth muscle spasm, mucus secretion, vasodilation, increased vascular permeability, activation of nociceptive neurons, platelet adherence, eosinophil activation, eosinophil chemotaxis	Wheeze, urticaria, angioedema, flush, itch, diarrhea, abdominal pain, hypotension, rhinorrhea, bronchorrhea
Neutral proteases: tryptase, chymase, carboxypeptidase, cathepsin G	Cleavage of complement components, chemoattractants for eosinophils and neutrophils, further activation and degranulation of mast cells, cleavage of neuropeptides, conversion of angiotensin I to angiotensin II	May recruit complement by cleaving C3; may ameliorate symptoms by invoking hypertensive response through angiotensin I–II conversion and by inactivating neuropeptides, although angiotensin II also may cause deleterious coronary artery vasoconstriction. Also, proteases can magnify response because of further mast cell activation
Proteoglycans: heparin, chondroitin sulfate	Anticoagulation, inhibition of complement, phospholipase A_2 binding, chemoattractant for eosinophils, cytokine inhibition, kinin pathway activation	Can prevent intravascular coagulation and recruitment of complement. Can recruit kinins, increasing severity of reaction
Chemoattractants: chemokines, eosinophil chemotactic factors	Summons cells to site	May be partly responsible for recrudescence of symptoms in late phase reaction or extension and protraction of reaction
Tumor necrosis factor-α activates nuclear factor κB	Produces platelet-activating factor (PAF)	Vascular permeability and vasodilation; PAF synthesized and released late, involved in late phase reactions

that characterize clinical anaphylaxis. Rapid systemic spread of immune activation and mediator release appears to be required for the development of severe anaphylaxis.[23] This may be due to mediators released by triggering mast cells directly affecting other mast cells and/or a complex "mast cell–leukocyte cytokine cascade" initially proposed in the context of allergic airway inflammation, but now supported by studies using mouse models of anaphylaxis and a human study of leukocyte gene activation in the early phase of anaphylaxis.[24] Recent data also indicate an important role for basophil activation in systemic allergic reactions, with a dose–response between the degree of activation and symptom severity.[25,26]

The activation of basophils and mast cells releases an array of biochemical mediators and chemotactic substances by degranulation of preformed mediators and *de novo* synthesis. Table 13.2 summarizes the main activities of these mediators and pathophysiologic consequences and clinical correlates. Additionally, low constitutional levels of regulatory enzymes such as PAF-acetylhydrolase (PAF-AH) may contribute to reaction severity in some patients.[23,27]

Mechanisms of Anaphylactic Shock

Box 13.2 summarizes likely key pathologic mechanisms of human anaphylactic shock. The balance of evidence from

---

BOX 13.2 Key Pathophysiologic Mechanisms of Human Anaphylactic Shock

Common/Clearly Demonstrated[a]

- Fluid extravasation and maldistribution, causing hemoconcentration, hypovolemia, and reduced venous return to the heart manifested as low filling pressures and reduction in stroke volume/cardiac output.

Likely[b]

- Venodilation and blood pooling, contributing to reduced venous return.
- Impaired myocardial contractility contributing, along with reduced venous return, to reduced cardiac output.
- Relative bradycardia (neurally mediated) in awake patients, contributing to reduced cardiac output.
- Early transient increase in pulmonary vascular resistance, contributing to reduced cardiac output by obstructing venous return to left side of heart.
- Early arteriolar dilation, manifested as a widened pulse pressure and contributing to hypotension. (However, an *increase* in systemic vascular resistance caused by increased arteriolar tone may predominate after this early phase.)

Uncommon/Postulated[c]

- Severe global depression of myocardial contractility, with nonspecific ST-segment electrocardiographic changes (unresponsive to adrenaline) possibly more likely in those with underlying cardiac disease or taking β-blockers.
- Severe arteriolar dilation as well as venous dilation.
- Coronary ischemia caused by coronary vasospasm and plaque ulceration.

Modified from Brown SGA. The pathophysiology of shock in anaphylaxis. Immunol Allergy Clin North Am 2007; 27:165–175.
[a] Supported by unambiguous observations of human anaphylaxis.
[b] Unproven but supported by animal studies, studies of histamine infusion in volunteers, known mediator actions, or indirect physiologic observations during human anaphylaxis.
[c] Based on case reports, speculation, and plausible mechanisms.

---

human observations and animal studies suggests that the main pathophysiologic features of anaphylactic shock are a profound reduction in venous tone and fluid extravasation.[28] The resulting mixed hypovolemic and distributive shock involves reduction in blood volume (hypovolemia) from extravasation and distribution of blood to the wrong areas. Both of these combine to cause reduced venous return to the heart and an empty ventricle. It was recently reported that significant fluid redistribution (and a consequence decrease in stroke volume) occurs independent of reaction severity during peanut-induced allergic reactions.[29] Furthermore, these data suggested that poor outcomes in anaphylaxis may occur as a result of a failure of the host to compensate for the allergic reaction. Animal models and a few human case reports also suggest that depressed myocardial function can be a factor in some cases, introducing a component of temporary cardiogenic shock as well. Electrocardiographic (ECG) changes are seen in some cases, but it is not known if this represents a mediator effect on the myocardium and/or arrhythmia generation, a reduction in coronary perfusion caused by low diastolic blood pressure (blood flow through coronary arteries occurs during diastole when the heart relaxes), coronary spasm (Kounis syndrome), or sometimes plaque rupture.

Arguably the most important human study to date is a series of 205 episodes of perioperative anaphylactic shock, in which the treating anesthesiologist was asked to provide detailed clinical and laboratory information immediately after the event.[30] Increases in hematocrit signaled extravasation of up to 35% of circulating blood volume within 10 minutes. A total of 46 patients with central or pulmonary artery catheters placed before or soon after onset of anaphylaxis had a significant fall in filling pressures, except in 9 of 11 patients with cardiac disease, who had elevated pressures. Even so, these patients appeared to need volume expansion to achieve a stable blood pressure. In all six patients with balloon pulmonary artery catheters, pulmonary pressure rose initially and then fell over the next 10 minutes.

In a case series of eight venom-induced anaphylaxis reactions that were closely monitored, hypotension was preceded by a fall in diastolic blood pressure (suggesting reduced systemic vascular resistance) with tachycardia. In all eight cases, the onset of hypotension was accompanied by a relative bradycardia, that is, rather than the heart rate further increasing to compensate for falling blood pressure, it fell as the blood pressure decreased.[31] This may have been caused by a neurocardiogenic reflex, triggered by cardiac mechanoreceptors, and enhanced by increased levels of mediators that are released during anaphylaxis and known to potentiate this reflex. However, bradycardia may also be a nonspecific feature of severe hypovolemic/distributive shock in awake animals.[28] Physiologic studies of awake mammals have identified two phases of response to hypovolemia, an initial phase of blood pressure maintenance by tachycardia and peripheral arteriolar constriction, followed by a second phase with more severe hypovolemia, characterized by bradycardia, reduced peripheral arteriolar tone, and a profound fall in blood pressure. However, bradycardia has not been reported as a feature of anaphylaxis under anesthesia, where tachycardia is the norm. This may be explained by the blunting of central reflexes that occurs under anesthesia and with different allergen routes and dosages.

Changes in posture, to upright or semirecumbent (sitting upright) positioning, have been associated with fatal anaphylaxis.[32,33] Movement from a supine to an upright or semiupright position reduces venous return to the heart and is likely to exacerbate all the pathophysiologic processes involved in anaphylaxis (reduced venous return, profound bradycardia with further reduction in cardiac output myocardial ischemia). Keeping a patient flat to maximize venous return to the heart is therefore a key component of the initial response to anaphylaxis.

CLINICAL FEATURES (PHENOTYPES)

Symptoms of an allergic reaction occur across a broad spectrum, from localized and clinically mild systemic (skin only) allergic reactions to severe life-threatening anaphylaxis. The clinical criteria that define anaphylaxis (Box 13.1) are based around the concept of a multisystem, severe reaction. This is helpful clinically, as it defines the need for urgent intervention, but is nevertheless somewhat artificial because essentially the same process (systemic effector cell activation triggered by allergen) may cause a mild reaction on one occasion but a life-threatening reaction on another occasion, even under controlled conditions within the same individual.

The main clinical manifestations of anaphylaxis are summarized in Table 13.3. Overall, the clinical similarities shared by patients in various published case series are striking. The most common manifestations are cutaneous, combined with

TABLE 13.3 Signs and Symptoms of Anaphylaxis: Frequency of Occurrence[a]

Signs/Symptoms	Percentage of Cases[b]
Cutaneous	>90
Urticaria and angioedema	85–90
Flush	45–55
Pruritus without rash	2–5
Respiratory	40–60
Dyspnea, wheeze	45–50
Upper airway angioedema	50–60
Rhinitis	15–20
Dizziness, syncope, hypotension	30–35
Abdominal	
Nausea, vomiting, diarrhea, cramping pain	25–30
Miscellaneous	
Headache	5–8
Substernal pain	4–6
Seizure	1–2

[a]Based on a compilation of 1784 patients reviewed in Lieberman P. Anaphylaxis and anaphylactoid reactions. In: Middleton E, editors. Allergy: principles and practice. 5th ed. St Louis: Mosby–Year Books; 1998, pp. 1079–1092.

[b]Percentages are approximations (see text).

respiratory, cardiovascular, and/or gastrointestinal features. Severe reactions tend to be either predominantly cardiovascular (hypotensive) or respiratory (hypoxemic/bronchospasm), although some (about 30%) display both.[23] Food-triggered reactions tend to involve predominantly respiratory symptoms,[34,35] which are consistent with data from the UK Fatal Anaphylaxis Registry in which the majority of food-triggered fatalities included respiratory involvement.[6] Older age and drug causation are risk factors for severe reactions; the latter may be related to administration via the parenteral route and/or the rapid absorption characteristics of oral drug formulations, causing rapid exposure to high doses of allergen.[23]

There are exceptions to the prototypical clinical presentation of skin features plus other organ involvement. For example, cardiovascular collapse with shock can occur immediately without any cutaneous or respiratory symptoms. The lack of cutaneous symptoms, specifically urticaria, in severe events, has also been noted in fatal reactions,[36] and may have contributed to delays in diagnosis and appropriate treatment. Even in food-triggered anaphylaxis reactions, cutaneous symptoms are absent in up to 10% of reactions.[1] The lack of cutaneous symptoms may be caused by an inability to manifest them due to profound hypotension and reduced cutaneous blood flow. Cardiovascular collapse is more common during perioperative anaphylaxis than in anaphylaxis episodes occurring outside the operating room. Cardiovascular collapse and bronchospasm are significantly more common during IgE-mediated perioperative anaphylaxis than those that are not IgE-mediated.

Anaphylaxis presents with a different pattern of signs and symptoms in infants, with nonspecific behavioral changes common, such as crying, fussing, irritability, and fright. Hoarseness and dysphonia with drooling and increased secretions, coughing, stridor, and choking can occur, as well as nasal congestion and gastrointestinal symptoms (e.g., regurgitation/vomiting within minutes of ingestion of an allergenic food, spitting up, loose stools, colicky pain). With severe reactions they may exhibit drowsiness and somnolence, followed by unresponsiveness and lethargy. Seizures can occur. Examination may show a weak pulse, pallor, and diaphoresis.

Characteristically, anaphylaxis is associated with a compensatory tachycardia that occurs in response to a decreased effective vascular volume.[29] However, bradycardia can also occur, as described in the section above on mechanisms. In a study of 21 healthy adults with systemic allergic reactions to insect venom, hypotension was always accompanied by an initial tachycardia followed by a relative bradycardia, which occurred with the onset of hypotension. In two subjects, this was severe enough for atropine to be given.[31] Myocardial depression with decreased cardiac output as a result of contractile depression can also occur and persist for several days. ECG abnormalities include ST-segment elevation, flattened T waves, inverted T waves, and arrhythmias (e.g., from heart block); cardiac enzyme elevations also occur. The mechanisms are uncertain, but may include mediator effects on the myocardium, coronary spasm, plaque ulceration (perhaps mediated by mast cells that are found in the coronary vasculature), and poor coronary blood flow secondary to hypotension and hypoxemia.

Anaphylaxis can present with unusual manifestations that make diagnosis difficult, especially when the episode has not been directly observed by a healthcare professional. Syncope without skin or respiratory manifestations can occur, sometimes with a seizure, especially if propped upright during hypotension, which further reduces cerebral blood flow and increases the risk of seizure from cerebral tissue hypoxia. This may be followed by a period of postictal confusion. In this situation, if a history of likely allergen exposure is missed, unnecessary cardiovascular and neurologic evaluations are often done before establishing the diagnosis of anaphylaxis.

Rarely, anaphylaxis can cause adrenal hemorrhage and thus prolonged hypotension. Profound anaphylactic episodes with hypotension can also result in clotting abnormalities. In some settings, it is also important to recognize coexistent coagulopathies, such as in anaphylactic reactions to snake venom and antivenoms (associated with snake venom–induced consumption coagulopathy) and in anaphylaxis to leech bites (heparin-like anticoagulant effect from the leech contents if they are squeezed into the body on leech removal).

An anaphylaxis episode can appear to resolve and then exhibit a recrudescence several hours later. This is often termed *biphasic anaphylaxis* but can also represent (and be difficult to distinguish from) protracted anaphylaxis with a temporary response to epinephrine. The exact incidence of biphasic reactions is uncertain. A recent systematic review and metaanalysis reported an estimated rate of 4.6% (95% confidence interval [CI] 4.0–5.3).[37] but is probably related to severity of the initial reaction. Delayed treatment of initial symptoms with epinephrine has also been reported to be a risk factor.[38] In a large prospective study, such delayed deteriorations treated with epinephrine occurred in 29 of 315 anaphylaxis cases (9.2%) and were more common after initially hypotensive reactions and in people with preexisting lung disease. In total, 22 of the 29 delayed deteriorations (76%) occurred within 4 hours of initial epinephrine treatment. Of the remaining seven cases, two were severe and occurred after initially severe reactions, within 10 hours.[23]

PATIENT EVALUATION, DIAGNOSIS, AND DIFFERENTIAL DIAGNOSIS

The diagnosis of anaphylaxis is a clinical one, based on the typical clinical features outlined above. However, for any episode of hypotension/shock or severe bronchospasm/hypoxemia in which the cause is not evident, a diagnosis of anaphylaxis should be considered and treatment with epinephrine initiated if there is an immediate threat to life.

The differential diagnosis of anaphylaxis is presented in Box 13.3. This first includes some consideration of the causes of anaphylaxis and then conditions that should be considered as potential alternate diagnoses. This process should start with the healthcare professional who sees the patient during the acute event, as careful and contemporaneous documentation of all clinical features and patient recollection of potential exposures and timing are important in reaching a correct diagnosis.

The healthcare professional must first consider the likely cause and timing of exposure. While some exposures are obvious (e.g., a common allergenic food being ingested with immediate oral allergy symptoms followed by anaphylaxis, a drug injection, or an insect sting), some may not be. Anaphylaxis may not start for several hours after ingestion of a NSAID (possibly related to the generation of metabolites) and monoclonal antibody

---

BOX 13.3   Differential Diagnosis of Anaphylaxis

Anaphylaxis
Anaphylaxis to exogenously administered agents
Physical factors
  Exercise
  Cold, heat, sunlight
Idiopathic

Vasodepressor Reactions
Flush syndromes
  Carcinoid
  Menopause
  Chlorpropamide, alcohol
Medullary carcinoma thyroid
Autonomic epilepsy

Restaurant Syndromes
Monosodium glutamate (MSG)
Sulfites
Scombroidosis

Other Forms of Shock
Hemorrhagic
Cardiogenic
Endotoxic

Excess Endogenous Production of Histamine Syndromes
Systemic mastocytosis
Urticaria pigmentosa
Basophilic leukemia
Acute promyelocytic leukemia (tretinoin)
Hydatid cyst

Nonorganic Disease
Panic attacks
Munchausen stridor
Vocal cord dysfunction syndrome
Globus hystericus
Undifferentiated somatoform anaphylaxis

Miscellaneous
Hereditary angioedema
Progesterone anaphylaxis
Urticarial vasculitis
Pheochromocytoma
Hyper-IgE, urticaria syndrome
Neurologic (seizure, stroke)
Pseudoanaphylaxis
Red man syndrome (vancomycin)
Capillary leak syndrome

injections. A similar delay in symptom onset occurs for food-allergic reactions triggered by the alpha-gal allergen in mammalian meat.[4] In the case of summative anaphylaxis, the triggering food alone does not result in anaphylaxis; anaphylaxis starts only when there is additional physical stress (typically physical exertion, although this can be moderate in activity). Where a trigger cannot be identified, or is known to be associated with nonanaphylaxis diagnoses (e.g., fish ingestion and scombroid poisoning, various drugs and flushing, angiotensin converting enzyme [ACE] inhibitors, and angioedema), and/or when the reaction is atypical, then careful consideration of differential diagnoses is required.

Perhaps the most common condition mimicking anaphylaxis is the vasodepressor reaction (vasovagal syncope), which is associated with vasodilatation, bradycardia, hypotension, and loss of consciousness. It often results from a threatening event or emotional trauma. Bradycardia and the absence of cutaneous manifestations are often used to distinguish these episodes but, as previously noted, bradycardia is also a feature of hypotensive anaphylaxis and skin features may not be evident during anaphylaxis.

It is also important to recognize the entities that can produce flushing. Flushing is a common phenomenon and can result from a variety of agents, including niacin, nicotine, catecholamines, ACE inhibitors, and alcohol (with and without associated drugs). Flushing is also seen in association with ingestion of spicy foods containing capsaicin; carcinoid syndrome; pancreatic tumors; medullary carcinoma of the thyroid; hypoglycemia; rosacea; pheochromocytoma; menopause; autonomic epilepsy; panic attacks; and systemic mastocytosis. A group of postprandial syndromes (restaurant syndromes) resembling anaphylaxis have been attributed to the ingestion of monosodium glutamate (MSG), sulfites, or histamine. Ingestion of MSG can produce chest pain, facial burning, flushing, paresthesia, sweating, dizziness, headaches, palpitations, nausea, and vomiting. Children can experience shivering and chills, irritability, screaming, and delirium. The occurrence of these symptoms has been termed "the Chinese restaurant syndrome." The mechanism is unknown, but MSG is thought to cause a transient acetylcholinosis. About 15% to 20% of the general population appear to be sensitive to small doses of MSG, but reactions can occur in any individual if the dose is large enough. Scombroidosis poisoning caused by the ingestion of histamine and other biogenic amines accumulating in spoiled fish, also causes flushing plus other typical signs and symptoms that include urticaria, angioedema, nausea, vomiting, diarrhea, wheeze, and hypotension.

Nonorganic disease can mimic anaphylaxis. Such episodes can be involuntary, such as in panic attacks, undifferentiated somatoform anaphylaxis, vocal cord dysfunction syndrome, and Munchausen stridor. Panic attacks are accompanied by tachycardia, flushing, gastrointestinal (GI) symptoms, and shortness of breath. Vocal cord dysfunction syndrome is caused by an involuntary adduction of the vocal cords that occludes the glottal opening. A bunching together of the false vocal cords produces obstruction in both inspiration and expiration; the patient is unaware of the process. The term *Munchausen stridor* was coined to describe patients who intentionally adduct their vocal cords and present to the emergency department (ED) with self-induced manifestations of laryngeal edema. This entity occurs in psychologically disturbed individuals and can be distinguished from vocal cord dysfunction syndrome by laryngoscopy during the acute episode. Also, patients with Munchausen stridor can be distracted from their vocal cord adduction by asking them to perform maneuvers such as coughing. "Undifferentiated somatoform anaphylaxis" is a term used to describe patients who present with manifestations that mimic idiopathic anaphylaxis but who lack objective confirmatory findings, do not respond to therapy, and exhibit psychologic signs of an undifferentiated somatoform disorder.

Other entities traditionally listed in the differential diagnosis of anaphylaxis include hereditary angioedema; progesterone anaphylaxis; anaphylaxis associated with recurrent and chronic urticaria; pheochromocytoma; neurologic disorders; tracheal foreign body; pseudoanaphylactic syndrome occurring after administration of procaine penicillin; and red man syndrome, often occurring after administration of vancomycin. Hereditary angioedema can cause laryngeal edema, abdominal pain, and an erythematous rash that can be confused with urticaria, although these two entities can usually be differentiated on clinical grounds without difficulty.

Laboratory Testing

In some patients, laboratory evaluations can help establish a diagnosis of anaphylaxis or exclude other conditions. Serum mast cell tryptase (MCT) is the only widely available assay used to confirm the diagnosis of anaphylaxis. Almost all human mast cells contain preformed tryptases in their granules; small amounts are also found in human basophils. Serum tryptase is specific to these cells, and released during anaphylaxis. The increase in serum concentrations of MCT levels seen during an anaphylactic event consists of the mature β-tryptase stored in mast cell granules; however, the only widely available assay measures total tryptase. Total tryptase is affected by the baseline release of constitutively secreted tryptase (a mixture of α- and β-protryptase). MCT peaks 60 to 90 minutes after the onset of anaphylaxis and persists for longer than plasma histamine. In some cases, a very high MCT found on one sample taken during a reaction may confirm a diagnosis of anaphylaxis, but a repeat sample is required several weeks later to exclude a diagnosis of mastocytosis, which may cause very high MCT concentrations.

A single MCT sampling approach is less sensitive than a multiple sampling approach at three time points: first assessment, 1 hour later, and then a convalescent sample at least 4 hours later (or the next day). MCT is relatively stable over time in an individual who is not experiencing anaphylaxis; serial sampling may detect a peak that would otherwise be missed by a single sample and also detects significant changes over time in an individual, sometimes within the normal range that applies to a single measurement. Various approaches to interpretation have been used and some caution is required because the specificity of serial MCT sampling (whether it is negative in other critical illnesses) has not been defined. Furthermore, this approach is expensive and is probably only required when there is clinical doubt about the diagnosis.[39]

It is sometimes also beneficial to obtain serum for the analysis of sIgE against suspected antigens (sIgE). For example, confirming the presence of sIgE to an insect venom species implicated in an anaphylactic event may streamline the subsequent decision to commence venom immunotherapy and the choice of venom extract, although caution is needed to exclude potential false positives.[40] However, in general sIgE testing is probably best left until follow-up after the acute event, when a careful history has identified potential allergens for appropriate testing, if needed. In some instances, skin testing is preferable and more sensitive for sIgE. However, skin responses to allergen are often suppressed following anaphylaxis; thus, skin testing for sIgE should be deferred until several weeks after the acute reaction. Most importantly, sIgE testing is nonspecific because many people have detectable sIgE without any history of anaphylaxis; test results should be interpreted in the proper context by an allergist before the result is used to inform subsequent treatments and allergen avoidance strategies.

TREATMENT

Life-threatening reactions often occur in response to accidental exposure or drug administration in a setting with practitioners who do not regularly treat this condition. The outcome of successful resuscitation will often be determined well before the patient reaches an ED or critical care environment staffed with highly experienced practitioners. A simple and easy-to-follow approach plus a one-page anaphylaxis emergency management plan (kept with resuscitation drugs) may assist. An example of this is the Australian Prescriber Anaphylaxis Wallchart, available at nps.org.au/assets/b3df19317d2acbf9-8dbd289b4af7-A3-Anaphylaxis-Wallchart-2018.pdf.

There is a paucity of high-level evidence to guide the emergency treatment of anaphylaxis, but there is a general consensus that the cornerstones are as follows[1]:

1. Basic life support (airway support, oxygen, ventilation support, and external chest compressions if cardiac arrest occurs).
2. Supine posture to prevent a deleterious reduction in venous return to the heart.
3. Early administration of epinephrine, which physiologically antagonizes most of the pathophysiologic manifestations of anaphylaxis.
4. If the blood pressure is low, intravenous (IV) fluid (volume) resuscitation to improve venous return to the heart.

Epinephrine (Adrenaline)

Intramuscular (IM) epinephrine at a dose of 0.01 mg/kg (max. 0.5 mg) is a sensible first-line option, even when the patient already has IV access. This dose can be repeated after 5 minutes if the response is inadequate. When given early before the onset of shock, the systemic absorption of IM epinephrine is rapid and an effect is seen within minutes, often negating the need for any further treatment. When given at this dose via the IM route, it is also remarkably safe with a relative tolerance for dosing errors. Conversely, IV bolus dosing of epinephrine is less safe and, in inexperienced hands, incorrect dosing has

been associated with serious adverse events, including acute pulmonary edema, ventricular arrhythmias, intracerebral hemorrhage, and death. Consequently, our preference is to reserve bolus IV dosing of epinephrine for cardiac arrest, in which case standard cardiac arrest dosing (1 mg IV bolus approximately every 3 min) is appropriate.

However, in severe anaphylaxis, poor muscle perfusion may result in slow absorption of epinephrine into the circulation. Furthermore, relatively high serum concentrations of epinephrine may be required for an adequate therapeutic effect in severe anaphylaxis where there is marked vasodilation. When a patient is severely shocked or has not responded to an initial dose of epinephrine, an IV infusion of epinephrine may be required and can be titrated to achieve the desired balance between efficacy and adverse effects. In particular, as soon as an adequate blood pressure has been achieved, the infusion can be scaled back to avoid excessive blood pressure surges. There are several infusion regimens available that have been designed for a rapid response to anaphylaxis. An example for practitioners who do not have an infusion pump available is given in the Australian Prescriber Wallchart, and uses 1 mg epinephrine in a 1 L bag of saline. In critical care environments, more concentrated infusions may be used. One approach is to use 1 mg in 100 mL, starting at 0.5 to 1 mL/kg per hour and titrated to response (Box 13.4).[31] This provides a fairly rapid response and sufficient epinephrine to complete the treatment of most reactions, compared with more concentrated infusions, which are given at low infusion rates for longer periods of time.

Whatever protocol is followed, it is important to note that:
1. There is typically a time lag of 5 to 10 minutes between a change in the epinephrine infusion rate and a new "steady state" serum concentration of epinephrine being achieved; therefore, if the infusion rate is rapidly escalated to counter life-threatening features, one must be aware of a delayed and rather sudden transition from therapeutic to toxic serum concentrations.
2. Increasing heart rate, pallor, sweating, and tachyarrhythmia in the setting of a normal or raised blood pressure are indicative of epinephrine toxicity, so the infusion rate should be reduced.
3. After 30 to 60 minutes, it is typical for a reaction to start resolving. It is appropriate to start turning the infusion down at this point (e.g., halving the rate) because as the reaction subsides, a previously therapeutic serum concentration can cause toxic effects.
4. Once the reaction has fully resolved clinically and remains so after halving the infusion rate, the infusion may need to be continued for another 1 to 2 hours (or longer) while the reaction continues to subside.

Intravenous Fluid (Volume) Resuscitation

If hypotension occurs, aggressive fluid (volume) resuscitation with isotonic crystalloid (normal saline or Hartman solution) is a critical component of therapy. Wide-bore IV access (16 gauge in adults) will facilitate this. Start with 20 mL/kg initially over 2 to 3 minutes, given under pressure. Repeat this dose again if necessary. As noted above, studies in humans monitoring changes

BOX 13.4 Adrenaline Infusion guideline for Anaphylaxis[31]

Adrenaline Infusion Guideline For Anaphylaxis

1 Preparation
- Requires continuous physiological monitoring (**ECG, SpO$_2$, BP 3–5 minutely**)
- Give via an **infusion pump** through a **dedicated line**, or piggybacked with **antireflux valves on all other lines** to prevent the adrenaline going back up into another fluid bag instead of into the patient
- BEWARE infusions on the same side as a BP cuff; frequent BP measurements may interfere with the infusion
- **FIRST BAG: 1 mg adrenaline in 100 mL saline = 0.01 mg/mL (1:100,000)**
  That is 1 mL/kg/hour gives the equivalent of a 0.01 mg/kg dose over 1 hour (0.17 ug/kg/min)

2 Initiation and Adjustment
- **Start at 0.5–1 mL/kg/h** (30–100 mL/h in adults) depending on reaction severity:
  Moderate severity: 0.5 mL/kg/h Severe (hypotensive or hypoxic): 1 mL/kg/h
- **Titrate** up or down according to response, aiming for the lowest effective infusion rate
  Allow for a short elimination half-life; steady state is reached 5–10 minutes after a change in the infusion rate
- **Tachycardia, tremor, and pallor with a normal or raised blood pressure are signs of adrenaline toxicity:**
  Reduce the infusion rate (if toxicity is severe, stop the infusion briefly before recommencing at a lower rate)
- **The safe maximum rate of adrenaline infusion** is unknown, but is probably <1 ug/kg/min (6 mL/kg/h of the above solution of 1 mg in 100 mL).

3 De-Escalation and Cessation
- **As the reaction resolves, an infusion that was previously therapeutic can start to have toxic effects:** Therefore, when features resolve begin reducing the infusion, aiming for around half the starting rate if possible
- 60 minutes after the resolution of all symptoms and signs, wean the infusion over another 30 minutes and stop; watch closely for reaction recurrence

with asthma and the known beneficial response of asthma to corticosteroids, corticosteroid therapy should also be considered.

- *Persisting hypotension/shock*: IV atropine may be required to treat profound bradycardia, but this will be of little use if fluid status is not corrected. Some patients may have profound vasodilation, so a trial of selective vasoconstrictor (e.g., metaraminol, vasopressin) may be warranted if blood pressure remains low despite the above measures. Also, because some patients have profound but reversible myocardial depression, urgent bedside echocardiographic assessment, glucagon/phosphodiesterase inhibitor inotropes (particularly if the patient is taking β-blockers), and mechanical circulatory support may be considered.
- *Persisting skin symptoms (itch)*: symptomatic treatment with an oral nonsedating antihistamine. There is no evidence for any beneficial effect of antihistamines other than relief of skin symptoms (which usually respond to epinephrine anyway). Conversely, there is evidence of potential harm from the use of parenteral antihistamines causing hypotension in patients who have not been given epinephrine.

Monitoring

Although the majority of reactions will respond promptly to a single dose of epinephrine, in severe reactions (hypotension or hypoxemia) around 40% will require multiple doses of epinephrine.[31] Therefore, close monitoring is required after the initial treatment. Patients with ongoing resuscitation requirements may require admission to intensive care. Around half of biphasic reactions occur within the first 6 to 12 hours following reaction.[1,37] An extended period of observation should be considered in those patients with more severe reactions, or anaphylaxis refractory to more than two doses of IM epinephrine, but there is currently no consensus as to how long this should be.[1] Overnight admission may be required.

ONGOING MANAGEMENT AND REFERRAL

All individuals experiencing anaphylaxis that have a risk for repeat accidental exposure should be prescribed an epinephrine autoinjector device prior to discharge from hospital. Training in the use of the device is mandatory, due to a high incidence of misuse resulting in no injection being administered. There is a discussion in the literature as to how many devices should be prescribed, with some healthcare professionals recommending at least two devices, in the event of misfiring of the first device, or a suboptimal response to the first injection. However, perhaps the most important counseling involves the recommendation to contact emergency medical services early, as refractory anaphylaxis will require intensive medical intervention, which cannot be delivered in the community. This recommendation is well-founded; around one-third of fatalities occur despite a first dose of epinephrine being given in a timely manner.[41]

Patients should be provided with a written management or action plan (e.g., from: http://www.allergy.org.au/health-professionals/anaphylaxis-resources/ascia-action-plan-for-anaphylaxis).

in hematocrit have shown that extravasation of up to 35% of circulating blood volume can occur within the first 10 minutes; on rare occasions, large volumes of isotonic crystalloid in the order of 50 mL/kg over the first 30 minutes have been needed. One caveat is that volume resuscitation is used to treat distributive/hypovolemic shock; if the patient is not hypotensive or is overloaded (e.g., distended neck veins are present), aggressive fluid resuscitation may be harmful.

Other Measures

- *Upper airway obstruction*: in addition to parenteral epinephrine, give nebulized epinephrine (5 mg/5 mL by nebulizer with oxygen at highest flow rate). Intubation or a needle cricothyrotomy/surgical airway may, very rarely, be required.
- *Severe bronchospasm*: in addition to parenteral epinephrine, give salbutamol (albuterol) by nebulizer or inhaler puffed directly into a ventilation circuit (if intubated). Given the diagnostic overlap of severe bronchospasm in this setting

Fatal anaphylaxis is rare but also unpredictable.[9] It is therefore difficult to identify those individuals who are most at risk of severe reactions. Risk factors include:

- *Dose of exposure*: the greater the exposure, the more severe the resulting allergic reaction may be.
- *Risk-taking behaviors*: these are considered to be important in teenagers and young adults, in whom compliance with dietary avoidance and carriage of epinephrine autoinjectors can be an issue.
- *Asthma*: although asthma is common (up to 50% of food-allergic children have asthma) the vast majority of people with asthma will never experience a severe anaphylaxis; the predictive value of asthma for severe anaphylaxis is thus poor. However, poorly controlled asthma may contribute to reaction severity and has been associated with pediatric deaths from anaphylaxis. Therefore, it is important to optimize asthma management/symptom control.
- *Delayed administration of rescue epinephrine or other medical treatments*: this highlights the need to contact emergency medical services early.
- *Presence of cofactors*: data from anaphylaxis registries and studies of immunotherapy have found that allergen exposure occurring together with cofactors (such as exercise, alcohol intake, use of antihypertensive medication, and/or NSAIDs) can increase symptom severity. Where possible, exposure to these cofactors should be minimized where they have been identified as a risk factor in previous reactions. Although some medications such as β-blockers and ACE inhibitors have been anecdotally associated with severe anaphylaxis, these medications also have demonstrated mortality reduction benefits for hypertension, heart disease, and stroke. Therefore, any decision to stop them or to use a substitute requires very careful consideration of these competing risks and benefits.
- *Severity of previous reactions*: for insect venom allergy, prior reaction severity tends to predict maximum subsequent reaction severity. However as noted above, this does not appear to be reliable for other forms of allergy.

Where exercise may have contributed to a food-allergic event, affected individuals should be advised to avoid exercise for 4 hours after ingestion.

Importantly, the degree of sensitization (demonstrated through allergy skin testing or blood tests for allergen-sIgE) does not reliably predict future severity of reactions, nor does a history of prior anaphylaxis. Evidence is emerging that individuals with sIgE to certain lipid transfer proteins (both in food and pollen) may be more at risk of severe reactions. Testing for these should be guided by an allergy specialist.

To provide some guidance to healthcare professionals, the European Academy of Allergy and Clinical Immunology (EAACI) suggests six absolute indications for provision of epinephrine autoinjectors[42]:

1. Previous anaphylaxis to food, latex, aeroallergens, for example, animals or other unavoidable triggers
2. Exercise-induced anaphylaxis
3. Previous idiopathic anaphylaxis
4. Coexistent unstable or moderate to severe, persistent asthma with food allergy
5. Venom allergy in adults with previous systemic reactions, who are not receiving venom immunotherapy
6. Underlying mast cell disorder and any previous systemic reaction

Where an episode occurs in someone with a known allergy, referral for specialist assessment and investigation may not be needed. Urgent referral is appropriate in the following situations:

- No clear trigger for the anaphylaxis exists
- First presentation of food allergy as anaphylaxis, so that appropriate dietary advice (including an assessment of potential cross-reactive allergens) can be provided, along with support strategies
- Features suggesting an underlying contributing pathology, such as mastocytosis

Referral should also be expedited where immunotherapy to prevent subsequent anaphylaxis is an option. This applies to most insect venom anaphylaxis and some drug anaphylaxis, where the agent is considered essential and an alternative drug is not available. For some food allergies, experimental immunotherapy research programs may be available locally as an option for the patient to consider.

CONCLUSIONS

Despite a significant increase in hospitalizations due to anaphylaxis over the past 20 years, the rate of fatal anaphylaxis has not increased and remains very low. However, while fatal anaphylaxis is rare at a population level, it is also unpredictable and in people at risk of severe anaphylaxis, the risk is higher and contributes to anxiety and social restrictions that impact significantly on quality of life measures. Management of acute anaphylaxis should follow a straightforward structured approach focusing on IM epinephrine, IV fluid (volume) resuscitation, and standard life-support measures. Follow-up is important in reducing the risk of repeat episodes; family and general physicians play an important role in allergen identification and risk reduction through a careful history, epinephrine autoinjector and action plan provision, and patient education. Specialist referral can assist with these, particularly with allergen identification, avoidance strategies and assisting with the management of comorbidities, and by providing access to immunotherapy where appropriate. Our ability to predict those most at risk of severe reactions is limited, and this remains the greatest challenge in improving management and patient outcomes. Work is ongoing to understand the mechanisms that predispose to severe anaphylaxis, in the hope that risk stratification of patients will be a realistic management strategy in the future.

REFERENCES

1. Cardona V, Ansotegui I, Ebisawa M, et al. World Allergy Organization anaphylaxis guidance 2020. World Allergy Organ J. 2020;13:100472.
2. Sampson HA, Muñoz-Furlong A, Campbell RL, Adkinson NF Jr, Bock SA, Branum A, et al. Second symposium on the definition and management of anaphylaxis: summary report—Second National Institute of Allergy and Infectious Disease/Food Allergy

and Anaphylaxis Network symposium. J Allergy Clin Immunol. 2006;117:391–397.

3. Simons FE, Ardusso LR, Bilò MB, et al. World allergy organization guidelines for the assessment and management of anaphylaxis. World Allergy Organ J. 2011;4(2):13–37.

4. Turner PJ, Worm M, Ansotegui IJ, et al. Time to revisit the definition and clinical criteria for anaphylaxis? World Allergy Organ J. 2019;12(10):100066.

5. Turner PJ, Campbell DE, Motosue MS, Campbell RL. Global trends in anaphylaxis epidemiology and clinical implications. J Allergy Clin Immunol Pract. 2020;8(4):1169–1176.

6. Turner PJ, Gowland MH, Sharma V, et al. Increase in anaphylaxis-related hospitalizations but no increase in fatalities: an analysis of United Kingdom national anaphylaxis data, 1992–2012. J Allergy Clin Immunol. 2015;135(4):956–963.

7. Liew WK, Williamson E, Tang ML. Anaphylaxis fatalities and admissions in Australia. J Allergy Clin Immunol. 2009;123(2):434–442.

8. Koplin JJ, Martin PE, Allen KJ. An update on epidemiology of anaphylaxis in children and adults. Curr Opin Allergy Clin Immunol. 2011;11(5):492–496.

9. Turner PJ, Baumert JL, Beyer K, et al. Can we identify patients at risk of life-threatening allergic reactions to food? Allergy. 2016;71(9):1241–1255.

10. Finkelman FD, Khodoun MV, Strait R. Human IgE-independent systemic anaphylaxis. J Allergy Clin Immunol. 2016;137(6): 1674–1680.

11. Leone R, Conforti A, Venegoni M, et al. Drug induced anaphylaxis: case/non-case study based on Italian pharmacovigilance database. Drug Saf. 2005;28:547–556.

12. Hetner D, Casdell SM. Latex allergy: an update. Anesth Analg. 2003;96:1219–1229.

13. Mertes P, Laxenaire M, Lienhart A, et al. Reducing the risk of anaphylaxis during anesthesia: guidelines for clinical practice. J Investig Allergol Clin Immunol. 2005;15:91–101.

14. Mertes PM, Alla F, Trechot P, et al. Anaphylaxis during anesthesia in France: an 8-year national survey. J Allergy Clin Immunol. 2011;128:366–373.

15. Cochran ST. Anaphylactoid reactions to radiocontrast media. Curr Allergy Asthma Rep. 2005;5:28–31.

16. Moffitt JE, Golden D, Reisman R, et al. Stinging insect hypersensitivity: a practice parameter update. J Allergy Clin Immunol. 2004;114:869–886.

17. Palmer K, Burks W. Current developments in peanut allergy. Curr Opin Allergy Clin Immunol. 2006;6:202–206.

18. Sicherer SH, Sampson HA. Food allergy. J Allergy Clin Immunol. 2006;117:S470–S475.

19. Moneret-Vautrin DA, Kanny G, Morisset M, et al. The food anaphylaxis vigilance network in France. Allergy Clin Immunol Int. 2003;15:155–159.

20. Ebo D, Bosmans J, Couttenye M, et al. Hemodialysis-associated anaphylaxis and anaphylactoid reactions. Allergy. 2006;61:211–220.

21. Webb L, Lieberman P. Anaphylaxis: a review of 601 cases. Ann Allergy Asthma Immunol. 2006;97:39–43.

22. Sala-Cunill A, Luengo O, Cardona V. Biologics and anaphylaxis. Curr Opin Allergy Clin Immunol. 2019;19(5):439–446.

23. Brown SGA, Stone SF, Fatovich DM, et al. Anaphylaxis: clinical patterns, mediator release, and severity. J Allergy Clin Immunol. 2013;132(5):1141–1149.

24. Stone SF, Bosco A, Jones A, et al. Genomic responses during acute human anaphylaxis are characterized by upregulation of innate inflammatory gene networks. PLoS One. 2014;9(7):e101409.

25. Korosec P, Turner PJ, Silar M, et al. Basophils, high-affinity IgE receptors, and CCL2 in human anaphylaxis. J Allergy Clin Immunol. 2017;140(3):750–758.e15.

26. Santos AF, Du Toit G, O'Rourke C, et al. Biomarkers of severity and threshold of allergic reactions during oral peanut challenges. J Allergy Clin Immunol. 2020;146(2):344–355.

27. Vadas P, Gold M, Perelman B, et al. Platelet-activating factor, PAF acetylhydrolase, and severe anaphylaxis. N Engl J Med. 2008;358(1):28–35.

28. Brown SG. The pathophysiology of shock in anaphylaxis. Immunol Allergy Clin North Am. 2007;27(2):165–175.

29. Ruiz-Garcia M, Bartra J, Alvarez O, et al. Cardiovascular changes during peanut-induced allergic reactions in human subjects. J Allergy Clin Immunol. 2020;147:633.

30. Fisher MM. Clinical observations on the pathophysiology and treatment of anaphylactic cardiovascular collapse. Anaesth Intensive Care. 1986;14(1):17–21.

31. Brown SGA, Blackman KE, Stenlake V, et al. Insect sting anaphylaxis; prospective evaluation of treatment with intravenous adrenaline and volume resuscitation. Emerg Med J. 2004;21(2):149–154.

32. Pumphrey RS. Fatal posture in anaphylactic shock. J Allergy Clin Immunol. 2003;112(2):451–452.

33. Mullins RJ, Wainstein BK, Barnes EH, Liew WK, Campbell DE. Increases in anaphylaxis fatalities in Australia from 1997 to 2013. Clin Exp Allergy. 2016;46(8):1099–1110.

34. Worm M, Moneret-Vautrin A, Scherer K, Lang R, Fernandez-Rivas M, Cardona V, et al. First European data from the network of severe allergic reactions (NORA). Allergy. 2014;69:1397–1404.

35. Pumphrey RS. Lessons for management of anaphylaxis from a study of fatal reactions. Clin Exp Allergy. 2000;30:1144–1150.

36. Sampson HA, Mendelson L, Rosen JP. Fatal and near-fatal anaphylactic reactions to food in children and adolescents. N Engl J Med. 1992;327(6):380–384.

37. Lee S, Bellolio MF, Hess EP, Erwin P, Murad MH, Campbell RL. Time of onset and predictors of biphasic anaphylactic reactions: a systematic review and meta-analysis. J Allergy Clin Immunol Pract. 2015;3(3):408–416.e162.

38. Lee S, Peterson A, Lohse CM, Hess EP, Campbell RL. Further evaluation of factors that may predict biphasic reactions in emergency department anaphylaxis patients. J Allergy Clin Immunol Pract. 2017;5(5):1295–1301.

39. Brown SGA, Stone SF. Laboratory diagnosis of acute anaphylaxis. Clin Exp Allergy. 2011;41(12):1660–1662.

40. Mittermann I, Zidarn M, Silar M, et al. Recombinant allergen-based IgE testing to distinguish bee and wasp allergy. J Allergy Clin Immunol. 2010;125(6):1300–1307.e3.

41. Pumphrey R, Sturm G. Risk factors for fatal anaphylaxis. In: Moneret-Vautrin DA, ed. Advances in anaphylaxis management. London: Future Medicine; 2014:32–48.

42. Muraro A, Roberts G, Worm M, et al. Anaphylaxis: guidelines from the European Academy of Allergy and Clinical Immunology. Allergy. 2014;69(8):1026–1045.

14

Occupational Allergy

Catherine Lemière and Hille Suojalehto

CHAPTER OUTLINE

SUMMARY OF IMPORTANT CONCEPTS

- Occupational allergic respiratory diseases represent a significant public health concern owing to their high prevalence and their long-term respiratory health consequences and socioeconomic costs for both the affected worker and society as a whole.
- Evaluation for occupational asthma (OA) and occupational rhinitis (OR) is indicated in all workers in whom asthma and/or rhinitis symptoms develop or worsen in relation to their work environment.
- The diagnosis of OA and OR should be established with the highest level of accuracy by performing a comprehensive investigation to avoid unwarranted socioeconomic costs.
- Complete avoidance of the causative agent remains the recommended management approach because available information indicates that reduction of exposure is a less beneficial management option.
- Continued exposure to the causative agent will result in substantial long-term respiratory morbidity because it is associated with a low rate of recovery, especially when the diagnosis is delayed.
- Primary prevention should be directed toward reducing exposure to levels below those known to induce the onset of asthma in all workers, irrespective of their individual susceptibility.

INTRODUCTION AND DEFINITIONS

Occupational Asthma

During the past decade, there has been growing recognition that work-related asthma is a major public health concern owing to its high prevalence and societal burden. *Work-related asthma* is a broad term indicating that asthma is caused or worsened by the workplace. Work-related asthma encompasses both *occupational asthma* (OA), which is asthma caused by a specific agent in the workplace, and *work-exacerbated asthma* (WEA), which is asthma worsened by nonspecific stimuli in the workplace but not caused by it.[1]

OA is a disease characterized by airway inflammation, variable airflow limitation, and bronchial hyperresponsiveness due to causes and conditions attributable to a particular occupational environment and not to stimuli encountered outside the workplace.[2] *Sensitizer-induced OA* is characterized by the development—after a latency period—of immunologically mediated specific bronchial hyperresponsiveness to an agent present in the workplace. By contrast, irritant-induced asthma (IIA), also called "OA without a latency period," encompasses a wide spectrum of clinical presentations.[3] The rapid onset of asthma within a few hours after a single exposure to very high levels of irritant substances (i.e., acute-onset IIA or *Reactive Airways Dysfunction Syndrome* (RADS) is the phenotype of IIA that has been the best characterized. Other clinical phenotypes, which occur after repeated inhalations of low doses of irritant agents, are mainly described in epidemiologic studies. The causal relationship between irritant exposures at the workplace and occurrence of respiratory symptoms is almost impossible to demonstrate at the individual level. In keeping with the focus of this book on allergic diseases, the scope of this chapter is restricted to sensitizer-induced OA.

Occupational Rhinitis

Occupational rhinitis (OR) has been defined as an inflammatory disease of the nose, which is characterized by intermittent or persistent symptoms (i.e., nasal congestion, sneezing, rhinorrhea, itching) and/or variable nasal airflow limitation and/or hypersecretion due to causes and conditions attributable to a particular work environment and not to stimuli encountered outside the workplace.[4]

As with work-related asthma (Fig. 14.1), the broad spectrum of rhinitis syndromes related to the work environment can be broken down into the following categories: (1) allergic OR; (2) non-allergic OR; and (3) work-exacerbated rhinitis.

EPIDEMIOLOGY

A pooled analysis of all epidemiologic studies published up to 2019 indicated that 16% of all cases of adult-onset asthma are attributable to workplace exposures.

Information on the incidence and prevalence of OR in the general population is largely lacking, although surveys of workforces exposed to sensitizing agents indicate that OR is two to four times more common than OA.

PATHOGENESIS AND ETIOLOGY

Agents Causing Occupational Asthma and Rhinitis

The workplace agents known to cause immunologically mediated OA and OR usually are categorized into high-molecular-weight (HMW; molecular mass >10 kDa) and low-molecular-weight (LMW; molecular mass <10 kDa) agents. HMW agents are (glyco)proteins of vegetable and animal origin, whereas LMW agents include reactive chemicals, transition metals, and wood dusts. The agents and occupations most commonly implicated are listed in Table 14.1. The main differences between HMW and LMW agents are summarized in Table 14.2. A very large number of substances (>400) used in the workplace have been documented as causing immunologic OA and OR (listed at www.asthme.csst.qc.ca). However, flour and isocyanates account for about half of the reported cases of OA in industrialized countries. The distribution of causative agents may vary across geographic areas, depending on the pattern of industrial activities.

Workers in occupations with the highest incidence rates of OA are bakers and pastry makers, other food processors, spray painters, hairdressers, wood workers, healthcare workers, cleaners, farmers, laboratory technicians, and welders. In more recent years, population-based studies conducted in various countries worldwide have consistently found that cleaning activities were associated with an excess risk of asthma and work-related asthma symptoms. Industrial and domestic cleaners are exposed to a wide variety of products containing irritant chemicals (e.g., detergents, acids, alkali, solvents, chelating compounds) as well as some potentially sensitizing substances, including biocides (e.g., quaternary ammonium compounds, aldehydes, chloramine-T), ethanolamines, enzymes, and latex gloves.

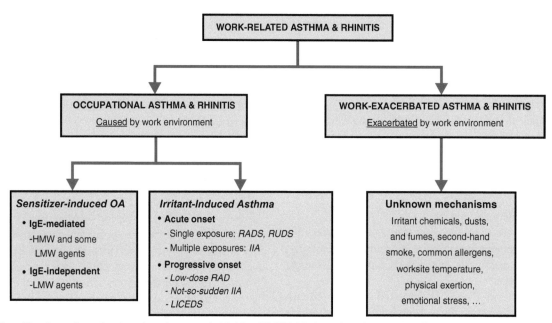

Fig. 14.1 Classification of work-related asthma and rhinitis. *HMW,* High-molecular-weight; *IIA,* irritant-induced asthma; *LICEDS,* low-intensity chronic exposure dysfunction syndrome; *LMW,* low-molecular-weight; *RADS,* reactive airways dysfunction syndrome; *RUDS,* reactive upper airways dysfunction syndrome.

TABLE 14.1   Principal Agents Causing Immunologic Occupational Asthma

Agent		Workers/Occupations at Risk
High-Molecular-Weight Agents		
Cereals (flour)	Wheat, rye, barley, buckwheat	Millers, bakers, pastry makers
Latex	Gloves	Healthcare workers, laboratory technicians
Animals	Mice, rats, cows, seafood	Laboratory workers, farmers, seafood processors
Enzymes	α-Amylase, maxatase, alcalase, papain, bromelain, pancreatin	Baking products manufacture, bakers, detergent production, pharmaceutical industry, food industry
Low-Molecular-Weight Agents		
Isocyanates	Toluene diisocyanate (TDI), methylene diphenyl-diisocyanate (MDI), hexamethylene diisocyanate (HDI)	Polyurethane production, plastic industry, molding, spray painters, insulation installers
Persulfate salts	Hair bleach	Hairdressers
Metals	Chromium, nickel, cobalt, platinum	Metal refinery, metal alloy production, electroplaters, welders
Biocides	Aldehydes, quaternary ammonium compounds	Healthcare workers, cleaners
Acrylates	Cyanoacrylates, methacrylates, di- and triacrylates	Manufacture of adhesives, dental and orthopedic materials, sculptured fingernails, printing inks, paints and coatings
Wood dusts	Red cedar, iroko, obeche, oak	Sawmill workers, carpenters, cabinet and furniture makers
Acid anhydrides	Phthalic, trimellitic, maleic, tetrachlorophthalic acids	Epoxy resin workers

TABLE 14.2   Main Differences Between High- and Low-Molecular-Weight Agents Causing Occupational Asthma

Feature	High-Molecular-Weight Agents	Low-Molecular-Weight Agents
Nature	(Glyco)proteins derived from plants and animals	Highly reactive chemicals, metals, and wood dusts
Immunologic mechanisms	IgE-mediated	Uncertain; specific IgE for some agents (e.g., platinum salts, reactive dyes, acid anhydrides)
Type of airway inflammation	Eosinophils	Eosinophils and sometimes neutrophils
Type of asthmatic reactions	Often early	Often late
Associated disorders		
Rhinoconjunctivitis	Common (~90%)	Less common (~50%)
Contact dermatitis	Rare, but protein contact dermatitis may occur (e.g., flour, seafood)	May occur (e.g., epoxy resins, acrylates, metals)
Urticaria and, anaphylaxis	Frequent with some agents (e.g., latex)	Rare

IgE, Immunoglobulin E.

Pathophysiology

The pathophysiology of sensitizer-induced OA and OR involves in most cases an immunoglobulin E (IgE)-dependent mechanism, especially for HMW agents, whereas in most cases of OA induced by LMW agents, the production of specific IgE antibodies or the upregulation of IgE receptors has not been identified.

Immunologic, IgE-Mediated

The pathophysiology of OA induced by IgE-dependent agents is similar to that of allergic asthma unrelated to work. HMW agents (proteinaceous products such as animal proteins and flour) act as complete antigens and induce the production of specific IgE antibodies. Certain LMW occupational agents, including platinum salts, acid anhydrides, reactive dyes, and some wood species, also induce specific IgE antibodies, probably by acting as haptens and binding with proteins to form functional antigens.

Immunologic, Non-IgE-Mediated

Many LMW chemicals, including isocyanates and plicatic acid (the agent causing Western red cedar asthma), cause OA but do not consistently induce specific IgE antibodies. Cell-mediated reactions are probably important in OA caused by LMW agents. While the predominant immune response to chemical respiratory allergens may be of the Th2 type, other cells are also likely to play important supportive or regulatory roles.

Risk Factors

Environmental Risk Factors

OA and OR result from the complex interaction between environmental and individual factors. The evidence supporting the role of potential risk factors is summarized in Table 14.3.

Level of Exposure. The intensity of exposure to sensitizing agents is currently the best characterized and the most important environmental risk factor for the development of OA (see Table 14.3). The timing of exposure may also play a role because the prevalence of onset of work-related asthma symptoms is consistently higher within the early period of exposure to the occupational agents, and exposure–response gradients

TABLE 14.3   Summary of Potential Risk Factors for Development of Occupational Asthma

Risk Factor	Evidence	Agents/Settings
High level of exposure	Strong	*HMW agents*: flour, enzymes, laboratory animals
	Moderate	*LMW agents*: platinum salts, acid anhydrides, isocyanates
Skin exposure	Weak	Isocyanates
Cigarette smoking	Moderate	*IgE sensitization*: laboratory animals, seafood, psyllium, green coffee, enzymes, acid anhydrides, platinum, reactive dyes
	Weak	*Clinical OA*: laboratory animals, enzymes
Atopy	Strong	*HMW agents*
	Weak	*LMW agents*: platinum, acid anhydrides
Work-related rhinitis	Strong	Laboratory animals
Preexisting nonspecific bronchial responsiveness	Moderate	HMW agents (laboratory animals, flour, latex)
Genetic markers:		
HLA class II alleles	Moderate	*LMW agents*: isocyanates, red cedar, acid anhydrides, platinum salts
Antioxidant enzymes[a]	Moderate	*HMW agents*: laboratory animals, latex
Alpha-T catenin SNPs	Moderate	Isocyanates
TLR4 SNPs	Weak	Isocyanates
IL-4 receptor α, IL-13 SNPs	Weak	Laboratory animals
TNFα, TGFB1, PTGS1, PTGS2 SNPs	Weak	Isocyanates
		Isocyanates
Gender (female)	Weak	Snow crab processors

HMW, High-molecular-weight; *IgE*, immunoglobulin E; *IL*, interleukin; *LMW*, low-molecular-weight; *OA*: occupational asthma; *SNPs*, single nucleotide polymorphisms; *TLR4*, toll-like receptor 4; *TNFα*, tumor necrosis factor α; *TGFB*, transforming growth factor-β; *PTGS*, prostaglandin-endoperoxide synthase.
[a]Glutathione-S-transferase and N-acetyltransferase.

are more clearly documented in those workers who develop these outcomes soon after the onset of exposure.

Smoking and Exposure to Other Pollutants. A number of studies have suggested that exposure to cigarette smoke can increase the risk of IgE-mediated sensitization to some HMW and LMW agents (see Table 14.3), but the evidence supporting an association between smoking and the development of clinical OA is still very weak.

Growing evidence indicates that environmental pollutants, such as ozone, nitrogen dioxide, tobacco smoke, diesel exhaust particles, and endotoxin, can act as adjuvants in allergic responses to common inhalant allergens. Only limited information, however, is available on the potential interactions between pollutants and sensitizing agents in the workplace.

Individual Risk Factors

Atopy. Atopy has consistently been demonstrated as an important host risk factor for the development of IgE-mediated sensitization, OA, and OR, due to HMW agents (see Table 14.3), whereas this association remains controversial for some LMW agents and absent for most other LMW agents. Preexposure sensitization to common allergens that are structurally related to workplace allergens, such as pets in the case of laboratory animal workers, could be a stronger predictor of OA than atopy.

Rhinitis. Epidemiologic studies have shown that OR is associated with an increased risk for the subsequent development of asthma and OA, particularly that caused by HMW agents. However, the proportion of subjects with OR who will develop OA remains uncertain. Among apprentices in animal health

technology, the predictive value of work-related nasal symptoms on the subsequent development of probable OA was only 11.4% over a follow-up period of 30 to 42 months (see Table 14.3). Prospective cohort studies of apprentices also have shown that rhinitis present before work exposure is an independent risk factor for IgE sensitization to HMW allergens.

Nonspecific Bronchial Hyperresponsiveness. Prospective cohort studies have shown that the presence of airway hyperresponsiveness and a physician's diagnosis of asthma before initiation of exposure to HMW occupational agents are associated with an increased risk of subsequent IgE sensitization and OA.

Genetic Susceptibility. Although genetic host factors in workers who develop OA has been identified (see Table 14.3), they are not sufficiently sensitive or specific for diagnostic or preventive purposes. In addition, environmental factors can interact with genetic determinants to affect disease susceptibility.

CLINICAL FEATURES

As in non–work-related asthma, the clinical features of OA include signs and symptoms of variable cough, wheezing, dyspnea associated with reversible airflow limitation, airway hyperresponsiveness, and airway inflammation. Some clinical features are more specifically related to OA. Typically, the affected worker initially complains of cough, wheeze, and dyspnea, either as soon as the work shift exposure starts or at the end of the work shift or even in the evening, after working hours, with remission during weekends and holidays. As the disease progresses, symptoms tend to occur earlier during the day and fail to remit during days off and long holidays. With further exposure, asthma symptoms may persist and become permanent, despite complete withdrawal from exposure. In these instances, even prolonged removal from exposure will result in only partial reversal of the asthma. It is therefore very important to establish the diagnosis of OA early and to remove the patient from exposure. Rhinitis is associated with respiratory symptoms in a majority of cases of OA and often precedes the occurrence of respiratory symptoms, especially with exposure to HMW agents.

PATIENT EVALUATION, DIAGNOSIS, AND DIFFERENTIAL DIAGNOSIS

Patient Evaluation and Diagnosis
History

OA should be suspected in every adult patient with new-onset asthma. The first diagnostic step is to confirm the presence of asthma and to exclude conditions with asthma-like manifestations such as vocal cord dysfunction, hyperventilation, and sick building syndrome.

A good occupational history, not only of the current job and exposure but also of past jobs and exposures, is essential. A scheme for addressing relevant points has been published and includes employment history (current and past jobs), symptoms (nature, temporal relationship to work, improvement while away from work), and potential risk factors. In many cases, the patient may not be aware of the exact chemical exposures at work; material safety data sheets (MSDSs) can be requested from the workplace and may be of help in clarifying the presence of a workplace sensitizer. If the content of the causative agent is <1%, it may not be listed in the MSDS. In such instances, the manufacturer must be contacted. It is often helpful to ask the worker to sketch the work site and the work process itself, and to indicate the locations where he or she works during the work shift. In addition to identifying potential high-risk agents, the exposure history should include the duration of exposure and the frequency and concentrations of exposure. The substances to which the worker is potentially exposed at work can be checked against a comprehensive list of agents recognized as causing OA, and the specific job for that worker checked against the list of at-risk occupations. These lists are available from various sources (websites and published tables). If available, the occupational health record and the industrial hygiene record from the company should be reviewed.

Assessment of Airway Hyperresponsiveness

The diagnosis of asthma needs to be confirmed by demonstrating a reversible airflow obstruction or the presence of airway hyperresponsiveness. A negative reaction to a histamine or methacholine challenge has a very high negative predictive value (95%)[5] when the patient is working, but does not exclude OA if such testing is performed when the patient is off work and free of symptoms. Thus, when the challenge test is performed while the patient is working and symptomatic, the diagnosis of OA can be reasonably excluded.

Immunological Testing

When possible, the sensitization to the suspected agent should be assessed by skin-prick tests (SPTs) or by measuring specific immunoglobulin E (sIgE). However, immunologic tests in the diagnosis of OA are limited by the lack of standardized commercially available reagents for skin and in vitro tests. A meta-analysis of studies published between 1967 and 2016[6] provided estimates for the assessment of serum sIgE: a pooled sensitivity of 74% (95% confidence interval [CI]: 66%–80%) and a specificity of 71% (95% CI: 63–77) for HMW allergens; a sensitivity of 28% (95% CI: 18–40) and a specificity of 89% (95% CI: 77%–95%) for LMW agents. Immunological tests alone are not able to confirm or exclude a diagnosis of OA in workers exposed to HMW agents with an appropriate level of confidence in the majority of cases. However, it has been demonstrated for some HMW agents that increasing the cut-off value for a positive sIgE test (i.e., $\geq$2.22 kU$_A$/L for wheat flour, $\geq$9.64 kU$_A$/L for rye flour, and $\geq$4.41 kU$_A$/L for natural rubber latex) increases both the specificity and positive predictive value above 95%.[7] Thus, a diagnosis of OA can be suspected with a high level of confidence in asthmatic workers with a suggestive history of OA who show very positive SPTs or high titers of specific IgE to the suspected agents.

In subjects exposed to LMW agents, the sensitivity of sIgE is low with a high specificity. These results suggest that, when available, the presence of sIgE against LMW agents, such as isocyanates or acid anhydrides, is associated with a high likelihood of OA. However, the very limited availability of these tests combined with a poor performance for ruling out a diagnosis of OA prevents them from being used as clinical tools.

Probability scores for the diagnosis of OA have been developed based upon statistical models, including age, presence of rhinoconjunctivitis, inhaled-corticosteroid use, agent type, airway hyperresponsiveness, and work-specific sensitization in patients exposed to HMW who are exposed to the suspected agents.[8] However, since the workers need to undergo a methacholine or histamine inhalation challenge as well as SPTs to occupational agents, the use of these scores in primary care is likely to be limited.

Serial Measurements of Functional Parameters

Cross-shift changes in forced expiratory volume in 1 second (FEV1) and peak expiratory flow (PEF) seem to show a low sensitivity for identifying OA (50%–60%),[9] but may have a high specificity (91%). However, the data supporting those findings are scarce.

Serial measurement of PEF with the subject at work and away from work is inexpensive and can be useful in obtaining objective information for the confirmation of OA.

However, compliance with PEF monitoring has been shown to be poor, especially when patients were asked to record values four times per day. The optimal duration of recording of PEF has not been established, but monitoring should include a minimum period of 2 weeks at work and exposed to the suspected causative agent and a similar period away from work, unless significant changes are recorded earlier at work. If the patient is using inhaled corticosteroids, it is important to keep the same dose throughout the period of monitoring. Inhaled bronchodilators should be used only when necessary, and the patient's self-dosing history should be recorded. PEF should be performed before use of bronchodilators.

No uniformly accepted criteria for the interpretation of PEF recordings have been established. Attempts have been made to develop such criteria, but the sensitivity and specificity of the diagnosis based on these objective criteria were no better than for the "eyeballing" method of experienced physicians. A computer-assisted diagnostic aid, observation and appraisal system (OASYS), has been developed to distinguish occupational from nonoccupational causes of airflow obstruction. This tool has a moderate sensitivity (82% [95% CI 76%–90%]) but a high specificity (88% [95% CI 80%–95%]) as compared to specific inhalation challenge (SIC) and seems therefore more reliable in confirming than excluding OA.[10]

Serial measurement of airway responsiveness at and away from work yields variable sensitivities (43%–62%) and specificities (52%–83%).[11,12] Although theoretically a decrease in airway hyperresponsiveness should occur after a period away from work, this has not been found to be a reliable means of confirming OA, probably because assessments are repeated after too short an interval of being away from work (usually 2 weeks). Combining those measurements with serial PEF monitoring only showed a slight improvement in sensitivity over serial PEF monitoring alone.[11]

Specific Inhalation Challenge Tests. SIC tests consist of exposing the subjects to the agent suspected to cause their asthma. These tests are considered to be the reference tests in investigation of OA.[13] Laboratory-specific challenge tests are time-consuming and require specialized facilities that are available in only a few clinical centers. Specific challenge tests are useful in the following circumstances: (1) when the diagnosis of OA remains in doubt after serial monitoring of PEF or airway responsiveness; (2) when a patient clearly has OA but it is necessary for management personnel to confirm or identify the causative agent at work; (3) when a new agent is suspected of causing OA; and (4) when the patient cannot be returned to the incriminated workplace.

Although SIC testing is still considered the gold standard for the diagnosis of OA, the potential for false-positive and false-negative responses is well recognized. A false-negative response may occur if the wrong agent is used (e.g., different types of diisocyanates), or if the exposure conditions are not comparable with those in the workplace. SIC testing at the workplace consists of serial spirometric measurements performed by a respiratory technologist, while the worker is doing his or her usual tasks. It can be useful to perform an SIC at the workplace when the SIC result in the laboratory is negative. SIC tests at the workplace have been shown to be positive in 22% of the subjects with a highly suggestive history and negative SIC reaction in the laboratory. However, they do not allow for the identification of the causative agent.

Serial Measures of Airway Inflammation

Sputum Cell Counts. Sputum eosinophil counts achieve the best diagnostic accuracy when performed serially during periods at and away from work or before and after exposure to an offending agent during SICs.[14] Approximately 70% of patients with OA show an increase of at least 3% in sputum eosinophil counts after exposure to the offending agent. An increase of at least 3% of sputum eosinophils after exposure to the offending agent achieves a 90% specificity for the diagnosis of OA.[14] An increase in sputum eosinophils can precede the occurrence of functional changes occurring after exposure to the occupational agent responsible for OA. Although a notable increase in the sputum eosinophil count in the absence of a fall in FEV_1 should incite pursuing the investigation, the lack of increase in sputum eosinophil counts after exposure to occupational agents should not rule out the diagnosis of OA. Interfering factors that can modify the sputum cell response such as corticosteroid treatment should be considered in the interpretation.

Exhaled Nitric Oxide. The measurement of a fractional nitric oxide (NO) concentration in exhaled breath (FeNO) is a quantitative, noninvasive, simple, and safe proxy for eosinophilic airway inflammation. Although the measurements of FeNO can be affected by a number of factors, it may be of interest in some cases to support the diagnosis of OA. A postchallenge increase in FeNO $\geq$13–17.5 ppb or >41% over baseline value shows a high specificity (90%–95%); however, the sensitivity is low (45%–50%) for predicting a positive SIC.[15-17] FeNO levels seem to increase more consistently in subjects with OA due to HMW agents than in subjects with OA due to LMW after exposure to those agents. The European Respiratory Society (ERS) Task Force *on SICs in the diagnosis of OA* (6) stated that the assessment of the FeNO levels during SIC may be useful in subjects who fail to provide suitable sputum samples, although changes in FeNO seem less discriminatory than those in sputum eosinophils. When the changes in FEV_1 are equivocal, an increase in FeNO 24 hours after the challenge supports a positive SIC.

Combination of Different Tests. A systematic review of studies on the diagnosis of OA assessed the sensitivity and specificity of the combination of various diagnostic tools: measure of airway responsiveness, SPT, and serum IgE.[18] For OA due to HMW agents, airway responsiveness, SPT, and serum-specific IgE had sensitivities >73% when compared with SIC, the reference test. High specificity was demonstrated for a positive result for airway responsiveness and SPTs alone (82.5%; 95% CI, 54.0–95.0) or in combination with specific IgE (74.3%; 95% CI, 45.0–91.0) versus SIC.

The highest sensitivity for the diagnosis of OA due to LMW agents occurred between combined airway responsiveness tests and SPTs versus SIC (100%; 95% CI, 74.1–100). When compared with SIC, specific IgE and SPT had similar specificities (88.9%; 95% CI, 84.7–92.1; and 86.2%; 95% CI, 77.4–91.9, respectively).

The combination of several biomarkers improves the accuracy of the diagnosis of OA. The combination of sputum eosinophil differential cell counts or FeNO levels with the measurement of airway responsiveness improves the sensitivity of the methacholine or histamine challenge alone. The combination of the changes in sputum eosinophil differential cell counts and airway responsiveness after exposure to the offending agents improves diagnostic accuracy for the diagnosis of OA. Making an accurate diagnosis of OA is crucial because of the significant social and financial consequences associated with this diagnosis. The validity of the different diagnostic tests and their practical limitations and advantages are summarized in Tables 14.4 and 14.5.

Fig. 14.2 shows the algorithm to be used in evaluating a patient suspected of having OA. The investigation may be carried out in two steps. The first step consists in assessing airway hyperresponsiveness and when possible the sensitization to the suspected agent. A negative methacholine/histamine challenge test performed while the patient is working can reasonably

TABLE 14.4 Validity of Objective Diagnostic Tests

Test	Sensitivity (%)	Specificity (%)
Single assessment of nonspecific bronchial responsiveness[a]	84 (69–93)	48 (26–72)
Immunologic tests:		
HMW agents (SPT)[a]	81 (70–88)	60 (42–75)
LMW agents (specific IgE antibodies)[a]	31 (23–41)	89 (85–92)
Serial measurements of PEF[a]	64 (43–80)	77 (66–85)
Serial measurements of PEF and nonspecific bronchial responsiveness[b]	84–92	61–67
Single assessment of sputum eosinophils[c]		
≥1%	50	67
≥3%	22	91
Serial assessments of sputum eosinophils at and away from work[d]:		
Increase >1%	65 (45–81)	76 (57–88)
Increase >2%	52 (33–71)	80 (61–91)
Increase >6.4%	26 (13–46)	92 (75–98)
Serial assessment[d]	50 (24–76)	75 (51–90)

Sensitivity and specificity of diagnostic tests are expressed as a percentage, with 95% confidence interval in parentheses when available. Sensitivity and specificity of combined diagnostic tests. *HMW*, High-molecular-weight; *LMW*, low-molecular-weight; *PEF*, peak expiratory flow; *SPT*, skin-prick test.
[a]Modified from Beach J, Russell K, Blitz S, et al. A systematic review of the diagnosis of occupational asthma. Chest 2007;131:569–78.
[b]Modified from Perrin B, Lagier F, L'Archevêque J, et al. Occupational asthma: validity of monitoring of peak expiratory flow rates and non-allergic bronchial responsiveness as compared to specific inhalation challenge. Eur Respir J 1992;5:40–8; and Côté J, Kennedy S, Chan-Yeung M. Sensitivity and specificity of PC20 and peak expiratory flow rate in cedar asthma. J Allergy Clin Immunol 1990;85:592–8.
[c]Modified from Malo JL, Cardinal S, Ghezzo H, et al. Association of bronchial reactivity to occupational agents with methacholine reactivity, sputum cells and immunoglobulin E-mediated reactivity. Clin Exp Allergy 2011;41:497–504.
[d]Difference between the percentage of eosinophils at work and away from work. Modified from Girard F, Chaboillez S, Cartier A, et al. An effective strategy for diagnosing occupational asthma: use of induced sputum. Am J Respir Crit Care Med 2004;170:845–50.

TABLE 14.5 Advantages and Limitations of Diagnostic Tests Used in the Investigation of Occupational Asthma (OA)

Diagnostic Test(s)	Advantages/Limitations
Assessment of airway responsiveness	Simple, low cost
	Allow to confirm the diagnosis of asthma
	Low specificity for diagnosis of OA. The lack of airway hyperresponsiveness does not allow discarding the diagnosis of OA in subjects who have been removed from the workplace
Immunologic tests	Easy to perform, low cost
	Commercial extracts are available (SPT or specific IgE for HMW agents)
	Lack of standardization for a majority of occupational allergens except latex
	Measure of specific IgE available for some LMW agents (anhydrides, acids, isocyanates, aldehydes), but low sensitivity
	Identify the sensitization but not the disease itself
PEF monitoring	Low cost
	Requires the worker's collaboration
	Low adherence (<60%)
	Possible falsification of the results
	Requires 2 weeks at and away from work, which are not always possible for the workers
	Impossible to perform when the worker has already been removed from exposure
	No standardized method for interpreting the results
	Interpretation of the results requires experience

(Continued)

TABLE 14.5 Advantages and Limitations of Diagnostic Tests Used in the Investigation of Occupational Asthma (OA)—cont'd

Diagnostic Test(s)	Advantages/Limitations
Specific inhalation challenges in the laboratory	Confirmation of the diagnosis of OA when the test is positive
	False-negative tests are possible
	Costly
	Available in a small number of centers worldwide
Specific inhalation challenges at the workplace	Exclude diagnosis if response is negative when performed in the usual work conditions
	Requires usual work condition
	Costly
Noninvasive measures of airway inflammation	Sputum cell counts
	Impossible to falsify
	Bring additional evidence to the diagnosis of OA
	Costly
	Not widely available
	Does not allow to confirm or discard the diagnosis of OA by itself
	Exhaled NO measurement
	Easy to perform
	Inconsistent results
	Difficult to interpret
	Affected by many different factors

HMW, High-molecular-weight; *IgE,* immunoglobulin E; *LMW,* low-molecular-weight; *NO,* nitric oxide; *PEF,* peak expiratory flow; *SPT,* skin-prick test.

exclude the diagnosis of OA. Very positive SPTs or high titers of specific IgE to the suspected agent have a high positive predictive value for the diagnosis of OA in asthmatic subjects with a suggestive history of OA. Outside of these scenarios, the second step assessing the relationship between work and asthma should be undertaken by performing serial measurements of PEF and/or assessments of airway responsiveness and/or noninvasive measures of airway inflammation at work and off work and/or SIC tests in the laboratory or at the workplace.[19]

Differential Diagnosis

The most challenging aspect of the differential diagnosis for OA is certainly the diagnosis of WEA.[1] In both conditions, the affected worker complains of a worsening of asthma symptoms when at work. Along with those symptoms, impairment of respiratory function, as evidenced by increased airflow limitation, increased airway hyperresponsiveness, and increased variability of serial PEF measurements, can be identified during periods at work, in comparison with periods away from work. Although workers with OA exhibited greater PEF variability during a period at work than workers with WEA, these differences in variability do not allow differentiation between the two conditions in clinical practice. The gold standard test to differentiate OA from WEA remains the SIC. Whereas the exposure to a specific occupational asthmagen induces a 15% to 20% fall in FEV_1 in workers with OA, no sustained fall in FEV_1 is observed in subjects with WEA. The occurrence of an eosinophilic inflammatory process on exposure to an occupational agent also favors the diagnosis of OA.

Eosinophilic bronchitis is a variant of asthma that represents 12% of the causes of chronic cough. It consists of cough or asthma-like symptoms related to an underlying eosinophilic inflammation without airflow obstruction or airway hyperresponsiveness. This condition is responsive to inhaled corticosteroids. Eosinophilic bronchitis can be caused by sensitization to occupational agents and has been labeled occupational eosinophilic bronchitis. The diagnostic criteria consist of the following: isolated chronic cough (lasting >3 weeks) that worsens at work; sputum eosinophilia with counts of ≥2.5% in either spontaneous or induced samples; increases in sputum eosinophilia related to exposure to the offending agent; spirometric parameters within normal limits and not significantly affected by exposure to the offending agent; absence of airway hyperresponsiveness to methacholine (provocative concentration of methacholine inducing a 20% fall in FEV1 [PC_{20}] >16 kDa mg/mL) both at work and away from work; other causes of chronic cough are ruled out.[20] Occupational eosinophilic bronchitis has been causally related to a number of occupational agents, including latex, wheat flour, α-amylase, egg lysozyme, isocyanates, acrylates, formaldehyde, chloramine-T, epoxy resin hardener, stainless steel welding fumes, and mushroom spores.

Exposure to specific occupational agents such as textile, grain dust, or aluminum can induce conditions that are considered as variants of OA (byssinosis, potroom asthma). Exposure to those agents can lead to partially reversible airflow obstruction with chronic airflow limitation.

OUTCOMES AND TREATMENT

Systematic reviews of existing data on the outcome of immunologic OA indicate that complete and definitive avoidance of exposure to the causative agent remains the optimal treatment for immunologic OA.[21] Almost all workers with immunologic

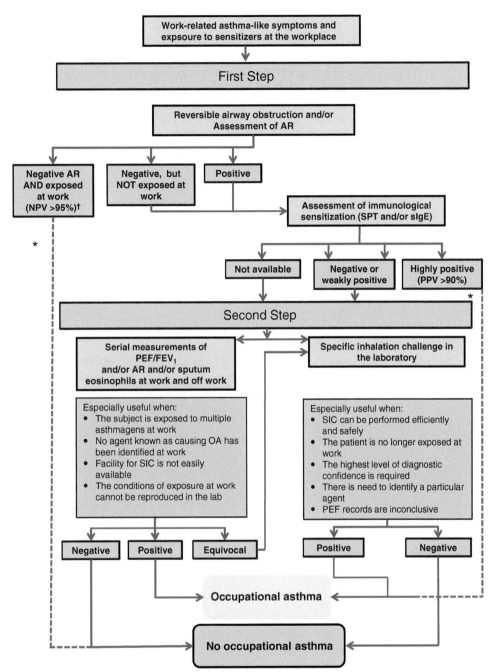

Fig. 14.2 Algorithm for the investigation of occupational asthma (OA). The absence of airway hyperresponsiveness in subjects exposed to the suspected agent makes the diagnosis of OA highly unlikely. A high level of sIgE against some high-molecular-weight (HMW) agents (i.e., wheat, rye, latex) provides a high specificity and positive predictive value, making the diagnosis of OA very likely in asthmatic patients with a suggestive history of OA. *AR*, Airway responsiveness; *FEV1*, Forced expiratory volume in 1 second; *NPV*, negative predictive value; *PEF*, peak expiratory flow; *PPV*, positive predictive value; *SIC*, specific inhalation challenge; *sIgE*, specific immunoglobulin E; *SPT*, skin-prick tests. *High negative and positive predictive values apply only to selected subjects with a high pretest probability of OA.
†Consider measurement of sputum eosinophil counts to identify occupational eosinophilic bronchitis or further investigation if the clinical history is highly suggestive of OA. (i.e., tertiary centres).
(Adapted from Vandenplas O, Suojalehto H, Cullinan P. Diagnosing occupational asthma. Clin Exp Allergy 2016;47: 6–18. Fig. 1. https://doi.org/10.1111/cea.12858).

OA who continue to be exposed to the causative agent will have persistent symptoms; they are at high risk for deterioration of asthma symptoms, airway obstruction, and airway hyperresponsiveness. Reduction of exposure to the agent causing OA through job modification is an alternative option to complete avoidance when elimination of exposure or accommodation of affected workers to unexposed jobs is not possible. This option is less beneficial than cessation of exposure, because it is associated with a lower likelihood of asthma improvement and a higher risk of worsening. This management approach should therefore be restricted to selected patients, and careful medical monitoring is required to ensure early identification of asthma worsening.

Clinicians should be aware that OA is not always reversible after cessation of exposure to the sensitizing agent. Asthma symptoms and airway hyperresponsiveness persist in approximately 70% of the patients with OA several years after their removal from the offending environment. Besides environmental interventions, the pharmacologic treatment of OA should follow the clinical practice guidelines for asthma. Systematic treatment with high-dose inhaled corticosteroids in addition to exposure cessation provides only a slight additional benefit. A few case reports suggest that the anti-IgE omalizumab could be beneficial in treating severe OA in patients with persistent symptoms despite maximum conventional therapy.

Follow-up studies consistently show that a better outcome of asthma after cessation of causal exposure is associated with a shorter symptomatic period before removal and with less severe disease at the time of diagnosis. These findings emphasize the need for early diagnosis and intervention.

The management of OR not only should aim at reducing nasal symptoms and their impact on quality of life but may also offer the opportunity to prevent the subsequent development of OA in keeping with the fact that OR is regarded as an early marker of OA. Complete cessation of exposure should be recommended to workers with OR. Only a few quantitative estimates of the risk of OA in workers with OR have been derived, however; accordingly, a reduction of exposure should be considered a reasonable option when complete avoidance would have important adverse socioeconomic consequences. Pharmacologic treatment of OR does not differ from that of non-OR. In some cases, when validated extracts are available, specific immunotherapy may be proposed.

PREVENTION

Primary prevention aims at blocking, or at least limiting, the development of immunologic sensitization and OA by excluding susceptible workers from at-risk jobs and minimizing exposure to potentially sensitizing substances. Primary preventive strategies for OA and OR should focus on the control of workplace exposures because strong evidence supports a dose–response relationship between the level of exposure to sensitizing agents and the occurrence of OA (see Table 14.3). Identifying susceptible persons at the time of preemployment examination to exclude them from employment or from high-risk jobs is inefficient and unduly discriminating. The currently identified markers of individual susceptibility (see Table 14.3) offer only a low positive predictive value for the development of OA, especially when these markers, such as atopy, are highly prevalent in the general population.

Secondary prevention of immunologic OA and OR involves detection of the disease process at an early (preferably preclinical) stage, to prevent the development of overt OA and to modify the disease process through appropriate interventions

to eliminate exposure. The rationale underlying secondary prevention is the consistent finding that the outcome of OA is better with an early diagnosis and milder disease at the time of removal from exposure. Increasing awareness of the disease among workers and healthcare professionals is a key step to enhance the recognition of OA because the condition still remains underdiagnosed and inappropriately investigated. Recent evidence suggests that appropriately designed surveillance programs are effective in identifying OA in subjects with less severe asthma and a more favorable outcome.

A few observational studies and historical data indicate that prevention is effective in reducing the incidence of OA and OR caused by natural rubber latex in healthcare workers, enzymes in the detergent industry, flour, laboratory animals, and isocyanates. However, available data do not distinguish among the relative effects of the diverse components of prevention strategies, because such strategies usually are implemented as multicomponent programs targeting education, control of exposure, and medical surveillance.

SOCIOECONOMIC IMPACT AND MEDICOLEGAL ASPECTS

Follow-up studies of workers with OA have consistently documented that the condition is associated with a high rate of prolonged unemployment, ranging from 18% to 69%, with a reduction in work-derived income in 44% to 74% of affected workers. Even with worker's compensation support, the income loss may be significant. Complete avoidance of exposure to the sensitizing agent, employment in smaller-sized companies, a lower level of education, older age, and lack of effective job retraining programs are associated with a worse socioeconomic outcome. Data derived from Quebec's Public Health Insurance Plan have shown that OA is associated with higher rates of physician visits, admission to an emergency department, and hospitalizations compared with asthma unrelated to work. Although medical resource utilization decreases after removal from exposure to the incriminated workplace, an excess rate of visits to physicians and emergency departments has been documented for such workers compared with other asthmatics. The socioeconomic impact of OR has rarely been investigated but is likely to be substantial.

Because bronchial hyperresponsiveness to occupational agents almost never completely disappears, workers with OA should be considered to be permanently and completely disabled for jobs involving exposure to the sensitizing agent that caused their OA. They should be thoroughly informed about the possibilities for compensation, and established cases should be reported to the appropriate public health authorities, in accordance with national regulations. Evaluation of physiologic impairment should take into account the characteristic features of asthma and should be based on the level of airway obstruction, the degree of airway hyperresponsiveness, the medication regimen required for controlling asthma, and the effects of asthma on quality of life.

WORK-RELATED ANAPHYLAXIS

The majority of work-related allergic symptoms are respiratory and cutaneous. Allergic symptoms are often reported in some occupations such as beauticians who are exposed to methacrylates by sculpting artificial nails, or healthcare workers exposed to chlorhexidine. Occupational agents can also induce anaphylactic reactions. Cases of anaphylaxis have been reported with several HMW and LMW agents encountered at the workplace. Beekeepers, gardeners, farmers, truck drivers, and masons are the occupations the most at risk of experiencing occupational venom allergy. Up to 32% of beekeepers and their family members had a history of insect sting anaphylaxis, which is much higher than in the general population (0.34%–7.5%). Latex has been responsible for cases of anaphylaxis in healthcare workers. Laboratory animal workers are also at risk to develop anaphylactic reactions.

Several cases of occupational anaphylaxis to different chemicals have also been reported; for example, nurses have developed an anaphylactic reaction after exposure to antibiotics. Exposure to cobalt has been associated with an anaphylactic reaction in a ceramic decorator. Therefore, clinicians need to be aware that severe allergic life-threatening reactions may occur in workers sensitized to proteinaceous or chemical occupational agents.

CONCLUSIONS

During the past decade, it has become apparent that OA and OR are highly prevalent and underdiagnosed diseases that impose a large medical and socioeconomic burden on affected workers and society in general. Because a late diagnosis of OA is associated with a poor outcome, and because prevention programs have been shown to decrease the incidence of new cases of OA, efforts should be made to increase the awareness of OA and OR in primary care practice. Evaluating the cost-effectiveness of preventive measures and compensation systems should become a priority for assisting policy-makers in elaborating rational strategies.

Current understanding of the pathophysiology of OA is limited, especially regarding OA induced by LMW agents. More research is needed to identify biologic markers, allowing an easier and more accurate way of diagnosing OA and OR, as well as developing effective surveillance programs for use in high-risk workforces.

Although additional tools such as noninvasive measures of airway inflammation have been made available for the investigation of OA in the past decade, the diagnosis remains difficult and requires a comprehensive investigation in order to avoid any misdiagnosis. Access to centers that offer a comprehensive investigation is limited. Furthermore, no current standardized approach to the investigation of OA has yet been established. Development and standardization of diagnostic procedures and consensus diagnostic algorithms for OA and OR would be helpful in formulating a consistent approach to the management of OA and OR worldwide. Determining the cost-effectiveness of different management options requires further investigations using the outcomes that have been validated for the evaluation of asthma and rhinitis, such as the level of disease control, disease-specific quality of life, and measurements of airway inflammation. Although the majority of work-related allergic symptoms are respiratory and cutaneous, work-related anaphylaxis can occur in workers exposed to HMW or LMW agents.

REFERENCES

1. Henneberger PK, Redlich CA, Callahan DB, et al. An official American Thoracic Society statement: work-exacerbated asthma. Am J Respir Crit Care Med. 2011;184(3):368–378.
2. Bernstein I, Bernstein D, Chan-Yeung M, et al. Definition and classification of asthma in the workplace. Asthma in the workplace. New York: Taylor & Francis; 2013:1–8.
3. Vandenplas O, Wiszniewska M, Raulf M, et al. EAACI position paper: irritant-induced asthma. Allergy. 2014;69(9):1141–1153.
4. Moscato G, Vandenplas O, Van Wijk RG, et al. EAACI position paper on occupational rhinitis. Respir Res. 2009;10:16.
5. Pralong JA, Lemière C, Rochat T, et al. Predictive value of nonspecific bronchial responsiveness in occupational asthma. J Allergy Clin Immunol. 2016;137(2):412–416.
6. Lux H, Lenz K, Budnik LT, et al. Performance of specific immunoglobulin E tests for diagnosing occupational asthma: a systematic review and meta-analysis. OEM. 2019;76(4):269–278.
7. Vandenplas O, Suojalehto H, Cullinan P. Diagnosing occupational asthma. Clin Exp Allergy. 2016;47:6–18.
8. Taghiakbari M, Pralong JA, Lemière C, et al. Novel clinical scores for occupational asthma due to exposure to high-molecular-weight agents. Occup Environ Med. 2019;76(7):495–501.
9. Park D, Moore VC, Burge CBSG, et al. Serial PEF measurement is superior to cross-shift change in diagnosing occupational asthma. Eur Respir J. 2009;34(3):574–578.
10. Moore VC, Jaakkola MS, Burge PS. A systematic review of serial peak expiratory flow measurements in the diagnosis of occupational asthma. Ann Resp Med. 2010;1:31–34.
11. Perrin B, Lagier F, L'Archeveque J, et al. Occupational asthma: validity of monitoring of peak expiratory flow rates and non-allergic bronchial responsiveness as compared to specific inhalation challenge. Eur Resp J. 1992;5(1):40–48.
12. Girard F, Chaboillez S, Cartier A, et al. An effective strategy for diagnosing occupational asthma. Am J Respir Crit Care Med. 2004;170(8):845–850.
13. Vandenplas O, Suojalehto H, Aasen TB, et al. Specific inhalation challenge in the diagnosis of occupational asthma: consensus statement. Eur Respir J. 2014;43(6):1573–1587.
14. Racine G, Castano R, Cartier A, et al. Diagnostic accuracy of inflammatory markers for diagnosing occupational asthma. JACI In Practice. 2017;5(5):1371–1377.
15. Lemiere C, Nguyen S, Francesco S, et al. Occupational asthma phenotypes identified by increased fractional exhaled nitric oxide after exposure to causal agents. J Allergy Clin Immunol. 2014;134(5):1063–1067.
16. Sastre J, Costa C, García del Potro M, et al. Changes in exhaled nitric oxide after inhalation challenge with occupational agents. J Investig Allergol Clin Immunol. 2013;23(6):421–427.
17. Walters GI, Moore VC, McGrath EE, et al. Fractional exhaled nitric oxide in the interpretation of specific inhalational challenge tests for occupational asthma. Lung. 2014;192(1):119–124.
18. Beach J, Russell K, Blitz S, et al. A systematic review of the diagnosis of occupational asthma. Chest. 2007;131:569–578.
19. Tarlo SM, Lemiere C. Occupational asthma. N Engl J Med. 2014;370(7):640–649.
20. Quirce S. Eosinophilic bronchitis in the workplace. Curr Opin Allergy Clin Immunol. 2004;4:87–91.
21. Vandenplas O, Dressel H, Wilken D, et al. Management of occupational asthma: cessation or reduction of exposure? A systematic review of available evidence. Eur Respir J. 2011;38(4):804–811.

15

Insect Allergy

David B.K. Golden

CHAPTER OUTLINE

SUMMARY OF IMPORTANT CONCEPTS

- Allergic reactions to insect stings can be large local reactions or systemic/anaphylactic reactions.
- Allergic reactions to stings can be prevented with venom immunotherapy (VIT).
- Large local reactions are not due to infection or cellulitis and do not require antibiotics or VIT.
- Absence of hives is associated with more severe anaphylaxis.
- Hypotension without hives suggests mastocytosis.
- Patients with symptoms and signs of hypotension should remain supine until recovered (upright posture is associated with sudden death).
- Avoid drinking from beverage containers or straws; a hidden yellow jacket can cause a sting on the tongue or throat.
- Honeybees always lose their stinger in the skin, but so do some common yellow jackets.
- Children do not always outgrow insect sting allergy. Those with mild (cutaneous) systemic reactions have only 3% chance of anaphylaxis to a future sting, but children who had more severe reactions have up to 30% chance of another reaction even 10 to 20 years later.
- The strength of the venom allergy (on skin test or serum test) predicts only the chance of systemic reaction, but not the severity of the reaction.
- Do not test people who have no history of systemic reaction to a sting because more than 20% of normal adults have positive tests for venom-IgE but do not have a high risk of future sting reaction.
- Protection from allergic reactions to stings is rapidly and almost completely effective (in a matter of weeks) with VIT.
- VIT gives a lasting tolerance in most patients after 5 years of treatment.
- VIT improves quality of life, epinephrine injectors do not.

STINGING INSECT ALLERGY

Insect stings are a common cause of allergic reactions, but also a common subject of misunderstanding. Both physicians and patients/caregivers often overestimate or underestimate the risk of sting anaphylaxis in cases of suspected insect allergy. Most primary care physicians are unaware that venom immunotherapy (VIT) is available, is rapidly protective, and is virtually curative for severe insect sting allergy. Current management is based on decades of epidemiologic, clinical, and laboratory research that have helped to characterize the natural history, risk factors, and mechanisms, and identify optimal treatment for insect sting allergy.[1,2] Our goal is to prevent both complacency and unnecessary fear, and thus prevent overtreatment or undertreatment.

HISTORICAL PERSPECTIVE

The potential for life-threatening allergic reactions to insect stings has been known since antiquity, but the first report of immunotherapy for insect sting allergy was in 1930. That study concluded falsely that body proteins were responsible for the allergy, and it was not until 50 years later that insect venoms were approved for clinical use in place of whole-body extracts, based on controlled clinical trials. Subsequent lengthy studies of large populations helped to clarify the natural history of the allergy in different groups, and the risk factors for severe sting reactions.[1-3]

EPIDEMIOLOGY

Insect sting allergy can occur at any age, often after a number of uneventful stings, and is more common than once thought. In the US, systemic allergic reactions are reported by up to 3% of adults, and almost 1% of children have a medical history of severe sting reactions. The frequency of large local reactions is less certain, but is estimated in the range of 5% to 15% of stings.

At least 40 fatal stings occur each year in the US, half of which occur in persons with no prior history of allergic reactions to stings. In postmortem blood samples, it has proved possible to document the presence of venom-specific immunoglobulin E (IgE) antibodies and elevated serum tryptase, suggesting a possible mechanism for some cases of unexplained sudden death. However, the presence of IgE antibodies to Hymenoptera venom is common even in those with no prior history of allergic reaction. More than 30% of adults who have been stung in the previous few months (with no abnormal reaction) will show venom-specific IgE antibodies on skin testing or immunoassay, and 10% to 20% of all adults demonstrate positive skin test or blood test results for yellow jacket or honeybee venom. Such asymptomatic sensitization is common with all known allergens.

Although insect sting allergy is sometimes familial, the vast majority of insect-allergic individuals have no family history of insect allergy. There is only a weak concordance with other allergic conditions, but the frequency of venom sensitization (regardless of history) is higher among individuals with sensitization to inhalant allergens (with or without symptoms).

ETIOLOGY

Allergic reactions can occur after insect stings or bites, but anaphylaxis is caused by stings and rarely by bites. Insect bite allergy is discussed at the end of this chapter. Stinging insects belong to the order Hymenoptera. The Hymenoptera of importance in allergy are from three families: Apidae, Vespidae, and Formicidae (Table 15.1). Selected representatives of these families are depicted in Fig. 15.1. Yellow jackets are the most frequent culprits in central and northern North America and Europe, whereas the *Polistes* species are more commonly implicated in the Gulf coast areas of the US and the Mediterranean coast of Europe. Common names in general usage can be misleading: the term *bee* can refer to honeybees only, or to all stinging insects. Similarly, *wasps* may refer to any of the social wasps (vespids) or only to the *Polistes* species. The stinging ants are an increasingly prevalent cause of anaphylaxis in the US, Asia, and Australia.

TABLE 15.1   Taxonomy of the Hymenoptera Insect Order

Family and Subfamily	Scientific Name	Common Name
Apidae	*Apis mellifera*	Honeybee
	Bombus spp.	Bumblebee
	Megabombus spp.	
	Halictus spp.	Sweatbee
	Dialictus spp.	
Vespidae		
Vespinae	*Vespula* spp.	Yellow jacket
	Dolichovespula arenaria	Yellow hornet
	Dolichovespula maculata	White-faced hornet
Polistinae	*Polistes* spp.	Paper wasp
Formicidae	*Solenopsis invicta*	Fire ant
	Myrmecia spp.	Jack jumper ant
	Pogonomyrmex spp.	Harvester ant
	Pachycondyla spp.	

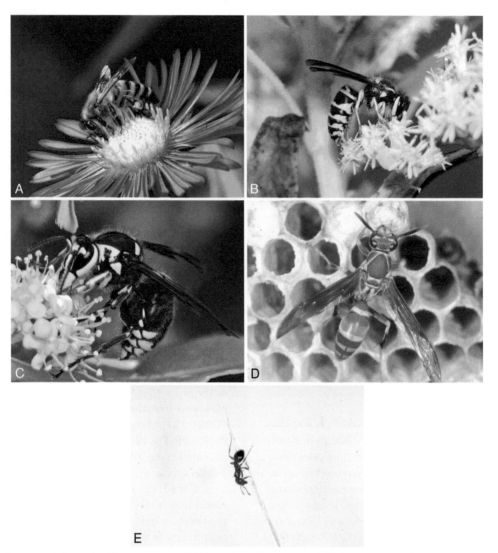

Fig. 15.1 Stinging insects of the order Hymenoptera. (A) Honeybee *(Apis mellifera)*. (B) Yellow jacket *(Vespula maculifrons)*. (C) White-faced hornet *(Dolichovespula maculata)*. (D) Paper wasp *(Polistes exclamans)*. (E) Imported fire ant *(Solenopsis invicta)*. (Reproduced by permission of ALK-Abelló A/S, Høsholm, Denmark © 2012 ALK.)

Apids

Honeybees are relatively docile and rarely sting or swarm without considerable provocation. Africanized honeybees look the same as other honeybees and deliver the same venom when they sting, but they have an unusual tendency to swarm and sting in large numbers. Delivery of large numbers of stings at one time can cause toxic reactions that have been fatal to livestock and humans; this has earned these insects the common name of *killer bees*.

Bumblebees, like honeybees, usually are not aggressive and do not usually sting. Allergic reactions to bumblebee stings *(Bombus* species) occur especially in greenhouse workers. Bumblebee venom shows very limited cross-reactivity with honeybee venom.

Vespids

Vespids use a wood pulp to construct nests that contain one or more layers of comb, each of which contains a large number of cells. These comb layers are attached in a vertical arrangement and usually are enclosed in *papier mâché* outer layers. The vespid sting apparatus usually has finer barbs than in the apids and does not commonly detach from the insect, so vespids are able to sting repeatedly. Some yellow jacket species do leave the sting apparatus in the skin, so this is not unique to the honeybee.

Yellow jackets (genus *Vespula*) are highly aggressive and may sting for no apparent reason, particularly in the autumn, when larger populations compete for limited food supplies. Yellow jacket nests are located in the ground or in cracks in buildings or residential landscape materials.

Yellow hornets and white-faced (bald-faced) hornets (genus *Dolichovespula*) are aerial nesting yellow jackets that are present in North America but not in Europe. They often build their nests in shrubs and trees, and their sensitivity to vibration can initiate their defensive sting behavior.

Paper wasps are primarily of the genus *Polistes*. The coloring of wasps varies greatly, and they can be black, brown, red, or striped. *Polistes* wasps are somewhat less aggressive than yellow jackets and hornets, but they sting readily when disturbed and can sting repeatedly without losing their sting apparatus.

Formicids

The ants of the Formicidae family have a true sting apparatus. Ants of the genus *Solenopsis* (imported fire ants) are widespread in the southeastern US, and stings occur so frequently that in many areas, as much as 50% of the population is stung each year.[4] In most cases, multiple ants each administer multiple stings, although they are not painful. The unique lesions form sterile pustules that can become infected if excoriated or opened.

Other genera of the formicid ants include the harvester ants (*Pogonomyrmex* spp.) found in western areas of the US, Canada, and Mexico; the Australian jack jumper ants (*Myrmecia* spp.); and Asian ants (*Pachycondyla* spp.), which have been reported to cause allergic reactions.

INSECT VENOMS

Commercial extracts are prepared from Hymenoptera venoms (honeybee, yellowjacket, yellow hornet, white-faced hornet, and *Polistes* wasp) and from imported fire ant bodies. Although imported fire ant venom is superior, their whole-body extracts contain sufficient quantities of venom allergens to be clinically useful.

Most of the native venoms contain vasoactive amines, acetylcholine, and kinins, which account for the localized burning, pain, and itching after a sting. Some venom components can cause toxic reactions, including neurologic complications. Within the vespid family, there is extensive cross-allergenicity of the venoms of different genera. This is not the case in the apid and formicid families. There is limited cross-reactivity of honeybee and bumblebee venoms, but most patients with bumblebee allergy do not show cross-reactivity to honeybee venom. There is significant cross-reactivity among the various fire ant *(Solenopsis)* species and among the harvester ant *(Pogonomyrmex)* species, but the two genera do not cross-react with each other. The venoms of different insect families have almost no cross-reactivity. There is limited and infrequent cross-reactivity between honeybee and vespid venoms, some of which may be related to cross-reacting carbohydrate determinants of uncertain clinical significance. Cross-reactivity can be distinguished from multiple sensitization by testing the serum in an inhibition immunoassay or measuring specific IgE using recombinant venom allergens.

CLINICAL FEATURES AND CLASSIFICATION OF REACTIONS

Insect stings cause reactions that are classified as local or systemic in distribution. Most large local reactions represent a late-phase, IgE-dependent reaction that is mild initially but that increases after 12 to 24 hours to a diameter often exceeding 10 to 20 cm. These reactions may manifest with a lymphangitic streak toward the axilla or the inguinal region, but this represents the drainage of inflammatory mediators rather than an infectious process (cellulitis). A large local reaction subsides after 5 to 10 days and is not dangerous except for potential local anatomic compression, especially on the head, neck, tongue, or throat.

A systemic reaction causes symptoms and signs in one or more anatomic systems distant from the site of the sting, usually representing IgE-mediated anaphylaxis. Patients may exhibit cutaneous signs (e.g., generalized urticaria, angioedema, flushing, pruritus), respiratory changes (e.g., throat tightness, dysphagia, dyspnea, stridor or dysphonia, chest tightness, wheezing), or a circulatory component (e.g., dizziness, hypotension, unconsciousness, shock). Less frequently, gastrointestinal complaints (e.g., cramps, diarrhea, nausea, vomiting) or uterine cramping occur. Cardiac anaphylaxis after insect stings can cause coronary vasospasm, tachyarrhythmias, or bradycardia, even with no underlying coronary or cardiac abnormality. Insect stings are among the reported causes of Kounis' syndrome—clinical and laboratory findings of classic angina pectoris caused by allergic reactions. The diagnosis of the acute reaction can be difficult when hypotension or cardiac manifestations occur with no other signs or symptoms. The absence of urticaria or angioedema is associated with more severe reactions to stings. Children have a higher frequency of isolated cutaneous reactions and a lower frequency of vascular symptoms or anaphylactic shock compared with adults.

Systemic reactions may be caused by underlying mast cell disorders in more than 2% of cases.[5] Up to 25% of patients with severe anaphylactic reactions to venom have elevated baseline serum tryptase. Hypotensive shock without urticaria after a sting is suggestive of mastocytosis. Systemic reactions may occasionally be caused by toxic effects from the vasoactive substances in a large number of stings. Massive envenomation from large numbers of stings can cause life-threatening reactions with renal failure, rhabdomyolysis, hemolysis, and acute respiratory distress syndrome or diffuse intravascular coagulation. Seizures have occurred, particularly after multiple fire ant stings. Unusual reactions of unknown mechanisms are usually delayed and include serum sickness-like reactions, encephalitis, peripheral and cranial neuropathies, glomerulonephritis, myocarditis, and Guillain–Barré syndrome.

PATIENT EVALUATION AND DIAGNOSIS

Diagnostic evaluation of patients for insect sting allergy includes historical inquiry as well as an array of laboratory tests that provide useful information about the diagnosis, the prognosis (relative risk of reaction), and long-term outcome with VIT (Table 15.2). The current approach to diagnosis of insect sting allergy is summarized in Box 15.1.[3] Diagnostic testing for venom-specific IgE antibodies by skin or serum tests is recommended in all individuals with a prior history of systemic reactions to insect stings, with the exception of those who had reactions limited to cutaneous manifestations. The rationale for diagnostic testing is to confirm the diagnosis in patients who are candidates for VIT based on their clinical history, and to identify the venoms to be included in treatment.

Clinical History

The diagnosis of insect sting allergy rests on the history as the primary evidence of allergic reactivity because venom-specific IgE antibodies are present in a large number of clinically

TABLE 15.2 Diagnostic Evaluation of Insect Sting Allergy

Variable	History	Skin Test	Specific IgE	BAT	Recombinant Allergen	RAST Inhibition	Tryptase Baseline
Diagnosis							
No reaction	X						
LLR	X						
Mild SR	X	X	X				
Anaphylaxis	X	X	X	X	X	X	X
Predict severe reaction (to stings or VIT)	X			X			X
Cross-reactivity (HB/YJ)					X	X	
Discontinue VIT	X			X			X

BAT, Basophil activation test; HB, honeybee; LLR, large local reaction; SR, systemic reaction; VIT, venom immunotherapy; YJ, yellow jacket.
From Golden DBK. Advances in diagnosis and management of insect sting allergy. Ann Allergy Asthma Immunol 2013;111:84–9.

BOX 15.1 Current Diagnosis

- History of systemic allergic reaction to a sting
- Positive test for venom-specific immunoglobulin E (IgE) (by serum or skin tests)
- Degree of sensitivity (by serum IgE or skin test) correlates with frequency but not severity of sting reaction
- Low risk if previous large local reaction only
- Low risk in patients with mild (cutaneous) systemic reactions
- Quality of life and frequency of exposure a consideration

nonreactive individuals. Physicians should inquire about severe reactions to insect stings when obtaining a complete medical history, because most affected individuals fail to mention the event during a routine history. The history should be reviewed in detail with respect to the location and timing of the stings, the time course of the reaction, and all associated symptoms and treatments. Concurrent medications, such as β-adrenergic blocking agents and angiotensin-converting enzyme inhibitors (ACEIs), may contribute significantly to the severity of the anaphylactic reaction.

It is most important, as with all allergy diagnostic tests, that the indication (pretest probability) should be clear before ordering the test. When the probability of anaphylaxis is low (mild or no reaction to previous stings, or never stung), a positive test will not improve the prediction of future anaphylaxis. This is in large part due to the high frequency of asymptomatic sensitization in the general population. A positive test can have a very negative impact on quality of life, and can lead to unnecessary treatment, or disqualification from professional and career activities.

Skin Tests

The standard method of skin testing employs the well-validated intradermal technique, using the five commercial Hymenoptera venom protein extracts at concentrations in the range of 0.001 to 1.0 µg/mL. Fire ant sensitivity can be tested with reasonable diagnostic accuracy using whole-body extracts of imported fire ants.

Skin test results are clearly positive for most patients with a convincing history, but they can be negative in more than 20% of cases. In the days or weeks after a sting reaction, 25% to 50% of patients have negative skin test attributed to a refractory (anergic) period: they should have skin tests repeated after 4 to 6 weeks. Negative skin test results for a history-positive patient may represent the loss of sensitivity in a person with a remote history of sting reaction. Some cases of sting anaphylaxis may be non–IgE-mediated or be attributable to subclinical (indolent) mastocytosis. Some persons with negative venom skin test results will have systemic reactions to subsequent stings. Most insect-allergic patients with negative venom skin test results have detectable venom-specific IgE antibodies in the serum. For these reasons, patients with negative skin test results and a convincing history of anaphylaxis should be further investigated with serologic testing, and if results remain negative, the skin tests should be repeated after 3 to 6 months. Baseline serum tryptase should also be measured.

Venom skin test sensitivities have different patterns. Because of cross-reactivity, almost all patients who have a positive skin test result in response to yellow jacket venom will also have positive skin tests to one or both of the hornet venoms, and approximately one-half will have positive tests to *Polistes* wasp venom. The degree of skin test sensitivity does not correlate reliably with the severity of sting reaction. The most reactive skin tests may occur in patients who have had only large local reactions and have a very low risk of anaphylaxis, whereas some patients who have had near-fatal anaphylactic shock show only weak skin test reactivity.

In Vitro Tests

The diagnosis of insect sting allergy by detection of allergen-specific IgE antibodies in serum has improved greatly over the past 10 years. A high level of venom-specific IgE is usually diagnostic, but low levels are of less clear clinical significance. Venom skin tests and venom-specific IgE assays correlate imperfectly. The latter produce negative results in up to 20% of skin test–positive subjects, and venom skin test results are negative for almost 10% of persons with elevated IgE antibodies. Neither test alone can detect all cases of insect sting allergy, and each test is useful as a supplement to the other. The clinical significance of a positive IgE antibody assay result with a negative skin test result is not known in all cases, but it is clearly associated with a risk of systemic reaction to a sting.

Sting Challenge Test

It has been assumed that the ultimate test of whether an individual will have a systemic reaction to a sting is to observe the outcome of a supervised live sting challenge. This procedure has been used as the gold standard in research studies of the efficacy of VIT and to determine the relapse rate after discontinuation of VIT. Sting challenge of untreated patients with a history of previous systemic reactions to stings and with positive venom skin test results has resulted in systemic reaction rates ranging between 30% and 65%. This variability in part reflects the variability of the culprit insect. The quantity of venom protein injected during a sting is relatively consistent for honeybees but varies greatly for vespids. The routine use of a live sting challenge as a diagnostic procedure for selection of patients for immunotherapy has been proposed, but there have been ethical and practical objections. Moreover, the lack of reaction to a single challenge sting has limited clinical significance, because a subsequent sting can still cause a systemic reaction in about 20% of cases.

TREATMENT OF ACUTE REACTIONS

Large local reactions, if severe or involving the head and neck, are best treated with a brief burst of an oral corticosteroid (e.g., initial dose of 40 to 60 mg of prednisone, tapering to 0 in 4 to 6 days). For best results, corticosteroids should be started within a few hours of the sting in patients with a known history of severe large local reactions to stings. Milder reactions may be treated conservatively, with cold compresses, and medication for pruritus or pain. Large local reactions can be mistaken for cellulitis, especially on the extremities, where intense inflammation can cause an apparent lymphangitis directed toward the axillary or inguinal lymph nodes. When such a reaction presents 24 to 48 hours after the sting, infection is very unlikely, and treatment may include ice and moderate-dose oral corticosteroids, but antibiotics are not necessary.

Systemic reactions require more urgent intervention and close monitoring. Urticaria may respond to H1-antihistamines alone, but anaphylactic reactions require epinephrine injection. Any sign of hypotension or respiratory obstruction should be treated promptly with aqueous epinephrine intramuscularly into the anterolateral aspect of the thigh, and should have full emergency medical attention and observation for 3 to 6 hours. The recommended dose of epinephrine is 0.3 to 0.5 mg (0.3–0.5 mL of 1:1000 weight/volume solution) for adults and 0.01 mg/kg for children to a maximum of 0.3 mg. After use of self-injectable epinephrine, the individual should be taken to an emergency department for observation and further treatment, if necessary. Some patients who have a history of rapid onset or very severe systemic reactions may warrant treatment immediately after the sting. Delay in the use of epinephrine has contributed to fatal reactions, and some individuals with anaphylactic shock are resistant to epinephrine. Patients taking β-blocker

medications may, for example, be resistant to the effects of epinephrine; glucagon injection can be beneficial in these cases. For a few patients, anaphylaxis is prolonged or recurrent for 6 to 72 hours, and it may require intensive medical care. The patient with hypotension should be kept supine with legs raised because upright posture has been associated with sudden death due to lack of venous return (i.e., empty ventricle syndrome).

Emergency treatment of anaphylaxis requires patient education before discharge. The risk of recurrence should be clearly described, and the use of self-injectable epinephrine requires consistent instruction and follow-up. Many patients are not specifically instructed about the need for self-injectable epinephrine, and they are not referred for an allergy consultation and preventive treatment. This is important because affected individuals often think the reaction was a chance occurrence and fail to inform their personal physicians.

PREVENTION OF ACUTE REACTIONS

Patients should avoid high-risk exposures such as yard and garden work, trash containers, and outdoor areas where food and drink are exposed. Food and flavored drinks in cans, bottles, and straws can be an unsuspected source of a sting to the tongue or throat (Box 15.2). Avoidance of wearing brightly colored clothes is of uncertain benefit, and insect repellents have little or no effect.

Epinephrine Kits

Epinephrine autoinjectors (0.3 mg EpiPen and 0.15 mg EpiPen Jr, Mylan NV, Canonsburg, PA; Auvi-Q 0.3 mg, 0.15 mg, and 0.1 mg, Kaleo Pharma, Richmond, VA; generic epinephrine autoinjector 0.3 mg and 0.15 mg, Impax Labs, Hayward, CA; Symjepi prefilled syringe 0.3 mg, Adamis Pharma, San Diego, CA) should be prescribed and explained to all patients at risk for anaphylaxis. The age at which to prescribe an adult-dose instead of pediatric-dose autoinjector is uncertain, but the question may be considered

---

BOX 15.2 Patient Information to Limit the Risk of Insect Stings

- Avoid drinking outdoors from cans or straws that may harbor stinging insects.
- Exercise caution when doing yard work, handling garbage, picnicking, swimming, bicycling, riding in open-air vehicles, boating, camping, or other outdoor activity.
- Always wear shoes outdoors.
- Look for insects in vehicles before driving, and keep vehicle windows closed.
- Avoid rapid or jerking movement around insects. Remain still. Most insects will not sting unless provoked.
- All nests or hives in the vicinity of the home should be removed by a professional exterminator and not by the insect-sensitive patient.
- Insect repellents do not deter stinging insects. Immunotherapy does not lessen the need for other measures of prevention.
- Wear an identification tag or bracelet at all times.
- Have an epinephrine injection kit available at all times, especially if at greater risk. Instruct family members and companions in its use.
- Seek medical attention immediately after emergency treatment is given.

From: Golden DBK. Insect allergy. In: DC Adelman, T Casale, J Corren, editors. Manual of Allergy and Immunology, 5th ed. Baltimore: Lippincott Williams & Wilkins; 2012, pp. 278–91.

TABLE 15.3 Risk of Systemic Reactions and Clinical Recommendations Based on Reaction to Previous Stings and Venom Skin Test or Serum IgE Test Results

Previous Sting Reaction	Skin and/or Serum IgE Test	CHANCE OF FUTURE SYSTEMIC STING REACTION		Clinical Recommendation
		Any	Severe	
None	Positive	10%–15%	5%	Avoidance
Large local	Positive	5%–10%	2%	Avoidance
Cutaneous systemic				
Child	Positive	1%–10%	<3%	Avoidance
Adult	Positive	10%–20%	<5%	Venom immunotherapy
Moderate systemic	Positive	30%–50%	10%	Venom immunotherapy
Anaphylaxis	Positive	50%–75%	30%	Venom immunotherapy
Anaphylaxis	Negative	5%–10%	30%	Repeat skin/serum venom-IgE test

From Golden DBK. Allergic Reactions to Hymenoptera. ACP Medicine 2011.

BOX 15.3 Patients With Low Risk for Anaphylaxis

- General population
- Asymptomatic sensitization
- Patients on venom immunotherapy
- Patients with only cutaneous systemic reactions
- Large local reactors
- Patients who completed 5 years of venom immunotherapy

TABLE 15.4 Predictors of Risk of Systemic Reaction to Insect Stings

Natural History	Screening Tests and Markers
Severity of previous reaction	Venom skin test
Insect species	Venom-specific IgE
Age, gender	Basophil activation test
No urticaria or angioedema	Baseline serum tryptase value
Medications	Platelet-activating factor (PAF) acetylhydrolase
Multiple or sequential stings	Angiotensin-converting enzyme (ACE)

when the child reaches a weight of 25 to 30 kg. Even when epinephrine kits are prescribed, patients often fail to carry the injector with them and delay or defer using them when they have a reaction. Patients, caretakers in homes and schools, and physicians need initial and follow-up education about the correct use of the device and how to recognize the expiration date on the unit and replace outdated units promptly.

The prescription of an epinephrine injector should always be considered when there is a known risk of anaphylaxis. However, the prescription itself creates fear in some people and reassurance in others. Studies have described the burden of epinephrine prescriptions, and the frequent negative impact on quality of life (compared to VIT which improves quality of life).[6] When VIT is indicated, epinephrine prescription is clearly indicated. In individuals at low risk for sting anaphylaxis (see Box 15.3), the prescription of an epinephrine injector is a matter of clinical judgment and may be discussed with the patient. There is some disagreement about whether epinephrine prescription is necessary when the chance it will be needed is relatively small, but once the risk is identified, it is reasonable to offer the epinephrine prescription and engage the patient in shared decision-making.

PREDICTORS OF RISK FOR STING ANAPHYLAXIS

Natural History

The prognosis for affected patients is based on the understanding of the natural history of the condition (Table 15.3) and on

specific clinical factors and biologic markers (Table 15.4). The chance that a future sting will cause an allergic reaction depends on the history and immunologic status of the patient. Because one in five healthy adults has detectable venom-specific IgE antibodies, testing of asymptomatic individuals is not recommended.

In patients with positive venom skin test results and previous systemic reactions, the outcome of the next sting is somewhat unpredictable because systemic reactions may occur on some occasions but not on others. The average frequency of systemic reaction to a subsequent sting has been 45% (range 30%–65%) in published studies. Even among patients who have no reaction to one challenge sting, 20% will have a systemic reaction to a subsequent sting.

The risk of recurrence is higher for those who are allergic to honeybee stings than for those with vespid allergies, higher for adults than for children, and higher for patients who had more severe systemic reactions previously than for those with milder systemic reactions. Contrary to popular belief, it is uncommon for patients to have more severe reactions with each subsequent sting.

There are a number of subtypes of people with positive tests for venom-IgE who are at low risk for sting anaphylaxis (Box 15.3). Most large local reactors consistently have similar reactions with repeated stings. The risk of a systemic reaction to future sting (not all of which are severe) in those with large local reactions is about 10%. The level of sensitivity shown by a venom skin test or specific IgE level does not predict the severity

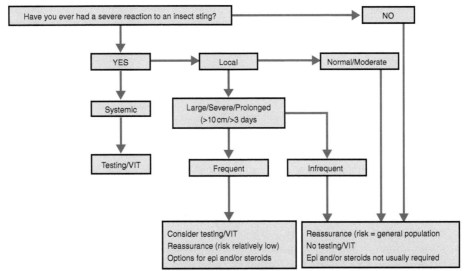

Fig. 15.2 Algorithm for large local reactions. (From Golden DBK. Large local reactions to insect stings. J Allergy Clin Immunol 2015;3:331–4.)

of future sting reactions, and no known clinical or laboratory characteristics differentiate patients who will progress to systemic reactions from those who will continue to have only large local sting reactions. Evaluation and treatment for large local reactions are summarized in Fig. 15.2.

In children with a history of systemic reactions to stings, the skin tests or specific IgE level became negative in 25% to 50% after an average of 10 years of follow-up without VIT. During 10 to 20 years of follow-up, children who had had strictly cutaneous systemic reactions had a 10% to 15% chance of subsequent systemic reactions (mostly milder than the previous reaction) and only about a 3% chance of more severe reactions with respiratory or circulatory symptoms. Those who had moderate or severe reactions in childhood had a significantly higher risk of reaction in adulthood, estimated to be 30%.[7]

The chance of progression from a mild (cutaneous) reaction to a more severe reaction has not been formally studied in adults. Some retrospective studies of field stings showed more frequent progression, but prospective sting challenge studies found a very low risk of progression (<3%).

Markers of Risk for Sting Anaphylaxis

Risk stratification is important to help prioritize the recommendation of resources (epinephrine injectors, venom skin tests, VIT) for optimal safety but without unnecessary concern or anxiety. Risk factors for severe reactions to insect stings, based on natural history and in vitro tests, are shown in Table 15.4. The history (i.e., severity and pattern of previous sting reactions) has been the most reliable predictor of the severity of subsequent sting reactions. The absence of urticaria or angioedema during anaphylaxis and rapid onset were associated with a higher frequency of severe reaction. Measurable markers that predict the risk of systemic reaction to a sting are summarized in Table 15.4. Results of skin tests and specific IgE tests correlate better with the frequency of sting reactions than with the severity of reactions. The baseline serum tryptase level correlates closely with the risk

of severe anaphylaxis from a sting. It is likely that abnormal measurements of other mast cell mediators will be found to reflect an increased risk of severe anaphylaxis. This is true for platelet-activating factor (PAF). The level of PAF correlates with the serum activity of PAF acetylhydrolase.

Another growing concern has been the effect of medications on the risk of reaction. β-blockers can increase the risk of anaphylaxis primarily by interfering with the effects of epinephrine. β-blockers should be avoided in all patients who are at risk for anaphylaxis, including those with insect sting allergy and those receiving allergen immunotherapy. However, risk analysis has suggested that in many patients with cardiovascular disease, stopping β-blockers can create greater risk than not stopping the drug during VIT. It is therefore acceptable, when necessary, to proceed with VIT in patients receiving β-blockers. Another concern has been the risk of anaphylaxis in patients taking ACEIs. As with beta-blockers, some reports have suggested a significant risk of more severe anaphylaxis, while others have not.

Baseline serum tryptase activity can predict the severity of sting anaphylaxis, and it has been useful as a predictor of systemic reactions during VIT, failure of VIT, and relapse of sting anaphylaxis after discontinuing VIT. Elevated baseline tryptase levels often indicate underlying mastocytosis, which occurs in approximately 2% of patients with sting anaphylaxis. Sting anaphylaxis is the most common cause of anaphylaxis in patients with indolent mastocytosis, and it can be the presenting sign of the disease,[6] typically in a male with rapid-onset hypotensive shock but no hives. Mastocytosis patients with positive tests for venom-IgE have a 93% frequency of anaphylaxis if they are stung, and the reactions are almost always life-threatening.

It is important to recognize that there are low-risk patients who should be reassured about their low risk for severe anaphylaxis to a sting, and who may consider not pursuing any intervention (epinephrine injector prescription, venom testing, VIT). These include patients with cutaneous systemic reactions (adults and children); large local reactors; individuals with asymptomatic sensitization (positive tests for venom-IgE but no history of allergic reaction); patients receiving VIT; and patients who have completed a course of VIT.

VENOM IMMUNOTHERAPY

Indications

VIT is the treatment of choice for prevention of systemic allergic reactions to insect stings, but it requires careful selection of patients[3] (Table 15.3). VIT is indicated in patients with a history of previous systemic allergic reaction to a sting and positive results on venom skin test or venom-specific IgE test. Those with recent and severe anaphylaxis are at highest risk (40%–70%) for systemic reaction to a future sting and require VIT. The lowest risk (<10%) has been found for children and adults with a history of large local reactions or systemic reactions limited to cutaneous signs and symptoms but with no respiratory or vascular manifestations. VIT is generally not required for patients with the lowest risk of anaphylaxis. Some low-risk patients request treatment because of their fear of reaction and its impact on their lifestyle. Quality of life is impaired in patients with a history of systemic reactions and is improved by VIT but not by prescription of self-injectable epinephrine. There is no test that predicts which patients will progress from large local or cutaneous systemic reactions to more severe anaphylactic reactions. There is evidence that VIT inhibits large local reactions to stings, which can benefit patients who have frequent and severe local reactions.

Safety

Adverse reactions to VIT are no more common than reactions during inhalant allergen immunotherapy. Systemic symptoms occur in 5% to 15% of patients during initial up-dosing, regardless of which of the two standard (Food and Drug Administration [FDA]-approved) schedules is used. There is an association between severe or repeated systemic reactions to injections and underlying mast cell disease (e.g., mastocytosis, urticaria pigmentosa, elevated baseline serum tryptase levels).

Systemic reactions to venom injections occur more frequently in patients treated with honeybee venom than in those treated with yellow jacket venom. Most systemic reactions are mild, and less than 5% of patients receiving VIT ever require epinephrine treatment for a reaction to an injection. These reactions are rare during maintenance VIT.

Pretreatment with antihistamines or a leukotriene modifier reduces the local reactions to injections. Antihistamines also reduce the frequency of systemic reactions to VIT and to subsequent stings. In the unusual case of recurrent systemic reactions to injections, therapy may be streamlined to a single venom and given in divided doses 30 minutes apart. In patients with recurrent systemic reactions to VIT, treatment with rush VIT and/or omalizumab has been successful. Large local reactions to venom injections occur in up to 50% of patients, but it may be necessary to advance the dose in the face of moderately severe local reactions in order to achieve the full maintenance dose.

Although large local reactions to venom injections have not predicted systemic reactions to subsequent doses, an association has been reported for fire ant immunotherapy. Like inhalant immunotherapy, maintenance VIT is considered acceptable during pregnancy.

Effectiveness

Clinical protection from anaphylactic reaction to a sting can be demonstrated as soon as the 100-mcg dose is reached, regardless of the build-up schedule. VIT with vespid venoms is 85% to 95% effective in preventing systemic reactions to stings, but honeybee VIT is only 75% to 85% effective. VIT with Jack Jumper ant venom was associated with complete protection from sting challenge in more than 95% of patients. Even in cases considered to be treatment failures, the repeat sting reactions are usually milder than pretreatment reactions. Treatment failure can be overcome with higher treatment doses (e.g., 200 μg). Failure of VIT occurs in 25% of patients with underlying mastocytosis.

VIT has been a model for the study of the mechanism of immunotherapy. Evidence supports the role of immunoglobulin G (IgG) in intercepting allergen and in facilitating lymphocyte responses. Immunotherapy induces suppression of venom skin test and specific IgE antibodies, and it reduces basophil release of histamine or leukotrienes. Studies of VIT have elucidated an important role for interleukin 10 (IL-10) in the suppression of the Th2 cytokines during VIT and suggest a role for regulatory T cells in the protective effects of VIT.[8] Additional investigation has identified more specific pathways of T cell regulation and identified a role for dendritic cells. Another novel pathway involves the role of IgG4 antibodies in facilitated antigen presentation to T cells and B cells that regulate the allergic response to venom.

Venom Species and Dose

The selection of venom extracts to be used for immunotherapy depends on the venom skin test reaction or venom-specific IgE antibody level to each venom. Therapy should include all venoms that elicit a positive response, because anaphylaxis to one venom may predispose to anaphylaxis to another venom. For this reason, the most common therapy for vespid sensitivities in the US is with the mixed vespid venoms preparation: 100 μg each of yellow jacket, yellow hornet, and white-faced hornet venoms. Although therapy with yellow jacket venom alone can protect against hornet stings because of the marked cross-reactivity of the *Vespula* venoms, treatment with mixed vespid venoms gives a more robust immune response and more reliable clinical protection. The skin test result is also positive to *Polistes* wasp venoms in at least 50% of vespid allergic patients, and treatment is usually given as a separate injection. Therapy with yellow jacket or mixed vespid venoms can protect against wasp stings, but this has been established only for patients whose wasp IgE showed complete cross-reactivity with yellow jacket venom as assessed by inhibition immunoassays. In patients with dual positivity to honeybee and yellow jacket venoms, serologic testing using recombinant venom component allergens can distinguish those with cross-reactivity (which may be due to the cross-reacting carbohydrate determinants on the native venoms) from those with true dual sensitization.

TABLE 15.5   Examples of Conventional Dosing Schedules for Venom Immunotherapy

SCHEDULE 1[a]			SCHEDULE 2[a]		
Week No.	Concentration (µg/mL)	Volume (mL)	Week No.	Concentration (µg/mL)	Volume (mL)
1	1.0	0.05	1a	0.01	0.1
			1b	0.1	0.1
			1c	1.0	0.1
2	1.0	0.1	2a	1.0	0.1
			2b	1.0	0.5
			2c	10	0.1
3	1.0	0.2	3a	10	0.1
			3b	10	0.5
			3c	10	1.0
4	1.0	0.4	4a	100	0.1
			4b	100	0.2
5	10	0.05	5a	100	0.2
			5b	100	0.3
6	10	0.1	6a	100	0.3
			6b	100	0.3
7	10	0.2	7a	100	0.4
			7b	100	0.4
8	10	0.4	8a	100	0.5
			8b	100	0.5
9	100	0.05	9	100	1.0
10	100	0.1	Monthly	100	1.0
11	100	0.2			
12	100	0.4			
13	100	0.6			
14	100	0.8			
15	100	1.0			
16	100	1.0			
18	100	1.0			
21	100	1.0			
Monthly	100	1.0			

[a]Injections are usually given weekly. Schedule 2 prescribes two or three doses, at 30-minute intervals for the first 8 weeks. When the maintenance dose is achieved, the interval may be advanced from weekly to monthly. Schedule 1 is based on the package insert for Hollister-Stier venom extracts (Spokane, Wash.). Schedule 2 is based on the package insert for ALK-Abelló venom extracts (Round Rock, Tex.).

The recommended maintenance dose for VIT is 100 µg of each venom. Data on the use of lower doses are limited, with various degrees of efficacy reported for adults. Patients who are not adequately protected with the 100-µg dose usually can be protected with higher doses. The treatment recommendations for children 3 years and older are the same as for adults. However, some studies have shown similar efficacy and long-term outcomes using a 50-µg maintenance dose in children.

Treatment Schedules

Initial VIT follows a schedule that can vary according to the recommendations of the source laboratory that prepared the allergen extract and the level of caution preferred by the clinician. Table 15.5 shows the recommended schedules for the two products that have been approved in the US. The modified rush regimen (ALK-Abelló, Round Rock, Texas; venom products no longer marketed in the US) is more rapid than the traditional regimen (Hollister-Stier Laboratories, Spokane, Washington), achieving maintenance dose in eight weekly injections instead of 15 weeks, respectively. These regimens show equal efficacy and safety. Once the full dose is achieved, it is usually repeated in 1 week, again after another 2 weeks, and then after another 3 weeks before beginning maintenance treatment every 4 weeks.

Rush VIT regimens administered over 2 to 3 days have been equally effective and safe, with adverse reactions occurring no more often than with traditional regimens. Ultrarush regimens, given over a period of hours, are associated with an increased risk of severe reactions.[9] Rush VIT has been used successfully in patients unable to achieve maintenance doses due to repeated systemic reactions using standard schedules. Use of rush regimens has become routine in Europe due to the regional availability of specialized treatment, and in the US military to hasten return to duty, and has been recommended as an option for routine VIT in the US.

Maintenance

Maintenance VIT is administered every 4 weeks for at least the first year. There are few studies on longer maintenance intervals, but clinical experience supports the practice of extending the maintenance interval to every 6 to 8 weeks over several years in most cases. VIT with a 12-week interval has been shown to be effective for extended maintenance treatment after several years of routine therapy. Maintenance evaluation should include a review of the dose and frequency of injections, all adverse reactions, any intervening stings, and all current medications. Repeat skin tests or immunoassays may be performed every 2 to 3 years, but usually show no change in the first few years. Venom skin test results become negative in at least 20% of patients after 5 years of treatment, and 50% to 60% had negative results after 7 to 10 years. Venom-specific IgE antibody levels usually remain detectable even after many years of treatment and even when skin tests become negative.

Discontinuation

Although the product package inserts recommend VIT indefinitely, the question is no longer whether VIT can be discontinued, but when and in which patients. Stopping VIT when venom skin test results or specific IgE antibody levels become negative has been successful, but only a small number of patients develop negative test results in the first 5 years of therapy.

Several studies have shown that 5 years of treatment was associated with better suppression of allergic sensitivity and lower risk of relapse than 3 years of VIT.[1,2,10] The chance of relapse was minimal initially, but increased 3 to 5 years after discontinuation and did not disappear during up to 13 years observation. There is an approximately 10% chance of systemic reaction with each sting after stopping treatment, with a cumulative risk of relapse of 15% to 20% after 10 years off treatment (because repeat stings increase the chance of reaction). Fortunately, most reactions are mild and much less severe than the pretreatment reaction, but patients who had very severe reactions before VIT can have severe reactions again if they do relapse after stopping treatment. Reactions have occurred even in patients who developed negative venom skin test or specific serum IgE test results.

Collectively, the published studies on discontinuing VIT suggest that treatment may be stopped after 5 years for most patients, with the exception of those treated for honeybee anaphylaxis, those who had systemic reactions to an injection or sting during VIT, those with elevated baseline serum tryptase levels, and those who had very severe sting reactions before treatment (Box 15.4). Mastocytosis has been associated with fatal reactions to stings after discontinuing a course of immunotherapy. Long-term extension of treatment may also be considered for patients who are not willing to accept the 10% to 20% chance of reaction to a subsequent sting, particularly if they have frequent exposures, which increases the cumulative risk of systemic reaction. In these cases, treatment at 12-week intervals can maintain protection.

BOX 15.4 Considerations in Discontinuing Venom Immunotherapy

- Severity of systemic reaction to stings
- Elevated baseline serum tryptase
- Honeybee sting allergy (beekeepers)
- Duration of venom immunotherapy
- Systemic reaction during venom immunotherapy (VIT) (to injection or sting)
- Frequency of exposure
- Persistent strong serum or skin test for venom IgE
- Age (child, adult, senior)
- Quality of life

Fire Ant Immunotherapy

The natural history of fire ant allergy is not as well described as for other Hymenoptera, but there is a clear need for effective immunotherapy. Although immunotherapy using whole-body extracts of imported fire ants has been reported to be effective in preventing systemic reactions to fire ant stings, there have been no placebo-controlled trials. The suggested materials, methods, regimens, and doses for fire ant immunotherapy have been reviewed.[4] The duration of fire ant immunotherapy is still uncertain, because attempts at discontinuation led to relapse within several years in a significant minority of cases.

BITING INSECT ALLERGY

There are few credible reports of allergic reactions to biting insects. Sensitization to salivary proteins may cause abnormal local swelling following insect bites, but anaphylaxis is rarely reported.

Triatoma (Kissing Bug, Cone-nose Bug)

The most common confirmed cause of systemic reactions to insect bites is the kissing bug (*Triatoma* spp.). The relevant species in the US are found throughout the arid areas of the southwest states and California. The allergens are salivary gland proteins, and they have little cross-reactivity between species. Immunotherapy with a salivary gland extract was effective in preventing anaphylaxis from *Triatoma* bites in a small number of patients.

Culicoidae (Mosquito)

Considering the widespread exposure to mosquitoes and the frequency of mosquito bites, it is remarkable that so few cases of anaphylaxis have been reported. There has been increased recognition of the clinical impact of large local reactions to mosquito bites in children (i.e., skeeter syndrome).[11] Unfortunately, the mosquito extracts commercially available in the US are of unreliable composition and activity and are not approved for therapeutic use.

The major allergens in mosquito extracts have been identified and recombinant allergens have been prepared. These studies demonstrated significant cross-reactivity of the major worldwide mosquito species. Immunotherapy with whole-body extracts has not been proven effective, and there have been no studies of immunotherapy with purified or recombinant allergens.

Tabanidae (Horsefly, Deerfly)

The tabanid species are large flies that suck blood and inflict painful bites. They have widespread distribution in rural and suburban areas. Allergic reactions to insect bites from horseflies and deerflies have been reported. The possibility of immunotherapy has been little studied.

Allergic Reactions to Other Biting Insects

There have been anecdotal reports of allergic (mostly local) reactions to a number of other biting insects. Fleas (order Siphonaptera) are an uncommon cause of allergy in humans. The most commonly encountered reaction to flea bites in humans is papular urticaria, a form of persistent papular inflammation. The reaction usually begins about the ankles and becomes generalized over a period of weeks, often persisting for months and resolving spontaneously.

INHALANT INSECT ALLERGY

Respiratory exposures to antigens from outdoor insects (e.g., caddis flies, midges, lake flies) or indoor insects (e.g., cockroaches, lady bugs) may cause allergic respiratory symptoms. In other cases, airborne insect antigens produce occupational disease.

CONCLUSIONS

Stinging insects are a common cause of allergic reactions ranging from large local reactions to life-threatening anaphylaxis. Clinical and immunologic features can predict the risk of future severe reactions to stings. Skin or serum tests for venom-specific IgE antibodies are useful to confirm sensitization to venom allergens. VIT is recommended for patients at moderate to high risk for systemic reactions to future stings, but it is not required for low-risk patients despite positive venom-IgE test results. VIT can rapidly achieve complete clinical protection from systemic reactions to stings in 75% to 95% of patients. VIT can be discontinued after 5 years in most patients but may be continued indefinitely in those at high risk for relapse. An elevated baseline serum tryptase level predicts the severity of reactions to stings, systemic reactions to VIT, limited protection with VIT, and chance of relapse if VIT is stopped after 5 years. Anaphylaxis is rare from biting insects, but large local reactions can be severe, especially with mosquito bites.

REFERENCES

1. Golden DBK. Advances in diagnosis and management of insect sting allergy. Ann Allergy Asthma Immunol. 2013;111:84–89.
2. Golden DBK. Insect allergy. In: Adkinson NF, Yunginger JW, Bochner BS, Busse WW, Holgate ST, Lemanske RF, Simons FER, eds. Middleton's allergy: principles and practice. 9th ed. Philadelphia: Mosby Elsevier; 2019.
3. Golden DBK, Demain J, Freeman T, Graft DF, Tankersley M, Tracy JM, et al. Stinging insect hypersensitivity: a practice parameter update 2016. Ann Allergy Asthma Immunol. 2017;118:28–54.
4. Steigelman DA, Freeman TM. Imported fire ant allergy: case presentation and review of incidence, prevalence, diagnosis and current treatment. Ann Allergy Asthma Immunol. 2013;111:242–245.
5. Golden DBK, Kagey-Sobotka A, Norman PS, Hamilton RG, Lichtenstein LM. Outcomes of allergy to insect stings in children with and without venom immunotherapy. New Engl J Med. 2004;351:668–674.
6. Niedoszytko M, de Monchy J, van Doormaal JJ, Jassem E, Oude-Elberink JNG. Mastocytosis and insect venom allergy: diagnosis, safety and efficacy of venom immunotherapy. Allergy. 2009;64:1237–1245.
7. Lerch E, Muller U. Long-term protection after stopping venom immunotherapy. J Allergy Clin Immunol. 1998;101:606–612.
8. Oude-Elberink JNG, de Monchy JGR, van der Heide S, Guyatt GH, Dubois AEJ. Venom immunotherapy improves health-related quality of life in yellow jacket allergic patients. J Allergy Clin Immunol. 2002;110:174–182.
9. Golden DBK. Rush venom immunotherapy: ready for prime time? J Allergy Clin Immunol Practice. 2017;5:804–805.
10. Ozdemir C, Kucuksezer UC, Akdis M, Akdis CA. Mechanisms of immunotherapy to wasp and bee venom. Clin Exp Allergy. 2011;41:1226–1234.
11. Simons FER, Peng Z. Skeeter syndrome. J Allergy Clin Immunol. 1999;104:705–707.

Internet Resources

Organization/Resource	Internet address
Professional organizations	
Allergy Academy	www.allergyacademy.org
American Academy of Allergy Asthma & Immunology	www.aaaai.org
American Academy of Pediatrics	www.aap.org
American Association of Immunologists	www.aai.org
American College of Allergy, Asthma & Immunology	www.acaai.org
American College of Chest Physicians	www.chestnet.org
American College of Physicians	www.acponline.org
American College of Rheumatology	www.rheumatology.org
American Medical Association	www.ama-assn.org
American Thoracic Society	www.thoracic.org
Asia Pacific Association of Allergy, Asthma and Clinical Immunology (APAAACI)	www.apaaaci.org
Australasian Society of Clinical Immunology and Allergy (ASCIA)	www.allergy.org.au
British Society for Allergy & Clinical Immunology (BSACI)	www.bsaci.org
British Thoracic Society	www.brit-thoracic.org.uk
Canadian Society of Allergy & Clinical Immunology	http://csaci.ca/
Clinical Immunology Society	www.clinimmsoc.org
European Academy of Allergy and Clinical Immunology (EAACI)	www.eaaci.org
Global Asthma Association	http://interasma.org
International Eosinophil Society, Inc.	www.eosinophil-society.org
Scottish Allergy and Respiratory Academy	http://scottishallergyrespiratoryacademy.org
World Allergy Organization	www.worldallergy.org
Government agencies	
Centers for Disease Control and Prevention (USA)	www.cdc.gov
Clinical Trials registry	www.clinicaltrials.gov
Global Initiative for Asthma	www.ginasthma.com
National Institute of Allergy and Infectious Diseases (USA)	www.niaid.nih.gov
National Heart, Lung, and Blood Institute (USA)	www.nhlbi.nih.gov
National Institutes of Health (USA)	www.nih.gov
National Institute of Health Research (UK)	www.nihr.ac.uk/
U.S. Food and Drug Administration	www.fda.gov
World Health Organization	www.who.org
Lay support organizations	
Allergy & Asthma Network/Mothers of Asthmatics	www.aanma.org
Allergy UK	www.allergyuk.org
American Partnership for Eosinophilic Disorders (APFED)	www.apfed.org
American Lung Association	www.lung.org

(Continued)

Organization/Resource	Internet address
Anaphylaxis Campaign (UK)	www.anaphylaxis.org.uk
Asthma and Allergy Foundation of America	www.aafa.org
Asthma UK	www.asthma.org.uk
European Federation of Allergy and Airways Diseases Patients Associations (EFA)	www.efanet.org
Food Allergy Research & Education (FARE)	www.foodallergy.org
Immune Deficiency Foundation	www.primaryimmune.org
The Mastocytosis Society, Inc. (TMS)	www.tmsforacure.org
Allergic Rhinitis and its Impact on Asthma MASK-AIR The App	https://www.euforea.eu/aria www.mask-air.com
American Partnership for Eosinophilic Disorders	http://apfed.org
Asthma and Allergic Disease Management Center	www.aaaai.org
Asthma Prevention Program and Guidelines	www.nhlbi.nih.gov/about/naepp/index.htm
Clinical Trials	https://clinical trials.gov
MedWatch: The FDA Safety Information and Adverse Event Reporting Program (USFDA)	www.fda.gov/medwatch
NLM Literature Searches (PubMed)	www.ncbi.nlm.nih.gov/sites/entrez?db=PubMed
Scientific resources	
Allergome Database (allergenic molecules)	www.allergome.org
Biocompare Buyer's Guide for Antibodies	www.biocompare.com/antibodies/
Human Cell Differentiation Molecules	http://hcdm.org
National Center for Biotechnology Information	www.ncbi.nlm.nih.gov
Web-based Protein Resources (NCBI)	www.ncbi.nlm.nih.gov/guide/proteins/
Credentialing organizations (USA)	
Accreditation Council for Graduate Medical Education	www.acgme.org
American Board of Allergy and Immunology	www.abai.org
American Board of Internal Medicine	www.abim.org
American Board of Medical Specialties	www.abms.org
American Board of Pediatrics	www.abp.org

INDEX

Page numbers followed by '*f*' indicate figures, '*b*' indicate boxes, and '*t*' indicate tables.